D1031779

HANDBOOK OF VITAMINS

FOOD SCIENCE AND TECHNOLOGY

A Series of Monographs, Textbooks, and Reference Books

1. Flavor Research: Principles and Techniques, *R. Teranishi, I. Hornstein, P. Issenberg, and E. L. Wick (out of print)*

2. Principles of Enzymology for the Food Sciences, *John R. Whitaker*

3. Low-Temperature Preservation of Foods and Living Matter, *Owen R. Fennema, William D. Powrie, and Elmer H. Marth*

4. Principles of Food Science
   Part I: Food Chemistry, *edited by Owen R. Fennema*
   Part II: Physical Methods of Food Preservation, *Marcus Karel, Owen R. Fennema, and Daryl B. Lund*

5. Food Emulsions, *edited by Stig Friberg*

6. Nutritional and Safety Aspects of Food Processing, *edited by Steven R. Tannenbaum*

7. Flavor Research: Recent Advances, *edited by R. Teranishi, Robert A. Flath, and Hiroshi Sugisawa*

8. Computer-Aided Techniques in Food Technology, *edited by Israel Saguy*

9. Handbook of Tropical Foods, *edited by Harvey T. Chan*

10. Antimicrobials in Foods, *edited by Alfred Larry Branen and P. Michael Davidson*

11. Food Constituents and Food Residues: Their Chromatographic Determination, *edited by James F. Lawrence*

12. Aspartame: Physiology and Biochemistry, *edited by Lewis D. Stegink and L. J. Filer, Jr.*

13. Handbook of Vitamins: Nutritional, Biochemical, and Clinical Aspects, *edited by Lawrence J. Machlin*

HANDBOOK OF VITAMINS

Second Edition, Revised and Expanded

edited by

Lawrence J. Machlin

Department of Vitamins and Clinical Nutrition
Hoffmann-La Roche, Inc.
Nutley, New Jersey

MARCEL DEKKER, INC.   **New York and Basel**

Library of Congress Cataloging--in--Publication Data

Handbook of vitamins / edited by Lawrence J. Machlin. -- -- 2nd ed., rev.
  and expanded.
      p.   cm. -- -- (Food science and technology; 40)
    Includes bibliographical references and index.
    ISBN 0-8247-8351-4
    1. Vitamins. 2. Vitamins in human nutrition. I. Machlin,
Lawrence J.   II. Series: Food science and technology
(Marcel Dekker, Inc.); 40.
QP771.H35   1990
612.3'99-- --dc20   90-41640
                                                     CIP

Marcel Dekker, Inc.
270 Madison Avenue, New York, New York 10016

Current printing (last digit):
10 9 8 7 6 5 4 3 2 1

Printed in the United States of America

Preface to the Second Edition

Since publication of the first edition of the *Handbook of Vitamins*, research and publications concerning vitamins have grown at an accelerating pace as evidenced by the publication of several international symposia on vitamin C (1), vitamin E (2), vitamin B_6 (3) and biotin (4) as well as an excellent review in German of all vitamins (5).

The first edition clearly filled a need and has been widely used as a text and reference. In order to continue its usefulness, it was necessary to update all the chapters to include the extensive research developed in the last six years. In view of the increased interest and importance of carnitine, a separate chapter on this nutrient is included. In addition, discussions of inositol, bioflavanoids, and vitamins B_6, E, and C have been expanded. The form and style have not been changed, and it is hoped the new edition will be of expanded value to the reader.

I would like to express my thanks to Dr. Adrianne Bendich and Dr. Hemmige N. Bhagavan for their excellent help in reviewing specific chapters and to my wife Ruth for her patience and understanding.

Lawrence J. Machlin

REFERENCES

1. J. J. Burns, J. M. Rivers, and L. J. Machlin, Third Conference on Vitamin C, *Ann. N.Y. Acad. Sci.*, *498* (1987).
2. A. T. Diplock, L. J. Machlin, L. Packer, and W. A. Pryor, Vitamin E: Biochemistry and Health Implications, *Ann. N.Y. Acad. Sci.*, *570* (1989).
3. J. E. Leklem and R. D. Reynolds, *Clinical and Physiological Applications of Vitamin B_6*, Alan R. Liss, New York, 1988.
4. K. Dakshinamurti and H. N. Bhagavan, Biotin, *Ann. N.Y. Acad. Sci.*, *447* (1985).
5. W. Friedrich, *Handbook Der Vitamine*, Urban & Schwarzenberg, Munich, 1987.

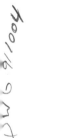

Preface to the First Edition

Vitamin deficiency diseases such as scurvy, beriberi, xerophthalmia, and pellagra have plagued the world at least since the existence of written records. The concept of a vitamin or "accessory growth factor" was developed in the early part of this century and for almost five decades there was an exciting era of isolation, identification, and synthesis of the vitamins. These discoveries led to the availability of inexpensive synthetic vitamins and to a dramatic reduction in overt vitamin deficiency disease. With the isolation of vitamin B_{12} in 1948 the period of vitamin discovery came to a close. Several excellent books (1–3) have summarized the significant information of those early decades of research. Since 1948, no new vitamins have been discovered and it is not likely that any will be identified in the future.

With the intense excitement of discovery at an end, some of the interest and romance in vitamins diminished. Nevertheless, many scientists have continued to carry out research on the nutritional effects of vitamins, their metabolism, their influence on disease resistance, and the numerous interactions of vitamins with other nutrients, drugs, alcohol, smoking, disease states, age, and environmental pollutants. Delicate techniques have been developed to determine when a person is at risk from a vitamin deficiency and with this technology has come an increased awareness and concern with the effects of marginal vitamin deficiencies. In addition, the use of high levels of vitamins to prevent or alleviate a number of diseases, and particularly to treat an increasing number of inherited metabolic disorders, is the subject of renewed interest. Significant vitamin deficiency problems that interfere with the economic production of farm animals are continually being identified.

As a result of this interest and research, a large body of information has accumulated in the last few decades. Some of this information is presented in books on individual vitamins (4–14). A number of good discussions of clinical and nutritional aspects of vitamins are also available (15–18). Two series, *The Vitamins* (19, 20) and *Vitamins and Hormones* (21), provide detailed discussions of a number of aspects of vitamin physiology. In all this literature, the information presented is too exhaustive and detailed, does not include discussions of all of the vitamins in one source, or does not include all of the many pertinent topics related to an intelligent understanding and utilization of the vitamins. In this book, we hope to provide a relatively brief but authoritative and comprehensive source of information on the vitamins for the human and animal nutritionist, the dietician, clinician, biochemist, and interested lay person. This includes a discussion of their chemistry, availability and content in food, metabolism, function, and deficiency symptoms; the methods for evaluating overt or marginal deficiencies; nutritional requirements; the interaction of vitamins with environmental and disease factors; and the efficacy and safety when used at high levels.

Vitamins have been defined as a group of organic substances present in minute amounts in natural foodstuffs which are essential to normal metabolism and lack of which in the diet causes deficiency diseases. There are many substances that according to this definition have erroneously been referred to as vitamins. For the sake of completeness, some of these substances are included in the book with a brief discussion of their history and potential importance in nutrition.

I would like to express my appreciation to Ms. Edda Gabriel for her excellent editorial assistance. In addition, my thanks extend to Dr. Hemmige Bhagavan, Dr. Myron Brin, Dr. Stanley Shapiro, Dr. George Cardinale, Dr. Zane Gaut, and Dr. Robert Rucker for their help in reviewing many of the manuscripts.

Lawrence J. Machlin

REFERENCES

1. H. R. Rosenberg, *Chemistry and Physiology of the Vitamins*, Interscience Pub., New York, 1942.
2. F. A. Robinson, *The Vitamin B Complex*, John Wiley, New York, 1951.
3. W. H. Eddy, *Vitaminology: The Chemistry and Function of the Vitamins*, Williams and Wilkins, Baltimore, 1949.
4. T. Moore, *Vitamin A*, Elsevier, New York, 1957.
5. L. E. Smith, *Vitamin B_{12}*, John Wiley, New York, 1957.
6. L. J. Machlin (Ed.), *Vitamin E: A Comprehensive Treatise*, Marcel Dekker, New York, 1980.
7. *Human Vitamin B_6 Requirements*, National Academy of Sciences, National Research Council, Washington, 1978.
8. *Folic Acid, Biochemistry and Physiology in Relation to the Human Nutrition Requirement*, National Academy of Sciences, National Research Council, Washington, 1977.
9. A. W. Norman (Ed.), *Vitamin D, Molecular Biology and Clinical Nutrition*, Marcel Dekker, New York, 1980.
10. G. G. Birch and K. Parker (Eds.), *Vitamin C*, John Wiley, New York, 1974.
11. J. N. Counsell and D. H. Hornig (Eds.), *Vitamin C Ascorbic Acid*, Applied Science Pub., Englewood, 1981.
12. P. A. Seib and B. M. Tolbert (Eds.), *Ascorbic Acid: Chemistry, Metabolism and Uses*, Advances in chemistry series 200. American Chemical Society, Washington, 1982.
13. S. Nobile and J. M. Woodhill (Eds.), *Vitamin C*, MTP Press, Boston, 1981.
14. S. Lewin (Ed.), *Vitamin C: Its Molecular Biology and Medical Potential*, Academic, New York, 1976.
15. B. M. Barker and D. A. Bender (Eds.), *Vitamins in Medicine*, William Heinemann Medical Books, London, Fourth ed., 1980.
16. H. F. De Luca and J. W. Suttie (Eds.), *The Fat Soluble Vitamins*, University of Wisconsin Press, Madison, 1970.
17. R. S. Goodhart and M. E. Shills, *Modern Nutrition in Health and Disease*, Fifth ed., Lea and Febiger, Philadelphia, 1973.
18. J. Marks, *A Guide to the Vitamins*, Medical and Technical Pub., 1977.
19. W. H. Sebrell, Jr. and R. S. Harris (Eds.), *The Vitamins: Chemistry, Physiology, Pathology, Methods*, Vols. I-V, Academic, New York, 1967–1972.
20. P. Gyorgy and W. N. Pearson (Eds.), *The Vitamins: Chemistry, Physiology, Pathology, Methods*, Vols. VI and VII, Academic, New York, 1973 to 1974.
21. R. S. Harris et al., *Vitamins and Hormones: Advances in Research and Application*, Vols. 1-34, Academic, New York, 1943 to 1977.

Contents

Contributors

Adrianne Bendich Department of Clinical Nutrition, Hoffmann-La Roche, Inc., Nutley, New Jersey

Jean-Pierre Bonjour Vitamins and Fine Chemicals, F. Hoffmann-La Roche, Ltd., Basel, Switzerland

Peggy R. Borum Department of Food Science and Human Nutrition, University of Florida, Gainesville, Florida

Tom Brody Department of Food Science and Human Nutrition, University of Hawaii at Manoa, Honolulu, Hawaii

Mabel M. Chan Department of Food, Nutrition, and Hotel Management, New York University, New York, New York

Mildred M. Cody Department of Nutrition and Dietetics, Georgia State University, Atlanta, Georgia

Elaine D. Collins Department of Biochemistry, University of California, Riverside, California

Bernard A. Cooper Departments of Medicine and Physiology, McGill University and Department of Hematology and Medical Oncology, Royal Victoria Hospital, Montreal, Quebec, Canada

Jack M. Cooperman Department of Community and Preventive Medicine, New York Medical College, Valhalla, New York

Leon Ellenbogen Medical Development, American Cyanamid Company, Lederle Laboratories, Pearl River, New York

Hazel Metz Fox† Department of Human Nutrition and Food Service Management, University of Nebraska, Lincoln, Nebraska

Clark Johnson Gubler Graduate Section of Biochemistry, Brigham Young University, Provo, Utah

---

†Deceased.

James E. Leklem   Department of Foods and Nutrition, Oregon State University, Corvallis, Oregon

Rafael Lopez*   Department of Community and Preventive Medicine, New York Medical College, Valhalla, New York

Lawrence J. Machlin   Department of Clinical Nutrition, Hoffmann-La Roche, Inc., Nutley, New Jersey

Ulrich Moser   Vitamins and Fine Chemicals, F. Hoffmann-La Roche, Ltd., Basel, Switzerland

Anthony W. Norman   Department of Biochemistry, University of California, Riverside, California

James Allen Olson   Department of Biochemistry and Biophysics, Iowa State University of Science and Technology, Ames, Iowa

J. W. Suttie   Departments of Biochemistry and Nutritional Sciences, College of Agricultural and Life Sciences, University of Wisconsin, Madison, Wisconsin

Jan van Eys   University of Texas, M. D. Anderson Cancer Center, Houston, Texas

---

*Present affiliation: Our Lady of Mercy Medical Center, Bronx, New York.

HANDBOOK OF VITAMINS

1
Vitamin A

James Allen Olson

Iowa State University of Science and Technology
Ames, Iowa

I. History

Probably the first nutritional deficiency disease to be clearly recognized was night blindness. The ancient Egyptians, as indicated in the Papyrus Ebers and later in the London Medical Papyrus, recommended that juice squeezed from cooked liver should be topically applied to the eye to cure night blindness. These writings date from 1500 B.C., but the observations probably are of much earlier origin. The Greeks, who depended heavily on Egyptian medicine, recommended both the ingestion of cooked liver as well as its topical application as a cure for night blindness, a tradition which has persisted in many societies to this day (1).

Although interesting references to vitamin A deficiency diseases and their cure can be found throughout history, the modern science of nutrition is only about a century old. The observation that experimental animals lose weight and die on purified diets was noted by many investigators towards the end of the nineteenth century. In the early part of this century, specific factors necessary for the growth and survival were beginning to be identified. Frederick Gowland Hopkins in England, for example, during the period 1906–1912, found that a growth-stimulating principle from milk was present in an alcoholic extract of milk rather than in the ash.

During the same period, Stepp in Germany identified one of these "minimal qualitative factors" as a lipid. Soon thereafter E. V. McCollum and Marguerite Davis in Wisconsin showed that butter or egg yolk, but not lard, contained a necessary lipid-soluble factor necessary for the growth of rats. In 1915 they coined the term "fat-soluble A," and thereby attributed for the first time the growth-stimulating property of these extracts to a single compound. Although approaching the problem in a very different way, Osborne and Mendel at Yale concomitantly found that cod liver oil or butter was an essential growth-promoting food for rats. The year 1915, therefore, was the beginning of the modern age of vitamin A exploration.

Many outstanding finds have been made during the past seven decades, of which only the most notable will be mentioned here. Inasmuch as both colorless extracts of liver as well as colored plant lipids showed biological activity, Steenbock in Wisconsin postulated in 1919 the interconversion of two forms of the vitamin. A decade later, Moore in England showed that β-carotene, the plant pigment, was converted to the colorless form of the vitamin in liver tissue. In the early 1920s, experimental vitamin A deficiency was well characterized by Wolbach and Howe in Boston, and the existence of vitamin A deficiency in children was noted by Bloch in Denmark. In 1930 Karrer and his colleagues in Switzerland determined the structure both of β-carotene and of vitamin A and shortly thereafter synthesized some of its derivatives. One of these derivatives was retinaldehyde, and in 1935 George Wald of Harvard, while working in Germany, proved that the retinene found in visual pigments of the eye was identical with Karrer's chemical compound retinaldehyde.

Of great importance for applied nutrition was the elegant synthesis of all-*trans* vitamin A from the inexpensive precursor β-ionone by Otto Isler and his collaborators in Basel in the late 1940s. Within a few years the price of vitamin A, which earlier had been painstakingly isolated from fish liver oils by molecular distillation, fell 10-fold, and the possibility of using vitamin A more generally in foods at reasonable cost was assured.

With the availability of radioative isotopes in the 1950s, many studies were initiated on the metabolism of vitamin A, and much of our present knowledge concerning it was defined. The details of the visual cycle involving rhodopsin in the eye were in large part worked out, and attention began to focus on the possible somatic function of vitamin A in growth and in cellular differentiation. In subsequent sections, the present state of knowledge relative to vitamin A will be summarized. Much of the early history of vitamin A is discussed in Moore's highly readable monograph (2).

II. CHEMISTRY

A. Isolation

In nature vitamin A is largely found as an ester, and consequently is highly soluble in organic solvents but not in aqueous solutions. The major provitamin carotenoid, β-carotene, has similar solvent properties. One of the riches sources of vitamin A is liver tissue, in particular the liver oils of marine fish and mammals. The esters can be directly isolated from these oils by molecular distillation at very low pressure, a procedure that has been used extensively for the commercial preparation of vitamin A-rich oils. Alternatively, vitamin A might be directly extracted with chloroform or with some other solvent combination, such as hexane together with ethanol, followed by purification of vitamin A by chromatographic means. In order to hydrolyze esters, not only of vitamin A and carotenoids but also of triglycerides and other lipids, saponification with KOH is commonly used, followed by extraction with organic solvents. Retinol or its esters can be readily crystallized at low temperature from a variety of organic solvents, including ethyl formate, propylene oxide, and methanol.

B.   Structure and Nomenclature

The structure of some major compounds in the vitamin A group are depicted in Figure 1, with their recommended names referenced in Table 1. The term vitamin A is employed generically for all derivatives of β-ionone (other than the carotenoids) that possess the biological activity of all-*trans* retinol or are closely related to it structurally (3). The parent substance of the vitamin A group is called all-*trans* retinol, the formula of which is given in Figure 1a and b. The numbering system for vitamin A derivatives commonly employed during the last 20 years and currently endorsed by IUPAC is given in Figure 1a. In the past, chemists sometimes considered the side chain as a substituent of the trimethyl cyclohexene ring, as shown in Figure 1b. Futhermore, in the case of retinoic acid derivatives, the carboxyl group carbon is conventionally denoted as C-1, with the trimethylcyclohexene ring as a substituent on C-9. For consistency, the numbering system depicted in formula a will be used in the present chapter.

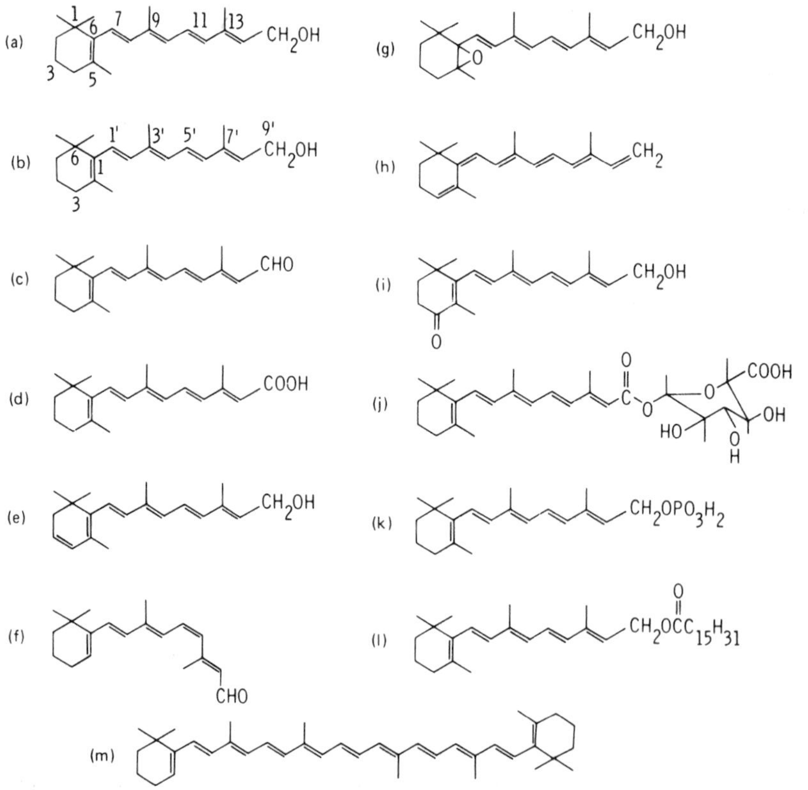

Figure 1   Formulas for retinol and its derivatives. The names of depicted compounds are referenced in Table 1.

Table 1 Nomenclature of Major Compounds in the Vitamin A Group

Recommended term[a]	Synonyms
Retinol (a,b)	Vitamin A_1 alcohol, axerophthol
Retinal, retinaldehyde (c)	Vitamin A_1 aldehyde, retinene
Retinoic acid (d)	Vitamin A_1 acid
3-Dehydroretinol (e)	Vitamin A_2
11-*cis*-Retinaldehyde (f)	11-*cis* or neo b Vitamin A aldehyde
5,6-Epoxyretinol (g)	5,6-Epoxy vitamin A alcohol
Anhydroretinol (h)	Anhydro vitamin A
4-Ketoretinol (i)	4-Keto vitamin A alcohol
Retinoyl β-glucuronide (j)	Vitamin A acid β-glucuronide
Retinyl phosphate (k)	Vitamin A phosphate
Retinyl palmitate (l)	Vitamin A palmitate
Retinyl acetate	Vitamin A acetate

[a]The formulas of most compounds are referenced (a,b, etc.) from Figure 1.

The recommended names for major compounds of the vitamin A group are given in Table 1. Esters of retinol are called retinyl esters, and the aldehyde form is termed retinal or retinaldehyde. Vitamin A with a terminal carboxyl group is called retinoic acid. A naturally occurring substance with significant biological activity is 3-dehydroretinol, initially called vitamin A_2.

Vitamin A and its derivatives belong to a much larger class of structurally related compounds, termed the *retinoids*. Retinoids, which include a wide variety of synthetic and natural compounds, have been used therapeutically to treat certain skin disorders and some forms of cancer. This chapter, which is primarily devoted to vitamin A, will consider their actions only briefly.

Of over 500 carotenoids that have been isolated from nature, only about 50 possess biological activity. An excellent summary of many aspects of carotenoid isolation, structure, and synthesis is given in the fine treatise edited by Isler (4). Thus, the term provitamin A is used as a generic indicator for all carotenoids that show the biological activity of vitamin A. The most active and quantitatively the most important of these provitamins is all-*trans* β-carotene (Fig. 1m). Generally, carotenoids must contain at least one β-ionone ring that is not hydroxylated in order to show vitamin A activity.

In addition to the all-*trans* form of vitamin A, all 15 of the other possible isomers have been prepared and characterized (5–7). The most interesting and important isomer is 11-*cis*-retinaldehyde, depicted in Figure 1f, which is the chromophore of the visual pigments rhodopsin and iodopsin. Similarly, 13-*cis*- retinaldehyde serves a similar function in bacteriorhodopsin of the Halobacteria. As the number of *cis* bonds increase, both the absorption maximum of the isomer and its absorbance tend to decrease. Thus, whereas all-*trans*- retinaldehyde has an absorption maximum and molecular extinction coefficient of 368 nm and 48,000 in hexane, respectively, the 9,11,13-*cis* isomer shows corresponding values of 302 nm and 15,500 (6,7). The tetra-*cis* isomer, 7,9,11,13-*cis*, of ethyl retinoate, retinal, and retinol show similar hypsochromic and hypochromic shifts relative to their all-*trans* analogs (5,6). Although the terms *cis* and *trans* have traditionally been used to denote various isomers of vitamin A, the current chemical notation is Z for *cis* and E for *trans*. Thus, 11-*cis*-retinal might equally well be termed 7E, 9E, 11Z, 13E-retinal. In

discussing the function of vitamin A, more will be said later about these fascinating interactions and the effects of light on them.

C.   Structures of Important Analogs, Antagonists, and Commercial Forms of Vitamin A

Interestingly, vitamin A has few structurally related antagonists; citral, a naturally occurring sesquiterpenoid aldehyde, has been reported to antagonize vitamin A action at high
doses, and fenretinamide (hydroxyphenylretinamide) inhibits acyl-coenyzme A:retinol tran-
sacylase (ARAT) and can cause night blindness in humans receiving daily high doses.
Because of the therapeutic action of vitamin A against certain skin diseases and some types
of experimental cancer, many analogs of vitamin A that possess therapeutic activity without
showing high toxicity have been synthesized during the past decade. Some of these analogs
are shown in Figure 2. 13-*cis*-Retinoic acid (Fig. 2), although a naturally occurring isomer
of retinoic acid, is largely used in high doses against certain kinds of skin disease and
cancer. Retinyl methyl ether (Fig. 2b) is not found naturally, but can be converted to vitamin
A by humans and experimental animals. 15-Dimethyl retinol (Fig. 2c), on the other hand,
cannot be converted into vitamin A in significant quantities in animals. The last five compounds (Figs. 2d–h) are all synthetic derivatives with variable protective activities against
carcinogen-induced tumors in experimental animals. The benzoic acid derivative (Fig.
2g) shows both significant biological activity in cellular differentiation as well as high
toxicity (8). A wide variety of other analogs, including methyl, fluoro, and chloro
derivatives, have also been synthesized, many of which are presently being tested against
various types of cancer.

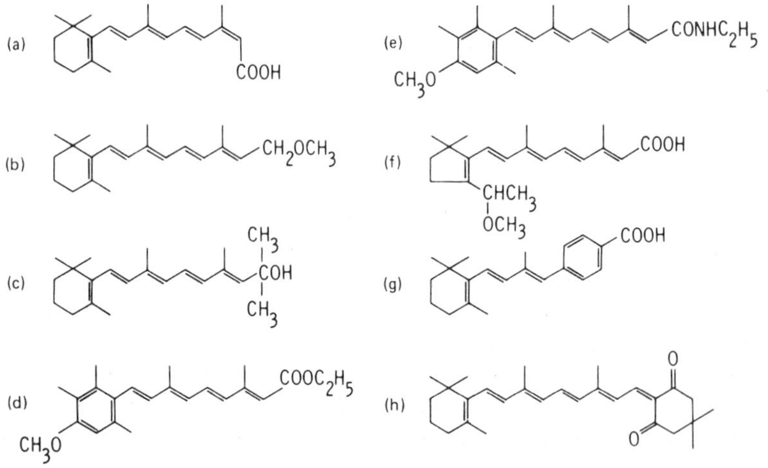

Figure 2   Formulas of vitamin A analogs (A 13-*cis*-retinoic acid, (B) retinyl
methyl ether, (C) 15-dimethylretinol, (D) the trimethylmethoxyphenol analog of
ethylretinoate, also termed Ro 10-9359, (E) the ethylamide analog of (D), also
termed Ro 11-1430, (F) the dimethylmethoxyethyl-cyclopentenyl analog of retinoic
acid, (G) an aryl triene analog of retinoic acid, (H) 2-retinylidene-5,
5-dimethyl-1,3-cyclohexanedione (retinylidene dimedone).

The major commercial forms of vitamin A are all-*trans*-retinyl acetate and all-*trans*-retinyl palmitate (Fig. 1l). The esters are generally produced because of their increased stability and better solubility in oils and other commercial preparations. The esters can also be incorporated into a gelatin matrix which protects them from oxidation over reasonable periods of time, even when subjected to cooking. These latter forms have been extensively used in the fortification of foods and animal feeds.

D. Synthesis

Since the complete elucidation of the structure of vitamin A by Karrer in 1930, intense effort has been expended in synthesizing vitamin A from a variety of precursors. As early as 1937, Kuhn and Morris (9) synthesized vitamin A, but their yield was only 7.5%. In most cases the starting material for the synthesis is β-ionone, which may be obtained inexpensively and in large quantities from natural sources, but even simpler starting materials, such as acetone and acetylene, can be employed. Of many possibilities, the two major synthetic procedures used commercially are those of Hoffmann-La Roche and of the Badische Anilin- und Sod-Fabrik (BASF). The Roche procedure involves as a key intermediate a C14 aldehyde and further requires the efficient reduction of acetylenic to olefinic bonds near the end of the synthesis. The BASF procedure, on the other hand, depends heavily on the Wittig reaction, by which a phosphonium ylid reacts with an aldehyde or ketone to give an olefin and phosphine oxide. The major steps in these two procedures are presented in Figure 3. An excellent summary of the major synthetic routes is given by Mayer and Isler in Isler (4) and by Frickel (10).

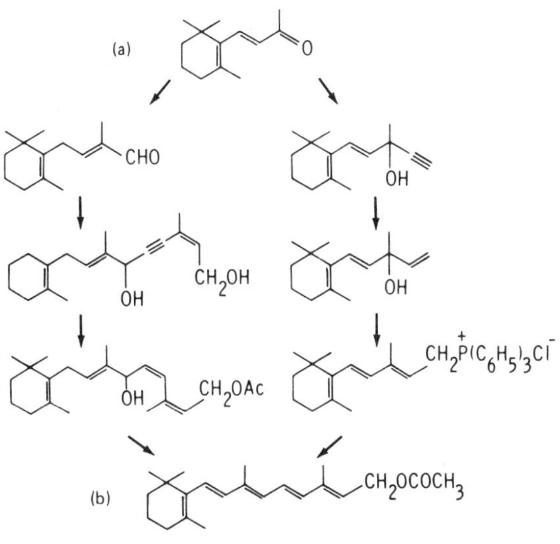

Figure 3 Major commercial routes to the synthesis of retinyl acetate (B) from β-ionone (A). The Isler (Roche) procedure is on the left, the Wittig (BASF) method on the right.

E. Chemical Properties

In concentrated solution, retinol and its esters are light yellow to reddish–hued oils that solidify when cooled and have a mild pleasant odor. As already mentioned, they are insoluble in water or glycerol but are readily miscible with most organic solvents. The formula, formula weights, melting points, and characteristics of the absorption and fluorescent spectra are summarized in Table 2. Indeed many other physiocochemical properties, including infrared spectra, polarography, proton magnetic reasonance, and the like, have also been studied (4,6,10). Nuclear magnetic resonance (NMR) spectra are particularly useful in characterizing various isomers of vitamin A (6,10). Vitamin A in crystalline form or in oil, if kept under a dry nitrogen atmosphere in a dark cool place, is stable for long periods. In contrast, vitamin A and its analogs are particularly sensitive to oxidation by air in the presence of light, particularly when spread as a thin surface film. In its natural form, whether present in liver or bound to protein in the plasma, vitamin A also is quite stable when stored in the frozen state, preferably at $-70\,°C$, in a hermetically closed container in the dark. On the other hand, upon extraction from biological materials, care must be taken to prevent both oxidation and isomerization of vitamin A.

Commercial firms have been successful in preparing several stabilized forms of vitamin A. For example, retinyl acetate, propionate or palmitate can be coated in the presence of antioxidants into a gelatin–carbohydrate matrix. The beadlets thus formed, upon being mixed in animal feeds or in human food, retain 90% or more of their activity for at least a 6-month period if kept under good storage conditions. In the presence of high humidity, heat, and oxygen, however, the loss is considerably greater.

III. ANALYTICAL PROCEDURES

A variety of methods may be used for determining the concentration of vitamin A in chemical or pharmaceutical preparations, tissues, and foods. Each of these methods will be considered in turn, with the advantages and constraints cited. As indicated in Table 2, vitamin A possesses a characteristic ultraviolet absorption spectrum. When the concentration of vitamin A is relatively high, measurement of the absorption at 325 nm in

Table 2   Physical Properties of All-*Trans*-Retinol and Its Esters

Property	Retinol	Retinyl acetate	Retinyl palmitate
Formula	$C_{20}H_{30}O$	$C_{22}H_{32}O_2$	$C_{36}H_{60}O_2$
Formula weight	286.46	328.50	524.88
Melting point (°C)	63–64	57–59	28–29
UV Absorption[a]			
λ_{max}	325	326	236
$E_{1cm}^{1\%}$	1820	1530	960
ϵ	52,140	50,260	50,390
Fluorescence			
Excitation λ_{max}	325	325	325
Emission λ_{max}	470	470	470

[a]In isopropanol. Values are similar in ethanol but differ in chloroform and other solvents. Absorbance values for retinol in hexane, for example, are essentially the same as in isopropanol, but for retinyl esters in hexane are about 3% higher.

ethanol, or the running of a complete UV spectrum, is a sensitive and relatively specific procedure. Indeed, in assaying reference solutions of vitamin A or its esters, the light absorption procedure should always be used. When extracts of vitamin A–rich tissues, such as liver, are studied, ultraviolet absorption might also be used, but a correction must be made for irrelevant absorption due to other compounds in the extract (11).

The most common method for analyzing vitamin A and its analogs in pharmaceutical preparations, feedstuffs, and tissues is high-pressure liquid chromatography (HPLC) combined with a UV-detector, usually set at 325 nm (12–14). Although many techniques have been described (13,14), new procedures continue to appear (15–18). Two major types of chromatographic columns are employed, so-called "straight-phase" and "reverse-phase" supports. In the former, hydrophobic compounds are eluted first and more polar compounds later, whereas in the latter, the reverse order of elution occurs. Isomers of a given retinoid are best separated on the former (19), whereas different retinyl esters are best resolved on the latter. Carotenoids can also be well resolved by HLPC, usually in conjunction with a UV-VIS detector set at 450 nm (13,20–22). Only a few of the available methods are cited here as a guide to the literature.

One of the most sensitive methods for measuring vitamin A is by its intense greenish-yellow fluorescence (Table 2). Because many other natural compounds fluoresce, of which the most troublesome is the polyene pigment phytofluene, chromatographic separation by HPLC or by other procedures is usually necessary to ensure adequate specificity in the response. The intense fluorescence of vitamin A has recently been used as well in separating liver cells containing large amounts of retinyl ester (stellate cells) from those containing smaller amounts by means of laser-activated flow cytometry (23,24).

Mass spectroscopy (MS) is also being increasingly used as a qualitative method for the analysis of retinoids and carotenoids (13,14). The combination of gas chromatography on selected capillary columns with MS (25) has been used to study the in vivo kinetics and the equilibration of deuterated retinol with endogenous reserves of vitamin A in humans (26,27). The new powerful technique, GC/MS, has also been employed, often in conjunction with HPLC, or even more effectively with supercritical fluid chromatography. both to identify and to quantitate retinoids and carotenoids in tissue extracts (28,29). Although now in their infancy, these new procedures will certainly have an important impact on the analysis of retinoids and carotenoids in the future.

The older conventional methods, such as the colorimetric measurement of the transient blue complex formed at 620 nm when vitamin A is dehydrated in the presence of Lewis acids and the decrease in absorbance at 325 nm when vitamin A in serum extracts is inactivated by ultraviolet light, remain of value. Currently, however, these procedures are the methods of choice primarily in field surveys where more sophisticated instrumentation is not available (30).

IV. BIOASSAY PROCEDURES

Biological tests have a utility which cannot be replaced by specific chemical or physical methods. The physiological response of a species to a given provitamin, a mixture of provitamins, or vitamin A can only be assessed by biological procedures. Indeed, the complexities of absorption, metabolism, storage, transport, and uptake by tissues is integrated into a meaningful whole only by biological tests.

The most commonly used biological methods for vitamin A are the classical growth response tests in vitamin A–deficient rats, liver storage assays in rats and chicks, and the vaginal smear technique. The requisite design and pitfalls of using the classical rat growth test have been well reviewed (31,32), and more recent applications of it to analogs of retinol might be cited (33,34). In the classical rat growth assay, sizable groups of rats are placed on graded doses of the unknown compound, and the growth response, as expressed in grams of weight gain per week, is plotted against the log of the dose. By comparing the growth response with that of groups of rats fed graded doses of all-*trans*-retinyl acetate, the biological activity can be calculated. Although useful information is gained, such assays tend to be very costly in terms of the number of animals required, animal care needed, and time.

In the last 15 years organ and cell culture systems have increasingly been used for assessing the biological activity of retinoids (35–37). For example, tracheal epithelium from vitamin A–deficient animals, which tends to be keratinized, or epidermal cells from newborn mouse skin are grown in a vitamin A–free tissue culture medium. The capacity of various vitamin A derivatives, when added to the medium in graded doses, either to reverse keratinization in the tracheal organ culture or to increase RNA synthesis in the epidermal cell culture is then assessed (35). A close relationship exists between the relative biological activity of many, but not all, vitamin A derivatives determined in these tests and that found by classical procedures. In addition, toxicity can be determined in the tracheal organ culture by measuring the amount of proteoglycan released into the culture median at different concentrations of a given vitamin A derivative. This procedure has been extensively used for screening retinoids for biological activity and toxicity (37).

In addition to determining the relative biological activity of a set of retinoids, another major focus in using cell and organ culture systems is to gain insight into the mechanisms by which retinoids induce the differentiation of cells and prevent the development of transformed, or neoplastic cells. Although a vast number of cell systems have been used in this regard, the F9 teratocarcinoma cell line, the HL-60 promyelocytic leukemic cell line, and keratinocytes have been particularly studied (38–40).

V. CONTENT IN FOOD

A. Tables of Food Content

Many tables have been compiled of the average content of so-called preformed vitamin A, i.e., retinol and its esters, and of total carotenoids, both in the United States and abroad (41). In 1949 the Food and Agricultural Organization of the United Nations published food composition tables for international use, and in 1961 specific tables for use in Latin America were jointly developed by the Institute of Nutrition for Central America and Panama and the Interdepartmental Committee on Nutrition for National Development (ICNND). Subsequently food composition tables for Africa and Asia were also published (41). A section-by-section revision of the U.S. tables is nearly complete (42). In the latter, both retinol equivalents (RE) as well as international unit (IU) are given for each food containing vitamin A and/or provitamin A carotenoids.

Common dietary sources of preformed vitamin A are various dairy products, such as milk, cheese, butter and ice cream, eggs, liver and other internal organs such as the kidney and heart, and many fish such as herring, sardines, and tuna. The very richest sources are liver oils of the shark, of marine fish, such as the halibut, and of marine mammals, such as the polar bear.

With respect to carotenoids, carrots and green leafy vegetables, such as spinach and amaranth, generally contain large amounts. Although the tomato contains some vitamin A active carotenoids, the major pigment is lycopene, which has no nutritional activity. Fruits like papaya and oranges have appreciable quantities of carotenoids. The cereal grains generally contain very little if any vitamin A, particularly when milled, an important consideration in dealing with the problem of vitamin A deficiency among very young children throughout the world. Yellow maize does have vitamin A–active carotenoids, however, whereas white maize, which is popular in many parts of Africa, does not. The richest source of carotenoids is red palm oil, which contains about 0.5 mg of mixed α- and β-carotene per ml. Thus, about 7 ml of red palm oil per day should meet the nutritional needs of a preschool child.

Unfortunately, dietary tables are not particularly useful in assessing the intake of vitamin A and carotenoids in a population. First of all, the amount of vitamin A in presumably good dietary sources, such as dairy products and liver, can vary tremendously depending on the diet of the cow or slaughtered animal. Second, vitamin A can be rapidly destroyed in foods unless the food processing technique is satisfactory. Third, the content of carotenoids in different vegetables and fruits can vary tremendously, depending on the species, growth conditions, mode of storage, and method of preparation. In many fruits and green leafy vegetables, for example, the biological oxidation of vitamin A–active carotenoids to inactive xanthophylls occurs rapidly during storage or senescence. Finally, past methods for analyzing carotenoids have not resolved nutritionally active from inactive compounds very well. By use of HPLC, more accurate values of provitamin A carotenoids are now being obtained (21,43).

The problem of interconverting the amounts of carotene found in a given food into retinol equivalents is also fraught with difficulty. At present 12 μg of mixed provitamin A carotenoids in a typical food or 6 μg of β-carotene is considered equivalent to 1 μg of retinol. The actual biological activity of the carotenoids in a given food may be considerably higher or lower than its analytically determined content, depending on the amount of carotenoid present, the nature of the meal, the presence of fat, the binding of the carotenoid within the food, the method of preparation of the food, and other factors (44). Although the 6:1 ratio of dietary β-carotene to vitamin A has been maintained in recent dietary recommendations (45,46), the actual provitamin A activity of a given dietary carotenoid clearly can vary significantly from the calculated value.

Needless to say, the best method of dietary assessment is actual chemical analysis of the foods eaten by specific members of a family and direct measurement of the amounts ingested over a significant (2–4-week) period. Such a procedure, however, is very costly and time consuming.

A summary of the established values of international units and of retinol equivalencies for humans is presented in Table 3. It should be pointed out, however, that the relative effectiveness of carotenoids as precursors of vitamin A will depend on the species considered (47).

B.   Stability of Vitamin A and Its Availability in Foods

As already mentioned, vitamin A is prone to oxidation, particularly when exposed to light and heat in a humid atmosphere in the absence of reducing agents or other stabilizers. When vitamin A is present together with natural antioxidants in an oil-rich state, such as in butter or in liver, it resists destruction quite well. When vitamin A is added in a

Table 3 International Units (IU) and Retinol Equivalents for Humans

Compound	μg/IU	IU/μg	Retinol equivalents/μg
all-*trans*-Retinol	0.300	3.33	1.000
all-*trans*-Retinyl acetate	0.344	2.91	—
all-*trans*-Retinyl palmitate	0.549	1.82	—
all-*trans*-β-Carotene	1.8[a]	0.56	0.167
Mixed carotenoids	3.6	0.28	0.083

[a]Since the rat uses small amounts of β-carotene with high efficiency under specific experimental conditions, an international unit for β-carotene was earlier set as 0.6 μg, twice that of retinol. Man utilized carotenoids less well, however (47), and consequently the given value of 1.8 μg/IU agrees with the convention of considering 6 μg β-carotene as 1 μg retinol equivalent.

stabilized commercial beadlet form, the total amount present in foods with low moisture content remains well above 90% for periods up to 6 months (48,49). As the temperature and the moisture content increases, however, vitamin A deteriorates somewhat more rapidly. Nonetheless, highly satisfactory beadlet forms of vitamin A are available for use in premixes and feeds for cattle and poultry.

Carotenoids in food products behave somewhat similarly to vitamin A. As already mentioned, carotenoids can be oxidized to inactive forms, either by enzymatic action during storage or by exposure to light and oxygen. In general the carotenoid content of hay falls approximately 7% per month during storage. By incorporating carotenoids into beadlets or emulsions in the presence of reducing agents, their destruction during processing and storage is much reduced, normally amounting to less than 20% over a one-year period (47–49). Carotenoids are somewhat less bioavailable than vitamin A in general, perhaps mainly because of their binding to highly organized structures within cells, their specific requirements for bile salts during absorption, and their relatively slow rate of cleavage to vitamin A in the intestine and in other tissues.

VI. METABOLISM

A. Absorption

After foods are ingested, preformed vitamin A of animal tissues and the provitamin carotenoids of vegetables and fruits are released from proteins by the action of pepsin in the stomach and of proteolytic enzymes in the small intestine. In the stomach the free carotenoids and retinyl esters tend to congregate in fatty globules, which then enter the duodenum. In the presence of bile salts, the globules are broken up into smaller lipid congregates, which can be more easily digested by pancreatic lipase, retinyl ester hydrolase, cholesteryl ester hydrolase, and the like. The resultant mixed micelles, which contain retinol, the carotenoids, sterols, some phospholipids, mono- and diglycerides and fatty acids, then diffuse into the glycoprotein layer surrounding the microvillus and make contact with the cell membranes. Various components of the micelles, except for the bile salts, are then readily absorbed into mucosal cells, mainly in the upper half of the intestine.

The bioavailability and the digestion of vitamin A and carotenoids, needless to say, are affected by the overall nutritional status of the individual and the integrity of the intestinal mucosa. Nutritional factors of importance are protein, fat, vitamin E, zinc, and probably iron (50,51). Some types of fiber, e.g., highly methoxylated pectins, markedly reduce carotenoid absorption (52).

Bile salts, which are detergents, promote the rapid cleavage of retinyl and carotenoid esters and assist in the transfer of these lipids into mucosal cells. Interestingly, carotenoid absorption has an absolute requirement for bile salts, independent of its dispersion in a suitable micelle, whereas vitamin A in any properly solubilized form is readily absorbed (53,54).

Within mucosal cells provitamin A carotenoids are oxidatively cleaved to retinal and, possibly in part, to a group of β-apocarotenals with a longer chain length than retinal (55,56). β-Carotenoid 15,15'-dioxygenase catalyzes the central cleavage of provitamin A carotenoids and the oxidative conversion of some β-apocarotenals to retinal. Other enzymes, although not yet characterized, might also convert carotenoids to β-apocarotenals (57). Major products of β-carotene cleavage found in tissues are retinol and retinoic acid (57a). Because carotenoid cleavage enzymes are unstable, they can be rapidly inactivated in cell-free preparations (58). The relative importance of these two pathways of cleavage in animals will profoundly affect the provitamin A activity of a given carotenoid; central cleavage yields two moles of retinal per mole of β-carotene consumed, whereas excentric cleavage would give only one mole of retinal. In the absence of any other characterized process, central cleavage is considered to be the predominant pathway. Carotenoid cleavage is responsive to nutritional conditions. In vitamin A–deficient rats, for example, the activity of intestinal β-carotenoid 15,15'-dioxygenase is significantly enhanced (59).

The retinal formed from carotenoids is mainly reduced to retinol by retinal reductase of the intestinal mucosa, and thereby merges with retinol derived from dietary preformed vitamin A. Intracellular retinol is then largely esterified (70–80%) with long-chain fatty acids in the mucosal cell. Two pathways for esterification have been defined: 1) esterification by an acyl-coenzyme A–independent pathway that involves a complex between retinol and cellular retinol-binding protein (type II), a distinct binding protein present in relatively high levels (1% of the total soluble protein) in absorptive cells of the jejunal mucosa but in traces, or not at all, in other adult organs (60), and 2) esterification by an acyl-coenzyme A–dependent pathway, in which retinol is probably bound to cellular proteins, but less specifically. The former pathway seems to show a higher affinity for retinol than the latter, which is catalyzed by acyl-coenzyme A:retinol acyl-transferase, or ARAT. The activity of intestinal ARAT is not observedly affected by vitamin A depletion but is significantly enhanced when large amounts of vitamin A are ingested (61,62). The predominant ester formed in tissues is the palmitate, together with smaller quantities of the oleate, stearate, and other fatty acyl esters (50). The esterified retinol, together with large amounts of triglyceride, some phospholipid, and a small amount of apolipoproteins, is released into the lymph in the form of chylomicra. The chylomicra also contain small amounts of unesterified retinol. Some unesterified retinol and retinoic acid may also be rapidly transported to the liver via the portal circulation (63).

The overall absorption of dietary vitamin A is approximately 80–90%, with somewhat less efficient absorption at very high doses. The efficiency of absorption of carotenoids from foods is 50–60%, depending on its bioavailability. The absorption efficiency of carotenoids decreases markedly at high intakes or doses (44,63a).

B. Transport

1. Lymph

During the transport of chylomicra from the lymph into the general circulation, the triglycerides are degraded by lipoprotein lipase of the plasma. The latter is activated by divalent metal ions and requires the presence of albumin as a fatty acid acceptor. After much of the triglyceride is digested and removed from the chylomicron, the resultant chylomicron remnant, which contains retinyl ester, cholesteryl ester, some other lipids, and several apoliproteins, is taken up primarily by the liver but also, to some extent, by other tissues (64). Uptake by liver involves interaction between *apo*-lipoprotein E in the chylomicron remnant and high affinity receptors on the cell surface of parenchymal cells (64).

2. Plasma

Whereas dietary retinol is transported to the liver largely as an ester in lipoproteins formed in the intestine, the mobilization of vitamin A from liver stores and its delivery to peripheral tissues is a highly regulated process. A precursor (pre-RBP) of a specific retinol-binding protein (RBP) is synthesized in liver parenchymal cells (65). After the removal of a 3500 dalton polypeptide, the resultant *apo*-RBP binds all-*trans* retinol, and the complex (*holo*-RBP) is secreted into the plasma. Human RBP, which was first isolated in the late 1960s (66), is a single polypeptide chain, has a molecular weight of 21,000 and posesses a single binding site for retinol. Under normal conditions of vitamin A nutriture, approximately 90% of retinol-binding protein is saturated with retinol. In children the usual level of RBP in plasma is approximately 1–1.5 μmol/l (20–30 μg/ml), which rises at puberty to adult levels of 2–2.5 μmol/l (40–50 μg/ml). In human plasma RBP forms a complex with transthyretin, a tetramer which also binds thyroid hormones, in a one-to-one molar complex. The association constant (K_a) between transthyretin and RBP is approximately 10^6 M. The amino acid sequence and three-dimensional structure of RBP have been determined (67,68), and a cDNA clone for it has been identified and studied (69).

Within RBP, retinol resides in a hydrophobic cleft, which protects it from oxidation or destruction during transport (Fig. 4). RBP has been isolated from the plasma of many other species, including the rat, monkey, rabbit, cow, dog, and chicken. In all of these species RBP is similar in size to that found in the human, and in most cases it forms a complex with transthyretin.

The formation of the larger transthyretin–RBP complex may minimize the loss of RBP in the urine during its passage through the kidney (66). In chronic renal disease, the levels of RBP and of plasma retinol are greatly elevated, whereas in severe protein calorie malnutrition, the amounts of both are reduced to approximately 50%. Thus, the steady-state concentrations of both vitamin A and RBP in the plasma are dependent on factors other than vitamin A status alone.

Under normal physiological conditions the turnover of *holo*-RBP in the plasma is quite rapid. When associated with transythyretin, its half-life is approximately 11 to 16 hr, whereas in the *apo* form, it is removed much more rapidly. These half-life values increase, i.e., turnover decreases, about 50% in severe protein calorie malnutrition.

The retinol ligand of *holo*-RBP in the plasma not only is taken up by peripheral target tissues, but also is recycled back to the liver. By use of in vivo kinetic analysis, Green et al. (70) estimated that about half of the retinol released as *holo*-RBP from the liver was taken up by peripheral tissues and about half was returned to the liver. While a

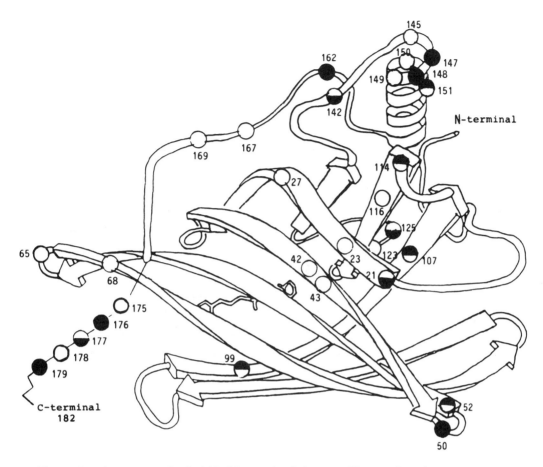

Figure 4 The structure of retinol-binding protein of plasma. Differences from the consensus sequence are denoted by ● (human), ◐ (rabbit), ○ (rat), and (all three species). Retinol is depicted within a barrel of β-sheets. (Reproduced with the permission of the *EMBO Journal*, Ref. 68.)

significant portion of the retinol recycled back to the liver seems to be in the form of a *holo*-RBP–transthyretin complex (70,71), other forms of vitamin A, e.g., retinyl ester and retinol carried by plasma lipoproteins, may also play a role in this process. The key point is that retinol is carefully conserved by the body and is not indiscriminately lost through excretion. Indeed, the irreversible daily loss of vitamin A in the feces and urine of vitamin A–depleted animals, and presumably of humans, is much reduced relative to the rate of loss in vitamin A–sufficient animals (72).

Of all processes relative to the uptake, storage, and transport of vitamin A, the combination of retinol with retinol-binding protein in the liver seems to be one of the most specific. Thus, the only ligand found under normal physiological conditions is all-*trans*-retinol. Other vitamin A analogs will combine with *apo*-retinol-binding protein in vitro, however, and 3-dehydroretinol, 15-methylretinol, and 15-dimethylretinol form *holo*-RBP analogs in vivo (33,73,74). Indeed, the abilities of specific analogs to saturate RBP in vivo can be closely related to their biological activities (33).

Retinoic acid is not transported on RBP, rather it is carried in the plasma on albumin and possibly on other proteins (66). Retinoic acid (75), as well as the water-soluble β-glucuronides of retinol and retinoic acid (76), are endogenous, albeit minor, components of human plasma.

C. Tissue Deposition and Storage

1. Cell-Surface Receptors for Plasma Retinol Binding Protein

The protein portion of *holo*-RBP, and not retinol itself, is recognized by cell-surface receptors on target tissues.

The tissue most studied in this regard is the retinal pigment epithelium of the vertebrate eye. The external surface of these cells, i.e., that in contact with plasma, contains a specific cell surface receptor for *holo*-RBP that it binds with great affinity, i.e., with a K_a of 2 $\times$ 10^{11} M (77). The estimated size of the receptor is 70–90 KDa. Transthyretin is not bound to the receptor, nor is a RBP-transthyretin complex necessary for binding. Each cell of the retinal pigment epithelium has about 50,000 cell-surface receptors for RBP. If other ligands, such as retinoic acid, are combined with chemically prepared *apo*-RBP in vitro, these ligands are also transferred into cells (78). It should be stressed, however, that the primary physiological ligand is all-*trans*-retinol. After complexing with the cell-surface receptor, *holo*-RBP, in all likelihood, is internalized within target cells by receptor-mediated endocytosis. Thereafter, retinol is released into the cytosol and the *apo*-RBP is either degraded or secreted from cells in a modified form (79). *Apo*-RBP is bound to surface receptors less tightly than *holo*-RBP.

Among the probable target tissues for retinol, such as the epithelium of the skin, the intestine, the adrenal gland, the testes, and the salivary gland, cell-surface receptors for *holo*-RBP have been identified thus far in the intestine, the skin (80), and the testes (81). Receptors seem to be present as well on stellate and parenchymal cells of the liver (71). Interestingly, receptors may well be absent in the well-known skin disease psoriasis (81). It is thus attractive to muse that many common skin diseases, which often respond positively to topical applications of vitamin A or its analogs, may result from the destruction or impaired synthesis of their cell-surface receptors for *holo*-RBP.

2. Intracellular Binding Proteins

Once retinol is transferred from RBP into the cell, it apparently is quickly bound by specific binding proteins in the cell cytosol. These proteins, called cellular retinol-binding proteins (CRBP), not only may protect retinol from oxidation within the cell, but also may serve as a carrier to its intracellular site of action (82). Cellular retinol-binding proteins have been detected in a large number of tissues, including the brain, eye, intestinal mucosa, testes, kidney, liver and lung, but not in heart or skeletal muscle.

CRBP from the testes and other tissues differs in many ways from RBP. Its molecular weight is 15,700 instead of 21,000. Furthermore, it is not immunologically cross-reactive with RBP, has no binding affinity for transthyretin, possesses an absorption spectra with peaks at 277 and 350 nm instead of at 280 and 330 nm, and has a greatly enhanced fluorescence emission with a peak at 470 nm instead of at 460 nm. The only similarities are that both are highly specific for all-*trans*-retinol and that both bind one mole of retinol per mole of protein. In normal animals, CRBP is about 40–70% saturated. Interestingly, vitamin A deficiency seems to have little effect on the concentration of CRBP within cells (83). CRBP has been highly purified from the testes and from several other tissues (82), and its amino acid sequence has been determined (84).

Cellular retinol-binding protein type II (CRBP II) is found primarily in the intestine of adult animals (85) The physical properties of the protein are similar to CRBP, except that it can be separated from it and from other retinoid-binding proteins by ion exchange chromatography (82). When bound to CRBP II, retinol is esterified by intestinal microsomes in the absence of acyl-coenzyme A (60). The pattern of retinyl esters formed is similar to that found in vivo. In association with CRBP II, retinol is also reversibly converted to retinal. Thus, CRBP II seems to play an important role in the metabolism, transport, and esterification of vitamin A in the intestine.

Another interesting intracellular binding protein is specific for retinoic acid. This binding protein, called cellular retinoic acid–binding protein (CRABP), is found in many of the same epithelial tissues in which CRBP is found, namely brain, eye, intestinal mucosa, skin, testes, etc., but not in the skeletal muscle or in the jejunal and ileal mucosa of adult animals. CRABP has a molecular weight of 12,000–18,000, depending on the species and organ (82). The amino acid sequence of bovine CRABP is known (86). CRABP can be differentiated from RBP by the same criteria as used for CRBP.

CRABP concentrations in some tissues vary considerably, depending on the age of the animal. Thus, CRABP is found in many fetal tissues but to a much smaller extent, if at all, in the corresponding adult tissues. In addition, CRABP has been identfied in many, but not all, epithelial cell tumors (82). Thus, the possibility exists that the antitumor action of some retinoids may be mediated through these proteins.

Two other retinoid-binding proteins are found solely in the eye. The first of these is cellular retinaldehyde-binding protein (CRALBP). CRALBP, which has a molecular weight of 33,000, is distinct from all other retinoid-binding proteins (87). It is found in the Müller cells of the retina and in the retinal pigment epithelia, but not in the rod outer segments. CRALBP binds both 11-*cis*-retinal and 11-*cis*-retinol with high stereospecificity (88). Indeed, these two ligands can be enzymatically interconverted when bound to the protein. Furthermore, 11-*cis*-retinal is protected from photoisomerization when bound to CRALBP (88).

The second retinoid-binding protein of the eye is interstitial (or interphotoreceptor) retinoid-binding protein (IRBP). IRBP, the most abundant protein of the interphotoreceptor matrix, has a molecular weight of 144,000 in the bovine and 138,000 in the chicken (89). IRBP is a glycoprotein, is synthesized in the neural retina, and is believed to transport all-*trans*- and probably 11-*cis*-retinol between the pigment epithelium and the rod and cone cells of the retina (90–92). IRBP is a flexible, elongated molecule (24 × 3–4 nm) that exists both in a straight and in a bent form (93). Human IRBP, which has recently been cloned, is associated with chromosome 10 (94).

3. Storage

Under normal conditions, over 90% of the vitamin A in the animal body is stored in the liver, although small quantities are also found in all other tissues. Thus, most attention has been given to elucidating the mechanism of its storage and release from the liver.

Endocytosed chylomicron remnants are initially located in light-density endosomes of parenchymal cells (62), where retinyl esters are hydrolyzed. Retinol is then translocated, presumably in a complex with CRBP, to the endoplastic reticulum, which is rich in *apo*-RBP and contains both acyl-CoA–independent retinyl ester synthase (RES) and acyl-CoA: retinol acyltransferase (ARAT). Retinol might either continue to circulate as *holo*-CRBP, be transferred to *apo*-RBP for release into the plasma, or be esterified to retinyl ester. Retinyl esters, which predominantly consist of palmitate with smaller amounts of stearate.

oleate, and linoleate, are then stored in vitamin A–containing globules (VAG) within the parenchymal cells. Parenchymal cells of the liver can be divided on the basis of their density into two major classes: "light" hepatocytes that contain much vitamin A and "heavy" hepatocytes that contain little (24). When liver reserves of vitamin A are low, parenchymal cells are the major storage site of vitamin A (95).

When liver reserves are adequate ($\geq$ 20 μg retinol/g), approximately 80% of the newly absorbed vitamin A is transferred from parenchymal cells to a specialized type of perisinusoidal cells, termed stellate cells (fat-storing cells, lipocytes, Ito cells (61,62,95–97). The mechanism of intercellular transport is not clear, although complexes of retinol with CRBP, RBP, and yet a new retinoid-binding protein have been postulated to serve as possible carriers. Within stellate cells, retinol is rapidly esterified to fatty acids in a pattern similar to that found in parenchymal cells. The resultant retinyl esters are stored in vitamin A–containing globules, which contain up to 60% retinyl esters, a significant amount of triglyceride, less phospholipid, and small amounts of cholesterol, cholesteryl esters, and α-tocopherol. Several proteins, which include retinyl ester synthase and hydrolase, are associated with these globules (98). Stellate cells also contain appreciable amounts of CRBP and CRABP, but little or no RBP or its mRNA (99). Circulating radiolabeled RBP, however, can be taken up by stellate cells (71). All other cells of the liver, including Kupffer cells, endothelial cells, and other nonparenchymal cells, contain very small amounts ($\leq$ 5%) of the total liver reserve of vitamin A.

In the storage of dietary vitamin A, the hydrolysis and formation of retinyl esters is important. Similarly, in the release of vitamin A from the liver as *holo*-RBP, hydrolysis of retinyl esters is a key step. In regard to the control of these processes, it is interesting that several forms of retinyl ester hydrolase exist in the liver (100) and that their activity is enhanced by a poor vitamin A status (101) and by vitamin E deficiency (102). The esterifying enzymes, on the other hand, are enhanced when large amounts of vitamin A are ingested (62,97,103). Thus, these enzymes should be included among factors that control vitamin A metabolism in vivo.

Stellate cells are not only found in rat liver, but also in many other tissues and in many other species (104,105). Besides storing vitamin A, stellate cells are highly active in synthesizing collagen and other structural proteins (96). Reasons underlying the association of these two important processes in stellate cells have not been clarified.

D. Metabolism

Major reactions in the metabolism of vitamin A are summarized in Figure 5. Dietary forms of vitamin A are retinyl esters, derived entirely from animal sources, and provitamin A carotenoids, derived largely from plant foods. Of the total carotenoids present in nature, however, less than 10% serve as precursors of vitamin A. These other nutritionally inactive carotenoids are metabolized primarily by oxidative reactions that have been considered in detail elsewhere (55,106).

Retinol is released from its dietary esters by the action of pancreatic hydrolases, which act in the presence of bile salts within the intestinal lumen. Within cells of many kinds, retinol is rapidly converted to retinyl esters. In most tissues, acyl-coenzyme A is the donor of acyl groups, but in the intestine and possibly in other tissues, the acyl groups may be transferred primarily from another lipid. Thus, at least two enzymes are involved in the esterification reaction.

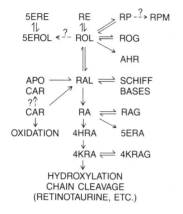

Figure 5 Metabolic transformation of vitamin A. Abbreviations: RE, retinyl ester; 5ERE, 5,6-epoxyretinyl ester; ROL, retinol; 5EROL, 5,6-epoxyretinol; RAL, retinaldehyde; RA, retinoic acid; RP, retinyl phosphate; RPM, retinyl-phosphate mannose; ROG, retinyl β-glucuronide; RAG, retinoyl β-glucuronide; 5ERA, 5,6-epoxyretinoic acid; 4HRA, 4-hydroxyretinoic acid; 4KRA, 4-ketoretinoic acid, 4KRAG, 4-ketoretinoyl β-glucuronide; AHR, anydroretinol; CAR, provitamin A carotenoids; APOCAR, β-apocarotenoids.

Retinyl esters are hydrolyzed by retinyl ester hydrolase, formerly called retinyl palmitate hydrolase:, At least three forms of this enzyme exist in the liver, and possibly in other organs as well. Because of the compartmentation of retinyl esters in different cells of the same tissue and in different subcellullar particles of a given cell, various isozymes of retinyl ester hydrolase may well be distributed differently and serve specific metabolic roles.

Retinol undergoes a number of other reactions. One of the most important, which is *not* indicated in Figure 5, is its combination with *apo*-RBP in the liver and its secretion into the plasma as *holo*-RBP. Although other tissues, such as the kidney, contain mRNA for *apo*-RBP, the physiological importance of *holo*-RBP release from other tissues is not yet clear. Nevertheless, much of the retinol released from the liver as *holo*-RBP does circulate back to the liver in some form (70).

Retinol also can react with uridine diphosphoglucuronic acid to form retinyl β-glucuronide (ROG) in the liver, intestine, kidney, and probably other tissues. Although originally thought to be mainly an excretory form of vitamin A because of its presence in the bile, its formation in many tissues and its high biological activity in growth and tissue differentiation indicate that it may play a physiological role per se. In tumor tissues, but rarely, if at all, in normal tissues, retinol can also be dehydrated to anhydroretinol (107). Retinol can also be phosphorylated, in the presence of ATP, to retinyl phosphate, and the latter can react with guanosine diphosphomannose in vitro to yield retinyl phosphomannose (RPM) (107,108). In vitro, RPM can transfer mannose to a glycoprotein receptor to give a mannosylated product. In vivo, however, the amount of retinyl phosphate formed is very small, and RPM has not been detected as an endogenous product (107,108). Thus, this interesting set of reactions does not seem to have major physiological significance (107,108).

Retinol is also reversibly oxidized to retinal by a NAD-dependent pathway in many tissues. Although alcohol dehydrogenase can catalyze this reaction, specific retinol dehydrogenases (retinal reductases) also exist.

Retinal is then irreversibly converted to retinoic acid in many tissues by aldehyde dehydrogenases and oxidases (109,110). The rate of conversion of retinal to retinoic acid is several fold faster than the oxidation of retinol to retinal (109,110). Retinoic acid is inactivated biologically either by hydroxylation at the C4 position or by epoxidation at the C5,6 positions (111). In animal tissues, both of these oxidative reactions are irreversible. 4-Hydroxyretinoic acid can be further oxidized to the 4-keto derivative, followed by a variety of oxidative, chain-cleaving, and conjugative reactions (111). One of the major conjugated cleavage products is retinotaurine, which appears in the bile in significant amounts (112).

Vitamin A also forms several β-glucuronides by interacting with UDP-glucuronic acid in the presence of glucuronyl transferases. The most interesting of these conjugates are retinyl β-glucuronide and retinoyl β-glucuronide, both of which retain high biological activity (34,113). Because both have now been synthesized chemically (34,113), further studies on them will be facilitated. Both are synthesized in the intestine, in the liver, and probably in other tissues in which they are found (114,115). Both are endogenous components of human blood (76,116) and, together with the glucuronides of 4-ketoretinoic acid and of other oxidized metabolites, appear in the bile (111).

When retinyl acetate or retinyl β-glucuronide is administered to rats, 5,6-epoxyretinyl ester is found in discrete amounts in the liver (117). Thus, epoxidation occurs at the level of retinol as well as of retinoic acid.

β-Carotene, as well as several other provitamin A carotenoids is converted by oxidative cleavage at the 15,15' double bond to yield two molecules of retinal. The enzyme catalyzing this reaction, 15,15' carotenoid dioxygenase, is found in the intestine, liver, kidney, and some other tissues (55). This enzyme will also convert β-apo-carotenoids found in plants and in trace amounts in some animal tissues to retinal (55). Although provitamin A carotenoids might also be converted to retinal in animal tissues via excentric cleavage of its central conjugated chain (55–58), no enzyme that acts excentrically has yet been clearly demonstrated. Apart from its cleavage, carotenoids are also oxidized in other ways (55,106).

Outside of the eye, where retinal is bound as a Schiff base to opsin and to CRALBP, retinal is present in very low concentrations in tissues. Its low concentration can be explained on kinetic grounds, namely, that the rate of conversion of retinal either to retinol or to retinoic acid greatly exceeds its rate of formation from retinol or from carotenoids. The metabolism of vitamin A and of carotenoids have been reviewed in the past several years (55,111,118,119).

E. Excretion

In a quantitative sense, ingested vitamin A is generally metabolized in the following way: 1) 10–20% is not absorbed, and hence is excreted within 1–2 days into the feces; 2) of the 80–90% absorbed, 20–60% is either conjugated or oxidized to products that are excreted within approximately one week in the feces or urine, with a small amount in expired CO_2; and 3) the remainder (30–60%) of the absorbed vitamin A is stored, primarily in the liver. When the initial liver reserves are depleted, however, the relative amount stored in the liver is much lower (120).

Stored vitamin A is metabolized much more slowly in the liver and peripheral tissues to conjugated and oxidized forms of vitamin A, which then are excreted. The half-life value for the overall depletion rate in humans is 128–156 days (45,121). As a general rule, derivatives of vitamin A with an intact carbon chain are excreted in the feces, whereas acidic chain–shortened products tend to be excreted in the urine. In the steady state, approximately equal amounts of metabolites are excreted in the feces and in the urine.

VII. BIOCHEMICAL FUNCTION

A. Vision

When a photon of light strikes the dark-adapted retina of the eye, the conformation of the visual pigment rhodopsin changes to yield a new transient photopigment, bathorhodopsin. That transient pigment in turn is converted in sequence to lumirhodopsin, to metarhodopsin I, and by deprotonation to metarhodopsin II. Another transient pigment formed directly from rhodopsin is hypsorhodopsin, which may be an obligatory nonprotonated intermediate in the formation of bathorhodopsin (122,123).

The primary photochemical event is the very rapid isomerization of 11-*cis*-retinal, present as a protonated Schiff base of a specific lysine residue in rhodopsin, to a highly strained *transoid* form in bathorhodopsin (122,123). These changes are summarized in Figure 6.

Rhodopsin contains hydrophilic and hydrophobic regions, has a molecular weight of approximately 38,000 in the cow, and is asymmetric, with a folded length of approximately 70°A. By use of both conventional sequencing and genetic cloning techniques, its complete amino acid sequence was determined (124–126). It contains an acetylated N-terminus, two oligosaccharides on asparagines 2 and 15, and retinal on lysine 296. Like several other transmembrane proteins, rhodopsin contains seven helical segments that extend back and forth across the disc membrane and make up approximately 60% of the total amino acid structure. In addition to loops between helical portions, less structured C-terminal and N-terminal portions extend into the cytosol and the intradisc space, respectively. The chromophore resides in a hydrophobic pocket formed by several transmembrane segments near to the cytosolic side of the disc membrane (124,127).

Metarhodopsin II, the penultimate conformation state of the light-activated visual pigment, reacts with transducin, a G-protein containing three subunits that is attached to the disc membrane (127). In response, the α-subunit of transducin binds GTP in place of endogenously associated GDP, thereby activating cGMP phosphodiesterase, which hydrolyzes cGMP to GMP. Because cGMP specifically maintains in an open state the sodium pore in the plasmalemma of the rod cell, a decrease in its concentration causes a marked reduction

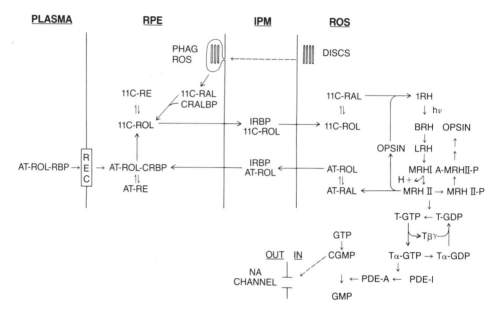

Figure 6   The visual cycle of vitamin A metabolism and photopigment formation in the retina of the eye. Abbreviations AT-ROL, all-*trans*- retinol; AT-RE, all-*trans*-retinyl ester, AT-RAL, all-*trans*-retinaldehyde; 11C-ROL, 11-*cis*-retinol; 11C-RE, 11-*cis*-retinyl ester; 11C-RAL, 11-*cis*-retinaldehyde; RBP, plasma retinol-binding protein; CRBP, cellular retinol-binding protein; CRALBP, cellular retinaldehyde-binding protein; IRBP, interstitial (interphotoreceptor) retinol-binding protein; RH, rhodopsin; BRH, bathorhodopsin; LRH, lumirhodopsin; MRH-I, metarhodopsin I; MRH-II, metarhodopsin II; T, transducin; Tα, Tβ and Tγ, subunits of transducin; A, arrestin; PDE-I and PDE-A, inhibited and activated forms of cGMP phosphodiesterase; ROS, rod outer segment; PHAG ROS, phagocytized rod outer segments; RPE, retinal pigment epithelial cells; IPM, interphotoreptor matrix; MRH II-P, phosphorylated metarhodopsin II.

in the influx of sodium ions into the rod outer segment. The membrane consequently becomes hyperpolarized:, which triggers the nerve impulse to other cells of the retina through the synaptic terminal of the rod cell.

The recovery from this activated state occurs in three ways: 1) The α-subunit of transducin, which also shows GTPase activity, hydrolyzes bound GTP to GDP, thereby leading to subunit reassociation to inactive transducin. As a consequence, cGMP phospodiesterase activity falls and the cGMP level increases back to a normal level, 2) metarhodopsin II is phosphorylated at sites in the C-terminal portion by ATP, which then reacts with arrestin to form a complex that no longer activates transducin, and 3) metarhodopsin II dissociates through metarhodopsin III to yield all-*trans*-retinal and opsin, which also does not activate transducin (127). These events are also summarized in Figure 6. Most aspects of retinal proteins and their photochemistry are considered in the proceedings of a recent conference (128).

Other metabolic events are also important in maintaining the visual process. All-*trans*-retinol, bound to RBP in the plasma, is taken up through a receptor-mediated process into the retinal pigment epithelium (RPE) (Fig. 6). All-*trans*-retinol can then be isomerized to 11-*cis*-retinol by all-*trans*:11-*cis*-retinol isomerase, a microsomal enzyme found predominantly, if not solely, in the RPE (129–131). Both isomers of retinol, bound to appropriate retinoid-binding proteins, can then be esterified to retinyl esters and stored in lipid globules (VAG) in the RPE. Alternatively, 11-*cis*-retinol can be transported on IRBP to the rod outer segment (ROS), where it is oxidized to 11-*cis*-retinal. Possibly, 11-*cis*-retinal might be transported directly from the RPE to the ROS. The latter spontaneously combines with opsin to yield rhodopsin.

After bleaching, the released all-*trans*-retinal is rapidly reduced to all-*trans*-retinol, which is ferried back to the RPE on IRBP. The overall transfer process is highly efficient, in that 11-*cis*-retinol does not accumulate in the RPE during regeneration of rhodopsin in the dark (19). Rather, 11-*cis*-retinal primarily bound to opsin in the ROS increases and all-*trans*-retinol in the ROS decreases to a similar extent (9).

Another, probably minor, source of 11-*cis*-retinol in the RPE is the 11-*cis*-retinal released by the digestion of phagocytized terminal discs of the ROS in the RPE (Fig. 6). Metabolic transformations of vitamin A in the eye have recently been reviewed (132).

B. Growth

The earliest assays for vitamin A were based on the growth response of rats fed a purified diet. The fact that maintenance of normal vision and enhancement of growth are two quite separate properties of the vitamin A molecule was dramatically demonstrated by the observation that retinoic acid stimulated growth but could not maintain vision (113). In nutritional studies the onset of vitamin A deficiency has often been detected by a so-called "growth plateau," which after several days is followed by a rapid loss of weight and ultimately death. In animals cycled on retinoic acid, i.e., given retinoic acid for 18 days followed by 10 days of deprivation, however, rats become exquisitely sensitive to the removal of retinoic acid from the diet (134). In these animals loss of appetite occurs within 1–2 days after the withdrawal of retinoic acid, which is closely followed by a depression in growth (135). Loss of appetite is therefore one of the first, if not the primary symptom, noted in all vitamin A–deficient animals.

Decreased food intake is not due in this case to impaired taste function, nor to the poor palatability of the deficient diet. Since many factors affect appetite, it has not been possible to define specifically the molecular effect of vitamin A on this process. Inasmuch as distortions in nitrogen metabolism and in amino acid balances within tissues and in the plasma occur concomitantly, the effect of vitamin A deficiency on appetite may well be related to these latter abnormalities (135).

C. Tissue Differentiation

In 1925, Wolbach and Howe (136) studied tissue changes that occurred in rats on a vitamin A–deficient diet. Many mucus-secreting tissues became keratinized, and a variety of other changes occurred in most epithelial tissues of the body. Tissues that were particularly sensitive to vitamin A deficiency were the trachea, the skin, the salivary gland, the cornea, and the testes. The cornea is of particular interest, inasmuch as its ulceration and ultimately its destruction in vitamin A–deficient children is a major cause of blindness among the very young (137).

Probably several factors contribute to corneal destruction. In vitamin A deficiency, goblet cell differentiation and the secretion of mucus are depressed in the glands around the eye. Consequently, tears have a lower concentration of mucus, which allows dry spots to form on the cornea. The small but significant concentration of vitamin A normally present in tear fluid is also markedly depressed in vitamin A deficiency (138). The thin layer of columnar epithelial cells on the cornea becomes keratinized, which disrupts their normal ordered architecture. Soon after corneal ulceration occurs, the activity of collagenases and other proteinases in the cornea also greatly increases (139). Furthermore, α_1-macroglobulin, a normal constituent of the plasma which is a collagenase inhibitor, is markedly decreased in severe vitamin A deficiency (140). And finally, the disrupted cell surface of the cornea may become infected (137). Thus, the destruction of the cornea due to vitamin A deficiency is probably a result of the synergistic action of several events, most of which are caused by the deficiency state.

An interesting case of modified differentiation as a result of vitamin A deficiency is the decreased prevalence of goblet cells in the crypts of Lieberkuhn in the intestine. In the vitamin A–deficient, retinoic acid–cycled rat, the number of goblet cells per crypt falls to approximately one-half within the first 2 or 3 days after withdrawal of retinoic acid from the diet, and then remains constant (141).

The mucus cells that remain in vitamin A deficiency respond normally to physiological stimulants and are equally able to synthesize mucus. Thus, vitamin A seems to block the differentiation of only one set of goblet cells from oligomucus cells and other precursors in the crypt (141). In contrast, most goblet cells in the conjunctiva of the eye are sensitive to vitamin A status (142). Indeed, a new method for evaluating mild vitamin A deficiency, termed conjunctival impression cytology (CIC), is based primarily on a reduced prevalence of conjunctival goblet cells (143).

Many attempts have been made to define in biochemical terms the manner in which vitamin A induces the differentiation of cells. Vitamin A deficiency has long been known to induce keratinized epithelial cells (136), and over 20 years ago, vitamin A was shown to stimulate RNA synthesis in the intestines of vitamin A–deficient rats (144). Although uncertainties still exist as to the precise manner in which vitamin A acts in cellular differentiation, one fairly general pathway increasingly seems to explain most of the disparate effects of various retinoids on different cell types. This pathway, first hypothesized by Chytil and Ong in 1979 (145), is summarized in Figure 7. As with other tissues and cells, *holo*-RBP delivers all-*trans*-retinol via a cell surface receptor to the cytosol of the cell. Retinol is subsequently oxidized via retinal to retinoic acid. Both retinol and retinoic acid are then bound by specific cellular retinoid-binding proteins, which migrate into the nucleus (82). Retinoic acid is then transferred to a nuclear retinoic acid receptor, termed RAR, which enhances the expression of specific regions of the genome (146–148). The retinoic acid receptor, which shows a molecular weight of approximately 54 KDa, belongs to a family of similar regulatory proteins, which include those for steroids, thyroid hormones, and 1,25-dihydroxyvitamin D_3 (147–148). RAR shows little or no homology with other retinoid-binding proteins. Although retinol and retinal also bind weakly to RAR, retinoic acid clearly is the primary ligand. Although not yet identified, a similar but distinct nuclear receptor for retinol probably exists as well (149).

Many new proteins appear during the retinoic acid–induced differentiation of cells. The difficulty has been to sort out those proteins that are induced in direct response to the signaling compound from those that appear later in the overall, complex process of differentiation. The mRNA for one such "early" protein that appears in response to retinoic acid in F9 teratocarcinoma cells is the so-called "Era" mRNA (150). As yet, the regulatory portion of the DNA that interacts with RAR has not been identified (147–149).

Other mechanisms may also exist for the vitamin A–induced differentiation of cells. Retinoic acid induces the granulocytic differentiation of HL-60 cells, for example, even

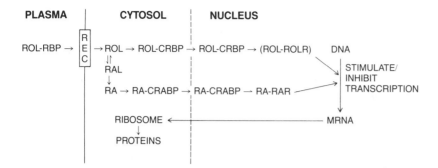

PLASMA | CYTOSOL | NUCLEUS

ROL-RBP → [REC] → ROL → ROL-CRBP → ROL-CRBP → (ROL-ROLR)   DNA

Figure 7 The Chytil-Ong hypothesis for the action of vitamin A in cellular differentiation. Abbreviations: ROL, retinol; RAL, retinal; RA, retinoic acid; RBP, plasma retinol-binding protein; CRBP, cellular retinol-binding protein; CRABP, cellular retinoic acid-binding protein; REC, cell-surface receptor for the ROL-RBP complex; RAR, the nuclear retinoic acid receptor; ROLR, the putative nuclear retinol receptor; mRNA, specific mRNA signaled by vitamin A; PROTEINS, specific proteins signaled by vitamin A.

though the latter lack detectable amounts of CRABP (151). The β-glucuronides of retinol and retinoic acid act similarly on HL-60 cells, apparently without being hydrolyzed to retinol and to retinoic acid, respectively (152–153). Indeed, retinyl β-glucuronide is a much better inducer than is retinol, which is relatively inactive in many cell culture systems. Retinoic acid also enhances the activity of three isozymes of phosphokinase C (154), suggestive of some mechanism involving second and/or third messengers. Finally, retinoic acid inhibits the phorbol ester–dependent release of fibronectin from enucleated as well as from nucleated 3T3 cells (155), indicative of a nucleus-independent action. Thus, we may well find that vitamin A may act in different ways depending on its specific chemical form, binding component, and cell type.

In vitamin A deficiency, glycoprotein synthesis is markedly depressed, and in the retinoid-induced differentiation of several cell types, glycoprotein synthesis is greatly enhanced (108,156). These changes are probably the result of increased levels of sugar transferases resulting from retinoid-induced cellular differentiation (157).

D. Proton Transfer Across Bacterial Membranes

In the past, it was thought that vitamin A was present only in species of the animal kingdom, whereas carotenoids, but not vitamin A, were generally found in bacteria and in plants. This generalization was upset in 1971 by the dramatic discovery of a new retinaldehyde-containing pigment, bacteriorhodopsin, in the membrane of the purple bacterium, *Halobacterium halobium* (158). Soon thereafter, its basic function was discovered, namely that, under the influence of light, protons are pumped from the inside to the outside of the bacterial cell. The chemiosmotic gradient thereby established may be used for the active transport of nutrients into the cell and for the formation of ATP and other energy-storage compounds.

Bacteriorhodopsin and rhodopsin are similar in many ways. Bacteriorhodopsin has a molecular weight of 26,000, 70% of which is in the form of an α-helix. Seven helical segments stretch back and forth across the membrane, each of which contains approximately 23 amino acid residues (125). The two chromophores of baceriorhodopsin are 13-*cis*- and all-*trans*-retinaldehyde, both of which are bound to the protein in approximately a 1:1 ratio at thermal equilibrium (42). In the light, the 13-*cis* isomer is converted to the all-*trans* form. In the dark-adapted pigment, as in the case of rhodopsin, the Schiff base is protected from reagents like hydroxylamine, but after exposure to light, reaction sites are exposed. After the absorption of a photon, a sequence of conformational changes occur in bacteriorhodopsin that are analogous to those seen with rhodospin.

In addition to bacteriorhodopsin, Halobacteria contain four other related pigments: halorhodopsin, which is involved in chloride transport, sensory photosystems PS565 and PS370, which control phototaxis, and slow-cycling rhodopsin (SR), the function of which is still unclear (159).

VIII. DEFICIENCY SIGNS

A. Animals

Whereas some signs of vitamin A deficiency occur early, such as reduced appetite, weight loss, a reduction in goblet cell number, and the reduced synthesis of some glycoproteins, ultimately vitamin A deficiency affects almost all tissues of the body. Commonly occurring signs are summarized in Table 4. The major causes of death are infection, twisting of the intestine, and urinary blockage.

Vitamin A deficiency has been diagnosed in many animals, birds, fish, and reptiles. In cattle a mild deficiency is associated with a scaly skin and roughened hair. As the deficiency deepens, the eyes become watery and the cornea becomes dry, soft, and cloudy. In calves the improper modeling of bone may constrict the optic nerve and result in blindness. The cerebrospinal fluid pressure rises, which may cause muscular incoordination and a staggering gait. Indeed, one of the early signs of vitamin A deficiency in growing calves is marked elevation of the cerebrospinal fluid pressure. In bulls used for breeding, vitamin A deficiency causes a decrease in sexual vigor as well as a fall in the motility and the number of mature spermatozoa.

In swine, vitamin A deficiency produces night blindness, a reduced growth rate, and an elevated cerebrospinal fluid pressure. Vitamin A deficiency can be disastrous for young pigs, who both fail to grow and develop abnormalities of the skeletal structure and the nervous system.

Table 4   Signs of Vitamin A Deficiency

Loss of appetite	Metaplastic and spongy bone
Retardation of growth	Cysts of endocrine and other glands
Nervous disorders	Keratinization of epithelial tissues
Skin disorders	Kupffer cell degeneration
Defective reproduction	Increased urinary calculi
Night blindness	Nephritis
Xerophthalmia	Fetal malformations and resorption
Blindness	Disorders of lactation
Increased infection	Death

In young, rapidly growing rams, symptoms of vitamin A deficiency may occur within 6 weeks. The signs consist of stiffness of the legs, an abnormal cocking of the head, muscular weakness, and an uncoordinated gait. Loss of appetite is common, and night blindness is prevalent.

In cats, the first sign of vitamin A deficiency is decreased food consumption followed by loss of weight. Muscular weakness and rigidity of the hindquarters as well as reproductive failure and degeneration of the retina have also been noted.

Poultry are very rapidly affected by vitamin A deficiency. Signs appear in growing chicks in 3-4 weeks. Loss of appetite and decreased growth rate are early signs, with general weakness, staggering gait, and ruffled plumage following. Birds become more susceptible to infection, and both egg production and hatchability are markedly reduced. The eyes are also affected, with an abnormal exudate and epithelial keratinization as typical signs (160,161).

B. Man

Needless to say, the major signs of vitamin A deficiency in man relate more to external, readily diagnosed changes than to abnormalities of tissue or cellular structure. Thus, throughout history night blindness has been closely associated with vitamin A deficiency (137,162–163). Another major sign of vitamin A deficiency is xerophthalmia, which includes various stages of conjunctival xerosis, Bitot's spots, and corneal involvement and ulceration (164–165). Bitot's spots, which are foamy white accumulations of sloughed cells that usually appear on the temporal quadrant of the conjunctiva, have conventionally been used as a clinical indicator of vitamin A deficiency in young children. Changes in the skin have also been observed, most specifically follicular hyperkeratosis. Although the signs of vitamin A deficiency have occasionally been noted among seemingly healthy adults, the most serious and dramatic manifestations are seen in very young children. In these cases, vitamin A deficiency is almost invariably associated with protein calorie malnutrition, a low intake of fats, gastrointestinal distress, and respiratory disease (2,162–165). Apart from clinical signs of deficiency, a marginal vitamin A status has been associated in children with increased morbidity and mortality, a decreased growth rate, and inefficient iron utilization (165a).

IX. METHODS OF NUTRITIONAL ASSESSMENT

A. Clinical

Vitamin A status can be classified into five categories: deficient, marginal, satisfactory, excessive, and toxic (Table 5). The deficient and toxic stages are characterized by clinical signs, whereas the other three states are not. The most commonly used indicator of clinical deficiency in surveys is the presence of xerophthalmia (164). Major eye signs and suggested cutoff points of public health significance (164,165) are given in Table 6. Of the signs listed, Bitot's spots (X1B) in preschool children has proven to be the most useful. Corneal involvement, although quite specific, is a relatively rare sign, and conjunctival xerosis (X1A) is fairly nonspecific. The disappearance of any reversible sign in response to vitamin A treatment, of course, strengthens its validity. Night blindness, which is difficult to evaluate in young children by direct measurement, can often be satisfactorily assessed by interviewing the mother (165).

Table 5 Indicators of Vitamin A Status for Preschool Children

Indicator	Deficient	Marginal	Satisfactory	Excessive	Toxic
Liver vitamin A (μg/g)	≪ 5	5– 20	20– 200	200– 300	≫ 300
Night blindness	+	±	—	—	—
Xerophthalmia	+	—	—	—	(+)[a]
Conjunctival impression cytology	+	±	—	—	—
Plasma vitamin A (μg/dl)	≪ 10	10– 20	20– 50	50– 100[b]	≫ 100[b]
Breast milk vitamin A[c] (μg/dl)	≪ 10	10– 20	20– 100	—	—
Diet (RE/day)	≪ 60	60–200	200–2000	2000–5000	≫ 5000
Relative dose response (%)	≫ 50	50– 20	≪ 20	—	—

[a]Conjunctivitis; different from xerophthalmia.
[b]An increasing portion of total plasma vitamin A is present as retinyl ester (≫20%) when large doses are ingested (264a).
[c]For nursing infants only.

A promising new procedure for measuring a state of mild deficiency, and presumably the lower part of the marginal state, is conjunctival impression cytology (CIC) (142,143). In this procedure, the relative numbers of goblet cells and of abnormal epithelial cells in a stained imprint of the conjunctiva are determined. The fewer the goblet cells and the greater the abnormal epithelial cells, the poorer the vitamin A status. Administration of a large dose of vitamin A to children with an abnormal conjunctiva corrects the condition. This procedure, which has given useful results in Indonesia and in a hospital-based study in France (166), is now being tested in other countries. In rural villages in Guatemala, however, where acute vitamin A deficiency was rare but conjunctivitis was common, the sensitivity of the method was low relative to biochemical indicators of a marginal vitamin A status (167,168).

In order to obtain useful information about the prevalence of vitamin A deficiency in a population, rigorous epidemiological techniques, which include the selection of an

Table 6 Xerophthalmia Classification and Public Health Criteria (1982)

Symbol	Sign	Critical prevalence
X1A	Conjunctival xerosis	Nonspecific
X1B	Bitot's spots with conjunctival xerosis	0.5%
X2	Corneal xerosis	
X3A	Corneal ulceration/keratomalacia involving ≪ ⅓ of the corneal surface	
X3B	Corneal ulceration/keratomalacia involving ≥ ⅓ of the corneal surface	0.01% total
XN	Night blindness	1%
XS	Corneal scars	0.05%
XF	Xerophthalmia fundus	Mainly of clinical interest

adequate sample size, carefully selected sampling areas, appropriate clinical and biochemical indicators, and "standardized" personnel, must be employed. Well-designed surveys, although expensive and time consuming, provide information of great value that cannot be obtained in other ways.

B. Biochemical

The five states of vitamin A nutriture can best be defined in terms of the total body reserve of vitamin A. The relationship between suggested indicators of vitamin A status for preschool children and the liver reserve, normally $\geq 90\%$ of the total body reserve, is summarized in Table 5. As the total body reserve decreases, however, the liver contains an increasingly smaller portion of the total vitamin A. Liver vitamin A values can be directly measured by biopsy, but only under specially justified conditions (169). Because liver vitamin A is quite stable, autopsy specimens also provide a useful indicator of vitamin A status (170). By use of tetradeuterated vitamin A, total body reserves can now be measured in humans by isotope-dilution (27). A similar approach, employing radiolabeled vitamin A, has previously been validated in rats and in several other species (120).

The relative dose response (RDR) assay measures the ratio of the difference in plasma retinol between 5 hours and zero time to the 5-hour value after a 450-μg dose of vitamin A in oil is given orally to children ((171,172). Expressed as a percentage, RDR values less than 20% are characteristic of satisfactory liver reserves of vitamin A ($\geq 20\ \mu g/g$), and values greater than 20% of lower liver concentrations. The relationship between RDR values and liver reserves of vitamin A has been validated in several studies (166,169,173). As a variant of the RDR, 3-dehydroretinyl acetate in oil (50 μg/kg body weight) can be given to children and a single blood sample taken at 4–5 hours. The ratio of 3-dehydroretinol to retinol in the plasma at 4–5 hours is inversely proportional to the liver reserves in experimental animals (74,174) and presumably in humans. The concentration of chlorinated analogs of ethyl retinoate in rat plasma 36 hours after an intraperitoneal dose is also inversely related to liver reserves (175). Thus, new biochemical procedures for evaluating a marginal vitamin A status in humans are now, or are becoming, available.

Plasma vitamin A values have long been used as a general guide to vitamin A status. Such values are particularly useful when they are very low, i.e., $\ll 10\ \mu g/dl$, or very high, i.e., $\gg 100\ \mu g/dl$. Very low values are indicative of depleted liver reserves and of a high risk of vitamin A deficiency in the individual (162), whereas very high values are suggestive of hypervitaminosis A. When liver reserves are adequate ($\geq 20\ \mu g/g$), plasma retinol values are homeostatically controlled in each individual at a level that is largely independent of total body reserves (176). In a healthy well-nourished population, the coefficient of variation of plasma retinol values is approximately 20% (177). Even in hypervitaminosis A, plasma retinol values, which are mainly determined by the concentration of *holo*-RBP, are only slightly increased (50). Besides the vitamin A status, plasma retinol values are lowered by protein-calorie malnutrition, infections, and parasitic infestations and raised by estrogenic contraceptive drugs and by kidney disease (54,163). As a consequence, plasma retinol values in the low to middle range (15–35 μg/dl) are not readily interpretable in regard to the vitamin A status of the individual. Mean plasma retinol values for children up to the age of puberty are approximately 50% that of adults (177).

In populations, however, mean plasma retinol values less than 20 μg/dl for preschool children (30) is often indicative of a marginal status. Supplementation of the population with vitamin A, e.g., by means of sugar fortification, increased the mean value of plasma retinol and normalized the distribution curve in children (30). In the United States the second percentile values of plasma retinol, starting from the bottom of the distribution, for children 3–5 years old and for adults 18–74 years old were approximately 19 μg/dl and 31 μg/dl, respectively (177). If a significantly larger portion of a given population show plasma retinol values below these values, a problem with vitamin A nutriture might be suspected.

The concentration of *holo*-RBP in the plasma is approximately 20–30 μg/ml in children, which then rises to 40–50 μg/ml in adults. In healthy, vitamin A–sufficient individuals, 80–90% of circulating plasma RBP is complexed with retinol (50). When the vitamin A status is poor, the total amount of RBP falls to approximately 50% of normal, most of which is present in the *apo* form. Several methods exist for the measurement of *holo*-RBP and of total RBP (30). Because the fluorescence of retinol is greatly enhanced by its binding to RBP, fluorescence assay of selected protein peaks eluted from size-exclusion columns is a simple, sensitive procedure for assaying plasma retinol levels (178).

C. Physiological

Night blindness is an early, common, and specific sign of vitamin A deficiency that can be measured quantitatively by determining the visual threshold after extensive dark adaptation. Generally, about 30 minutes are required for the eye to be completely dark adapted, at which point defective adaptation is very evident. In normal clinical practice the detection of very low levels of illumination is made subjectively by the patient, but might also be measured quantitatively by use of an electroretinogram. These procedures, which are usually conducted in a physiological laboratory, are much less adaptable to field use, particularly with children. Thus, night blindness in children can best be detected by interviewing the mother, particularly in societies that have coined specific terms for this condition (137). An ingenious procedure, termed the rapid dark adaptation test, has been effectively used in a hospital setting to detect incipient vitamin A deficiency in adults suffering from alcoholic liver disease (179). The test, which consists of sorting differently colored discs in dim light, is based on a shift in the rod-cone break time as a result of vitamin A deprivation. In a field setting, however, the test results suffered from a large variance and a lack of association with plasma retinol values (180).

D. Dietary

As already discussed under the section on the content of vitamin A and carotenoids in food, dietary surveys have limited usefulness relative to vitamin A. They are highly indicative in two particular cases: 1) when the diet is relatively simple and is clearly devoid of vitamin A and carotenoids, and 2) when the diet contains many vitamin A- and carotenoid-containing foods.

Quantitation of the average dietary intake of vitamin A and carotenoids is difficult. Because liver, a major source of vitamin A in the American diet, is eaten rarely, the day-to-day variation in the vitamin A intake of an individual is large. Thus, the commonly used 24-hour recall method can be very misleading relative to the average intake of an individual. Indeed, the ratios of the intraindividual variance to interindividual variance in the dietary intakes of vitamin A and β-carotene in 24 men over a 4-week period were 2.6 and 3.4, respectively (181). Thus, 9–26 independent 24-hour recalls would be needed to discriminate medium differences in intake (181). The longer the period selected, of course, the better the estimate of average dietary intakes. Food-frequency methods seem to provide more reliable estimates of the average vitamin A intakes, providing that portion size and other aspects of data collection are standardized (182).

The use of overall per capita intake data is also not very helpful, inasmuch as the high-risk group of preschool children often have a diet quite different from that of older children and adults. A good example is the Salvador region of the State of Bahia in Brazil where red palm oil is extensively used in cooking. Although the per capita intake of vitamin A exceeds 100% of the recommended dietary intake (RDI), many children die with very low liver reserves of vitamin A (183).

Perhaps the greatest use of dietary data is not in assessing the intake of a given nutrient, but rather in providing a general picture of the types of food that individuals eat and the way in which these foods are prepared. In any attempt to improve the nutrition of families or larger social groups, such information is crucial for the formulation of corrective strategies.

X. NUTRITIONAL REQUIREMENTS

A. General Considerations

A nutritional requirement, whether for animals or humans, must be defined operationally in terms of nutrient-specific indicators. If a different indicator is selected, the value of the requirement may well change. Thus, the presumed requirement will progressively increase as survival, prevention of clinical signs of deficiency, reproductive performance, and longevity are used as endpoints. As a conseqeunce, several tiers of requirements might be defined, based on the physiological level of satisfactory performance that is desired. Many vitamins, including vitamin A, also show biological *actions*, some beneficial and some adverse, at yet higher levels, e.g., the adjuvant effect of large doses of vitamin A in stimulating the immune system. These effects, which are pharmacological in nature, should *not* be considered in setting the nutritional requirement. Some responses to nutrients, however, which fall between clearly nutritional and clearly pharmacological effects, can be difficult to classify.

Strictly speaking, the nutritional requirement for a population, as defined by a given selected indicator, should be expressed as the mean requirement, i.e., where 50% of those in the population show satisfactory values and 50% show unsatisfactory values of a given indicator. Because the objective of nutritional analysis is the maintenance of a satisfactory status in most individuals in a population, however, the recommended dietary intake (RDI), a term used worldwide (183a), or recommended dietary allowance (RDA), as used in the United States and in a few other countries, has been defined as the average intake over time that theorectically would meet or exceed the nutritional needs of 97.7% (mean + 2 SD) of a selected healthy population group, or, more pragmatically, of "nearly all" members of the group. Although reliable data on the frequency distribution of requirements for many species are not available, a coefficient of variation of 20% seems to apply to several vitamins in humans and in other species.

Often, the dietary content of a nutrient is set at a level generously above that which provides for any possible physiological need but significantly lower than that which causes toxic effects. In such cases, a "safety factor," usually selected rather arbitrarily, is included in the calculation of the desired nutrient level.

Because all of the above procedures have been used in setting recommended intakes of vitamin A, a range of recommended values exists. In selecting an appropriate level for a given application, the basis of various recommendations must consequently be probed.

Another aspect of nutritional requirements that merits comment is the concept of a single "optimal" intake. Little evidence favors such a view. Rather, most studies indicate that a broad range of satisfactory intakes exists between a low level that prevents deficiency and a high level that causes toxicity. The "satisfactory range" viewpoint is inherent in the establishment of a "safe and adequate range " for several nutrients (184) and in the persuasive writings of George Beaton (185).

The most suitable indicator of vitamin A nutriture, as indicated earlier, is its total body reserve. The status of many other nutrients, such as iron, folic acid, vitamin B_{12}, and vitamin C, can also be related to their total body reserves. The relation of various indicators of nutritional status to the total body reserve and the selection of a total body reserve that meets specified operational criteria of adequacy are essential for the future definition of more scientifically based nutritional requirements and recommendations.

B. Animals

Two approaches have been taken relative to satisfactory vitamin A intakes: 1) to define the amount of vitamin A needed per kilogram body weight to promote normal growth in young animals, and 2) to provide an adequate concentration of vitamin A or β-carotene in the feed. Since the efficiency of conversion of carotene to vitamin A differs with the species, each major species must be considered individually. At periodic intervals the National Academy of Sciences (U.S.) defines or updates the nutrient needs of various animals. Since 1974 the following species have been considered: dogs, sheep, beef cattle, rabbits, warm-water fishes, poultry, cats, dairy cattle, horses, small laboratory animals, and nonhuman primates. Whereas no attempt will be made here to define the specific recommended levels per kilogram body weight or per kilogram feed for a wide variety of domestic and farm animals, some general guidelines might be given. Doses that cure deficiencies in many adult species are 3–8 μg retinol/kg/day, whereas those that ensure maximal growth and longevity for many animals fall in the range of 30–60 μg retinol (100–200 IU) per kilogram body weight per day. With respect to vitamin A concentrations in the feed, values from 4,000 to 10,000 IU per kilogram generally are used in the United States to ensure good vitamin A nutrition (160,161). In Europe, the recommended amounts in the feed of a variety of domestic animals are roughly twofold higher (160,161).

C. Humans

Several dietary recommendations (46,184,186) are given in Table 7 as a function of age, sex and physiological state. Of particular interest in the FAO/WHO recommendations (46) is the definition of two tiers of values, a *basal* RDI, which is an intake level that prevents signs of vitamin A deficiency and ensures normal growth in nearly all persons in a population, and a *safe level of intake*, which provides as well a suitable body reserve of vitamin A to meet periods of low intake and stress in nearly all members of a population. In the case of vitamin A, a satisfactory liver reserve of 20 μg/g, i.e., 0.07 μmol/g, was selected, primarily because plasma retinol levels are fully maintained at this liver level and an adult is protected for approximately 4 months if ingesting a diet low in vitamin A (46). The same approach was used to define RDI values of vitamin A for a U.S. population (45,186), which are equivalent on a weight basis to the "safe levels of intake" used by the FAO/WHO (46). The calculated RDI values for adult populations in the United States (45,186) are

Table 7 Dietary Recommendations for Vitamin A in Retinol Equivalents[a]

Group	Age	WHO/FAO (1988) Basal	WHO/FAO (1988) Safe	Olson (1987)	NRC-US (1989)
Infants	0– 0.5 yr	180	350	375	375
	0.5– 1 yr	180	350	375	375
Children	1– 2 yr	200	400	375	400[b]
	2– 6 yr	200	400	500	500[c]
	6–10 yr	250	400	500	700[d]
Males	10–12 yr	300	500	600	1000[e]
	12–70+ yr	300[f]	600	700	1000
Females	10–70+ yr	270[f]	500	600	800[g]
Pregnancy	0–3 mo	+100	+100	+0	+0
	3–6 mo	+100	+100	+0	+0
	6–9 mo	+100	+100	+200	+0
Lactation	0–6 mo	+180	+350	+400	+500
	⩾ 6 mo	+180	+350	+320	+400

[a]A retinol equivalent is defined as 1 μg retinol. 6 μg β-carotene or 12 μg of mixed provitamin A carotenoids are considered to be equal to 1 μg retinol.
[b]1–3 years.
[c]4–6 years.
[d]7–10 years.
[e]11–14 years.
[f]18–70+ years.
[g]11–70+ years.

approximately 15% higher than the FAO/WHO levels for adults solely on the basis of the weights of selected reference individuals. In the United States, the weights of the reference male and female were 76 kg and 62 kg, respectively, whereas the corresponding FAO/WHO reference weights are 65 kg and 55 kg, respectively. Since the need for vitamin A is presumed to be determined largely by mass, a value of 9.3 μg retinol equivalents per kg body weight was used in both cases. The present U.S. recommendations of the National Research Council (184), termed recommended dietary allowances, are based on a different approach. The relative merits of these approaches have been discussed (45).

XI. FACTORS THAT INFLUENCE VITAMIN A STATUS

A. Drugs and Other Organic Compounds

The metabolism of vitamin A is not appreciably affected by most common antibiotics, pain relievers, or other frequently employed drugs. Neomycin sulfate, however, which precipitates fatty acids and bile acids, disrupts lipid micelles within the lumen of the small intestine and reduces vitamin A absorption (187). When given in repeated doses, cortisone also significantly reduces the liver stores of vitamin A. Phenobarbital, caffeine and alcohol in modest amounts tend to lower somewhat vitamin A reserves.

Oral contraceptive agents are known to affect the metabolism of several vitamins and minerals, including that of vitamin A. Routine usage of an estrogen-progestagen combination-type oral contraceptive markedly increases the level of *holo*-RBP in women and rats (188–190). The estrogen component of the mixed contraceptive agent apparently stimulates protein synthesis in the liver, which give rise to heightened *holo*-RBP levels in the plasma. Concomitantly, the liver reserves of vitamin A are slightly decreased. Although the use of contraceptive agents cannot be considered as hazardous with respect to vitamin A nutrition, supplementation of the diets of women using them with small amounts of vitamin A is advisable (190).

The fact that vitamin A metabolism and transport is markedly affected by chlorinated hydrocarbons was dramatically illustrated by the case of X disease in cattle. This condition was first observed by Olafson in New York State in 1941. Two heifers, although suffering from emaciation and a thick hyperkeratotic skin, refused to accept food. The inducing agent was traced to a processed wheat concentrate which contained substantial quantities of pentachloronaphthalene as a contaminant. One of the early signs of X disease is a dramatic fall in the level of vitamin A, both in the plasma and in the liver. Other halogenated hydrocarbons, such as DDT, chlordane, lindane, dieldrin, polychlorobiphenyl, methoxychlor, and dioxin, when fed in significant doses, all reduce the liver concentration of vitamin A (191–193).

The mechanism by which polyhalogenated hydrocarbons deplete liver stores is not fully known. The fecal and urinary excretion of vitamin A metabolites after a single dose of dioxin or hexabromobiphenyl, however, is increased (193,194). Although the intestinal absorption of vitamin A and plasma retinol levels are not demonstrably affected (194,195), the ability of the liver to store vitamin A is markedly depressed (195). Furthermore, a higher proportion of administered vitamin A is found in the kidney in the form of retinyl esters. Finally, the activities of both acyl-CoA:retinol acyltransferase (ARAT) and retinyl ester hydrolase (REH) in the liver are depressed (195). Thus, polychlorinated aromatic hydrocarbons are clearly disruptive of storage and conservation mechanisms for vitamin A while not immediately affecting the maintenance of plasma retinol levels (195).

B. Disease

Diseases influence vitamin A status by altering its absorption, storage, tissue utilization, and conservation or recycling. As mentioned earlier, the absorption both of carotenoids and of vitamin A depends on the formation of bile salt containing micelles, on the cleavage of esters with pancreatic lipases or esterases, and on the transfer of the lipid moieties of the micelle into the mucosal cell. Consequently, chronic lipid malabsorption syndromes will markedly reduce the intestinal absorption of carotenoids and, to a somewhat lesser extent, of preformed vitamin A. These syndromes include pancreatitis, pancreatic insufficiency, biliary cirrhosis, cholestasis, and sprue. Chronic diarrhea and severe protein-calorie malnutrition also reduce the absorption of carotenoids and vitamin A.

The efficient storage and transport of vitamin A depend greatly on the integrity of the liver. Consequently, liver disease of various kinds, including hepatitis, cirrhosis, and liver cancer, all reduce both absorption and storage. Liver poisons such as carbon tetrachloride disrupt the membrane systems of liver and have dramatic effects on vitamin A status as well. In cystic fibrosis both the plasma levels of vitamin A and the liver stores are markedly reduced. This rather complex condition is characterized by poor lipid absorption and impaired hepatic function.

Inasmuch as the kidneys are mainly responsible for the tubular reabsorption of *holo*-RBP and the metabolism of *apo*-RBP, tubular or glomerular dysfunction will markedly influence the control of vitamin A metabolism within the organism. Indeed, the markedly increased plasma retinol levels characteristic of renal failure are often associated with a hypervitaminosis A–like syndrome (196).

Susceptibility to infection also increases markedly in vitamin A deficiency. In addition, various infections also affect the transport and utilization of vitamin A (197). Hepatitis, measles, and upper respiratory infections reduce vitamin A and RBP levels of the plasma to a signifiant degree. Severe diarrhea, on the other hand, tends to raise plasma retinol and RBP values, presumably due to the marked dehydration and hemoconcentration that occurs in that disease. Needless to say, many other diseases also affect vitamin A levels both in the plasma and in the liver. In these latter cases, however, the effects are probably secondary to the overall stress on the organism and the general disruption of metabolism that ensues. The effects of disease on vitamin A metabolism and status have been thoroughly reviewed (198).

C. Parasites

Parasitic infestation influences both plasma retinol values as well as overall vitamin A status (199–203). Human adults infested with intestinal flukes have mean plasma values only one-third those of normals, whereas hookworm and liver fluke infestations lower plasma retinol levels by about one-fourth. Children and adults suffering from ascariasis or giardiasis show an impaired absorption of vitamin A. Adults suffering from liver schistosomiasis, which is often associated with chronic salmonella infection, absorb vitamin A poorly and have very low liver stores (183,201). Intestinal schistosomiasis and malarial parasitemia lower serum retinol levels in children (203) and exacerbate vitamin A deficiency in rats (202). Thus, intestinal parasites seem to act mainly by reducing the absorption of vitamin A and carotenoids, whereas liver flukes and schistosomes impair liver function and vitamin A storage.

D. Alcohol

Alcohol, either in a single acute dose or repeated chronic doses, reduces vitamin A levels in the liver (204). Plasma retinol and retinyl ester levels transiently rise (204,205), and vitamin A levels in peripheral tissues increase (204). Alcohol also stimulates collagen formation by stellate cells (206), quite possibly accompanied by either the release of retinyl esters or a reduced storage capability. Retinyl ester hydrolase is stimulated by ethanol in vitro (207), although its activity in vivo after the administration of a large acute dose of ethanol is depressed (205). Chronic ethanol ingestion induces P450-mediated oxidative reactions as well as a microsomal pathway for retinol oxidation (204). Thus, after ethanol ingestion, retinol in liver cells seems to be oxidized more rapidly to retinoic acid and to yet more oxidized, nutritionally inactive metabolites. Interestingly, ethanol does not seem to affect the intestinal absorption of vitamin A (208), the release of *holo*-RBP from the liver, or the homeostatic maintenance of plasma retinol levels, at least until liver stores are severely depleted (204). Zinc status also influences the effects of alcohol on vitamin A metabolism (209). Chronic abuse of ethanol, besides depleting liver reserves of vitamin A, can lead to cirrhosis and increases the risk of hepatic cancer. These longer-term adverse effects of alcohol have been thoughtfully reviewed (204).

E. Heavy Metals

Because of their general toxicity, heavy metals affect vitamin A metabolism as well as other metabolic reactions of the body. Only in the cases of cadmium and copper, however, have dramatic effects been noted. In chronic cadmium poisoning in humans, tubular reabsorption in the kidney is impaired, which results in the urinary excretion of large amounts of RBP, vitamin A, and other low molecular weight proteins (210). In spite of this considerable drain of RBP and vitamin A, however, the levels of RBP and plasma vitamin A rather surprisingly tend to be maintained within the normal range.

In rats given cadmium (50 ppm) for 8 months, the only change noted was a significant decrease in serum vitamin A with a concurrent increase in liver stores (211). In sheep, but apparently not in rats, the ingestion of copper also markedly reduces plasma concentrations of retinol (212). Because these metals act nonspecifically on many organs, their toxic effects on vitamin A are only a small part of their general adverse effects.

F. Smoking

Smoking is a major risk factor for cancer of the lung (213). Although the frequency of intake of carotenoid-rich foods did not differ appreciably among current smokers, ex-smokers and nonsmokers in recent studies conducted in Japan (214) and the United States (215), plasma β-carotene and α-carotene levels in nondrinkers varied inversely with smoking. Plasma lycopene and, in the U.S. study, α-tocopherol levels were little affected. Smoking is not known to influence plasma retinol levels or liver reserves of vitamin A. More detailed biochemical studies on the effects of smoking on the metabolism of carotenoids and vitamin A are warranted.

G. Age

Children are much more sensitive to vitamin A deficiency then are adults. Indeed, the incidence of blindness due to vitamin A deficiency is almost exclusively limited to children from 6 months to 6 years of age. The reasons for this effect are quite clear: 1) children at birth have very low stores of vitamin A, 2) the growth and rapid differentiation of cells during the first 2 years of age are particularly affected by the lack of vitamin A, and 3) the metabolism of the very young, and hence the turnover of nutrients, is more rapid than in persons of greater age.

Plasma retinol levels (177,216) and carotenoid levels (214,217) in humans increase moderately with age. Males in the United States show higher plasma retinol values than females to the age of 60 (216), and women in Japan show higher carotenoid intakes and plasma values than men to the age of 80 (214,217). The intestinal absorption of vitamin A may be *more* efficient in older than in younger rats, probably because of a thinner unstirred water layer (218), and the rate of storage of intravenously injected vitamin A in mice is inversely related to age (219). The rate of dark-adaptation, which is slower in older rats, is further decreased by vitamin A deprivation, although the ultimate threshold in all cases in similar (220). The amount and type of retinyl esters in the eye is also affected by age (221). In healthy elderly persons, however the intakes of vitamin A, plasma retinol concentrations, and liver reserves are similar to those found in younger adults 222). Although physiological processes clearly are affected by age, such changes do not seem to impact significantly on vitamin A nutriture in the absence of chronic disease or of bizarre food habits (222).

H. Genetics

Familial retinol-binding protein deficiency has been reported in Japan (223). Although presumably well nourished, a mother and her two daughters showed plasma retinol and

RBP values of 31–32 μg/dl and of 20–23 μg/ml, respectively, whereas the father and other close relatives showed RPB values of 33–63 μg/ml. The plasma retinol and RBP levels of one daughter (19 mo.), who developed keratomalacia in association with measles, were not increased by treatment with vitamin A administered topically and orally (223). In response to the suggestion that zinc or protein malnutrition might have caused the low RBP levels (224), Matsuo and his colleages (225) indicated that low RBP levels persisted in the patient during a 6-month recovery period on a diet adequate in vitamin A and protein and that plasma zinc values, lipid absorption, and the growth rate in the patient were normal.

On a different tack, two siblings who presumably ingested normal amounts of vitamin A showed persistent high plasma retinyl ester values (500–2500 μg/dl) and signs of hypervitaminosis A (226). Indeed, one sibling died of renal failure with a syndrome of hypervitaminosis A. Although the molecular defect was not identified, the clearance of retinyl ester from the plasma seems to be impaired. A few similar cases in children have been reported earlier. Some young children who ingest normal amounts of baby food also seem to have difficulty in clearing carotenoids from the plasma. The state of hypercarotenosis that develops, although benign, can be mistaken for jaundice. This condition, however, seems to disappear with age.

I. Stress

Stresses of various kinds, such as extremes of temperature (227), physical immobilization (228), fever, forced exercise, burn injury, and chronic infections (229), tend to lower plasma retinol levels and to enhance vitamin A catabolism in both experimental animals and in humans. Thymus weights fall in response to several kinds of stress, whereas both the weight and the vitamin A content of the adrenals increase as a result of immobilization stress (228). Underwood (198) has suggested that the increased thyroid activity induced by stress may stimulate the catabolism of vitamin A. Stress will also enhance corticoid secretion from the adrenals. Indeed, large doses of cortisone markedly lower the weights of the thymus and adrenals as well as reduce the concentrations of vitamin A in the plasma, liver, thymus, and adrenals (230). The stress-induced hormonal response is depressed by vitamin A depletion (231). Thus, stress reduces total body stores of vitamin A and causes some tissue redistribution of vitamin A, whereas vitamin A depletion seems to blunt the hormonal response to stress.

J. Other Nutrients

Acute *protein* deficiency interferes both directly and indirectly with vitamin A metabolism (51,198). Direct effects include a reduction in carotenoid dioxygenase of the intestinal mucosa (232) and decreases in both RBP and prealbumin synthesis. Since most children with protein-calorie malnutrition depend largely on carotenoids as a source of vitamin A, a reduction in the formation of retinaldehyde from carotenoids has great practical significance. Similarly, because of the rapid turnover of RBP in the plasma and its high content of aromatic and other essential amino acids, the transport of vitamin A to the tissues in severe protein-calorie malnutrition is clearly impaired.

Indirect effects largely concern the synthesis and release of proteolytic and lipolytic enzymes of the gut and pancreas. With a reduced amount of such enzymes, the hydrolysis of carotenoid and retinyl esters are slower, and the formation and diffusion of micelles to the mucosal cell membrane are impaired. Thus, in protein-calorie malnutrition, the rates of digestion, absorption, carotenoid cleavage, and plasma transport are all reduced.

Fat in the diet markedly stimulates the absorption of carotenoids and vitamin A, not only by enhancing gall bladder contraction but also by providing a lipid vehicle for vitamin A transport and absorption (51,198). In many areas of the world, the daily fat intake by preschool children is 5 grams or less per day, which unquestionably interferes with carotenoid and vitamin A absorption. Indeed, supplementation of the typical low-fat diet (7% of calories) ingested by African boys with 20 ml of olive oil increased carotenoid absorption from <5% to 25% (233).

Iron status is significantly influenced by vitamin A nutriture (51,198). The hemoglobin level, albeit of a single male adult, fell significantly during the ingestion of a vitamin A-free, iron-sufficient diet (234). Whereas supplementation with iron gave only a modest transient response, treatment with β-carotene plus iron rapidly increased hemogloblin levels to normal (234). In vitamin A deficiency, the intestinal absorption of iron is not affected, but plasma iron levels fall, tissue iron deposits increase, and the incorporation of iron into hemoglobin decreases (51). In children with a marginal or deficient vitamin A status, vitamin A supplements alone significantly increase blood hemoglobin levels (235,236). Although the mechanism is not clear, vitamin A might well affect both the release of iron from tissue reserves into the plasma and the differentiation of red blood cells from its precursor cells in the bone marrow.

Zinc deficiency markedly influences vitamin A metabolism (51,198). Plasma vitamin A values fall, liver vitamin A values may increase, the activity of zinc-dependent alcohol dehydrogenase of several, but not all, tissues decreases, night blindness develops, and the amount of rhodopsin in the eye falls. Furthermore, zinc and vitamin A deficiencies are synergistic in producing fetal malformations in rats (237). Quite apart from any direct relationship with vitamin A, zinc is an inherent component of many enzymes that are involved in most major metabolic pathways, including protein and nucleic acid synthesis. Finally, because both zinc deficiency and vitamin A deficiency are characterized by markedly reduced food intake in experimental animals, generalized malnutrition tends to be present as a confounding influence in most studies, even when pair-feeding or equalized-weight regimens are imposed.

Initially, two possible sites of action of zinc deficiency on vitamin A metabolism were postulated: 1) a defect in the release of *holo*-RBP from the liver, and 2) a defect in the interconversion of retinol and retinal in the eye. It now seems likely that the lower *holo*-RPB levels in zinc deficiency are due to a lower rate of nucleic acid and protein synthesis in the liver, exacerbated by a generalized state of malnutrition (51,198). Similarly, a reduced intake of vitamin A by the eye and an impaired synthesis of opsin seem to be the primary rate-limiting steps in the observed reduced levels of rhodopsin in the eye and consequent night blindness (238). Clinical interactions between zinc and vitamin A have been carefully reviewed (239).

Vitamin E protects carotenoids and vitamin A from oxidation during the digestive process (51,198), is associated with retinyl ester in the vitamin A-containing storage globules of liver cells (98), and prevents a rapid breakdown of stored vitamin A in the liver (240). The latter action seems to be specific, inasmuch as other chemical antioxidants are not effective (240). Quite possibly, retinyl ester hydrolase is regulated by the vitamin E status, i.e., activated in vitamin E deficiency and inhibited in vitamin E sufficiency (102,241). In a practical context, children who are at high risk of vitamin A deficiency often show very low plasma vitamin E levels and plasma vitamin E/lipid ratios (242,243). Vitamin

E, together with other antioxidants, is also crucially involved in preventing oxidative damage to membranes in the retina and retinal pigment epithelium (244). Large doses of vitamin E seem to protect animals from some signs of vitamin A toxicity (51,245). On the other hand, in animals they also inhibit the intestinal absorption of carotenoids, but not of vitamin A, and exacerbate the testicular derangements caused by hypervitaminosis A (245). Thus both inadequate and excessive intakes of vitamin E can adversely affect vitamin A nutriture.

In addition to those interactions discussed above, relationships have been described between vitamin A and vitamin C, vitamin K, vitamin D, calcium, copper, and iodine (51,198).

XII. EFFICACY OF PHARMACOLOGIC DOSES

McLaren (246) first suggested that large oral doses of vitamin A might be used prophylactically in infants at risk of vitamin A deficiency. First developed as a public health measure in Hyderabad, India (247), a dose of 200,000 IU of retinyl palmitate in oil (60 mg of retinol equivalents) has been administered 1–3 times annually during the past 20 years to tens of millions of preschool children, primarily in Asia (248). This approach has been used extensively in India (247), Indonesia (249), and Bangladesh (250), and to a lesser degree in several other countries where vitamin A deficiency is a public health problem (248).

The use of massive doses of vitamin A to prevent vitamin A deficiency is feasible because of several unique physiological and practical considerations: 1) the high efficiency of absorption and storage, which is largely independent of dose, 2) the ability of the liver to store efficiently very large amounts of vitamin A and to release it at a relatively slow rate, 3) the infrequency of manifestations of hypervitaminosis A at the dosage given, 4) the relatively low cost of a large dose of vitamin A, and 5) its ease of administration (251). The major difficulty in this program is one of logistics, namely that doses must be given individually to children by a trained individual. Thus, the task of treating very large numbers of children by this method is both costly and time consuming. Furthermore, the percentage of children at risk who receive treatment tends to fall significantly with repeated rounds of administration (248). In Bangladesh, the efficacy of protection against potentially binding corneal lesions was estimated to be 63% (250). Thus, other health interventions, such as the fortification of commodities (49) and nutrition education (252), might either be used separately or combined with dosing, depending on the nature and extent of the problem in a given country.

A large family of synthetic retinoids (4,10) as well as vitamin A have been tested for efficacy against both skin disorders as well as induced and spontaneous tumors. This vast literature has been summarized in part in recent reviews (253–255), chapters (256,257), and monographs (258–261). As a general summary, many retinoids, particularly 13-*cis*-retinoic acid (Fig. 2a), etretinate (Fig. 2d), and hydroxyphenylretinamide, show marked therapeutic efficacy, either used alone or in combination with other treatments, against severe acne, some forms of psoriasis, several other skin disorders, and some types of cancer. Because relatively high doses of retinoids (0.2–1.5 mg/kg/day) are required for maximal effectiveness, toxic side effects are frequent. As a consequence, the ratio of acceptable risk to benefit is a key concern relative to the selection of a given retinoid and of its dosage schedule.

Esters of vitamin A are also efficacious in treating some skin disorders and cancers. Because vitamin A, unlike the largely acidic retinoids, are stored in the liver, hepatotoxicity becomes of concern with long-term chronic usage. Some relatively nontoxic water-soluble forms of vitamin A currently show promise in the prevention of neoplastic changes in breast tissue (262).

XIII. HAZARDS OF HIGH DOSES OF VITAMIN A

In 1944 Josephs described for the first time hypervitaminosis A in a child (2). A 3-year-old boy who had received about 240,000 IU of vitamin A daily for over 2 years suffered from enlargement of the liver and spleen, hypoplastic anemia, leukopenia, precocious skeletal development, clubbing of the fingers, and coarse sparse hair. The vitamin A level in his plasma was about 270 μg/dl. When the excessive dosing of vitamin A was terminated, the plasma vitamin A level fell dramatically and most of the symptoms disappeared within 1–2 weeks, except for a lingering abnormality in bone growth and a slowly subsiding enlargement of the liver and spleen.

Since that time, over 600 individual cases have been described in over 200 clinical reports (163,263). Hypervitaminosis A may be considered as two related toxic conditions, acute and chronic (263,264). Acute toxicity is due to a single dose or a limited number of large doses taken during a short period, whereas chronic toxicity is caused by moderately high doses taken frequently, usually daily, over a span of months or years. Reported signs of hypervitaminosis A are given in Table 8 (163). When large doses of vitamin A are routinely ingested, plasma retinyl ester values rise dramatically, whereas plasma retinol concentrations increase only slightly, if at all (264a). The relative amount of retinyl ester in fasting plasma is usually < 10% of the total plasma vitamin A. In hypervitaminosis A, higher concentrations of retinyl ester are present (264a).

Oral doses of vitamin A that cause toxic manifestations, based primarily on Bauernfeind's thorough review (263), are summarized in Table 9. Some comments on this table are appropriate. First of all, the ranges for each listed category are very broad. This wide range includes both mild and severe forms of toxicity, which clearly is dose-dependent. Furthermore, cited intakes in medical papers, which depend primarily, if not solely, on the patient's statements, can include instances both of gross over- and underreporting. In

Table 8 Toxic Manifestations Associated with Acute and Chronic Hypervitaminosis A

Alopecia	Exanthema	Nausea
Anemia	Fatigue	Negative N balance
Anorexia	Fever	Nervous ailments
Ataxia	Fontanelle bulging	Papilledema
Bone pain	Headache	Petechiae
Brittle nails	Hepatomegaly	Polydipsia
Cheilitis	Hepatotoxicity	Premature epiphyseal closure
Conjunctivitis	Hypercalcemia	Pruritus
Dermatitis	Hyperlipemia	Pseudotumor cerebri
Diarrhea	Hyperostosis	Skin desquamation
Diplopia	Insomnia	Skin erythema
Dysuria	Irritability	Skin rash
Edema	Membrane dryness	Skin scaliness
Elevated CSF pressure	Menstrual irregularities	Vomiting
Epistaxis	Muscular pain	Weight loss

Table 9 Toxicity of Vitamin A in Humans

Category	Age	Reported dosage range
Acute	Adults	1–30 $\times 10^6$ IU[a]
	Children (1–6 yr)	0.2– 0.6 $\times 10^6$
	Infants ($\ll$ 1 yr)	0.1– 0.75 $\times 10^6$
Chronic	Adults	50–1000 $\times 10^3$
	Adolescents	50– 300 $\times 10^3$
	Infants ($\ll$ 1 yr)	12– 220 $\times 10^3$
Embryotoxic	Adult women	25– 500 $\times 10^{3}$[b]

[a]1 IU = 0.30 μg all-*trans*-retinol. The current RDA for adult men and women (184), in terms of preformed vitamin A only, is 3333 IU and 2677 IU, respectively.
[b]This range is based on case reports, not on established cause-effect relationships in humans.

chronic toxicity, clinical signs appear earlier at higher doses and later at lower doses within the toxic range. All such cases are included in this compilation. Finally, not all reported cases are included within the range. As indicated below, hypersensitivity to vitamin A (vitamin A intolerance) might well occur in a few persons, probably as a result of genetically based abnormalities in vitamin A metabolism. Furthermore, little data exist about individuals who ingest large doses of vitamin A *without* showing toxic signs of such severity that they consult a physician. Most acute and chronic signs of toxicity disappear within weeks after discontinuation of dosing.

The possibility that hypersensitivity to vitamin A exists is based on a very few literature reports. As mentioned earlier, two siblings showed signs of hypervitaminosis A and extremely high plasma retinyl ester levels on usually nontoxic dietary intakes of vitamin A (226). In another case, a 10-year-old boy showed signs of vitamin A intoxication after being supplemented with only 1500 IU of vitamin A daily over a 5-year period (265). Unfortunately, dietary intake data were not obtained in that case. The few reported cases of possible vitamin A intolerance have recently been summarized (266). When new cases are reported, particular efforts should be made to clarify the metabolic basis of the defects.

The most serious consequences of an excessive intake of vitamin A unquestionably are its embryotoxicity and teratogenicity. That large intakes of vitamin A cause abortion and birth defects in experimental animals has been known for a very long time (2,267). To induce such effects in rats and mice, very larges doses, i.e., 100,000 IU per kg body weight, are often requried. The water-soluble glucuronides of vitamin A, however, unlike retinol and retinoic acid, are not teratogenic in rats at similar high doses (268). The observation that doses of 13-*cis*-retinoic acid (0.5–1.5 mg/kg/day) induced a high incidence (a relative risk of 25.6) of abortions and birth defects in the progeny of pregnant women (269) has stimulated reexamination of the teratogenic effects of vitamin A itself in humans.

Unquestionably, the acidic retinoids, both synthetic and natural, are more powerful teratogens than are retinol and its esters (270a). Because retinol is converted at a limited rate in vivo to retinoic acid, which is rapidly metabolized to other products, the amount of both 13-*cis*-and all-*trans*-retinoic acid found in tissues in the steady state is low. Furthermore, ingested retinol, unlike the acidic retinoids, is rapidly converted into retinyl esters that are stored in the liver and in other tissues. As a consequence, retinol and its esters should be considered separately in this context from the retinoids that are used in large doses as drugs.

On the other hand, 17 cases of birth defects, including unpublished reports to the Food and Drug Administration from physicians, have been reported with the daily ingestion of >25,000 IU of vitamin A early in pregnancy (270). One additional case was associated with the daily ingestion of 18,000 IU (270), and another with a possibly lower intake (270b). The most common daily dosage in this group was 25,000–50,000 IU (270). In considering the possible teratogenic actions of vitamin A, the Teratology Society (277) has stated:

> Almost all of the FDA cases are brief, retrospective reports of malformed infants or fetuses exposed to supplements of 25,000 IU/day or more of vitamin A during pregnancy. The biases that contributed to the decision to report or publish these cases of malformed vitamin A-exposed infants are unknown but are probably substantial. Some of these infants have malformations similar to those found among isotretinoin-exposed infants; the malformations of the others were quite different. At best, it can be said that the malformations of some of the vitamin A-exposed infants fit the pattern of malformation seen among infants exposed to isotretinoin. There are no epidemiologic studies that provide the data necessary to quantitate the risk for major malformation following daily fetal exposure to supplements of any dose of vitamin A.

Thus, the number of abortions and birth defects that have been associated with excessive use of vitamin A is very small indeed, despite the extensive use of supplements of vitamin A in the United States (271).

In experimental animals, vitamin A can cause permanent learning disabilities in the progeny at 10–50% the dose that induces gross birth defects (272–275). Because vitamin A and other retinoids seem to act, at least in part, on the neural crest cells in the developing embryo, the probability of similar effects in humans at doses that do not cause gross fetal deformities is high.

In recognition of the fact that a deficiency of vitamin A in the mother can also cause abortion and fetal abnormalities, the International Vitamin A Consultative Group (IVACG) has recommended that the average daily diet of pregnant women should supply 620 μg retinol equivalents (276), in keeping with FAO/WHO recommendations (46). In areas of the world where this level of intake does not occur and little opportunity exists for dietary improvement, or in emergency situations in which food supplies are disrupted, however, IVACG recommends that daily supplements of 3000 μg retinol equivalent (10,000 IU) can be given safely anytime during pregnancy (165,263,276). They do not suggest, by the way, that well-nourished women take supplements.

Responding to concerns about the teratogenicity of vitamin A, the Teratology Society recommended that women who might become pregnant limit their daily intake of preformed vitamin A to 8,000 IU and ingest provitamin A carotenoids as a primary source of dietary vitamin A (277). Furthermore, they recommended that the unit dose of commercially available vitamin A be limited to 5000–8000 IU and that the hazards of excessive intakes of vitamin A be indicated on the labels of such products (277). Similarly, the American Institute of Nutrition, the American Society for Clinical Nutrition, and the American Dietetic Association recently issued a formal statement that supplements of vitamins and minerals were not needed by well-nourished, healthy individuals, including pregnant women, except in some specific cases (278). The Council for Responsible Nutrition has also advised that pregnant women, while needing to ensure an adequate intake of vitamin A, should prudently limit their intake of nutritional supplements of vitamin A to 5,000–10,000 IU

(279). Subsequently, they recommended that the unit dosage of retinol in commercial vitamin A preparations be limited to 10,000 IU.

To summarize, well-nourished healthy women of reproductive potential should include carotenoid-rich fruits and vegetables in their diet. They should also avoid taking supplements of preformed vitamin A during the first trimester of pregnancy, during which increased nutritional demands are small and the risk of fetal abnormalities is high. If supplements of vitamin A are subsequently taken, the daily dose should be carefully limited to 5,000–10,000 IU.

XIV. CAROTENOIDS

Unlike retinoids, including vitamin A, carotenoids are generally nontoxic. Individuals who routinely ingest large amounts of carotenoids, either in tomato or carrot juice or in commercial supplements of β-carotene, however, can develop hypercarotenosis, which is characterized by a yellowish coloration of the skin and a very high concentration of carotenoids in the plasma. This benign condition, although resembling jaundice, gradually disappears upon correcting the excessive intake of carotenoids. The only known toxic manifestation of carotenoid intake is canthaxanthin retinopathy, which can develop in patients with erythropoietic porphyria and related disorders who are treated with large daily doses (50–100 mg) or canthaxanthin, the 4.4′ diketo derivative of β-carotene, for long periods (280,281). Canthaxanthin-containing supplements are not currently available in the United States. β-Carotene at similar doses is not known to cause retinopathy. Carotenoids, even when ingested in large amounts, are not known to cause birth defects nor to cause hypervitaminosis A, primarily because the efficiency of their absorption from the intestine falls rapidly as the dose increases and because their conversion to vitamin A is not sufficiently rapid to induce toxicity (282).

Quite apart from their function as precursors of vitamin A, carotenoids are distributed widely in mammalian tissues (283), can quench singlet oxygen and serve an antioxidant action in tissues, particularly under conditions of low oxygen tension (284), can stimulate the immune response (285), can protect against some types of induced cancer (286) but not others (287), and are components of foods the ingestion of which is associated with a lower incidence of lung cancer and possibly of other neoplasms (288).

Thus, by using provitamin A activity as the nutritional function and singlet oxygen-quenching and antioxidant activity as the biological action (289), four classes of carotenoids might be defined; namely, those that are both nutritionally and biologically active, such as β-carotene, those that are nutritionally active and biologially inactive, such as 14′-β-apo-carotenal, those that are nutritionally inactive but biologically active, such as lycopene and violaxanthin, and those that are both nutritionally and biologically inactive, such as phytoene. A symposium on the biological actions of carotenoids (282–289) and a state-of-the-art review of this subject (290) have recently appeared.

Because over 90% of the 600 characterized carotenoids in nature are not precursors of vitamin A, the biological effects that they show in mammalian physiology, independent of their provitamin A activity, will be followed with interest.

ACKNOWLEDGMENTS

This study has been supported in part by grants from the National Institutes of Health (DK-32793, DK-39733, CA-46406, and EY-03677), the USDA (CRG-87-CRCR-1-2320), the Thrasher Research Fund (2800-8), the World Food Institute of Iowa State University (No. 0124), the Wilfred S. Martin Fund, and the Allen Whitfield Memorial Cancer Fund.

REFERENCES

1. Wolf, G., Historical note on mode of administration of vitamin A for cure of night blindness. *Am. J. Clin. Nutr., 31*:290–292 (1978).

2. Moore, T., *Vitamin A.* Elsevier, Amsterdam, 1957.

3. Nomenclature Policy: Generic descriptors and trivial names for vitamins and related compounds. *J. Nutr., 117*:7–14 (1987).

4. Isler, O. (ed.), *Carotenoids.* Birkhauser Verlag, Basel, 1971.

5. Asato, A. E., A. Kim, M. Denny, and R. S. H. Liu, 7-*cis*-,9-*cis*, 11-*cis*-Retinal, all-*cis*-vitamin A, and 7-*cis*,9-*cis*,11-*cis*-12-fluororetinal. New geometric isomers of vitamin A and carotenoids. *J. Am. Chem. Soc., 105*:2923–2924 (1983).

6. Liu, R. S. H., and A. E. Asato, Photochemistry and synthesis of stereoisomers of vitamin A. *Tetrahedron, 40*:1931–1969 (1984).

7. Knudsen, C. G., S. C. Carey, and W. H. Okamura, [1,5]-Sigmatropic rearrangement of vinyl allenes: A novel route to geometric isomers of the retinoids possessing 11-*cis* linkages including 9-*cis*,11-*cis*,13-*cis* retinal. *J. Am. Chem. Soc., 102*:6355–6356 (1980).

8. Stephens-Jarnegan, A., D. A. Miller, and H. F. DeLuca, The growth supporting activity of a retinoidal benzoic acid derivative and 4,4-difluororetinoic acid. *Arch. Biochem. Biophys., 237*:11–16 (1985).

9. Kuhn, R., and C. J. O. R. Morris, Synthesis of vitamin A. *Chem. Ber., 70*:853–858, (1937).

10. Frickel, F., Chemistry and physical properties of retinoids. In *The Retinoids*, Vol. 1, M. B. Sporn, A. B. Roberts, and D. S. Goodman (eds.). Academic Press, Orlando, FL, 1984, pp. 7–145.

11. Olson, J. A., A simple dual assay for vitamin A and carotenoids in human liver. *Nutr. Rep. Intern.., 19*:807–813 (1979).

12. Bieri, J. G., T. J. Tolliver, and G. L. Catignani, Simultaneous determination of α-tocopherol and retinol in plasma or red cells by high pressure liquid chromatography. *Am. J. Clin. Nutr., 32*:2143–2149 (1979).

13. Taylor, R. F., and M. Ikawa. Gas chromatography, gas chromatography-mass spectrometry, and high-pressure liquid chromatography of carotenoids and retinoids. *Meth. Enzymol., 67*:233–261 (1980).

14. Frolik, C. A., and J. A. Olson. Extraction, separation and chemical analysis of retinoids. In *The Retinoids*, Vol. 1, M. B. Sporn, A. B. Roberts, and D. S. Goodman (eds.). Academic Press, Orlando, FL, 1984, pp. 181–233.

15. Furr, H. C., O. Amedee-Manesme, and J. A. Olson, Gradient reversed-phase high pressure liquid chromatographic separation of naturally occurring retinoids. *J. Chromatog., 309*:299–307 (1984).

16. Furr, H. C., D. A. Cooper, J. A. Olson, Separation of retinyl esters by non-aqueous reversed-phase high-pressure liquid chromatography. *J. Chromatog., 378*:45–53 (1986).

17. Biesalski, H., H. Greiff, K. Brodda, and G. Hafner, Rapid determination of vitamin A (retinol) and vitamin E (alpha-tocopherol) in human serum by isocratic absorption HPLC. *Int. J. Vitam. Nutr. Res., 56*:319–327 (1986).

18. Peng, Y-M., M-J. Xu, and D. S. Alberts, Analyses and stability of retinol in plasma. *J. Natl. Cancer Inst., 78*:95–99, (1987).

19. Landers, G. M., and J. A. Olson, Rapid simultaneous determination of isomers of retinaldehyde, retinal oxime, and retinol by high-performance liquid chromatography. *J. Chromatog, 438*:383–392 (1988).

20. Broich, C. R., L. E. Gerber, and J. W. Erdman, Jr., Determination of lycopene, α- and

β-carotene and retinyl esters in human serum by reverse-phase high-performance liquid chromotography. *Lipids, 18*:253–258 (1983).

21. Khachik, F., G. R. Beecher, and N. F. Whittaker, Separation, identification, and quantification of the major carotenoid and chlorophyll constituents in extracts of several green vegetables by liquid chromatography. *Agr. Food Chem., 34*:603–616 (1986).

22. Vecchi, M., E. Glinz, V. Meduna, and K. Schiedt, HPLC separation and determination of astacene, semiastacene, astaxanthin, and other keto-carotenoids. *J. High Res. Chromatogr.: Chromatogr. Commun., 10*:348–351 (1987).

23. Tanaka, Y., R. Hirata, Y. Minato, Y. Hasumura, and J. Takeuchi, Isolation and higher purification of fat-storing cells from rat liver with flow cytometry. In *Cells of the Hepatic Sinusoids*, Vol. I, A. Kien, D. L. Knook, and E. Wisse (eds.). The Kupffer Cell Foundation, Rijswijk, The Netherlands, 1986, pp. 473–747.

24. Batres, R. O., and J. A. Olson, Separation of rat liver hepatocytes with high and low vitamin A concentration by flow cytometry. *J. Cell Biol., 105*:303a (1987).

25. Clifford, A. J., A. D. Jones, Y. Tondeur, H. C. Furr, and J. A. Olson, Assessment of vitamin A status of humans by isotope dilution GC/MS. *Proc. Conf. Mass Spectrom. Allied Topics,34*:327–328 (1986).

26. Furr, H. C., A. J. Clifford, A. D. Jones, H. R. Bergen III, and J. A. Olson, In vivo kinetic pattern of ingested tetradeuterated vitamin A in the serum of an adult human. *Federation Proc., 46*:1335 (1987).

27. Furr, H. C., O. Amedee-Manesme, A. J. Clifford, H. R. Bergen III, A. D. Jones, D. P. Anderson, and J. A. Olson, Relationship between liver vitamin A concentration determined by isotope dilution assay with tetradeuterated vitamin A and by biopsy in generally healthy adult humans. *Am. J. Clin. Nutr., 49*:713–716 (1989).

28. Clifford, A. J., A. D. Jones, H. C. Furr, and J. A. Olson, Tandem mass spectrometry of retinyl esters. *Federation Proc., 46*:580 (1987).

29. Taylor, R. F. HPLC and HPLC/MS analysis of carotenoids. *Proc. Eight Intern. Symp. Carotenoids*, Boston, MA, 1987, p. 5.

30. Arroyave, G., C. O. Chichester, H. Flores, J. Glover, L. A. Mejia, J. A. Olson, K. L. Simpson, and B. A. Underwood, *Biochemical Methodology for the Assessment of Vitamin A Status*, International Vitamin A Consultative Group (IVACG), Nutrition Foundation, Washington, DC, 1982.

31. Embree, N. D., S. R. Ames, R. W. Lehman, and P. L. Harris, Vitamin A assay. *Meth. Biochem. Anal., 4*:43–98 (1957).

32. Harris, P. L. Bioassay of vitamin A compounds. *Vitam. Horm., 18*:341–370 (1960).

33. Tosukhowong, P., and J. A. Olson, The syntheses, biological activity and metabolism of 15-methyl retinone, 15-methyl retinol and 15-dimethyl retinol in rats. *Biochem. Biophys. Acta., 529*:438–453, (1978).

34. Barua, A. B., and J. A. Olson, Chemical synthesis and growth promoting activity of all - *trans*-retinyl beta-D-glucuronide. *Biochem J., 244*:231–234 (1987).

35. Sporn, M. B., N. M. Dunlop, D. L. Newton, and W. R. Henderson, Relationship between structure and activity of retinoids. *Nature* (London), *263*:110–113 (1976).

36. Shapiro S. S. Retinoids and epithelial differentiation. In *Retinoids and Cell Differentiation*, M. I. Sherman (ed.). CRC Press, Boca Raton, FL, 1986, pp. 29–59.

37. Roberts, A. B., and M. B. Sporn, Cellular biopsy and biochemistry of the retinoids. In *The Retinoids*, Vol. 2, M. B. Sporn, A. B. Roberts, and D. S. Goodman (eds.). Academic Press, Orland, FL, 1984, pp. 209–286.

38. Jetten, A. M., Induction of differentiation of embryonal carcinoma cells by retinoids. In *Retinoids and Cell Differentiation*, M. I. Sherman (ed.). CRC Press, Boca Raton, FL, 1986, pp. 105–136.

39 Imaizumi, M., and T. R. Breitman, Retinoic acid-induced differentiation of the human promyelocytic leukemia cell line HL-60 and fresh human leukemia cells in primary culture—

a model for differentiation-inducing therapy of leukemia. *Eur. J. Haematol.*, *38*:289–302 (1987).

40. Buckley, A., and M. C. Middleton, Retinoic acid alters the keratinization of cultured rat sublingual keratinocytes in vitro, *Arch. Derm. Res.*, *279*:257–265 (1987).

41. Watt, B. K., and A. L. Merrill, *Composition of Foods-Raw, Processed, Prepared*, Handbook 8 (rev.), USDA, Washington, DC 1963; Food Composition Tables for International Use, FAO, UN, Rome 1949, 1954; Food Composition Table for Use in Latin America, INCAP/ICNND, 1961; Food Composition Table for Use in Africa, FAO, UN/USPHS, US, 1968, Food Composition Table for Use in East Asia, FAO, UN/USPHS, US, 1972.

42. USDA, Consumer and Food Economics Institute: Comparison of Foods, *Agriculture Handbook No. 8-1 to 8-12*, U.S. Government Printing Office, Washington, DC, 1976–1984.

43. Quackenbush, F. W., Reverse phase HPLC separation of *cis* carotenoids and *trans* carotenoids and its application to beta carotenes in food materials. *J. Liq. Chrom.*, *10*:643–653 (1987).

44. Brubacher, G., and H. Weiser, The vitamin A activity of beta-carotene. *Intern. J. Vitam. Nutr. Res.*, *55*:5–15, (1985).

45. Olson, J. A., Recommended dietary intakes (RDI) of vitamin A in humans. *Am. J. Clin. Nutr. 45*:704–716 (1987).

46. Food and Agriculture Organization/World Health Organization. Requirements of vitamin A, iron, folate and vitamin B12. Report of a joint Food and Agriculture Organization/World Health Organization expert committee. Rome, Italy: Food and Agriculture Organization, FAO Food and Nutrition Series, Report No. 23, 1988.

47. Bauernfeind, J. C., and W. M. Cort, Nutrification of foods with added vitamin A. *CRC Crit. Rev. Food Technol.*, *4*:337–375 (1974).

48. Bauernfeind, J. C. Vitamin A: Technology and applications. *World Rev. Nutr. Dietet.*, *41*:110–199 (1983).

49. Bauernfeind, J. C., and G. Arroyave, Control of vitamin A deficiency by the nutrification of food approach. In *Vitamin A Deficiency and Its Control*, J. C. Bauernfeind (ed.). Academic Press, Orland, FL, 1986, pp. 359–388.

50. Goodman, D. S., and W. S. Blaner, Biosynthesis, absorption and hepatic metabolism of retinol. In *Retinoids*, Vol. 2, M. B. Sporn, A. B. Roberts, and D. S. Goodman (eds.). Academic Press, Orlando, FL, 1984, pp. 1–39.

51. Mejia, L. A. Vitamin A–nutrient interrelationships. In *Vitamin A Deficiency and Its Control*, J. C. Bauernfeind (ed.). Academic Press, Orland FL, 1986, pp. 69–100.

52. Erdman, J. W., G. C. Fahey, and C. B. White, Effects of purified dietary fiber sources on β-carotene utilization by the chick. *J. Nutr.*, *116*:2415–2423 (1986).

53. Olson, J. A., The conversion of radioactive β-carotene into vitamin A by the rat intestine in vivo. *J. Biol. Chem.*, *236*:349–356 (1961).

54. El-Gorab, M. I., B. A. Underwood, and J. D. Loerch, Role of bile salts in the uptake of β-carotene and retinol by rat everted gut sacs. *Biochem. Biophys. Acta, 401*:265–277 (1975).

55. Olson, J. A., Formation and function of vitamin A. In *Biosynthesis of Isoprenoid Compounds*, Vol. 2, J. W. Porter and S. L. Spurgeon (eds.). John Wiley and Sons, New York, 1983, pp. 371–412.

56. Ganguly, J., and P. S. Sastry, Mechanism of conversion of β-carotene into vitamin A—central cleavage versus random cleavage. *Wld. Rev. Nutr. Dietet.*, *45*:198–220 (1985).

57. Goswami, B. C., and G. Britton, Mechanisms of the conversion of β-carotene into vitamin A. *Proc Eighth Intern. Symp. Carotenoids*, Boston, MA, 1987, p. 38.

57a. Napoli, J. L., and K. R. Race, Biogenesis of retinoic acid from beta-carotene. *J. Biol. Chem.*, *263*:17372–17377 (1988).

58. Hansen, S., and W. Maret, Retinal is not formed in vitro by enzymatic central cleavage of beta-carotene. *Biochem.*, *27*:200–206 (1988).

59. Villard, L., and C. J. Bates, Carotene dioxygenase (EC 1.13.11.21) activity in rat intestine—

effects of vitamin A deficiency and of pregnancy. *Am. J. Clin. Nutr.*, *56*:115–122 (1986).

60. Ong, D. E., B. Kakkad, and P. N. MacDonald, Acyl-CoA-independent esterification of retinol bound to cellular retinol-binding protein (type II) by microsomes from rat small intestine. *J. Biol. Chem.*, *262*:2729–2736 (1987).

61. Norum, K. R., R. Blomhoff, M. H. Green, J. B. Green, K-O. Wathne, T. Gjoen, M. Botilsrud, and T. Berg, Metabolism of retinol in the intestine and liver. *Biochem. Soc. Trans.*, *14*:923–925 (1986).

62. Blomhoff, R., T. Berg, and K. R. Norum, Absorption, transport and storage of retinol. *Chim. Scripta*, *27*:169–177 (1987).

63. Yeung, P. L., and M. J. Veen-Baigent. Compartmentation of endogenous and newly absorbed vitamin A in the rat. *Can. J. Physiol. Pharmacol.*, *52*:583–589 (1974).

63a. Nageswara Rao, C., and B. S. Narasinga Rao, Absorption of dietary carotenes in human subjects. *Am. J. Clin. Nutr.*, *23*:105–109 (1970).

64. Blomhoff, R., Hepatic retinol metabolism: Role of the various cell types. *Nutr. Rev.*, *45*:257–263 (1987).

65. Soprano, D. R., C. B. Pickett, J. E. Smith, and D. S. Goodman, Biosynthesis of plasma retinol-binding protein in liver as a larger molecular weight precursor. *J. Biol. Chem.*, *256*:8256–8258 (1981).

66. Goodman, D. S., Plasma retinol-binding protein. In *The Retinoids*, Vol. 2, M. B. Sporn, A. B. Roberts, and D. S. Goodman (eds.). Academic Press, Orlando, FL, 1984, pp. 41–88.

67. Rask, L., W. Anundi, J. Fohlman, and P. A. Peterson, The complete amino acid, sequence of human serum retinol-binding protein. *Uppsala J. Med.*, *92*:115–146 (1987).

68. Newcomer, M. E., T. A. Jones, A. Aquist, J. Sundelin, U. Eriksson, L. Rask, and P. A. Peterson, The three-dimensional structure of retinol-binding protein. *EMBO J.*, *3*:1451–1454 (1984).

69. Colantuoni, V., V. Romano, G. Bensi, C. Santoro, F. Costanza, G. Raugei, and R. Cortese, Cloning and sequencing of a full length cDNA for human retinol-binding protein. *Nucleic Acid Res.*, *11*:7769–7776 (1983).

70. Green, M. H., L. Uhl, and J. B. Green, A multi-compartmental model of vitamin A kinetics and rats with marginal liver vitamin A stores. *J. Lipid Res.*, *26*:806–818 (1985).

71. Gjoen, T., T. Bjerkelund, W. K. Blomhoff, K. R. Norum, T. Berg, and R. Blomhoff, Liver takes up retinol-binding protein from plasma, *J. Biol. Chem.*, *262*:10926–10930 (1987).

72. Green, M. W., J. B. Green, and K. C. Lewis, Variation in retinol utilization rate with vitamin A status in the rat. *J. Nutr.*, *117*:694–703 (1987).

73. Wilson, T. C. M., and G. A. J. Pitt, 3,4-Didehydroretinol (vitamin A_2) has vitamin A activity in the rat without conversion to retinol. *Biochem. Soc. Trans.*, *14*:950 (1986).

74. Tanumihardjo, S. A., A. B. Barua, and J. A. Olson, Use of 3,4-didehydroretinol to assess vitamin A status in rats. *Intern. J. Vitamin. Nutr. Res.*, *57*:127–132 (1987).

75. DeRuyter, M. G., W. E. Lambert, and A. P. De Leenheer, Retinoic acid: An endogenous compound of human blood. Unequivocal demonstration of endogenous retinoic acid under normal physiological conditions. *Anal. Biochem.*, *98*:402–409 (1979).

76. Barua, A. B., and J. A. Olson, Retinyl β-glucuronide: An endogenous compound of human blood. *Am. J. Clin. Nutr.*, *43*:481–485 (1986).

77. Bok, D., and J. Heller, Transport of retinol from the blood to the retina: An autoradiographic study of the retinal pigment epithelial cell surface receptor for plasma retinol-binding protein. *Exp. Eye Res.*, *22*:395–402 (1976).

78. Chen, C. C., and J. Heller, Uptake of retinol and retinoic acid from serum retinol-binding protein by retinal pigment epithelial cells. *J. Biol. Chem.*, *252*:5216–5221 (1977).

79. Chen, W. Y. J., H. O. James, and J. Glover, Retinol transport proteins. *Biochem. Soc. Trans.*, *14*:925–928 (1986).

80. Rask, L., and P. A. Peterson, In vitro uptake of vitamin A from the retinol-binding plasma protein to mucosal epithelial cells from the monkey's small intestine. *J. Biol. Chem.*, *251*:

6360–6366 (1976).

81. McGuire, B. W., M. C. Orbegin-Crist, and F. Chytil, Auto-radiographic localization of serum retinol-binding protein in rat testes. *Endocrinol.*, *108*:658–667 (1981).

82. Chytil, F., and D. Ong, Intracellular vitamin A-binding proteins, *Ann. Rev. Nutr.*, *7*:321–335 (1987).

83. Kato, M., W. S. Blaner, J. R. Mertz, K. Das, K. Kato, and D. S. Goodman, Influence of retinoid nutritional status on cellular retinol- and cellular retinoic acid-binding protein concentrations in various rat tissues. *J. Biol. Chem.*, *260*:4832–4838 (1985).

84. Sundelin, J., H. Anundi, L. Tragardh, U. Eriksson, P. Lind, H. Ronne, P. A. Peterson, and L. Rask, The primary structure of rat liver cellular retinol-binding protein. *J. Biol. Chem.*, *260*:6488–6493 (1985).

85. Ong, D. E., A novel retinol-binding protein from rat: Purification and partial characterization. *J. Biol. Chem.*, *259*:1476–1482 (1984).

86. Sundelin, J., S. R. Das, U. Eriksson, L. Rask, and P. A. Peterson, The primary structure of bovine cellular retinoic acid-binding protein. *J. Biol. Chem.*, *260*:6494–6499 (1985).

87. Stubbs, G. W., J. C. Saari, and S. Futterman, 11-*cis* Retinal-binding protein from rat retina. Isolation and partial characterization. *J. Biol. Chem.*, *254*:8529–8533 (1979).

88. Saari, J. C., and D. L. Bredberg, Photochemistry and stereo selectivity of cellular retinal-binding protein from bovine retina. *J. Biol. Chem.*, *262*:7618–7622 (1987).

89. Bridges, C. D. B., R. A. Alvarez, S-L. Fong, G. I. Liou, and R. J. Ulshafer, Rhodopsin, vitamin A, and interstitial retinol-binding protein in the rd chicken. *Invest. Ophthalmol. Vis. Sci.*, *28*:613–617 (1987).

90. Fong, S-L., G. I. Liou, R. A. Landers, R. A. Alvarez, F. Gonzalez-Fernandes, P. A. Glazebrook, DM-K. Lam, and C. D. B. Bridges, The characterization, localization and biosynthesis of an interstitial retinol-binding protein in the human eye. *J. Neurochem.*, *42*:1667–1676 (1984).

91. Adler, A. J., and K. J. Martin, Retinol-binding proteins in bovine interphotoreceptor matrix. *Biochem. Biophys. Res. Commun.*, *108*:1601–1608 (1982).

92. Redmond, T. M., B. Wiggert, F. A. Robey, N. Y. Ngugen, M. S. Lewis, L. Lee, and G. J. Chader, Isolation and characterization of monkey interphotoreceptor retinoid-binding protein, a unique extracellular matrix component of the retina. *Biochem.*, *24*:787–793 (1985).

93. Adler, A. J., W. F. Stafford III, and H. S. Slater, Size and shape of bovine interphotoreceptor retinoid-binding protein by electron microscopy and hydrodynamic analysis. *J. Biol. Chem.*, *262*:13198–13203 (1987).

94. Liou, G. I., S-L. Fong, J. Gosden, P. van Tuinen, D. H. Ledbetter, S. Christie, D. Rout, S. Bhattacharya, R. G. Cook, Y. Li, C. Wang, and C. D. B. Bridges, Human interstitial retinol-binding protein (IRBP): Cloning, partial sequence and chromosomal localization. *Somatic Cell Mol. Genet.*, *13*:315–323 (1987).

95. Batres, R. O., and J. A. Olson, A marginal vitamin A status alters the distribution of vitamin A among parenchymal and stellate cells in rat liver. *J. Nutr.*, *117*:874–879 (1987).

96. Hendriks, H. F. J., A Brouwer, and D. L. Knook, The role of hepatic fat-storing cells (stellate cells) in retinoid metabolism. *Hepatology, 7*:1368–1371 (1987).

97. Knook, D. L., A. M. Seffelaar, and A. M. De Leeuw, Fat-storing cells of the rat liver: Their isolation and purification. *Exp. Cell. Res.*, *139*:468–471 (1982).

98. Gunning, D. B., and J. A. Olson, Lipid and protein composition of vitamin A-containing globules of rat liver. *Federation Proc.*, *46*:1191 (1987).

99. Yamada, M., W. S. Blaner, Soprano, J. L. Dixon, H. M. Kjeldbye, and D. S. Goodman, Biochemical characteristics of isolated rat liver stellate cells. *Hepatology, 7*:1224–1229 (1987).

100. Cooper, D. A., and J. A. Olson, Hydrolyses of *cis* and *trans* isomers of retinyl palmitate by retinyl ester hydrolase of pig liver *Arch. Biochem. Biophys.*, *260*:705–711 (1988).

101. Cooper, D. A., H. C. Furr, and J. A. Olson, Factors influencing the level and interanimal variability of retinyl ester hydrolase activity in rat liver. *J. Nutr.*, 117:2066–2071 (1987).

102. Napoli, J. L., A. M. McCormick, B. O'Meara, and E. A. Dratz, Vitamin A metabolism: α-Tocopherol modulates tissue retinol levels *in vivo* and retinyl palmitate hydrolysis *in vitro*. *Arch. Biochem. Biophys.*, *230*:194–202 (1984).

103. Ball, M. C., H. C. Furr, and J. A. Olson, Enhancement of acyl coenzyme A:retinol acyl transferase in rat liver and mammary tumor tissue by retinyl acetate and its competitive inhibition by *N*-(4-hydroxphenyl) retinamide. *Biochem. Biophys. Res. Commun.*, *128*:7–11 (1985).

104. Wake, K., Perisinusoidal stellate cells (fat-storing cells, interstitial cells, lipocytes), their related structure in and around the liver sinusoids, and vitamin A storing cells in extrahepatic organs. *Int. Rev. Cytol.*, *66*:303–353 (1980).

105. Wake, K., K. Motomatsu, and H. Senoo, Stellate cells storing retinol in the liver of adult lamprey, *Lampetra Japonica*. *Cell Tissue Res.*, *249*:289–299 (1987).

106. Simpson, K. L., and C. O. Chichester, Metabolism and nutritional significance of carotenoids. *Annu. Rev. Nutr.*, *1*:351–374 (1981).

107. De Luca, L. M. and K. E. Creek, Vitamin A and the liver. *Prog. Liver Disease, 81*:81–98 (1986).

108. De Luca, L. M, C. S. Silverman-Jones, D. Rimoldi, and K. E. Creek, Retinoids and glycosylation. *Chem. Scripta*, *27*:193–198 (1987).

109. Napoli, J. L., and K. R. Race, The biosynthesis of retinoic acid from retinol by rat tissues in vitro. *Arch. Biochem. Biophys.*, *255*:95–101 (1987).

110. Anonymous, Retinoic acid biosynthesis from retinol. *Nutr. Rev.*, *46*:30–31 (1988).

111. Frolik, C. A. Metabolism of retinoids. In *The Retinoids*, Vol. 2, M. B. Sporn, A. B. Roberts, and D. S. Goodman (eds.). Academic Press, Orlando, FL, 1984, pp. 177–208.

112. Skare, K. L., H. K. Schnoes, and H. F. DeLuca, Biliary metabolites of all-*trans* retinoic acid: Isolation and identification of a novel polar metabolite. *Biochem.*, *21*:3308–3317 (1982).

113. Barua, A. B., and J. A. Olson, Chemical synthesis of all-*trans* retinoyl β-glucuronide. *J. Lipid Res.*, *26*:1277–1282 (1985).

114. Silva, Jr., D. P., and H. F. DeLuca, Metabolism of retinoic acid *in vivo* in the vitamin A-deficient rat. *Biochem. J.*, *206*:33–41 (1982).

115. Silva, Jr., D. P., C. R. Valliere, and H. F. DeLuca, The biological activity of metabolites of all-*trans* retinoic acid, *Federation Proc.*, *46*:1012 (1987).

116. Barua, A. B., R. O. Batres and J. A. Olson, Characterization of retinyl β-glucuronide in human blood, *Am. J. Clin. Nutr.*, *50*:370–374 (1989).

117. Barua, A. B., R. O. Batres, and J. A. Olson, Synthesis and metabolism of all-*trans* [11-^{3}H] retinyl β-glucuronide in rats *in vivo*. *Biochem. J.*, *252*:415–420 (1988).

118. Olson, J. A. Metabolism of vitamin A. *Biochem. Soc. Trans.*, *14*:928–930 (1986).

119. Olson, J. A. The storage and metabolism of vitamin A. *Chem. Scripta*, *27*:179–183 (1987).

120. Rietz, P., O. Wiss, and F. Weber, Metabolism of vitamin A and the determination of vitamin A status. *Vitam. Horm.* (N.Y.), *32*:237–249 (1974).

121. Sauberlich, H. E., R. E. Hodges, D. L. Wallace, H. Kolder, J. E. Canham, J. Hood, N. Raica, Jr., and L. K. Lowry, Vitamin A metabolism and requirements in the human studied with the use of labelled retinol. *Vitam. Horm.* (N.Y.), *32*:251–275 (1974).

122. Birge, R. R., C. M. Einterz, H. M. Knapp, and L. P. Murray, The nature of the primary photochemical events in rhodopsin and isorhodopsin. *Biophys. J.*, *53*:367–385 (1988).

123. Sandorfy, C., and D. Vocelle, The photochemical event in rhodopsin. *Can. J. Chem.*, *64*:2251–2266 (1986).

124. Ovchinnikov, Y. A., Structure of rhodopsin and bacteriorhodopsin. *Photochem. Photobiol.*, *45*:909–914 (1987).

125. Khorana, H. G., Rhodopsin, the visual pigment, and bacteriorhodopsin. *Ann. N. Y. Acad. Sci.*, *471*:272–288 (1986).

126. Dratz, E. A., and P. A. Hargrave, The structure of rhodopsin and the rod outer segment disc membrane. *Trends Biochem. Sci.*, *8*:128–131 (1983).

127. Stryer, L., *Textbook of Biochemistry*, 3d ed. W. H. Freeman, New York, 1988, pp. 1027–1038.

128. Ovchinnikov, Y. A. (ed.), *Retinal Proteins*. VSP Press, Utrecht, The Netherlands, 1987.

129. Bernstein, P. S., W. C. Law, and R. R. Rando, Isomerization of all-*trans* retinoids to 11-*cis* retinoids in vitro. *Proc. Natl. Acad. Sci. (U.S.), 84:*1849–1853 (1987).

130. Bernstein, P. S., W. C. Law, and Robert R. Rando, Biochemical characterization of the retinoid isomerase system of the eye. *J. Biol. Chem., 262:*16848–16857 (1987).

131. Bridges. C. D. B., and R. A. Alvarez, The visual cycle operates via an isomerase acting on all-*trans* retinol in the pigment epithelium. *Science, 236:*1678–1680 (1987).

132. Bridges, C. D. B. Retinoids in photo sensitive systems. In *The Retinoids*, M. B. Sporn, A. B. Roberts, and D. S. Goodman (eds.). Academic Press, Orlando, PL, 1984, pp. 125–176.

133. Dowling, J. E., and G. Wald, The role of vitamin A acid. *Vitam. Horm.* (U.S.), *18:*515–541 (1960).

134. Lamb, A. J., P. Apiwatanaporn, and J. A. Olson, Induction of rapid synchronous vitamin A deficiency in the rat, *J. Nutr., 104:*1140–1148 (1974).

135. Anzano, M. A., A. J. Lamb, and J. A. Olson, Growth, appetite, sequence of pathological signs and survival following the induction of rapid synchronous vitamin A deficiency in the rat. *J. Nutr., 109:*1419–1431 (1979).

136. Wolbach, S. B., and P. R. Howe, Tissue changes following deprivation of fat-soluble vitamin A. *J. Exp. Med., 43:*753–757 (1925).

137. Sommer, A. *Nutritional Blindness.* Oxford University Press, Oxford, 1982.

138. Ubels, J. L., K. M. Foley, and V. Rismondi, Retinol secretion by the lacrimal gland. *Inv. Opthalmol. Vis. Sci., 27:*1261–1268 (1986).

139. Pirie, A., Z. Werb, and M. C. Burleigh, Collagenase and other proteinases in the cornea of retinol-deficient rats. *Br. J. Nutr., 34:*297–309 (1975).

140. Wolf, G., T. C. Kiorpes, S. Masushige, J. B. Schreiber, M J. Smith, and R. S. Anderson, Recent evidence for the participation of vitamin A in glycoprotein synthesis. *Federation Proc., 38:*2540–2543 (1979).

141. Rojanapo, W., A. J. Lamb, and J. A. Olson, The prevalence, metabolism, and migration of goblet cells in rat intestine following the induction of rapid synchronous vitamin A deficiency. *J. Nutr., 110:*178–188 (1980).

142. Hatchell, D., and A. Sommer, Detection of ocular surface abnormalities in experimental vitamin A deficiency. *Arch. Ophthalmol, 102:*1389–1393 (1984).

143. Natadisastra, G., J. R. Wittpenn, K. P. West, H. Muhilal, and A. Sommer, Impression cytology for detection of vitamin A deficiency. *Arch. Ophthalmol., 105:*1224–1228 (1987).

144. Zachman, R. D., The stimulation of RNA synthesis in vivo and in vitro by retinol (vitamin A) in the intestine of vitamin A-deficient rats. *Life Sciences, 6:*2207–2213 (1967).

145. Chytil, F., and D. Ong, Cellular retinol- and retinoic acid-binding proteins in vitamin A action. *Fed. Proc., 38:*2510–2514 (1979).

146. Daly, A. K., and P. F. Redfern, Characterization of a retinoic acid-binding component from F9 embryonal carcinoma cell nuclei, *Euro. J. Biochem., 168:*133–139 (1987).

147. Petkovich, M., N. J. Brand, A. Krust, and P. Chambon, A human retinoic acid receptor which belongs to a family of nuclear receptors. *Nature, 330:*444–450 (1987).

148. Giguere, V., E. S. Ong, P. Segui, and R. M. Evans, Identification of a receptor for the morphogen retinoic acid. *Nature, 330:*624–629 (1987).

149. Robertson, M., Towards a biochemistry of morphogenesis. *Nature, 330:*420–421 (1987).

150. LaRosa, G. J., and L. J. Gudas, An early effect of retinoic acid: cloning of a mRNA (ERa-1) exhibiting rapid and protein synthesis-independent induction during teratocarcinoma stem cell differentiation. *Proc. Natl. Acad. Sci., 85:*329–333 (1988).

151. Davies P. J. A., M. P. Murtaugh, W. T. Moore, Jr., G. S. Johnson, and D. Lucas, Retinoic acid-induced expression of tissue transglutaminase in human promyelocytic leukemia (HL-60) cells, *J. Biol. Chem., 260:*5166–5174 (1985).

152. Zile, M. H., M. E. Cullum, R. U. Simpson, A. B. Barua, and D. A. Swartz, Induction of

differentiation of human promyelocytic leukemia cell line HL-60 by retinoyl glucuronide, a biologically active metabolite of vitamin A. *Proc. Natl. Acad. Sci. U.S.A. 84*:2208–2212 (1987).

153. Gallup, J. M., A. B. Barua, H. C. Furr, and J. A. Olson, Effects of retinoid β-glucuronides and N-retinoyl amines on the differentiation of HL-60 cells in vitro. *Proc. Soc. Exp. Biol. Med., 186*:269–274 (1987).

154. Makowske, M., R. Ballester, and O. M. Rosen, Immunochemical evidence that three protein kinase C isozymes increase in abundance during HL-60 differentiation induced by dimethyl sulfoxide and retinoic acid. *J. Biol. Chem., 263*:3402–3410 (1988).

155. Bolmer, S. D., and G. Wolf, Retinoids and phorbol esters alter release of fibronectin from enucleated cells. *Proc. Natl. Acad. Sci. U.S.A., 79*:6541–6545 (1982).

156. Lotan, R., and T. Irimura, Enhanced glycosylation of a melano cell-surface glycoprotein by retinoic acid: Carbohydrate chain analysis by lectin binding. *Cancer Biochem. Biophys., 9*:211–221 (1987).

157. Cummings, R. D., and S. A. Mattox, Retinoic acid-induced differentiation of the mouse teratocarcinoma cell line F9 is accompanied by an increase in the activity of UDP-galactose:β-D-galactosyl-α1,3-galactosyltransferase. *J. Biol. Chem., 263*:511–519 (1988).

158. Stoeckenius, W., and R. A. Bogomolni, Bacteriorhodopsin and related pigments of halobacteria. *Annu. Rev. Biochem., 51*:587–616 (1982).

159. Dencher, N. A., The five retinal-protein pigments of halobacteria: bacteriorhodopsin, halorhodopsin, P565, P370, and slow-cycling rhodopsin. *Photochem. Photobiol., 38*:753–767 (1983).

160. Maddy, K. H., *Vitamin A.* BASF Wyandotte Corp., New York, 1978.

161. *Vitamin Compendium.* Hoffmann-La Roche and Co., Basel, 1976.

162. *Vitamin A Deficiency and Xerophthalmia.* Tech. Rpt. Series 590, World Health Organization, Geneva, 1976.

163. Olson, J. A., Vitamin A, retinoids, and carotenoids. In *Modern Nutrition in Health and Disease*, 7th ed., M. E. Shils and V. R. Young (eds.). Lea and Febiger, Philadephia, 1988, pp. 292–327.

164. Sommer, A. *Field guide to the detection of control of xerophthalmia*, 2nd ed. World Health Organization, Geneva, 1982, p. 58.

165. *Control of vitamin A deficiency and xerophthalmia.* Tech Report Series 672, World Health Organization, Geneva, 1982, pp. 70.

165a. Sommer, A., New imperatives for an old vitamin (A). *J. Nutr., 119*:96–100 (1989).

166. Amedee-Manesme, O., R. Luzeau, J. R. Wittpenn, A. Hanck, and A. Sommer. Impression cytology detects subclinical vitamin deficiency. *Am. J. Clin. Nutr., 47*:875–878 (1988).

167. Kjolhede, C. L., A. M. Gadomski, J. Wittpenn, J., Bulux, A. R. Rosas, N. W. Solomons, K. H. Brown, and M. R. Forman, Field trial of conjunctival impression cytology to detect subclinical vitamin A deficiency. Part I: Feasibility. *Am. J. Clin. Nutr., 49*:490–494 (1989).

168. Gadomski, A. M., C. L. Kjolhede, J. Wittpenn, J. Bulux, A. R. Rosas, and M. R. Forman, Field trial of conjunctival impression cytology (CIC) to detect subclinical vitamin A deficiency. Part II: Comparison of CIC with biochemical measurements. *Am. J. Clin. Nutr., 49*:495–500 (1989).

169. Amedee-Manesme, O., D. Anderson, and J. A. Olson, Relation of the relative dose response to liver concentrations of vitamin A in generally well-nourished surgical patients. *Am. J. Clin. Nutr., 39*:898–902 (1984).

170. Olson, J. A., D. B. Gunning, and R. A. Tilton, Liver concentrations of vitamin A and carotenoids, as a function of age and other parameters, of American children who died of various causes. *Am. J. Clin. Nutr., 39*:39–910 (1984).

171. Loerch, J. D., B. A. Underwood, and K. C. Lewis, Response of plasma levels of vitamin A to a dose of vitamin A as an indicator of hepatic vitamin A reserves in rats. *J. Nutr., 109*:778–786 (1979).

172. Flores, H., F. Campos, C. R. C. Araujo, and B. A. Underwood, Assessment of marginal vitamin A deficiency in Brazilian children using the relative dose response. *Am. J. Clin. Nutr.*, *40*:1281–1289 (1984).

173. Amedee-Manesme, O., S. Mourey, A. Hanck, and J. Therasse, Vitamin A relative dose response test: Validation by intravenous injection in children with liver disease. *Am. J. Clin. Nutr.*, *46*:286–289 (1987).

174. Tanumihardjo, S. A., and J. A. Olson, A modified relative dose-response assay employing 3,4-didehydroretinol (vitamin A$_2$) in rats. *J. Nutr.*, *118*:598–603 (1988).

175. Burri, B. J., and R. A. Jacob, Vitamin A analogs as tests for liver vitamin A status in the rat. *Am. J. Clin. Nutr.*, *47*:458–462 (1988).

176. Olson, J. A., Serum levels of vitamin A and carotenoids as reflectors of nutritional status. *J. Natl. Cancer Inst.*, *73*:1439–1444 (1984).

177. Pilch, S. M., Assessment of the vitamin A nutritional status of the U.S. population based on data collected in the health and nutrition examination surveys, Life Science Research Office, Federation of American Societies for Experimental Biology, Washington, DC, 1985.

178. Furr, H. C., and J. A. Olson, A direct microassay for serum retinol (vitamin A alcohol) by using size-exclusion high-pressure liquid chromatography with fluorescence detection. *Anal. Biochem.*, *171*:360–365 (1988).

179. Vinton, N. E., and R. M. Russell, Evaluation of a rapid test of dark adaptation *Am. J. Clin. Nutr.*, *34*:1961–1966 (1981).

180. Favaro, R. M. D., N. V. De Souza, H. Vannucchi I. D. Desai, and J. E. D. De Oliveira, Evaluation of rose bengal staining test and rapid dark-adaptation test for the field assessment of vitamin A status of preschool children in Southern Brazil. *A. J. Clin. Nutr.*, *43*:940–945 (1986).

181. Tangney, C. C., R. B. Shekelle, W. Raynor, M. Gale, and E. P. Betz, Intra- and interindividual variation in measurements of β-carotene, retinol, and tocopherols in diet and plasma. *Am. J. Clin. Nutr.*, *45*:764–769 (1987).

182. Hankin, J. H., L. N. Kolonel, and M. W. Hinds. Dietary history methods for epidemiologic studies: Application in a case-control study of vitamin A and lung cancer. J. Natl. Cancer Inst., 73:1417–1422 (1984).

183. Olson, J. A., Liver vitamin A reserves of neonates, preschool children and adults dying of various causes in Salvador, Brazil. *Archiv. Latinoamer. Nutr.*, *29*:521–545 (1979).

183a. Truswell, A. S., Recommended dietary intakes around the world. *Nutr. Abstr. Rev.*, *53*:939–1015, 1075–1119 (1983).

184. *Recommended Dietary Allowances*, 10th ed. National Research Council, National Academy of Sciences Press, Washington, DC, 1989, p. 284.

185. Beaton, G. H., Toward harmonization of dietary, biochemical and clinical assessments: The meanings of nutritional status and requirements. *Nutr. Rev.*, *44*:349–358 (1986).

186. Shils, M. E., and V. R. Young (eds.), *Modern Nutrition in Health and Disease*, 7th ed. Lea and Febiger, Philadelphia, 1988, Appendix: Table A-1a-A. Some Recommended Dietary Intakes, p. 1490.

187. Barrowman, J. A., A. D. Mello, and A. Herxheimer, A single dose of neomycin impairs absorption of vitamin A (retinol) in man. *Euro. J. Clin. Pharm.*, *5*:199–202 (1973).

188. Gal, I., and C. E. Parkinson. Changes in serum vitamin A levels during and after oral contraceptive therapy. *Contraception*, *8*:13–25 (1973).

189. Supopark, W., and J. A. Olson, Effect of Ovral, a combination type oral contraceptive agent, on vitamin A metabolism in rats. *Intern. J. Vitam. Nutr. Res.*, *45*:113–123 (1975).

190. Ahmed, F., and M. S. Bamji, Vitamin supplements of women using oral contraceptives. *Contraception*, *14*:309–318 (1976).

191. Phillips, W. E. J., and G. Hatina, Effect of dietary organochlorine pesticides on liver vitamin A content of weanling rats. *Nutr. Reports Intern.*, *5*:357–362 (1972).

192. Kato, N., M. Kato, T. Kimura, and A. Yoshida, Effect of dietary addition of PCB, DDT or BHT and dietary protein on vitamin A and cholesterol metabolism. *Nutr. Reports Intern.*, *18*:437–445 (1978).

193. Hakansson, H., and U. G. Ohlborg, The effect of 2,3,7,8-tetrachloro-dibenzo-para-dioxin on the uptake, distribution, and excretion of a single oral dose of [11,12 $^{-3}$H] retinyl acetate and on the vitamin A status in the rat. *J. Nutr.*, *115*:759–771 (1985).

194. Cullum, M. E., and M. H. Zile, Acute polybrominated biphenyl toxicosis alters vitamin A homeostasis and enhances degradation of vitamin A. *Toxicol. Appl. Pharmacol.*, *81*:177–181 (1985).

195. Jensen, R. K., M. E. Cullum, J. Deyo, and M. H. Zile, Vitamin A metabolism in rats chronically treated with 3,3′, 4,4′, 5.5′-hexabromobiphenyl. *Biochem. Biophys. Acta, 926*:310–320 (1987).

196. Gleghorn, E. E., L. D. Eisenberg, S. Hack, P. Parton, and R. J. Merritt, Observations of vitamin A toxicity in three patients with renal failure receiving parenteral alimentation. *Am. J. Clin. Nutr.*, *44*:107–112 (1986).

197. Arroyave, G., and M. Calcano, Depression of serum levels of retinol and of retinol-binding protein (RBP) during infections. *Archiv. Latinoamer. Nutr.*, *29*:233–260 (1979).

198. Underwood, B. A., Vitamin A in animal and human nutrition. In *The Retinoids*, Vol. 1, M. B. Sporn, A. B. Roberts, and D. S Goodman (eds.). Academic Press, Orlando, FL, 1984, pp. 281–392.

199. Mahalanabis, D., T. W. Simpson, M. L. Chakraborty, C. Ganguli, A. K. Bhattacharjee, and K. L. Mukherjee, Malabsorption of water-miscible vitamin A in children with giardiasis and ascariasis. *Am. J. Clin. Nutr.*, *32*:313–318 (1979).

200. Mansour, M. M., M. M. Mikhail, Z. Farid, and S. Bassily, Chronic salmonella septicemia and malabsorption of vitamin A. *Am. J. Clin. Nutr.*, *32*:319–324 (1979).

201. DeLuca, L. M., J. Glover, Heller, J. A. Olson, and B. Underwood, Recent advances in the metabolism and function of vitamin A and their relationship to applied nutrition. International Vitamin A Consultative Group, The Nutrition Foundation, New York, 1979.

202. Stolzfus, R., M. C. Nesheim, and P. Harvey, Vitamin A deficiency and *P. berghei* infection in rats. *FASEB J.*, *2*:A1195 (1988).

203. Sturchler, D., M. Tanner, A. Hanck, B. Betschart, K. Gantschi, N. Weiss, E. Burnier, G. Del Giudice, and A. Degrémont, A longitudinal study on relations of retinol with parasitic infections and the immune response in children of Kikwawila Village, Tanzania. *Acta Tropica, 44*:213–227 (1987).

204. Lieber, C. S., A. Garro, M. A. Leo, K. M. Mak, and T. Worner, Alcohol and cancer. *Hepatol., 5*: 1005–1019 (1986).

205. Erdman, J. W., Jr., H. C. Furr, J. M. Dietz, D. B. Gunning, and J. A. Olson, Effect of acute ethanol dosing on vitamin A metabolism. *FASEB J., 2*:A1426 (1988).

206. Horn, T., J. Junge, and P. Christoferson, Early alcoholic liver injury—activation of lipocytes in acinar zone 3 and correlation to degree of collagen formation in the Disse space. *Hepatol., 3*:333–340 (1986).

207. Friedman, H., S. Mobarhan, J. Hupert, D. Lucchesi, C. Henderson, P. Langenberg, and T. J. Layden, In vitro stimulation of rat liver retinyl ester hydrolase by ethanol. *Arch. Biochem. Biophys., 269*:69–74 (1989).

208. Grummer, M. A., and J. W. Erdman, Jr., Effect of chronic alcohol consumption and moderate fat diet on vitamin A status in rats fed either vitamin A or β-carotene. *J. Nutr., 113*:350–364 (1983).

209. Anonymous, The interaction of alcohol, vitamin A, and zinc in rats. *Nutr. Rev., 45*:62–64 (1987).

210. Kanai, M., T. Iwanaga, V. Hagino, and Y. Muto, Retinol-binding protein in tubular proteinuria of patients with Itai-Itai disease. *World Rev. Nutr. Dietet., 31*:31–36 (1978).

211. Sugawara, C., and N. Sugawara, Effect of cadmium on vitamin A metabolism. *Toxicol. Appl. Pharmacol.*, *56*:19–27 (1978).

212. Moore, T., I. M. Sharman, J. R. Todd, and R. H. Thompson, Copper and vitamin A concentrations in the blood of normal and copper-poisoned sheep. *Brit. J. Nutr.*, *28*:23–30 (1972).

213. Kromhout, D., Essential micronutrients in relation to carcinogenesis. *Am. J. Clin. Nutr.*, *45*:1361–1367 (1987).

214. Aoki, K., Y. Ito, R. Sasaki, M. Ohtani, N. Hamajima, and A. Asano, Smoking, alcohol, drinking, and serum carotenoid levels. *Jpn. J. Cancer Res.*, *78*:1049–1056 (1987).

215. Stryker, W. S., L. A. Kaplan, E. A. Stein, M. J. Stampfer, A. Sober, and W. C. Willett, The relation of diet, cigarette smoking, and alcohol consumption to plasma β-carotene and α-tocopherol levels. *Am. J. Epidemiol.*, *127*:283–296 (1988).

216. Garry, P. J., W. C. Hunt, J. C. Bandrofchak, D. Vander Jagt, and J. S. Goodwin, Vitamin A intake and plasma retinol levels in healthy elderly men and women. *Am. J. Clin. Nutr.*, *46*:989–994 (1987).

217. Ito, Y., R. Sasaki, M. Minohara, M. Otani, and K. Aoki, Quantitation of serum carotenoid concentrations in healthy inhabitants by high-performance liquid chromatography. *Clin. Chem. Acta, 169*:197–208 (1987).

218. Hollander, D., and D. Morgan, Aging—its influence on vitamin A intestinal absorption in vivo by the rat. *Exp. Gerontol.*, *14*:301–305 (1979).

219. Sundboom, J., and J. A. Olson, Effect of aging on the storage and catabolism of vitamin A in mice. *Exp. Gerontol.*, *19*:257–265 (1984).

220. Bankson, D. D., J. K. Ellis, and R. M. Russell, Effects of a vitamin A-free diet on visual function and tissue vitamin A concentration in aging rats. *Federation Proc.*, *45*:710 (1986).

221. Katz, M. L., C. M. Drea, and W. G. Robison, Jr., Age-related alterations in vitamin A metabolism in the rat retina. *Exp. Eye Res.*, *44*:939–949 (1987).

222. Suter, P. M., and R. M. Russell, Vitamin requirements of the elderly. *Am. J Clin. Nutr.*, *45*:501–512 (1987).

223. Matsuo, T., N. Matsuo, F. Shiraga, and N. Koide, Familial retinol-binding protein deficiency. *Lancet, 2*:402–403 (1987).

224. Thuluvath, P. J., Familial retinol-binding protein deficiency? *Lancet, 2*:910 (1987).

225. Matsuo, T., Further studies on familial retinol-binding protein deficiency. *Lancet 2*:910 (1987).

226. Carpenter, T. O., J. M. Pettifor, R. M. Russell, J. Pitha, S. Mobarhan, M. S. Ossip, S. Warner, and C. S. Anast, Severe hypervitaminosis in siblings: Evidence of variable tolerance to retinol intake. *J. Pediatr., 111*:507–512 (1987).

227. Sundaresan, P. R., V. G. Winters, and D. G. Therriault, Effect of low environmental temperature on the metabolism of vitamin A (retinol) in the rat. *J. Nutr.*, *92*:474–478 (1967).

228. Morita, A., and K. Nakano, Effect of chronic immobilization stress on tissue distribution of vitamin A in rats fed a diet with adequate vitamin A. *J. Nutr.*, *112*:789–795 (1982).

229. Campos, F. A. C. S., H. Flores, and B. A. Underwood, Effect of an infection on vitamin A status of children as measured by the relative dose response. *Am. J. Clin. Nutr.*, *46*:91–94 (1987).

230. Atukorala, T. M. S., T. K. Basu, and J. W. T. Dickerson, Effect of cortisone on the plasma and tissue concentrations of vitamin A in rats. *Ann. Nutr. Metab.*, *25*:234–238 (1981).

231. Nakano, K., and R. Mizutani, Decreased responsiveness of pituitary-adrenal axis to stress in vitamin A-depleted rats. *J. Nutr. Sci. Vitaminol.*, *29*:353–363 (1983).

232. Gronowska-Senger, A., and G. Wolf, Effect of dietary protein on the enzyme from rat and human intestine which converts beta-carotene into vitamin A. *J. Nutr.*, *100*:300–308 (1970).

233. Roels, O. A., M. Trout, and R. Dujacquier, Carotene balances on boys in Ruanda where vitamin A deficiency is prevalent. *J. Nutr.*, *65*:115–127 (1958).

234. Hodges, R. E., H. E. Sauberlich, J. E. Canham, D. L. Wallace, R. B. Rucker, L. Mejia, and M. Mohanram, Hematopoietic studies in vitamin A deficiency. *Am. J. Clin Nutr.*, *31*:876–885 (1978).

235. Mejia, L. A., and F. Chew, Hematological effect of supplementing vitamin A alone and in combination with iron to anemic children. *Am. J. Clin. Nutr., 48*:595–600 (1988).

236. Muhilal, H., D. Permeisih, Y. R. Idjradinata, Muherdiyantiningsih, and D. Karyadi, Impact of vitamin A fortified MSG on health, growth and survival of children: A controlled field trial. *Am. J. Clin. Nutr., 48*:1271–1276 (1988).

237. Duncan, J. R., and L. S. Hurley, An interaction between zinc and vitamin A in pregnant and fetal rats. *J. Nutr., 108*:1431–1438 (1978).

238. Dorea, J. G., and J. A. Olson, The rate of rhodopsin regeneration in the bleached eyes of zinc-deficient rats in the dark. *J. Nutr., 116*:121–127 (1986).

239. Solomons, N. W., and R. M. Russell, The interaction of vitiman A and zinc: implications for human nutrition. *Am. J. Clin. Nutr., 33*:2031–2040 (1980).

240. Sondergaard, E., The influence of vitamin E on the expenditure of vitamin A from the liver. *Experimentia, 28*:773–774 (1972).

241. Napoli, J. L., and C. D. Beck, Alpha-tocopherol and phylloquinone as noncompetitive inhibitors of retinyl esters hydrolysis. *Biochem. J., 223*:267–270 (1984).

242. McLaren, D. S., E. Shirajian, M. Tchalian, and G. Khoury, Xerophthalmia in Jordan. *Am. J. Clin. Nutr., 17*:117–130 (1965).

243. Bergen, H. R., Jr., G. Natadisastra, H. Muhilal, A. Dedi, D. Karyadi, and J. A. Olson, The vitamin A and vitamin E status of rural preschool children in West Java, Indonesia, and their response to oral doses of vitamin A and of vitamin E. *Am. J. Clin. Nutr., 48*:279–285 (1988).

244. Handelman, G. J., and E. A. Dratz, The role of antioxidants in the retina and retinal pigment epithelium and the nature of prooxidant-induced damage. *Adv. Free Radical Biol. Med., 2*:1–89 (1986).

245. Arnrich, L., and V. Arthur, Interactions of fat-soluble vitamins in hypervitaminosis. *Ann. N.Y. Acad Sci., 355*:109–118 (1980).

246. McLaren, D. S., Xerophthalmia: A neglected problem, *Nutr. Rev., 22*:289–291 (1964).

247. Reddy, V., Vitamin A deficiency control in India. In *Vitamin A Deficiency and its Control*, J. C. Bauernfeind (ed.). Academic Press, Orlando, FL, 1986, pp. 389–404.

248. West, K. P., Jr., and S. T. Pettiss, Control of vitamin A deficiency by the vitamin A periodic oral dosing approach. In *Vitamin A Deficiency and its Control*, J. C. Bauernfeind (ed.). Academic Press, Orlando FL, 1986, pp. 325–357.

249. Tarwotjo, I., R. Tilden, I. Satibi, and H. Nedrawati, Vitamin A deficiency control in Indonesia. In *Vitamin A Deficiency and its Control*, J. C. Bauernfeind (ed.). Acaemic Press, Orlando, FL, 1986, pp. 445–460.

250. Cohen, N., H. Rahman, M. Mitra, J. Sprague, S. Islam, E. L. de Regt, and M. A. Jalil, Impact of massive doses of vitamin A on nutritional blindness in Bangladesh. *Am. J. Clin. Nutr., 45*:970–976 (1987).

251. Olson, J. A., The prevention of childhood blindness by the administration of massive doses of vitamin A. *Israel J. Med. Sci., 8*:1199–1206 (1972).

252. Solon, M. A. Control of vitamin A deficiency by education and the public health approach. In *Vitamin A Deficiency and its Control*, J. C. Bauernfeind (ed.). Academic Press, Orlando, FL, 1986, pp. 285–318.

253. Orfanos, C. E., R. Ehlert, and H. Gollnick. The retinoids: A review of their clinical pharmacology and therapeutic use. *Drugs, 24*:459–503 (1987).

254. Lippman, S. M., J. F. Kessler, and F. L. Meyskens, Jr., Retinoids as preventative and therapeutic anticancer agents, Parts I and II. *Cancer Treat. Rep., 71*:391–405, 493–515 (1987).

255. Birt, D. F., Update on the effects of vitamins A, C, and E and selenium on carcinogenesis. *Proc. Soc. Exp. Biol. Med., 183*:311–320 (1986).

256. Moon, R. C., and L. M. Itri, Retinoids and cancer. In *The Retinoids*, Vol. 2, M. B. Sporn, A. B. Roberts, and D. S. Goodman (eds.). Academic Press, Orlando, FL, 1984, pp. 327–371.

257. McCormick, D. L., and R. C. Moon, Vitamin A status and cancer induction. In *Vitamin A Deficiency and its Control*, J. C. Bauernfeind (ed.). Academic Press, Orlando, FL, 1986, pp. 245–284.

258. Orfanos, C. E. (ed.), *Retinoids: Advances in Basic Research and Therapy*. Springer Verlag, Berlin, 1981, p. 527.

259. Poirier, L. A., P. M. Newberne, and M. W. Pariza (eds.). *Essential Nutrients in Carcinogenesis*. Plenum Press, New York, 1986, p. 562.

260. Meyskens, F. L., Jr., and K. N. Prasad (eds.), *Vitamins and Cancer*. Humana Press, Clifton, NJ, 1986, p. 481.

261. Moon, R. C., *Oncology Overview: Selected Abstracts on Retinoids, β-Carotene and Cancer*. National Institutes of Health, Public Health Service, Washington, DC, 1986, p. 152.

262. Mehta, R. G., A. B. Barua, J. A. Olson, and R. C. Moon, Effects of retinoid glucuronides on the mouse mammary gland in vitro. *Am. Assoc. Cancer Res.*, 28:50 (1987).

263. Bauernfeind, J. C., *The Safe Use of Vitamin A*. International Vitamin A Consultative Group, Nutrition Foundation, Washington, DC, 1980, p. 44.

264. Olson, J. A., Adverse effects of large doses of vitamin A and retinoids. *Seminars Oncol.*, 10:290–293 (1983).

264a. Smith, F. R., and D. S. Goodman, Vitamin A transport in human vitamin A toxicity. *N. Engl. J. Med.*, 294:805–808 (1976).

265. Schurr, D., J. Herbst, E. Habibi, and A. Abrahamov, Unusual presentation of vitamin A intoxication: Case report. *J. Pediatr. Gastroenterol. Nutr.*, 2:705–707 (1983).

266. Olson, J. A., Upper limits of vitamin A in infant formulas, with some comments on vitamin K. *J. Nutr.*, 119:1820–1824 (1989).

267. Geelen, J. A. G., Hypervitaminosis A-induced teratogenesis. *CRC Crit. Rev. Toxicol.*, 6:351–375 (1979).

268. Gunning, D. S., A. B. Barua, and J. A. Olson, Retinoid beta-glucuronides are not teratogenic in rats. *FASEB J.*, 3:A467 (1989).

269. Lammer, E. J., D. T. Chen, R. M. Hoar, N. D. Agnish, P. J. Benke, J. T. Braun, C. J. Curry, P. M. Fernhoff, A. W. Grix, I. T. Lott, J. M. Richard, and S. C. Sun, Retinoic acid embryopathy. *N. Engl. J. Med.*, 313:837–841 (1985).

270. Rosa, F. W., A. L. Wilk, and F. O. Kelsey, Vitamin A congeners. *Teratology*, 33:355–364 (1986).

270a. Howard, W. B., and C. C. Willhite, Toxicity of retinoids in humans and animals. *J. Toxicol. Toxin Rev.*, 5:55–94 (1986).

270b. Lungarotti, M. S., D. Marinelli, T. Mariani, and A. Calabro, Multiple congenital anomalies associated with apparently normal intake of vitamin A: A phenocopy of the isotretinoin syndrome? *Am. J. Med. Genet.*, 27:245–248 (1987).

271. Stewart, M. L., J. L. McDonad, A. S. Levy, R. E. Schucker, and D. R. Henderson, Vitamin/mineral supplement use: A telephone survey of adults in the United States. *J. Am. Diet. Assoc.*, 85:1585–1590 (1985).

272. Vorhees, C. V., and R. E. Butcher, Behavioral teratology. In *Development Toxicology*, K. Snell (ed.). Croom Helm Press, London, 1982, pp. 247–265.

273. Hutchings, D. E., J. Gibbon, and M. A. Kaufman, Maternal vitamin A excess during the early fetal period: Effects on learning and development in the offspring. *Develop. Psychobiol.*, 6:445–457 (1973).

274. Vorhees, C. V. Some behavioral effects of maternal hypervitaminosis A in rats. *Teratol.*, 10:269–274 (1974).

275. Nolan, G. A. The effect of prenatal retinoic acid on the viability and behavior of the offspring. *Neurobehav. Toxicol. Teratol.*, 8:643–654 (1986).

276. Underwood, B. A. *The safe Use of Vitamin A by Women During the Reproductive Years*. International Vitamin A Consultative Group, ILSI-Nutrition Foundation, Washington, DC, 1986.

277. Recommendations for vitamin A use during pregnancy: Teratology Society position paper. *Teratol.*, *35*:269–275 (1987).

278. Callaway, C. W., K. W. McNutt, R. S. Rivlin, A. C. Ross, H. H. Sandstead, and A. P. Simopoulos, Statement on vitamin and mineral supplements, The Joint Public Information Committee of the American Institute of Nutrition and the American Society for Clinical Nutrition. *J. Nutr.*, *117*:1649 (1987).

279. *Safety of Vitamins and Minerals: A Summary of Findings of Key Reviews*. Council for Responsible Nutrition, Washington, DC, 1986, p. 12.

280. Weber, U., G. Goerz, R. Hennekes, Carotenoid retinopathy I. Morphological and functional findings. *Klin. Monatsbl. Augenheilkd.*, *186*:351–354 (1985).

281. Daicker, B., K. Schiedt, J. J. Adnet, and P. Bermond, Canthaxanthin retinopathy: An investigation by light and electron microscopy and physicochemical analysis. *Graefe's Arch. Clin. Exp. Ophthalmol.*, *225*:189–197 (1987).

282. Olson, J. A. The provitamin A function of carotenoids. *J. Nutr.*, *119*:105–108 (1989).

283. Parker, R. S., Carotenoids in blood and tissues. *J. Nutr.*, *119*:101–104 (1989).

284. Burton, G., Antioxidant actions of carotenoids. *J. Nutr.*, *119*:109–111 (1989).

285. Bendich, A., Carotenoids and the immune response. *J. Nutr.*, *119*:112–115 (1989).

286. Krinsky, N. I. Carotenoids and cancer in animal models. *J. Nutr. 119*:123–126 (1989).

287. Moon, R. C., Comparative aspects of carotenoids and retinoids as chemopreventive agents for cancer. *J. Nutr.*, *119*:127–134 (1989).

288. Ziegler, R., Epidemiologial studies of carotenoids and cancer. *J. Nutr.*, *119*:116–122 (1989).

289. Olson, J. A., Introduction to a symposium on the biological actions of carotenoids. *J. Nutr.*, *119*:94–95 (1989).

290. Bendich, A., and J. A. Olson, Biological actions of carotenoids. *FASEB J.*, *3*:1927–1932 (1989).

2
Vitamin D

Elaine D. Collins and Anthony W. Norman
University of California
Riverside, California

I. INTRODUCTION

Vitamin D designates a group of closely related compounds that possess antirachitic activity. The two most prominent members of this group are ergocalciferol (vitamin D_2) and cholecalciferol (vitamin D_3). Ergocalciferol is derived from a common plant steroid, ergosterol, and is the usual form employed for vitamin D fortification of foods. Cholecalciferol is the form of vitamin D obtained when radiant energy from the sun strikes the skin and converts the precursor 7-dehydrocholesterol into vitamin D_3. Since the body is capable of producing cholecalciferol, vitamin D does not meet the classical definition of a vitamin. A more accurate description of vitamin D is that it is a prohormone; that is, vitamin D is metabolized to a biologically active form that functions as a steroid hormone (1–3). However, since vitamin D was first recognized as an essential nutrient, it has historically been classified among the lipid-soluble vitamins. Even today it is thought of by many as a vitamin, although it is now known that there exists a vitamin D endocrine system.

Together with two peptide hormones, calcitonin and parathyroid hormone (PTH), vitamin D functions to maintain calcium homeostasis and plays an important role in phosphorus homeostasis (4). Calcium and phosphorus are required for a wide variety of biological processes (see Table 1). Calcium is necessary for muscle contraction, nerve pulse transmission, blood clotting, and membrane structure. It also serves as a cofactor for such enzymes as lipases and ATPases and is needed for eggshell formation in birds. Phosphorus is an important component of DNA, RNA, membrane lipids, and the intracellular energy-transferring ATP system. Additionally, the phosphorylation of proteins is important for regulating many metabolic pathways. Furthermore, the maintenance of serum calcium and phosphorus levels within narrow limits is important for normal bone mineralization. Any perturbation in these levels will result in bone calcium accretion or resorption. Disease states, such as rickets, can develop if the serum ion product is not maintained at a level consistent with that required for normal bone mineralization. Maintaining a homeostatic state for these two elements is of considerable importance to a living organism.

Recently $1,25(OH)_2D_3$ has been shown to act on novel target tissues, not related to calcium homeostasis. There have been reports characterizing $1,25(OH)_2D_3$ receptors and activities in such diverse tissues as brain, pancreas, pituitary, skin, muscle, immune cells, and parathyroid (Table 2). These studies suggest that $1,25(OH)_2D_3$ is important for insulin and prolactin secretion, muscle function, immune and stress response, melanin synthesis, and cellular differentiation of skin and blood cells.

II. HISTORY

Rickets, a deficiency disease of vitamin D, appears to have been a problem in ancient times. There is evidence that rickets occurred in Neanderthal man about 50,000 B.C. The first scientific description of rickets was written by Dr. Daniel Whistler in 1645 and by

Table 1 Biological Calcium and Phosphorus

Calcium	Phosphorus
Utilization	
Body content: 70-kg man has 1200 g Ca^{2+}	Body content: 70-kg man has 770 g P
Structural: bone has 95% of body Ca	Structural: Bone has 90% of body P_i
Plasma $[Ca^{2+}]$ is 2.5 mM, 10 mg%	Plasma $[P_i]$ is 2.3 mM, 2.5–4.3 mg%
Muscle contraction	Intermediary metabolism (phosphorylated
Nerve pulse transmission	intermediates)
Blood clotting	Genetic information (DNA and RNA)
Membrane structure	Phospholipids
Enzyme cofactors	Enzyme/protein components
(amylase, trypsinogen, lipases, ATPases)	(phosphohistidine, phosphoserine)
Eggshell (birds)	Membrane structure
Daily requirements (70-kg man)	
Dietary intake: 700[a]	Dietary intake:1200[a]
Fecal excretion: 300–600[a,b]	Fecal excretion: 350–370[a,b]
Urinary excretion: 100–400[a,b]	Urinary excretion: 200–600[a,b]

[a]Values in milligrams per day.
[b]Based on the indicated level of dietary intake.

Table 2   Tissue Distribution of the $1,25(OH)_2D_3$ Receptor

Normal mammalian tissues/cell types that contain the $1,25(OH)_2D_3$ receptor:
   Intestine
   Kidney (proximal and distal tubules)
   Bone (osteoblasts)
   Parathyroid glands
   Thyroid (c-cells)
   Skin (epidermal cells and fibroblasts)
   Skeletal muscle (myoblasts)
   Cardiac muscle
   Cartilage (chondrocyte)
   Mammary tissue
   Testes
   Ovary
   Uterus
   Placenta
   Pituitary gland
   Pancreas (B-cell)
   Colon
   Parotid gland (B-cell)
   Thymus
   Circulating lymphocytes (activated)
   Circulating monocytes
$1,25(OH)D_2D_3$ receptors in malignant tissues/cancer cell lines
   Osteosarcoma
   Melanoma
   Breast carcinoma
   Colon carcinoma
   Medullary thyroid carcinoma
   Myeloid/lymphocytic leukemia
   Pancreatic adenocarcinoma
   Transitional cell bladder carcinoma
   Cervical carcinoma
   Fibrosarcoma
Additional studies in the chick have reported the presence of the $1,25(OH)_2D_3$ receptor in the
avian ultimobranchial gland, oviduct, and egg-shell gland.

Source: From Refs. 38 and 143.

Professor Francis Glisson in 1650. Rickets became a health problem in northern Europe, England, and the United States during the industrial revolution when many people lived in urban areas with little sunlight and air pollution. Prior to the discovery of vitamin D, theories on the causitive factors of rickets ranged from heredity to syphilis (2).

   Some of the important scientific discoveries leading to the understanding of rickets include the first formal description of bone by Marchand (1842), Bibard (1844), and Friedleben (1860). In 1885, Pommer wrote the first pathological description of the rachitic skeleton. In 1849, Trousseau and Lasque recognized that osteomalacia and rickets were different manifestations of the same disorder. In 1886 and 1890, Hirsch and Palm did a quantitative geographical study of the worldwide distribution of rickets and found that the incidence of rickets paralleled the incidence of lack of sunlight (5). This was substantiated in 1919 when Huldschinsky demonstrated that ultraviolet rays were effective in healing rickets (6).

In the early 1900s nutrition emerged as an experimental science, and the existence of vitamins as a concept was developed. In 1914, Professor C. Funk recognized that rickets only occurred when certain substances were lacking in the diet (5). Sir Edward Mellanby followed up on this idea by feeding synthetic diets to over 400 dogs over a 5-year period and was able to experimentally produce rickets in puppies. He further showed that addition of cod liver oil or butterfat to the feed prevented rickets. He postulated that the nutritional factor preventing rickets was vitamin A, since butterfat and cod-liver oil were known to contain vitamin A (7).

The distinction between the antixerophthalmic factor, vitamin A, and the antirachitic factor, vitamin D, was made in 1922 when McCollum's laboratory showed that the antirachitic factor in cod liver oil could survive both aeration and heating to 100 °C for 14 hr, whereas the activity of vitamin A was destroyed by this treatment. McCollum named the new substance vitamin D (8).

Although it was known that ultraviolet (UV) light and vitamin D were both equally effective in preventing and curing rickets, the close interdependence of these two factors was not immediately recognized. Then, in 1924, Steenbock and Black discovered that food that was irradiated and fed to rats could cure rickets, whereas food that was not irradiated could not cure rickets (9). In 1925, Hess and Weinstock demonstrated that a factor with antirachitic activity was produced in the skin upon UV irradiation (10–12). Both groups demonstrated that the antirachitic agent was in the lipid fraction. The action of the light appeared to produce a permanent chemical change in some component of the diet and the skin. They postulated that a provitamin D existed that could be converted to vitamin D by ultraviolet light absorption. Much more work ultimately demonstrated that the antrachitic activity resulted from the irradiation of 7-dehydrocholesterol.

The isolation and characterization of vitamin D was now possible. In 1932, the structure of vitamin D_2 was simultaneously determined by Windaus in Germany, who named it vitamin D_2 (13), and by Askew in England, who named it ergocalciferol (14). In 1936, Windaus identified the structure of vitamin D found in cod liver oil, vitamin D_3 (15). Thus the "naturally" occurring vitamin is vitamin D_3, or cholecalciferol. The structure of vitamin D was determined to be that of a steroid, or more correctly, a secosteroid. However, the relationship between its structure and its mode of action was not realized for another 30 years.

Vitamin D was believed for many years to be the active agent in preventing rickets. It was assumed that vitamin D was a cofactor for reactions that served to maintain calcium and phosphorus homeostasis. However, when radioisotopes became available, more precise measurements of metabolism could be made. Using radioactive $^{45}Ca^{2+}$, Lindquist found that there was a "lag period" between the administration of vitamin D and the initiation of its biological response (16). Stimulation of intestinal calcium absorption required 36–48 hr for a maximal response. Other investigators found delays in bone calcium mobilization and serum calcium level after treatment with vitamin D (17–25). The duration of the lag and the magnitude of the response were proportional to the dose of vitamin D used (18).

One explanation for the time lag was that vitamin D had to be further metabolized before it was active. With the development of radioactively labeled vitamin D, it became possible to study the metabolism of vitamin D. Norman et al. were able to prepare tritiated vitamin D_3 with high specific activity (7.3 mCi/mmol) (26). With this they were able to detect three metabolites that possess antirachitic activity (27). One of these metabolites was identified as the 25-hydroxy derivative of vitamin D_3 [25(OH)D_3] (28,29). 25(OH)D_3 was found to have 1.5 times more activity than vitamin D in curing rickets in the rat, so it was first thought that this metabolite was the biologically active form of vitamin D (30). However, in 1968, Haussler et al. reported a more polar metabolite, which was found in the nuclear fraction of the intestine of chicks given tritiated vitamin D_3 (31). Biological studies demonstrated that this new metabolite was 13–15 times more effective than vitamin D in stimulating intestinal calcium absorption and 5–6 times more effective in elevating serum calcium levels. The new metabolite was also as effective as vitamin D in increasing growth rate and bone ash. In 1971, the structural identity of this metabolite was reported to be the 1,25-dihydroxy derivative of vitamin D [1,25(OH)$_2D_3$] (32–34), the biologically active metabolite of vitamin D.

In 1970, the site of production for 1,25(OH)$_2D_3$ was demonstrated to be the kidney (35). This discovery together with the finding that 1,25(OH)$_2D_3$ is found in the nuclei of intestinal cells suggested that vitamin D was functioning as a steroid hormone (36). Much evidence has been reported in support of this concept and with the recent cloning and sequencing of the cDNA to the human 1,25(OH)$_2D_3$ receptor (37), the relationship between vitamin D and the other steroid hormones has been clearly established (38). The discovery that the biological actions of vitamin D could be explained by the classical model of steroid hormone action marked the beginning of the modern era of vitamin D.

III. CHEMISTRY

A. Structure

As previously mentioned, vitamin D refers to a family of compounds that possess antirachitic activity. Members of the family are derived from the cyclopentanoperhydrophenanthrene ring system (Fig. 1A), which is common to other steroids. However, vitamin D has only three intact rings; the B ring has undergone fission of the 9,10-carbon bond resulting in the conjugated triene system of double bonds that is possessed by all the D vitamins. The structure of vitamin D_3 is shown in Figure 1A. Naturally occurring members of the vitamin D family differ from each other only in the structure of their side chains; the side chain structures of the various members of the vitamin D family are given in Table 3.

From the x-ray crystallographic work of the Nobel laureate Crowfoot-Hodgkin et al., it is now known that the diene system of vitamin D that extends from C-5 to C-8 is transoid and nearly planar (39,40). However, the C-6 to C-19 diene system is cisoid and is not planar. The C-10 to C-19 double bond is twisted out of the plane by 60°. As a result, the A ring exists in one of two possible chair conformations. It is also known that the C and D rings are rigid and that the side chain prefers an extended configuration. In 1974, Okamura et al. reported that vitamin D and its metabolites have a high degree of conformational mobility (41). Using nuclear magnetic resonance (NMR) spectroscopy they were able to detect that the A ring undergoes rapid interconversion between the two chair conformations, as is shown on Fig. 1B. This conformational mobility is unique to the vitamin D molecule and is not observed for other steroid hormones. It is a direct consequence of the breakage of the 9,10-carbon bond of the B ring, which serves to "free" the A ring. As a result of this mobility, substituents on the A ring are rapidly and continually alternating beween the axial and equatorial positions. This is likely to present special problems for vitamin D receptors that are not encountered by the receptors for other steroid hormones.

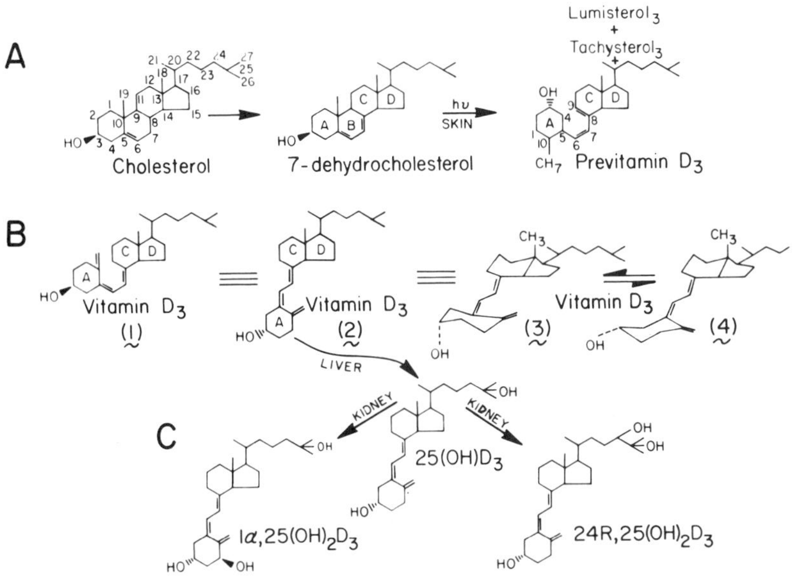

Figure 1 Key vitamin D sterol structures. (A) Vitamin D_3 and its metabolites are structurally related to cholesterol (the numbering of the carbon atoms is identical). Vitamin D_3 is formed in the skin from 7-dehydrocholesterol by the UV-mediated photochemical reaction. Previtamin D_3 thermally equilibrates into vitamin D_3. (B) Summary of the conformational representations of vitamin D_3. Structures 3 and 4 show the A ring chair-chair conformer equilibrium present in all vitamin D metabolites in solution. (C) Structures of the three principal metabolites of vitamin D_3.

Table 3 Side Chains of Provitamin D^a

Provitamin trivial name	Vitamin D produced upon irradiation	Empirical formula (complete steroid)	Side chain Structure
Ergosterol	D_2	$C_{28}H_{44}O$	
7-Dehydrocholesterol	D_3	$C_{27}H_{44}O$	
22,23-Dihydroergosterol	D_4	$C_{28}H_{46}O$	
7-Dehydrositosterol	D_5	$C_{29}H_{48}O$	
7-Dehydrostigmasterol	D_6	$C_{29}H_{46}O$	
7-Dehydrocampesterol	D_7	$C_{28}H_{46}O$	

^{a}Note that 22,23-dihydroergosterol and 7-dehydrocampesterol are epimers at C-24.

B. Nomenclature

Vitamin D is named according to the new revised rules of the International Union of Pure and applied Chemists (IUPAC). Since vitamin D is derived from a steroid, the structure retains its numbering from the parent steroid compound. Vitamin D is designated seco because its B ring has undergone fission. Assymmetric centers are named using R,S notation and Chen's rules of priority. The configuration of the double bonds are notated E, Z:E for *trans*, Z for *cis*. The formal name for vitamin D_3 is 9,10-seco(5Z,7E)-5,7,10(19)-cholestatriene-3β-ol and for vitamin D_2 is 9,10-seco (5Z,7E)-5,7,10(19),21-ergostatetraene-3β-ol.

C. Chemical Properties

1. Vitamin D_3 ($C_{27}H_{44}O$)

Three double bonds
Melting point, 84–85 °C
UV absorption maximum at 264–265 nm with a molar extinction coefficient of
  18,300 in alcohol or hexane, $\alpha_D{}^{20}$ + 84.8 ° in acetone
Molecular weight, 384.65
Insoluble in H_2O
Soluble in benzene, chloroform, ethanol, and acetone
Stable to heat, acid, and alkali
Unstable in light
Will undergo oxidation if exposed to air 24–72 hr
Best stored in evacuated ampules at 0 °C

2. Vitamin D_2 ($C_{28}H_{44}O$)

Four double bonds
Melting point, 121 °C
UV absorption maximum at 265 nm with a molar extinction coefficient of 19,400 in
  alcohol or hexane, $\alpha_D{}^{20}$ + 106 ° in acetone.
Same solubility and stability properties as D_3

D. Isolation

Many studies that have led to our understanding of the mode of action of vitamin D have involved the tissue localization and identification of vitamin D and its various metabolites. Since vitamin D is a steroid, it can best be isolated from tissue by methods that extract total lipids. The technique most frequently used for this extraction is the method of Bligh and Dyer (42).

Over the years a wide variety of chromatographic techniques have been used to separate vitamin D and its metabolites. These include paper, thin-layer, column, and gas chromatographic methods. Paper and thin-layer chromatography usually require long development times and yield unsatisfactory resolutions and have limited capacity. Column chromatography, using alumina, Floridin, celite, silica acid, and Sephadex LH-20 as supports, has been used to rapidly separate many closely related vitamin D compounds (2). However, none of the above methods are capable of resolving and distinguishing vitamin D_2 from vitamin D_3. Gas chromatography is able to separate these two compounds. However, in the process vitamin D is thermally converted to pyrocalciferol and isopyrocalciferol and these are chromatographed, resulting in two peaks. High-pressure liquid chromatography has become the method of choice for the separation of vitamin D and its metabolites. This powerful technique is very rapid and gives good recovery with high resolution.

E. Synthesis

1. Photochemical Production

In the 1920s, it was recognized that provitamins D were converted to vitamins D upon treatment with ultraviolet (UV) radiation (see Fig. 1a). The primary structural requirement for a provitamin D is a sterol with a C-5 to C-7 diene double-bond system in ring B. The conjugated double bond system is a chromaphore which, upon UV irradiation, initiates a series of transformations resulting in the production of the vitamin D secosteroid structure. The two most abundant provitamins D are ergosterol (provitamin D_2) and 7-dehydrocholesterol (provitamin D_3).

2. Chemical Synthesis

There are two basic approaches to the synthesis of vitamin D. The first involves the chemical synthesis of a provitamin that can be converted via UV radiation to vitamin D. The second is a total chemical synthesis.

Since vitamin D is derived from cholesterol, the first synthesis of vitamin D resulted from the first chemical synthesis of cholesterol. Cholesterol is easily converted to 7-dehydrocholesterol. Cholesterol was first synthesized by two groups in the 1950s. The first method involves a 20-step conversion of 4-methyoxy-2,5-toluquinone to a progesterone derivative, which is then converted in several more steps to progesterone, testosterone, cortisone, and cholesterol (43). The other method used the starting material 1,6-dihydroxynaphthalene. This was converted to the B and C rings of the steroid. A further series of chemical transformations led to the attachment of the A ring and then the D ring. The final product of the synthesis was epiandrosterone, which could be converted to cholesterol (44). The cholesterol was then converted to 7-dehydrocholesterol and UV irradiated to give vitamin D.

The first pure chemical synthesis of vitamin D, without any photochemical irradiation steps, was accomplished in 1967 (45). This continuing area of investigation allows for the production of many vitamin D metabolites and analogs without the necessity of a photochemical step. The yield of vitamin D from photochemical conversion is normally less than 10%. Pure chemical synthesis also allows for the synthesis of radioactive vitamin D and metabolites for the study of the metabolism of vitamin D.

F. Structures of Important Analogs

Neither vitamin D nor $25(OH)D_3$ is able to elicit a significant biological response when administered in physiological doses to nephrectomized animals (46,47) since the kidney is the site of $1,25(OH)_2D_3$ production. Also, it was noted in the 1940s and 1950s that dihydrotachysterol, (a 5,6-*trans* analog of vitamin D_3) was biologically active under circumstances where the parent vitamin D demonstated little or no biological activity. These findings raise the question of the functional importance of structural elements of the vitamin D molecule. Attempts to answer this question have been made by synthesizing various structural analogs of vitamin D and its metabolites. The ability of these analogs to increase intestinal calcium absorption (ICA) and bone calcium mobilization (BCM) and to promote cellular differentiation are then determined. Analogs prepared so far have involved modifications of the A ring and alterations of the side chain. Recent advances in new vitamin D syntheses may allow analogs to be made with alterations in the C and D rings (48).

The importance of the configuration of the A ring has been studied by synthesizing 5,6-*trans* analogs. Because of the rotation of the A ring, these analogs cannot undergo 1-hydroxylation and have been found to be only 1/1000 as biologically effective as $1,25(OH)_2D_3$. The relative significance of the 3β-hydroxyl group has been assessed by preparing analogs, such as the 3-deoxy-$1,25(OH)_2D_3$. Although this analog is active in vivo, it is interesting in that it preferentially stimulates intestinal calcium absorption over bone calcium mobilization (49). Of all the analogs synthesized, only a few show such selective biological activity (see Fig. 2).

The effect of altering the length of the side chain has been studied. The 27-*nor*-$25(OH)D_3$ and $26,27$-bis-*nor*-$25(OH)D_3$ are reportedly able to stimulate intestinal calcium absorption and bone calcium mobilization in both normal and anephric rats but are 10–100 times less active than $25(OH)D_3$ (50). The 24-*nor*-$25(OH)D_3$ was found to have no biological activity (51), although it was able to block the biological response to vitamin D, but not to $25(OH)D_3$ or $1,25(OH)_2D_3$. This suggests that it might have anti–vitamin D activity.

One of the most interesting side-chain analogs of $1,25(OH)_2D_3$ is $1\alpha(OH)D_3$. This metabolite appears to have the same biological activity in the chick as $1,25(OH)_2D_3$ (52) and is approximately half as active in the rat (53). In an attempt to determine if the biological activity of $1\alpha(OH)D_3$ is the result of in vivo 25-hydroxylation, the 25-fluoro-$1\alpha(OH)D_3$ derivative was prepared (54). The fluorine on C-25 prevents this carbon from becoming hydroxylated. The fluoro- compound was found to be 1/50 as active as $1,25(OH)_2D_3$, suggesting that $1\alpha(OH)D_3$ has some activity even without 25-hydroxylation.

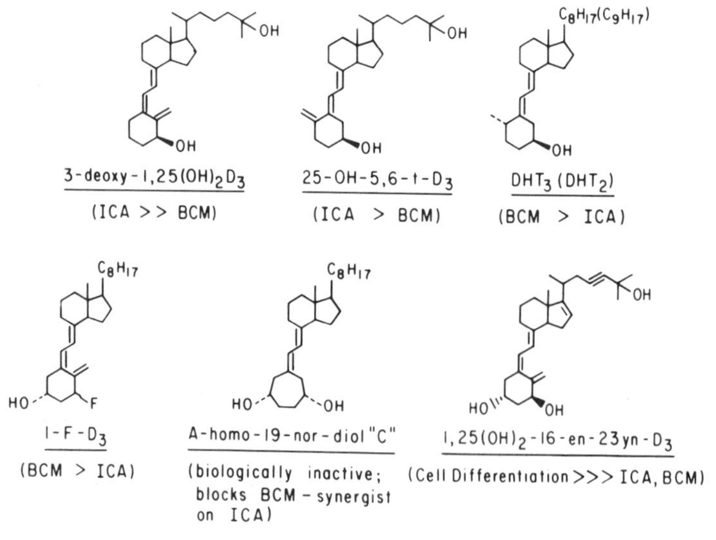

Figure 2 Vitamin D analogs known to possess selective biological activity. ICA = intestinal calcium absorption; BCM = bone calcium mobilization.

From such studies, the particular attributes of the structure of 1,25(OH)$_2$D$_3$ that enable it to elicit its biological responses are now being defined. It is now known that the 3β-hydroxy group does not appear to be as important for biological activity as the 1α- or 25-hydroxyl groups; the *cis* configuration of the A ring is preferred over the *trans* configuration; and the length of the side chain appears critical, as apparently there is no tolerance for its being shortened or lengthened.

IV. METABOLISM

The elucidation of the metabolic pathway by which vitamin D is transformed into its biologically active form is one of the most important advances in our understanding of how vitamin D functions. It is now known that both vitamin D$_2$ and vitamin D$_3$ must be hydroxylated at the C-1 and C-25 positions (see Fig. 1C) before they are able to produce their biological effects. The activation of vitamin D$_2$ occurs via the same metabolic pathway as does the activation of vitamin D$_3$, and the biological activities of both vitamin D$_2$ and vitamin D$_3$ have been shown to be identical in all animals except birds and the New World monkey. Apparently these animals have the ability to discriminate against vitamin D$_2$ (55).

A. Absorption

Vitamin D can be obtained from the diet, in which case it is absorbed, with the aid of bile salts, in the small intestine (56–58). In the rat and human, the specific mode of vitamin D absorption is via the lymphatic system and its associated chylomicrons. It has been reported that only about 50% of a dose of vitamin D is absorbed (59). However, considering that sufficient amounts of vitamin D can be produced daily by exposure to sunlight, it is not surprising that the body has not evolved a more efficient mechanism for vitamin D absorption from the diet

Although the body can obtain vitamin D from the diet, the major source of this prohormone is its production in the skin from 7-dehydrocholesterol. The 7-dehydrocholesterol is located primarily in the Malpighian layer of the skin. Upon exposure to ultraviolet light, it is photochemically converted to previtamin D, which then isomerizes to vitamin D over a period of several days (60). Once formed, the vitamin D is preferentially removed from the skin into the circulatory system by the blood transport protein for vitamin D, the vitamin D–binding protein (DBP).

B. Transport

Like other steroids that circulate in the plasma, vitamin D and its metabolites are protein-bound to the vitamin D–binding protein (DBP). Although the precise molecular function of these binding proteins is unknown, it is thought that they serve in the transportation of the hydrophobic steroid molecules through the aqueous media of the plasma. In general, the uptake of the steroid by the protein is rapid and occurs with high affinity.

The actual site of transfer of vitamin D from the chylomicrons to its specific plasma carrier protein is unknown. After an oral dose of radioactive vitamin D, the radioactivity becomes associated with the lipoprotein fraction of the plasma (61). As time passes, there is a progressive shift from this fraction to the α-globulin fraction (62). It has been shown that the electrophoretic mobility of the vitamin D-binding protein is identical to α_2-globulins and albumins (63–65).

In mammals, vitamin D, $25(OH)D_3$, $24,25(OH)_2D_3$, and $1,25(OH)_2D_3$ are transported on the same protein (66). The vitamin D–binding protein is a globulin protein with a molecular weight of 58,000 daltons in humans. It binds $25(OH)D_3$ with high affinity and other metabolites with somewhat lower affinity. Sequence analysis of the cDNA for vitamin D–binding-protein, which is also known as the group-specific protein (Gc protein), indicates that the vitamin D–bindng protein shares homology with serum albumin and α-feto protein (67). It is believed that DBP may help in the internalization of vitamin D sterols and that levels of DBP influence the concentration of "bound" and "free" hormone in the plasma. The concentration of the "free hormone" may be important in determining the biological activity of the hormone (68,69).

C. Storage

Vitamin D is rapidly taken up by the liver. Since it was known that the liver serves as a storage site for retinol, another fat-soluble vitamin, it was thought that the liver also functioned as a storage site for vitamin D. However, it has since been shown that blood has the highest concentration of vitamin D when compared to other tissues (70–72). From studies in rats it was concluded that no rat tissue can store vitamin D or its metabolites against a concentration gradient (73). The persistence of vitamin D in animals during periods of vitamin D deprivation may be explained by the slow turnover rate of vitamin D in certain tissues, such as skin and adipose. During times of deprivation, the vitamin D in these tissues is released slowly, thus meeting the vitamin D needs of the animal over a period of time.

On the other hand, Mawer et al. carried out studies in humans on the distribution and storage of vitamin D and its metabolites (74). In human tissue, adipose tissue and muscle were found to be major storage sites for vitamin D. Their studies also indicated that adipose tissue serves predominantly as the storage site for vitamin D_3 and that muscle serves as the storage site for $25(OH)D_3$.

D. Metabolism

Before vitamin D can exhibit any biological activity, it must first be metabolized by the body to its active forms. $1,25(OH)_2D_3$ is the most active metabolite known, but there is evidence that $24,25(OH)_2D_3$ is required for some of the biological responses attributed to vitamin D (75). Both these metabolites are produced in vivo following carbon-25 hydroxylation of the parent vitamin D molecule.

1. 25(OH)D₃

In the liver, vitamin D undergoes its initial transformation which involves the addition of a hydroxyl group to the 25-carbon. The metabolite thus formed is $25(OH)D_3$, which is the major circulating form of vitamin D. Although there is evidence that this metabolite can be formed in some other tissues such as intestine and kidney, it is generally accepted that the formation of $25(OH)D_3$ occurs predominantly in the liver.

The production of $25(OH)D_3$ is catalyzed by the enzyme vitamin D 25-hydroxylase. The 25-hydroxylase is found in liver microsomes and mitochondria. It is a P_{450}-like enzyme that is poorly regulated. Therefore, circulating levels of $25(OH)D_3$ are a good index of vitamin D status, i.e., a reflection of the body content of the parent vitamin D_3. Recent studies have suggested that the 25-hydroxylation of vitamin D is partially regulated by $1,25(OH)_2D_3$ (76). Other studies suggest that 25-hydroxylation is dependent on intracellular calcium levels. The extent, nature, and physiological significance of any regulatory mechanism of this step in the metabolism of vitamin D remains uncertain.

2. $1,25(OH)_2D_3$

From the liver, $25(OH)D_3$ is returned to the circulatory system where it is transported to the kidney. In the kidney, a second hydroxyl group can be added at the C-1 position. The enzyme responsible for the 1-α-hydroxylation of $25(OH)D_3$ is 25-hydroxyvitamin D_3-1-α-hydroxylase (1-hydroxylase). There is some evidence that some species may have an extra-renal source of the 1-hydroxylase.

The 1-hydroxylase is located in the mitochondria of the proximal tubules in the kidney. The enzyme belongs to a class of enzymes known as mitochondrial mixed-function oxidases. Mixed function oxidases use molecular oxygen as the oxygen source, instead of water. The 1-hydroxylase is composed of three proteins that are integral components of the mitochondrial membrane; they are the renal ferredoxin reductase, the renal ferredoxin, and the cytochrome P_{450}.

The most important point of regulation of the vitamin D endocrine system occurs through the stringent control of the activity of the renal-1-hydroxylase. In this way the production of the hormone $1,25(OH)_2D_3$ can be modulated according to the calcium needs of the organism. Several regulatory factors have been identified that modulate 1-hydroxlase activity, but some are functional only in certain species and under certain experimental conditions. The major factors are $1,25(OH)_2D_3$ itself, PTH, and the serum concentrations of calcium and phosphate.

Probably the most important determinant of 1-hydroxylase activity is the vitamin D status of the animal. When circulating levels of $1,25(OH)_2D_3$ are low, the production of $1,25(OH)_2D_3$ in the kidney is high, and when circulating levels of $1,25(OH)_2D_3$ are high, synthesis of $1,25(OH)_2D_3$ is low. The changes of enzyme activity induced by $1,25(OH)_2D_3$ can be inhibited by cyclohexamide and actinomycin D (77), which suggests that $1,25(OH)_2D_3$ is acting at the level of transcription. Another modulator of renal $1,25(OH)_2D_3$ production is parathyroid hormone (PTH). PTH is released when plasma calcium levels are low, and in the kidney it stimulates the activity of the 1-hydroxylase and decreases the activity of the 24-hydroxylase. $1,25(OH)_2D_3$ and $24,25(OH)_2D_3$ also operate in a feedback loop to modulate and/or reduce the secretion of PTH. Other modulators of renal $1,25(OH)_2D_3$ production are shown in Figure 3.

3. $24,25(OH)_2D_3$

A second dihydroxylated metabolite of vitamin D is produced in the kidney, namely $24,25(OH)_2D_3$. Also, virtually all other tissues that have receptors for $1,25(OH)_2D_3$ can also produce $24,25(OH)_2D_3$. There is some controversy concerning the possible unique biological actions of $24,25(OH)_2D_3$. However, there is some evidence that $24,25(OH)_2D_3$ plays a role in the suppression of parathyroid hormone secretion and in the mineralization of bone (78,79). Other studies demonstrated that the combined presence of $24,25(OH)_2D_3$ and $1,25(OH)_2D_3$ are required for normal egg productivity, fertility, and hatchability in chickens (80) and quail (81). From these studies it was apparent that only combination doses of both compounds were capable of eliciting the same response as the parent vitamin D. Thus, it appears that both $1,25(OH)_2D_3$ and $24,25(OH)_2D_3$ may be required for some of the known biological responses to vitamin D.

The enzyme responsible for the production of $24,25(OH)_2D_3$ is the 25-hyroxyvitamin D_3-4-hydroxylase (24-hydroxylase). Experimental evdience suggests that this enzyme is

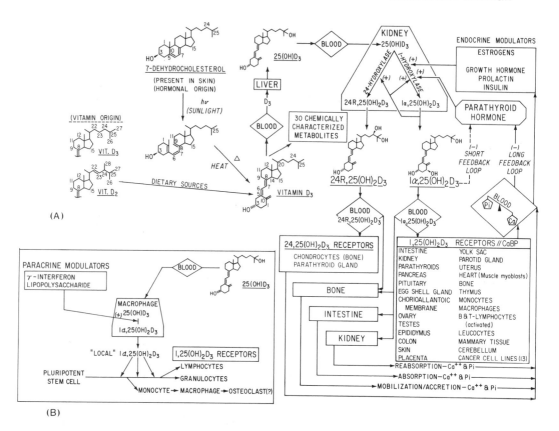

Figure 3 Overview of the vitamin D endocrine and paracrine systems.

also a mixed-function oxidase. The activity of this enzyme is regulated so that when $1,25(OH)_2D_3$ levels are low, the activity of the 24-hydroxylase is also low, but when $1,25(OH)_2D_3$ levels are high the activity of the 24-hydroxylase is high. Under normal physiological conditions both $1,25(OH)_2D_3$ and $24,25(OH)_2D_3$ are secreted from the kidney and circulated in plasma of all classes of vertebrates.

In addition to these three metabolites, many other vitamin D_3 metabolites have been chemically characterized, and the existence of others appears likely. The chemical structures of 30 known metabolites are shown in Figure 4. Most of these metabolites appear to be intermediates in degradation pathways of $1,25(OH)_2D_3$. None of these other metabolites have yet been shown to have biological activity except for the $1,25(OH)_2D_3$-26,23-lactone. The lactone is produced by the kidney when the plasma levels of $1,25(OH)_2D_3$ are very high. The metabolite appears to be antagonistic to $1,25(OH)_2D_3$, since it mediates a decrease in serum calcium levels in the rat. Recent experiments suggest that the lactone inhibits bone resorption and blocks the resorptive action of $1,25(OH)_2D_3$ on the bone (82), perhaps functioning as a natural antagonist of $1,25(OH)_2D_3$ to prevent toxic effects from overproduction of $1,25(OH)_2D_3$.

The metabolism of vitamin D_2 has not been studied as much as the metabolism of vitamin D_3. The chemical structures of the known metabolites of vitamin D_2 are shown in Figure 5.

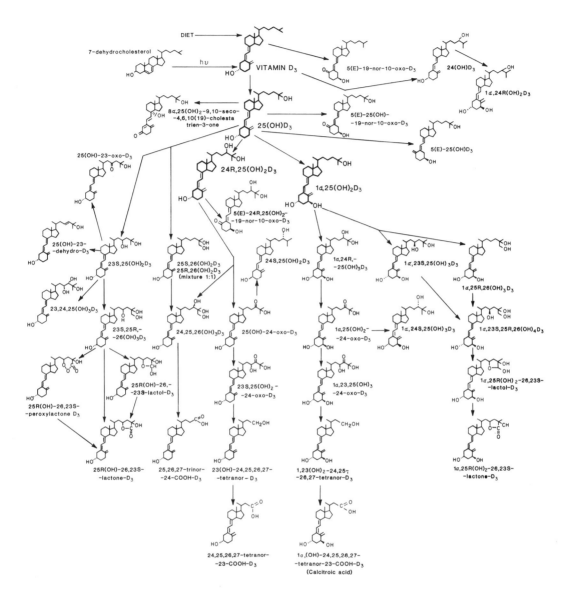

Figure 4 Summary of the metabolic transformations of vitamin D_3. The structures of all known chemically characterized metabolites are shown.

E. Catabolism and Excretion

Several pathways exist in man and animals to further metabolize $1,25(OH)_2D_3$. These include oxidative cleavage of the side chain, 24-hydroxylation to produce $1,24,25(OH)_3D_3$, formation of $24\text{-oxo-}1,25(OH)_2D_3$, formation of $1,25(OH)_2D_3\text{-}26,23\text{-lactone}$, and formation

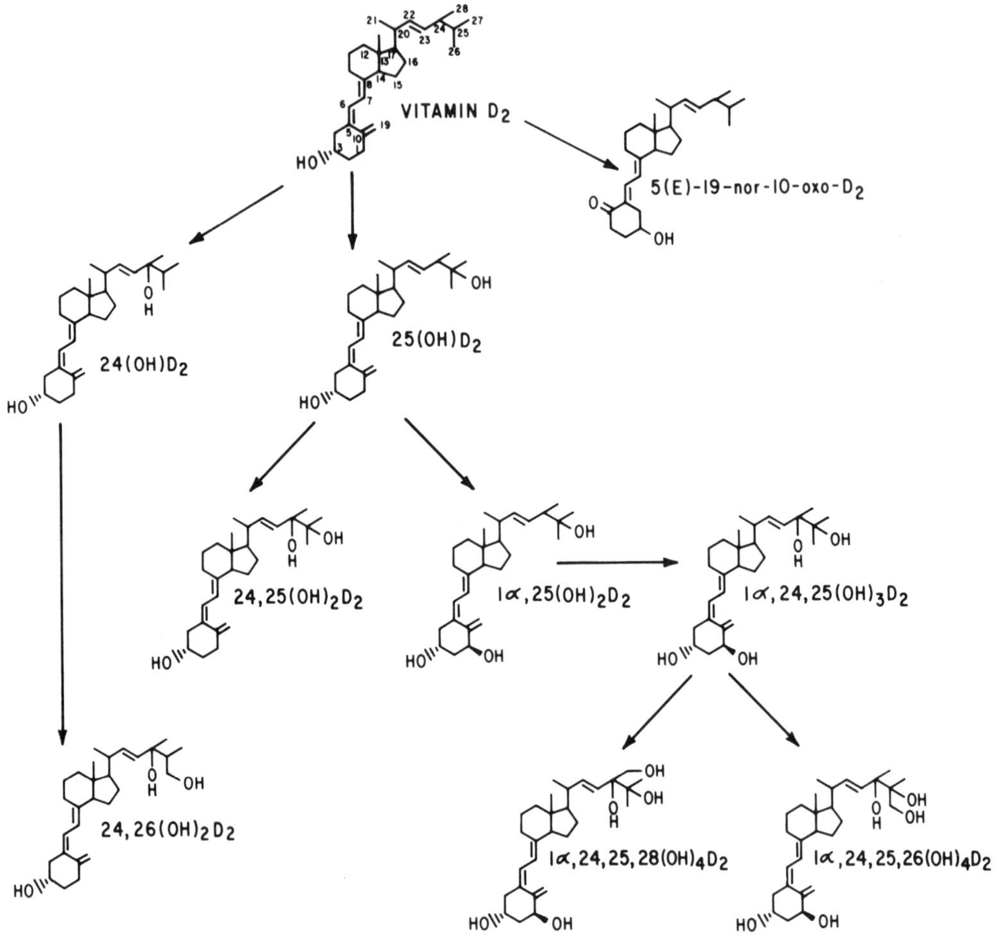

Figure 5 Summary of the metabolic transformations of vitamin D_2. The structures of all known chemically characterized metabolites are shown.

of $1,25,26(OH)_2D_3$ (see Fig. 4). It is not known which of these pathways are involved in the breakdown or clearance of $1,25(OH)_2D_3$ in man.

The catabolic pathway for vitamin D is obscure, but it is known that the excretion of vitamin D and its metabolites occurs primarily in the feces with the aid of bile salts. Very little appears in the urine. Studies in which radioactively labeled $1,25(OH)_2D_3$ was administered to humans have shown that 60–70% of the $1,25(OH)_2D_3$ was eliminated in the feces as more polar metabolites, glucuronides and sulfates of $1,25(OH)_2D_3$. The half-life of $1,25(OH)_2D_3$ in the plasma has two components. Within 5 minutes only half of an administered dose of radioactive $1,25(OH)_2D_3$ remains in the plasma. A slower component of elimination has a half-life of about 10 hours. $1,25(OH)_2D_3$ is catabolized by a number of pathways, which result in its rapid removal from the organism (83).

V. BIOCHEMICAL MODE OF ACTION

The major physiological effects of vitamin D are to increase the active absorption of Ca^{2+} from the proximal intestine and to increase the mineralization of bone. Vitamin D, through its daughter metabolite $1,25(OH)_2D_3$, functions in a manner homologous to that of steroid hormones. A model for steroid hormone action is shown in Figure 6. The hormone is produced by an endocrine gland in response to physiological stimuli. Small quantities of the steroid hormone circulate in the blood, usually bound to some carrier protein, i.e., DBP, and are transported to the target tissue. In the target tissue, the hormone enters the cell and binds to a cytosolic receptor or a nuclear receptor. The receptor–hormone complex becomes localized in the nucleus, undergoes some kind of activation, and becomes associated with the chromatin, modulating the transcription of hormone-sensitive genes. The modulation of gene transcription results in either the induction or repression of specific mRNAs, ultimately resulting in changes in protein expression needed to produce the required biological response. Genes that have been shown to be regulated by $1,25(OH)_2D_3$ at the level of mRNA accumulation are listed in Table 4.

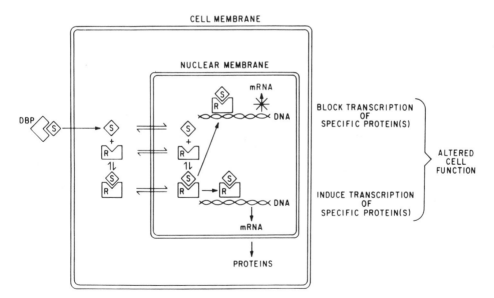

Figure 6 General model for the mechanism of action of steroid hormones illustrated using $1\alpha,25(OH)_2D_3$ as the steroid hormone. Target tissues contain receptors for the steroid which confer upon them the ability to modulate genomic events. S = steroid; R = receptor protein, which may be present inside the cell in either the cytosol or nuclear compartment; SR = steroid–receptor complex; DBP = serum vitamin D–binding protein, which functions to transport the steroid hormone from the endocrine gland to its various target tissues.

Table 4 Genes Regulated by $1,25(OH)_2D_3$ at the Level of mRNA Accumulation

Gene	Tissue	Direction
PreproPTH	rat parathyroid glands	↓
Calcitonin	rat thyroid gland	↓
Type I collagen	rat fetal calvaria	↓
Fibronectin	human fibroblast line	↑
Bone matrix GLA protein	rat osteosarcoma cells	↑
Interleukin-2	activated human lymphocytes	↓
Interferon-γ	activated human lymphocytes	↓
GM-CSF	activated human lymphocytes	↓
c-myc	human HL-60 myeloid leukemia	↓
c-fos	human HL-60 myeloid leukemia	↑
c-fms	human HL-60 myeloid leukemia	↑
$1,25(OH)_2D_3$-receptor	mouse fibroblasts	↑
Calbindin-D_{28K}	chick intestinal mucosa	↑
Calbindin-D_{9K}	rat intestinal mucosa	↑
Prolactin	rat pituitary cells	↑

An effect on $1,25(OH)_2D_3$ on transcription has thus far been demonstrated only for the genes encoding preproPTH, calcitonin, c-myc, and calbindins D_{9K} and D_{28K}. $1,25 (OH)_2D_3$ modified GM-CSF mRNA posttranscriptionally and also has posttranscriptional effects on mRNA expression of both calbindins. In the other cases, it is not known if $1,25(OH)_2D_3$ modulates gene transcription or induces other factors which alter mRNA accumulation posttranscriptionally.

Source: Ref. 143.

The $1,25(OH)_2D_3$ receptor has been extensively characterized, and the cDNA for the human receptor has been recently cloned (37). The $1,25(OH)_2D_3$ receptor is a protein with a molecular weight of about 67,000 daltons. It has a high affinity for $1,25(OH)_2D_3$ with a K_D in the range of $1-50 \times 10^{-11}M$. The receptor binds vitamin D metabolites and analogs with a specificity that parallels the biological activity of these compounds. The sequence data indicate that the $1,25(OH)_2D_3$ receptor is homologous to other steroid hormone receptors, the thyroid hormone receptor, and the retinoic acid receptor. Tissues that have been shown to possess $1,25(OH)_2D_3$ receptors are listed in Table 2.

One of the major effects of $1,25(OH)_2D_3$ in many of its target tissues is the induction of a calcium-binding protein, named calbindin-D. In the mammalian kidney and brain and in the chick, a larger from of the protein is expressed, calbindin-D_{28K}, while in the mammalian intestine and placenta a smaller form is expressed, calbindin-D_{9K} (84). The expression of calbindins in various tissues and species appears to be regulated to differing degrees by $1,25(OH)_2D_3$.

Early experiments showed that actinomycin D and α-amanitin, transcriptional inhibitors, could block the induction of calbindin-D_{28K} by $1,25(OH)_2D_3$ (85). Later experiments showed that $1,25(OH)_2D_3$ was able to stimulate total RNA synthesis in the chick intestine (86) in addition to specifically inducing the mRNA for calbindin-D_{28K} (87). Nuclear transcription assays have shown that transcription of calbindin-D_{28K} mRNA is directly induced by $1,25(OH)_2D_3$ in the chick intestine and is correlated to the level of occupied $1,25(OH)_2D_3$ receptors (88). The gene for calbindin-D_{28K} has now been cloned and sequenced, and the analysis of its promoter will allow a better understanding of how $1,25(OH)_2D_3$ induces this gene (89).

Recent studies (90) suggest that not all of the actions of $1,25(OH)_2D_3$ can be explained by receptor–hormone interactions with the genome. $1,25(OH)_2D_3$ can stimulate the intestinal transport of calcium within 4–6 minutes, too quickly to involve genome activation. The rapid transport of calcium mediated by $1,25(OH)_2D_3$ in the intestine has been termed "transcaltachia." Transcaltachia is not inhibited by actinomycin D but is inhibited by colchicine, an antimicrotubule agent, and by leupeptin, an antagonist of lysomal cathespin B. Transcaltachia induced by $1,25(OH)_2D_3$ in the intestine appears to involve the internalization of calcium in endocytic vesicles at the brush border membrane, which then fuse with lyzosomes and travel along microtubules to the basal lateral membrane where exocytosis occurs. Therefore, some of the actions of $1,25(OH)_2D_3$ may be mediated at the cell membrane or by extranuclear subcellular components, not only by genomic interactions.

A. $1,25(OH)_2D_3$ and Mineral Homeostasis

The classical target tissues for $1,25(OH)_2D_3$ are those tissues that have been found to be directly involved in the regulation of mineral homeostasis. Together with PTH, $1,25(OH)_2D_3$ exerts its actions on the intestine, kidney, bone, and parathyroid gland.

$1,25(OH)_2D_3$ maintains serum calcium and phosphate levels and provides minerals for bone formation mainly through its actions in the intestine. One of the best characterized effects of $1,25(OH)_2D_3$ is the stimulation of intestinal lumen-to-plasma flux of calcium and phosphate (75,91–92). Although extensive evidence exists showing that $1,25(OH)_2D_3$, interacting with its receptor, upregulates calbindin-D in a genome mediated fashion, the relationship between the calbindins-D and calcium transport is not clear. In the vitamin D–deficient state, both mammals and birds have severely decreased intestinal absorption of calcium with no detectable levels of calbindin. Also, there is a linear correlation between the increased cellular levels of calbindin-D and calcium transport. When $1,25(OH)_2D_3$ is given to vitamin D–deficient chicks, the transport of calcium reaches maximal rates at 12–14 hr, while calbinin-D does not reach its maximal levels until 48 hr. Also, intestinal absorption of calcium begins to decrease while calbindin-D levels are still maximal (90). $1,25(OH)_2D_3$ treatment is also known to alter the biochemical and morphological characteristics of the intestinal cells. The size of the villus and the size of the microvilli increases upon $1,25(OH)_2D_3$ treatment. The brush border undergoes noticeable alterations of structure and composition of cell surface proteins and lipids, occurring in a time frame corresponding to the increase in Ca^{2+} transport mediated by $1,25(OH)_2D_3$ (93). However despite extensive work, the exact mechanisms involved in the vitamin D-dependent intestinal absorption of calcium remain unknown.

The kidney is the major site of synthesis of $1,25(OH)_2D_3$ and of several other hydroxylated vitamin D derivatives. Probably the most important effect $1,25(OH)_2D_3$ has on the kidney is the inhibition of $25(OH)D_3$-1α-hydroxylase activity, which results in a decrease in the synthesis of $1,25(OH)_2D_3$ (94,95). Simultaneously, the activity of the $25(OH)D_3$-24-hydroxylase is stimulated. The actions of vitamin D on calcium and phosphorus metabolism in the kidney have been controversial, and more research is needed to clearly define the actions of $1,25(OH)_2D_3$ on the kidney.

Although vitamin D is a powerful antirachitic agent, its primary effect on bone is the stimulation of bone resorption leading to an increase in serum calcium and phosphorus levels (96). With even slight decreases in serum calcium levels, parathyroid hormone is synthesized, and it stimulates the synthesis of $1,25(OH)_2D_3$ in the kidney. Both of these hormones stimulate bone resorption. Maintaining constant levels of calcium in the blood is crucial, whether calcium is available from the diet or not. Therefore, the ability to release calcium from its largest body store, the bone, is vital. Bone is a dynamic tissue which is constantly being remodeled. Under normal physiological conditions, bone formation and bone resorption are tightly balanced. The stimulation of bone growth and mineralization by $1,25(OH)_2D_3$ appears to be an indirect effect due to the provision of minerals for bone matrix incorporation through an increase of intestinal absorption of calcium and phosphorus.

Parathyroid hormone is an important tropic stimulator of $1,25(OH)_2D_3$ synthesis by the kidney. High circulating levels of $1,25(OH)_2D_3$ have been shown to decrease the levels of PTH by two different mechanism: an indirect mechanism due to the resulting increase in serum calcium levels, which is an inhibitory signal for PTH production, and a direct mechanism involving the interaction of $1,25(OH)_2D_3$ and its receptor, which directly suppresses the expression of the preprothyroid hormone gene.

During pregnancy and lactation, large amounts of calcium are needed for the developing fetus and milk production. Hormonal adjustments in the vitamin D endocrine system are critical to prevent depletion of minerals leading to serious bone damage for the mother. Although receptors for $1,25(OH)_2D_3$ have been found in placental tissue and in the mammary gland, the role vitamin D plays is not clear.

B. Vitamin D in Nonclassical Systems

In the past 10 years, receptors for $1,25(OH)_2D_3$ have been found in a wide range of tissues and cells (Table 2) by far extending the classical limits of vitamin D actions on calcium homeostasis. In many of these systems, it is not yet clear what effect vitamin D has on the tissue or its mode of action.

In the pancreas, $1,25(OH)_2D_3$ has been found to be essential for normal insulin secretion. Experiments with rats have shown that vitamin D increases insulin release from isolated perfused pancreas, both in the presence or absence of normal serum calcium levels (97). Human patients with vitamin D deficiency, even under conditions of normal calcemia, exhibit impaired insulin secretion but normal glucagon secretion, suggesting that $1,25(OH)_2D_3$ is directly effecting β-cell function (98).

Receptors for $1,25(OH)_2D_3$ have been found in some sections of the brain. However, the role of $1,25(OH)_2D_3$ in the brain is not well understood. Both calbindins-D have been found in the brain, but the expression of neither calbindin-D_{28K} nor calbindin-D_{9K} appears to be modulated directly by vitamin D (99,100). In the rat, $1,25(OH)_2D_3$ appears to increase the activity of choline acetyltransferase (CAT) in specific regions of the brain (99). Other steroid hormones have also been shown to affect the metabolism of specific brain regions.

Skeletal muscle is also a target organ for $1,25(OH)_2D_3$. Clinical studies have shown the presence of muscle weakness or myopathy during metabolic bone diseases related to vitamin D deficiency (101). In addition, there are electrophysiological abnormalities in muscle contraction and relaxation in vitamin D deficiency (102). These abnormalities can be reversed with vitamin D therapy. Experimental evidence has shown that $1,25(OH)_2D_3$ has a direct effect on Ca^{2+} transport in cultured myoblasts and skeletal muscle tissue. Furthermore, there is evidence that the action of $1,25(OH)_2D_3$ on skeletal muscle may be important for the calcium homeostasis of the entire organism since the sterol induces a rapid release of calcium from muscle into serum of hypocalcemic animals. $1,25(OH)_2D_3$ receptors have been detected in myoblast cultures, and the changes in calcium uptake have been shown to be RNA and protein synthesis-dependent, suggesting a genomic mechanism.

In the skin, $1,25(OH)_2D_3$ appears to exert effects on cellular growth and differentiation. Receptors of $1,25(OH)_2D_3$ have been found in human and mouse skin. $1,25(OH)_2D_3$ inhibits the synthesis of DNA in mouse epidermal cells (103). The hormone induces changes in cultured keratinocytes which are consistent for terminal differentiation of nonadherent cornified squamous cells. (104). Additional experiments have shown that human neonatal foreskin keratinocytes produce $1,25(OH)_2D_3$ from $(25(OH)_3$ under in vitro conditions (105) suggesting that keratinocyte-derived $1,25(OH)_2D_3$ may affect epidermal differentiation locally.

$1,25(OH)_2D_3$ also promotes the differentiation of leukemic myeloid precursor cells towards cells with the characteristics of macrophages (106). Subsequent experiments have shown that $1,25(OH)_2D_3$ does not alter the clonal growth of normal myeloid precursors, but it does induce the formation of macrophage colonies preferentially over the formation of granulocyte colonies (107). In addition, macrophages derived from different tissue are able to synthesize $1,25(OH)_2D_3$ when activated by γ-interferon (108). Also, $1,25(OH)_2D_3$ can suppress immunoglobulin production by activated B-lymphocytes (109) and inhibit DNA synthesis and proliferation of both activated B and T lymphocytes (110,111). These findings suggest that a vitamin D paracrine system exists involving activated macrophages and activated lymphocytes (see Fig. 3).

VI. BIOLOGICAL ASSAYS

With the exception of vitamin B_{12}, vitamin D is the most potent of the vitamins (as defined by the amount of vitamin required to elicit a biological response). Consequently, biological samples and animal tissues usually contain only very low concentrations of vitamin D. For example, the circulating plasma level of vitamin D_3 in humans is only 10–20 ng/ml, or $2–5 \times 10^{-8}$ M (112). In order to be able to detect such low concentrations of vitamin D, assays that are specific for and sensitive to vitamin D and its biologically active metabolites are required.

A. Rat Line Test

From 1922 to 1958, the only official assay for the determination of the vitamin D content of pharmaceutical products or food was the rat line test. The term "official" indicates that the reproducibility and accuracy of the assay are high enough that the results of the test can be accepted legally. This assay, which is capable of detecting 1–12 IU (25–300 ng) of vitamin D [1 IU (International Unit) = 0.025 μg vitamin D], is still widely used today to determine the vitamin D content of many foods, particularly milk. The rat line test for vitamin D employs recently weaned rachitic rats; these rats are fed a rachitogenic diet for 19–25 days until severe rickets develops. The rats are then divided into groups of 7–10 animals and are fed diets that have been supplemented either with a graded series of known amounts of vitamin D_3 as standards or with the unknown test sample. (Although vitamin D oils can be directly assayed, milk, vitamin tablets, and vitamin D–fortified foods must be saponified and the residue taken up into a suitable oil vehicle prior to assay.) The rats are maintained on their respective diets for a period of 7 days. The animals are sacrificed and their radii and ulnae dissected out and stained with a silver nitrate solution.

Silver is deposited in areas of bone where new calcium has been recently deposited. The regions turn dark when exposed to light. Thus, the effects of the unknown sample on calcium deposition in the bone can be determined by visual comparison with the standards.

B. AOAC Chick Assay

Since the rat line test is done in rats, it is unable to discriminate between vitamin D_2 and vitamin D_3. In the chick, vitamin D_3 is 10 times more potent than vitamin D_2 so it is important to accurately determine the amount of vitamin D_3 in poultry feeds. The AOAC (Association of Official Agricultural Chemists) chick test was developed to specifically measure vitamin D_3.

Groups of 20 newly hatched chicks are placed on D-deficient diets containing added levels of vitamin D_3 (1–10 IU) or the test substance. After 3 weeks on the diet, the birds are sacrificed and the percentage of bone ash of their tibia is determined. A rachitic bird typically has 25–27% bone ash, whereas a vitamin D–supplemented bird has 40–45% bone ash. This assay is not used frequently since it is time-consuming and expensive.

C. Intestinal Calcium Absorption

Other biological assays have been developed that make use of the ability of vitamin D to stimulate the absorption of calicum across the small intestine. Two basic types of assays measure this phenomenon: those that measure the effect of the test substance on intestinal calcium uptake in vivo and those that employ in vitro methods. Each is capable of detecting physiological quantities, i.e., 2–50 IU (50–1250 ng; 0.13–3.2 nmol), of vitamin D.

1.   In Vivo Technique

The in vivo technique for measuring intestinal calcium absorption uses rachitic chicks that have been raised on a low-calcium (0.6%) rachitogenic diet for 3 weeks. The birds are then given one dose of the test compound either orally, intraperitoneally, or intracardially. The chicks are anesthetized 12–48 hr later, and 4.0 mg of $^{40}CA^{2+}$ and approximately 6×10^6 dpm $^{45}Ca^{2+}$ are placed in the duodenal loop. Thirty minutes later, the chicks are killed by decapitation and serum is collected. Aliquots of serum are measured for $^{45}Ca^{2+}$ in a liquid scintillation counter.

2.   In Vitro Technique

The general design of this technique is the same as the in vivo technique, since vitamin D activity is being measured in terms of intestinal calcium transport. In these assays, a vitamin D standard or test compound is given orally or intraperitoneally 24–48 hr before the assay. At the time of the assay, the animals are killed, and a 10-cm length of duodenum is removed and turned inside out. A gut sac is formed by tying off the ends of the segment so that the mucosal surface is on the outside and the serosal surface on the inside. The everted intestinal loop is incubated with solutions of $^{45}Ca^{2+}$. The mucosal surface of the intestine will actively transport the calcium through the tissue to the serosal side. The ratio of calcium concentration on the serosal versus the mucosal side of the intestine is a measure of the "active" transport of calcium . In a vitamin D–deficient animal this ratio is 1:2.5; in a vitamin D–dosed animal this ratio can be as high as 6:7. The chick in vivo assay is usually preferred because of the tedious nature of preparing the everted gut sacs. The in vitro technique is used primarily for studies with mammals rather than birds.

D. Bone Calcium Mobilization

Another assay for vitamin D activity often performed simultaneously with the chick in vivo intestinal calcium absorption assay is the measurement of the vitamin D– mediated elevation of serum calcium levels. If 3-week-old rachitic chicks are raised on a zero-calcium diet for at least 3 days before the assay and then given a compound with vitamin D activity, their serum calcium levels will rise in a highly characteristic manner, proportional to the amount of steroid given. Since there is no dietary calcium available, the only calcium source for elevation of serum calcium is bone. By carrying out this assay simultaneously with the intestinal calcium absorption assay, it is possible to measure two different aspects of the animal's response to vitamin D at the same time.

E. Growth Rate

The administration of vitamin D to animals leads to an enhanced rate of whole body growth. An assay for vitamin D was developed in the chick using the growth-promoting properties of the steroid. One-day-old chicks are placed on a rachitogenic diet and given standard doses of vitamin D_3 or the test compound three times weekly. The birds are weighed periodically, and weight is plotted versus age. In the absence of vitamin D the rate of growth essentially plateaus by the fourth week, whereas 5–10 IU of vitamin D_3 per day is sufficient to maintain a maximal growth rate in the chick. The disadvantage of this assay is the 3–4 week time period needed to accurately determine the growth rate.

F. Radioimmunoassay and Enzyme-Linked Immunosorbent Assay for Calbindin-D_{28K}

Additional biological assays utilize the presence of calbindin-D_{28K} protein as an indication of vitamin D activity. Calbindin-D_{28K} is not present in the intestine of vitamin D–deficient chicks and is only synthesized in response to the administration of vitamin D. Therefore, it is possible to use the presence of calbindin-D_{28K} to determine vitamin D activity. A radioimmunoassay (RIA) and an enzyme-linked immunosorbent assay (ELISA), both capable of detecting nanogram quantities of calbindin-D_{28K}, have been developed (113).

A comparison of the sensitivity and working range of the biological assays for vitamin D is given in Table 5.

VII. ANALYTICAL PROCEDURES

Although considerable progress has been made in the development of chemical or physical means to measure vitamin D, these methods at present generally lack the sensitivity and selectivity of the biological assays. Thus, they are not adequate for measuring samples that contain low concentrations of vitamin D. However, these physical and chemical means of vitamin D determination have the advantage of not being as time-consuming as the biological assays and so are frequently used on samples known to contain high levels of vitamin D.

A. Ultraviolet Absorption

The first techniques available for quantitating vitamin D were based on the measurement of the ultraviolet absorption at 264 nm. The conjugated triene system of double bonds

Table 5 Comparison of Sensitivity and Working Range of Biological Assays for Vitamin D

Assay	Time required for assay	Minimal level detectable in assay		Usual working range
		ng	nmol	
Rat line test	7 days	12	0.03	25–300 ng
AOAC chick	21 days	50	0.13	50–1250 ng
Intestinal Ca^{2+} absorption				
In vivo				
^{45}Ca^{2+}	1 day	125	0.33	0.125–25 g
^{47}Ca^{2+}	1 day	125	0.33	0.125–25 g
In vitro				
Everted sacs	1 day	250	0.65	250–1000 ng
Duodenal uptake of ^{45}Ca^{2+}	1 day	250	0.65	250–1000 ng
Bone CA^{2+} mobilization				
In vivo	24 hr	125	0.32	0.125–25 g
Body growth	21–28 days	50	0.06	50–1250 ng
Immunoassays for calcium-binding protein	1 day	1	0.0025	1–ng

in the vitamin D secosteroids produces a highly characteristic absorption spectra (Fig. 7). The absorption maxima for vitamin D occurs at 264 nm, and at this wavelength the molar extinction coefficient for both vitamin D$_2$ and D$_3$ is 18,300. Thus, the concentration of an unknown solution of vitamin D can be calculated once its absorption at 264 nm is known. Although this technique is both quick and easy, it suffers from the disadvantage that the sample must be scrupulously purified prior to assay in order to remove potential UV-absorbing contaminants.

B. Colorimetric Methods

Several colorimetric methods for the quantitation of vitamin D have been developed over the years. Among these various colorimetric assays is a method based on the isomerization of vitamin D to isotachysterol. This procedure, which employs antimony trichloride, can detect vitamin D in the range of 1–1000 μg. Because it can detect such large amounts of vitamin D, this assay is now used primarily to determine the vitamin D content of pharmaceutical preparations and has become the official USP colorimetric assay for vitamin D$_3$.

In this assay three types of assay tubes are normally prepared: one containing the standard vitamin D or unknown sample plus the color reagent; one containing only the solvent, ethylene chloride, and a third containing ethylene chloride, acetic anhydride, and the color reagent. The absorbance at 500 nm is measured 45 seconds after the addition of the color reagent. The concentration of vitamin D in the assay tube is proportional to its absorbance, which is corrected for the solvent blank and for the tube containing the acetic anhydride. This procedure has been found to follow Beer's law for solutions containing 3.25–6.5 nmoles vitamin D per milliliter assay solution. The major disadvantage to this assay is that the copresence of vitamin A, which is often present in pharmaceutical samples along with vitamin D, will interfere with the assay. Thus, purification procedures that include absorption chromatography and partition chromatography are required,

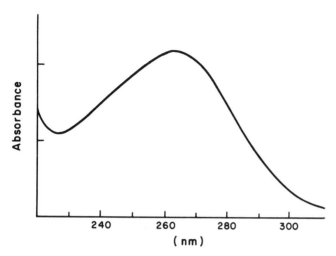

Figure 7 Ultraviolet spectrum of vitamin D. The absorption maxima occurs at 264 nm.

making this assay procedure rather laborious and time-consuming. Another disadvantage is the necessity for careful timing of the reaction because of the short time required for the appearance of maximal intensity of color. However, since this is the only direct chemical method routinely available, it enjoys widespread industrial application.

C. Fluorescence Spectroscopy

There have been two reports in the literature describing assays that depend on the reaction of vitamin D with a substance capable of fluorescing (114,115). Both of these procedures are based on the fact that an acetic anhydride–sulphuric acid solution containing vitamin D is capable of fluorescence if the solution is activated by light of the correct wavelength. The lower limits of detectability of this assay are the same as those of the antimony trichloride colorimetric assay, and the same compounds that interfere with the colorimetric assay also interfere with this fluorescence assay. As a result, this assay is not normally used for the analytical determination of vitamin D concentration.

D. Gas Chromatography–Mass Spectrometry

One of the most powerful modern techniques available to steroid chemists for the analytical determination of samples containing mixtures of steroids is mass spectrometry, or mass spectrometry coupled with prior separation by gas chromatography. The gas chromatography–mass spectrometry (GC-MS) technique can be coupled to an online computer that collects information on the fragmentation patterns of steroids in the mass spectrometer. In this way a sophisticated quantitative assay can be developed with a sensitivity and selectivity approaching that of radioimmunoassay. There have recently appeared several GC-Ms procedures applicable to vitamin D secosteroids (116), but they are not yet widely employed.

E. High-Pressure Liquid Chromatography

Several papers that describe the separation of vitamin D and its various metabolites by high-pressure liquid chromatography (HPLC) have appeared (117,118). This separation process has an exceedingly high resolving capability due to the large number of theoretical plates present in a typical column. Of equal importance to this technique is the sensitivity of the detector used for observing the separated compounds. The published procedures for the separation of vitamin D by HPLC have all used a UV detector, and so their sensitivity is limited to approximately 5 ng. The chief advantages of using the HPLC are the reduced labor and time required to separate vitamin D and its metabolites. In the present official USP method for the determination of vitamin D, two prepurification steps, requiring up to 8 hr, are necessary before the colorimetric analysis can be performed. However, with HPLC, reproducible separation of closely related compounds can be achieved in less than 1 hr. HPLC has great potential once a more sensitive detection method is developed.

F. Competitive Binding Assays

Various competition assays that can specifically quantitate the levels of $25(OH)D_3$, $24,25(OH)_2D_3$, or $1,25(OH)_2D_3$ in a sample are now available. Such assays were developed as a consequence of the discovery of specific vitamin D–binding proteins in the serum and tissue of mammals and birds, along with the availability of high specific activity tritiated $25(OH)D_3$ and $1,25(OH)_2D_3$. Since these steroid competition assays are sensitive (they are capable of detecting picogram quantities), they are now routinely used to measure vitamin D metabolite levels in plasma.

Two different types of steroid competition assays have been developed for the detection of $1,25(OH)_2D_3$. The first employs incubation of intestinal mucosal cytosol plus the nuclear chromatin fractions with standardized amounts of tritiated $1,25(OH)_2D_3$. The $1,25(OH)_2D_3$ in the sample competes with the tritiated hormone for the binding sites of the $1,25(OH)_2D_3$ receptors present in the cytosol and chromatin fractions. By measuring the amount of tritiated $1,25(OH)_2D_3$ that was able to bind to the receptor, the amount of $1,25(OH)_2D_3$ in the sample can be determined. The first such assay developed that could be used to measure $1,25(OH)_2D_3$ levels in plasma was that of Brumbaugh and Haussler (119). Their technique requires a minimum of 10 ml plasma and involves a laborious three-stage chromatographic procedure. The final $1,25(OH)_2D_3$ peak is then assayed. Separation of bound from free steroid is achieved by filtration of the incubation media through glass filters. The steroid associated with the chromatin-cytosol receptor is specifically bound to these filters. A similar assay has been described by Proscal et al., except that separation of the bound from free steroid is achieved by high-speed differential centrifugation (120).

The second type of competition assay involves using calf thymus cytosol as the source of binding protein. Reinhardt et al. developed a radioreceptor assay for vitamin D_2, vitamin D_3, and their metabolites that does not require HPLC (121). Their technique includes the use of a stable $1,25(OH)_2D_3$ receptor preparation from calf thymus, nonequilibrium assay conditions, and solid-phase extraction of vitamin D metabolites from serum or plasma samples. This procedure requires 0.2–1.0 ml plasma. $1,25(OH)_2D_3$ is removed from the plasma on a C18-Silica cartridge. The cartridge is first reversed phase eluted and then switched to normal phase elution (122). The $1,25(OH)_2D_3$ is recovered and incubated with

[^{3}H]-1,25(OH)$_2$D$_3$ and reconstituted thymus receptor. Separation of receptor-bound hormone from free hormone is achieved by the addition of dextran-coated charcoal. Similar assays have been developed for 25(OH)D$_3$ and 24,25(OH)$_2$D$_3$ (123). This assay has a sensitivity of 0.7 pg.

VIII. NUTRITIONAL REQUIREMENTS FOR VITAMIN D

A. Humans

The vitamin D requirement for healthy adults has never been precisely defined. Since vitamin D$_3$ is produced in the skin upon exposure to sunlight, the human does not have a requirement for vitamin D when sufficient sunlight is available. However, vitamin D does become an important nutritional factor in the absence of sunlight. In addition to geographical and seasonal factors, ultraviolet light from the sun may be blocked by many means. Air pollution succeeds in blocking ultraviolet rays. It is not a coincidence that as air pollution became prevalent during the industrial revolution, the incidence of rickets became widespread in industrial cities. It is now known that this rickets epidemic was partly caused by lack of sunlight due to air pollution. Thus, rickets has been called the first air pollution disease. Man's tendency to wear clothes, to live in cities where tall buildings block adequate sunlight from reaching the ground, to live indoors, to use sunscreens that block ultraviolet rays, and to live in geographical regions of the world that do not receive adequate sunlight all contribute to the inability of the skin to biosynthesize sufficient amounts of vitamin D. Under these conditions vitamin D becomes a true vitamin, in that it must be supplied in the diet on a regular basis.

Since vitamin D can be endogenously produced by the body and since it is retained for long periods of time by vertebrate tissue, it is difficult to determine minimum daily requirements for this substance. The requirement for vitamin D is also dependent on the concentrations of calcium and phosphorus in the diet, the physiological stage of development, age, sex, degree of exposure to the sun, and the amount of pigmentation in the skin.

In 1970, the Expert Committee of the FAO/WHO reviewed the data that showed that, in full-term infants, greater absorption of calcium and faster growth rates occur in those children given 400 IU [1 IU (International Unit) = 0.025 μg vitamin D] per day over those given 100 IU/day, although 100 IU/day is enough to prevent rickets. The current allowance of vitamin D recommended by the National Research Council is 400 IU/day, but this is an arbitrary figure and may represent the upper limit of vitamin D required. Since rickets is more prevalent in preschool children, the FAO/WHO committee recommended that children receive 400 IU/day until the age of 6, after which the recommended daily allowance is 100 IU/day.

In the United States adequate amounts of vitamin D can readily be obtained from the diet and from casual exposure to sunlight. For example, in the summer in the United States, the human skin synthesizes 6 IU vitamin D/cm^2/hour and the rate decreases to one fourth of that in winter. More than 2 hours of exposure of the face would be required in winter to provide 200 IU for an adult. At higher latitudes more time would be required. Therefore, in some parts of the world where food is not routinely fortified and sunlight is often limited, obtaining adequate amounts of vitamin D becomes more of a problem. As a result, the incidence of rickets in these countries is higher than in the United States.

B. Animals

The task of assessing the minimum daily vitamin D requirement for animals is no easier than it is for humans. Such factors as the dietary calcium–phosphorus ratio, physiological stage of development, sex, the amount of fur or hair, color, and perhaps even breed, all affect the daily requirement for vitamin D in animals. Also, some animals, such as chickens and turkeys, do not respond as well to vitamin D_2 as to vitamin D_3. As with humans, animals that are maintained in sunlight can produce their own vitamin D so that dietary supplementation is not really necessary. For animals that are kept indoors or that live in climates where the sunlight is not adequate for vitamin D production, the vitamin D content of food becomes important. Suncured hays are fairly good sources of vitamin D, but dehydrated hays, green feeds, and seeds are poor sources. A brief list of the recommended daily allowances for animals is given in Table 6.

IX. FOOD SOURCES OF VITAMIN D

For the most part, vitamin D is present in unfortified foods in only very small and variable quantities (Table 7). The vitamin D that naturally occurs in unfortified foods is generally derived from animal products. Saltwater fish, such as herring, salmon, and sardines, contain substantial amounts of vitamin D, and fish-liver oils are extremely rich sources.

Table 6 Vitamin D Requirements of Animals

Animal	Daily requirements (IU)
Chickens, growing	90[a]
Dairy cattle	
Calves	660[b]
Pregnant, lactating	5000–6000[c]
Dogs	
Growing puppies	22[d]
Adult maintenance	11[d]
Ducks	100[a]
Monkey, growing rhesus	25[d]
Mouse, growing	167[d]
Sheep	
Calves	300[e]
Adults	250[e]
Swine	
Breed sows	550[c]
Lactating sows	1210[c]
Young boars	690[c]
Adult boars	550[c]
Turkeys	400[a]

[a]IU required per pound of feed.
[b]IU required for 100 kg body weight.
[c]IU required per animal.
[d]IU required per kilogram body weight.
[e]IU required for 45 kg body weight.
Source: Published information by the Committee of Animal Nutrition, Agricultural Board (National Research Council).

Table 7 Vitamin D Content of Unfortified Foods

Food source	Vitamin D (IU/100 g)
Beefsteak	13
Beet greens	0.2
Butter	35
Cabbage	0.2
Cheese	12
Cod	85
Cod liver oil	10,000
Corn oil	9
Cream	50
Egg yolk	25
Herring (canned)	330
Herring liver oil	140,000
Liver	
Beef (raw)	8–40
Calf (raw)	0–15
Pork (raw)	40
Chicken (raw)	50–65
Lamb (raw)	20
Mackerel	120
Milk	
Cow (100 ml)	0.3–4
Human (100 ml)	0–10
Salmon (canned)	220–440
Sardines (canned)	1,500
Shrimp	150
Spinach	0.2

Source: From Refs. 2 and 124.

However, eggs, veal, beef, unfortified milk, and butter supply only small quantities of the vitamin. Plants are extremely poor sources of vitamin D; fruits and nuts contain no vitamin D, and vegetable oils contain only negligible amounts of the provitamin. As a consequence, in the United States dietary requirements for vitamin D are met by the artificial fortification of suitable foods. Among these fortified foods are milk, both fresh and evaporated; margarine and butter; cereals; and chocolate mixes. Milk is fortified to supply 400 IU vitamin D per quart, and margarine usually contains 2000 IU or more per pound. A complete listing of the vitamin D values of food is given by Booher et al. (124).

X. SIGNS OF VITAMIN D DEFICIENCY

A. Humans

A deficiency of vitamin D results in inadequate intestinal absorption and renal reabsorption of calcium and phosphate. As a consequence, serum calcium and phosphate levels fall and serum alkaline phosphatase activity increases. In response to these low serum calcium levels, hyperparathyroidism occurs. Parathyroid hormone, along with whatever

$1,25(OH)_2D_3$ is still present at the onset of the deficiency, results in the demineralization of bone. This ultimately leads to rickets in children and osteomalacia in adults. The classical skeletal symptoms associated with rickets, i.e., bowlegs, knock-knees, curvature of the spine, and pelvic and thoracic deformities (Fig. 8), result from the application of normal mechanical stress to demineralized bone. Enlargement of the bones, especially in the knees, wrists, and ankles, and changes in the costochondral junctions also occur. Since in children

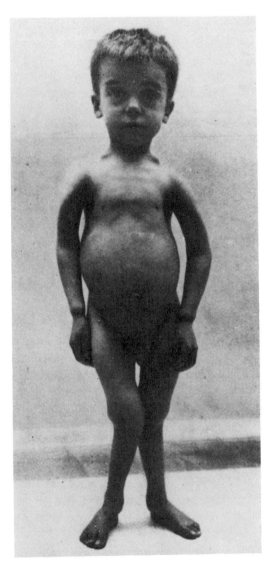

Figure 8   Classic appearance of rickets in a child.

bone growth is still occurring, rickets can result in epiphyseal abnormalities not seen in adult osteomalacia. Rickets also results in inadequate mineralization of tooth enamel and dentin. If the disease occurs during the first 6 months of life, convulsions and tetany can occur. Few adults with osteomalacia develop tetany.

Low serum calcium levels in the range of 5–7 mg per 100 ml and high serum alkaline phosphatase activity can be used to diagnose rickets and osteomalacia. Also, a marked reduction in circulating $1,25(OH)_2D_3$ levels in individuals with osteomalacia has been reported (125). Radiographic changes are also evident and can be used in diagnosis.

B. Animals

The response to vitamin D deficiency in animals closely resembles that in humans. Among the first symptoms of the deficiency is a decline in the plasma concentrations of calcium and phosphorus. This is followed by an abnormally low growth rate and the characteristic alteration of bones, including faulty calcification of the bone matrix. As the disease progresses, the forelegs bend sideways and the joints become swollen. In laying birds, the eggs are thin-shelled, egg production declines, and the hatchability is markedly reduced (126); classic symptoms of rickets develop, followed by tetany and death.

XI. HYPERVITAMINOSIS D

Excessive amounts of vitamin D are not available from natural sources. However, vitamin D intoxication is a concern in those patients being treated with vitamin D or vitamin D analogs for hypoparathyroidism, vitamin D–resistant rickets, renal osteodystrophy, osteoporosis, psoriasis, some cancers, or in those who are taking supplemental vitamins. Hypervitaminosis D is a serious problem as it can result in irreversible calcification of the heart, lungs, kidneys, and other soft tissues. Therefore, care should be taken to detect early signs of vitamin D intoxication in patients receiving pharmacological doses. Symptoms of intoxication include hypercalcemia, hypercalciuria, anorexia, nausea, vomiting, thirst, polyuria, muscular weakness, joint pains, diffuse demineralization of bones, and disorientation. If allowed to go unchecked, death will eventually occur. The minimum toxic dose has been estimated to be 50,000 IU for most adults and 1000–2000 IU for infants and for adults with certain infections and metabolic diseases (126a).

Vitamin D intoxication is thought to occur as a result of high 25(OH)D levels rather than high $1,25(OH)_2D$ levels. Patients suffering from hypervitaminosis D have been shown to exhibit a 15-fold increase in plasma 25(OH)D concentration as compared to normal individuals. However, their $1,25(OH)_2D$ levels are not substantially altered (127). Furthermore, anephric patients can still suffer from hypervitaminosis D even though they are for the most part incapable of producing $1,25(OH)_2D$. It has also been shown that large concentrations of 25(OH)D can mimic the actions of $1,25(OH)_2D$ at the level of the receptor (119).

In the early stages of intoxication, the effects are usually reversible. Treatment consists of merely withdrawing vitamin D and perhaps reducing dietary calcium intake until serum calcium levels fall. In more severe cases treatment with glucocorticoids, which are thought to antagonize the action of vitamin D, may be required to facilitate correction of hypercalcemia. Since calcitonin can bring about a decline in serum calcium levels, it may also be used in treatment.

XII. FACTORS THAT INFLUENCE VITAMIN D STATUS

A. Disease

In view of the complexities of the vitamin D endocrine system, it is not surprising that many disease states are vitamin D–related. Figure 9 classifies some of the human disease states believed to be associated with vitamin D metabolism according to the metabolic step where the disorder occurs.

1. Intestinal Disorders

The intestine functions as the site of dietary vitamin D absorption and is also a primary target tissue for the hormonally active $1,25(OH)_2D_3$. Impairment of intestinal absorption of vitamin D can occur in those intestinal disorders that result in the malabsorption of fat. Patients suffering from such disorders as tropical sprue, regional enteritis, and multiple jejunal diverticulosis often developed osteomalacia because of what appears to be a malabsorption of vitamin D from the diet (128). Surgical conditions, such as gastric resection and jenunal-ileal bypass surgery for obesity, may also impair vitamin D absorption. Also, patients receiving total parenteral nutrition in the treatment of the malnutrition caused by profound gastrointestinal disease often develop bone disease (129).

On the other hand, intestinal response to vitamin D can be affected by certain disease states. Patients suffering from idiopathic hypercalciuria exhibit an increased intestinal absorption of calcium that may result from an enhanced intestinal sensitivity to $1,25(OH)_2D_3$

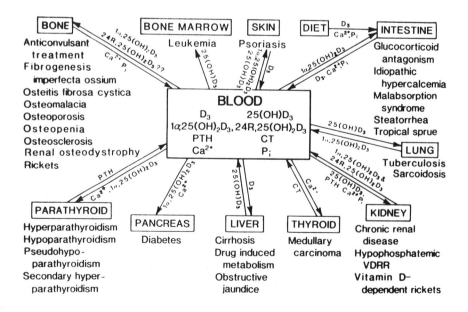

Figure 9 Human disease states related to vitamin D

or from an overproduction of $1,25(OH)_2D_3$. The disease state sarcoidosis also results in enhanced sensitivity to vitamin D. Sarcoidosis is characterized by hypercalcemia and hypercalciuria in patients receiving only modest amounts of vitamin D. Experiments have shown that these patients have elevated levels of serum $1,25(OH)_2D_3$. The excess $1,25(OH)_2D_3$ is likely of extrarenal origin and therefore not regulated by circulating levels of PTH (130). Other experiments have shown that macrophages from patients with sarcoidosis can produce $1,25(OH)_2D_3$ (131).

Other disease states that can result in extrarenal production of $1,25(OH)_2D_3$ are tuberculosis (132), leprosy (133), and some lymphomas (134).

2. Liver Disorders

The liver plays an important role in the vitamin D endocrine system; not only is it the primary site for the production of $25(OH)D$, it is also the source of bile salts, which aid in the intestinal absorption of vitamin D. Furthermore, it is likely that the liver is the site where the binding of $25(OH)D$ by vitamin D–binding protein occurs, and it may even be the location where this binding protein is synthesized. Hence, malfunctions of the liver can possibly interfere with the absorption, transport, and metabolism of vitamin D. Malabsorption of calcium and the appearance of bone disease have been reported in patients suffering from either primary biliary cirrhosis or from the prolonged obstructive jaundice. The disappearance of radioactive vitamin D from the plasma of these patients is much slower than in normal humans (135), and their plasma $25(OH)D$ levels are reduced (136). Although these patients respond poorly to vitamin D treatment, they immediately respond if treated with $25(OH)D_3$. Thus, it appears that the bone disease experienced by these patients results from their inability to produce $25(OH)D$.

3. Renal Disorders

The kidney functions as the endocrine gland for $1,25(OH)_2D_3$. Thus, disease states that affect the kidney can concomitantly alter the production of this calcium homeostatic hormone. It is well known that patients suffering from renal failure also often suffer from skeletal abnormalities. Termed renal osteodystrophy, these skeletal abnormalities include growth retardation, osteitis fibrosa, osteomalacia, and osteosclerosis. It became apparent with the discovery that under normal conditions $1,25(OH)_2D_3$ is produced in the kidney that these skeletal abnormalities result from the failure of the patients to produce $1,25(OH)_2D_3$. Support for this theory came from studies on the metabolism of radioactively labeled vitamin D in normal persons versus patients with chronic renal failure. From these studies, anephric or uremic individuals appeared unable to produce $1,25(OH)_2D_3$. Direct evidence for this came from the observation that circulating levels of $1,25(OH)_2D_3$ in the normal subject are in the range of 30–35 pg/ml, whereas in chronic renal failure the levels have been reported as low as 3–6 pg/ml (137). However, after a successful renal transplant, $1,25(OH)_2D_3$ levels return to the normal range. Also, the administration of $1,25(OH)_2D_3$ to these patients results in the stimulation of intestinal calcium absorption and an elevation of serum calcium levels (138).

4. Parathyroid Disorders

As previously outlined, PTH influences the production of $1,25(OH)_2D_3$. So, any disease that affects the secretion of PTH may, in turn, have an effect on the metabolism of vitamin D. Hyperactivity of the parathyroid glands, as in primary hyperparathyroidism, results in the appearance of bone disease resembling osteomalacia. Circulating $1,25(OH)_2D_3$ levels in these subjects have been reported to be significantly elevated (139), as is their intestinal calcium transport (140). On the other hand, in hypoparathyroidism, hypocalcemia occurs. In these patients a slight reduction in circulating $1,25(OH)_2D_3$ levels has been reported (141). When these patients are treated with $1,25(OH)_2D_3$, their serum levels are increased to normal.

For a review on the role of vitamin D in disease see Reichel et al. (142,143).

B. Genetics

Vitamin D–resistant rickets (hypophosphatemic rickets) appears to be an X-linked, dominant genetic disorder. Winters et al. presented evidence that this disease is almost always inherited and is usually congenital (144). Males are usually more severely affected by this disease than are females. Associated with the disease are skeletal abnormalities, such as rickets or osteomalacia, and a diminished renal tubular reabsorption of phosphate that results in hypophosphatemia. Individuals with this disease do not respond to physiological doses of vitamin D. Also, treatment with $25(OH)D_3$ and $1,25(OH)_2D_3$ are also ineffective, although an increase in intestinal calcium absorption does occur (145). These patients have also been reported to have normal serum $1,25(OH)_2D_3$ levels. Thus, it appears that this disorder does not result from an alteration in the metabolism of vitamin D or from an impaired intestinal response to $1,25(OH)_2D_3$ but rather from a specific defect in renal tubular reabsorption of phosphate.

A specific genetic defect that interferes with vitamin D metabolism has also been suggested in vitamin D–dependent rickets-type I. This ailment differs from rickets in that it appears in children who are receiving adequate amounts of vitamin D and it requires pharmacological doses of vitamin D or $25(OH)D_3$ to reverse the harmful effect this disease has on bone. However, the disease is responsive to physiological amounts of $1,25(OH)_2D_3$, which suggests that the defect occurs in the metabolism of $25(OH)D_3$ to $1,25(OH)_2D_3$ (146). This disease state appears to be the result of an autosomal recessively inherited genetic defect (147). It is not known how this defect affects the metabolism of $1,25(OH)D_3$.

Vitamin D–dependent rickets-type II also has a genetic basis. This ailment is similar to type I-vitamin D–dependent rickets except that children do not respond to large doses of vitamin D, $25(OH)D_3$, or $1,25(OH)_2D_3$. The combination of symptoms, i.e., defective bone mineralization, decreased intestinal calcium absorption, hypocalcemia, and increased serum levels of $1,25(OH)_2D_3$, suggest end-organ resistance to the action of $1,25(OH)_2D_3$. Experiments have shown that these children have defective receptor-effector systems for $1,25(OH)_2D_3$ (148).

C. Drugs

Recent evidence suggests that prolonged use of anticonvulsant drugs, such as diphenylhydantoin or phenobarbitol, can result in an impaired response to vitamin D; this results in an alteration of calcium metabolism and the appearance of rickets or osteomalacia. Serum $1,25(OH)D_3$ levels in patients receiving these drugs have been reported to be markedly reduced (149). Also, studies in animals suggest that these drugs stimulate the hepatic microsomal cytochrome P_{450} enzymes, which could lead to an increased catabolism of $1,25(OH)D_3$ (150). However, $1,25(OH)_2D_3$ levels have been shown to be normal or even increased after drug treatment (151). It appears that this drug-induced osteomalacia may not be the result of an effect of the drug on vitamin D metabolism. Studies on rat and chick duodena in organ culture indicate that anticonvulsant drugs may act on the gastrointestinal tract and affect the absorption of calcium (152). Anticonvulsant drugs have also been shown to inhibit calcium reabsorption in organ-culture mouse calvaria (153). Further research is needed to determine the mechanism by which these anticonvulsant drugs affect calcium metabolism.

Another drug reported to affect the status of various vitamins is the oral contraceptive. Persons taking this type of drug have been found to have slightly elevated levels of the fat-soluble vitamins A and E. It has been reported that these individuals also have slightly elevated $1,25(OH)_2D_3$ levels (154).

D. Alcohol

Persons suffering from chronic alcoholism exhibit a decrease in plasma $1,25(OH)D_3$ levels and in intestinal calcium absorption and bone mineral content. This is observed in patients with and without cirrhosis of the liver. Current evidence indicates that the impairment of intestinal calcium absorption is the result of low $25(OH)D_3$ levels (155). However, how chronic alcoholism results in low $25(OH)D_3$ levels is at present not understood.

E. Age

The fact that changes in the metabolism of vitamin D may occur with aging has been suggested by the observation that the ability to absorb dietary calcium decreases with age (156). In addition, loss of bone increases in the elderly, and an age-related hypoplasia of bone cells occurs. $1,25(OH)_2D_3$ levels in the plasma decrease with age, possibly due to an age-related reduction of epidermal concentrations of 7-dehydrocholesterol, resulting in less photochemical production of $1,25(OH)_2D_3$ by the skin. Also, the 1α-hydroxylase enzyme is less responsive to induction by PTH due to the decrease in glomular filtration with age (157).

F. Sex Differences

Gray et al. demonstated that men and women differ in their metabolism of vitamin D in response to various physiological stimuli (158). In women, they observed that dietary phosphate deprivation resulted in a decrease in serum phosphorus levels with a concomitant increase in plasma $1,25(OH)_2D_3$ concentrations. However, no change of either of these parameters was noted in men. Thus, the mechanism by which men and women respond to dietary phosphate deprivation seems to differ.

XIII. EFFICACY OF PHARMACOLOGICAL DOSES

Several ailments are known to respond to massive doses of vitamin D. For example, the intestinal malabsorption of calcium that results from chronic renal failure and the subsequent development of rickets or osteomalacia can be overcome by administration of 100,000–300,000 IU vitamin D per day (159). Patients suffering from hypoparathyroidism can usually be treated by giving 80,000–100,000 IU vitamin D per day (160). Also, children afflicted with vitamin D–dependent rickets-type I can be treated with 10,000–100,000 IU per day (2). The therapeutic effect of such massive doses can be explained by the fact that $25(OH)D$ in sufficiently high concentrations will mimic the action of $1,25(OH)_2D_3$ at the receptor. However, as mentioned earlier, the administration of such pharmacological doses of vitamin D to patients over a prolonged period of time carries with it the danger of vitamin D toxicity.

Experiments are in progress now to develop $1,25(OH)_2D_3$ analogs that will be active in stimulating cell differentiation but do not have the hypercalcemic action of $1,25(OH)_2D_3$. These drugs would could be very beneficial in the control of some forms of psoriasis and some leukemias (161,162).

XIV. CONCLUSION

Vitamin D, through its hormonally active metabolite $1,25(OH)_2D_3$, is known to act on bone and intestine to maintain calcium homeostasis. However, the actions of $1,25(OH)_2D_3$ are much broader than was thought originally. There is evidence that $1,25(OH)_2D_3$ is involved in the physiology of tissues not related to calcium homeostasis such as skin, pancreas, pituitary, muscle, and hematopoietic cells. Figure 3 demonstrates the complexity of the vitamin D endocrine system as it is understood today. Although many advances have been made in the past decade, much still remains to be learned about vitamin D and its metabolites.

REFERENCES

1. A. W. Norman (Ed.), *Vitamin D: Molecular Biology and Clinical Nutrition*. Marcel Dekker, New York, 1980.
2. A. W. Norman, *Vitamin D: The Calcium Homeostatic Steroid Hormone*. Academic Press, New York, 1979.
3. H. F. DeLuca, *Vitamin D Metabolism and Function*. Springer-Verlag, New York, 1979.
4. H. E. Harrison and H. C. Harrison, *Disorders of Calcium and Phosphate Metabolism in Childhood and Adolescence*. Saunders Company, Philadelphia, 1979.
5. A. E. Hess, *Rickets, Osteomalacia, and Tetany*. Lea and Febiger, Philadelphia, 1929.
6. K. Huldschinsky, *Dtsch. Med. Wochenschr.*, *45*:712 (1919).
7. E. Mellanby, *Medical Research Council*, Special Reports, Series SRS-61.
8. E. V. McCollum, N. Simmonds, J. E. Becker, and P. G. Shipley, *J. Biol. Chem.*, *53*:293 (1922).
9. H. Steenbock and A. Black, *J. Biol. Chem.*, *61*:405 (1924).
10. A. F. Hess and M. Weinstock, *J. Biol. Chem.*, *64*:181 (1925).
11. A. F. Hess and M. Weinstock, *J. Biol. Chem.*, *64*:193 (1925).
12. A. F. Hess and M. Weinstock, *J. Biol. Chem.*, *64*:1181 (1925).
13. A. Windaus, O. Linsert, A. Leittringhaus, and A. Weidlich, *Justus Liebigs Ann. Chem.*, *429*:276 (1932).
14. F. Askew, R. G. Bourdillon, H. M. Bruce, R. K. Callow, J. Philpot, and T. A. Webster, *Proc. R. Soc. Lond. [Biol.]*, *109*:448 (1932).
15. A. Windaus, R. Schenck, and F. von Werder, *Hoppe-Seylers Z. Physiol. Chem.*, *241*:100 (1936).
16. B. Lindquist, *Acta Paediatr. Scand. (Suppl.)*, *41*:86 (1952).
17. B. B. Migicovsky, *Can. J. Biochem. Physiol.*, *35*:1267 (1957).
18. A. W. Norman, *Am. J. Physiol.*, *211*:829 (1966).
19. J. E. Zull, E. Czarnowska-Misztal, and H. F. DeLuca, *Proc. Natl. Acad. Sci. USA*, *55*:177 (1966).
20. D. Schachter, D. V. Kimberg, and H. Schenker, *Am. J. Physiol.*, *200*:1263 (1961).
21. E. B. Dowdle, D. Schachter, and H. Schenker, *Am. J. Physiol.*, *198*:269 (1960).
22. H. E. Harrison and H. C. Harrison, *Am. J. Physiol.*, *208*:370 (1965).
23. A. Carlsson, *Acta Physiol. Scand.*, *26*:212 (1952).
24. A. Carlsson and G. Holleinger, *Acta Physiol. Scand.*, *31*:317 (1954).

25. V. W. Thompson and H. F. DeLuca, *J. Biol. Chem.*, *239*:984 (1964).

26. A. W. Norman and H. F. DeLuca, *Biochemistry, 2*:1160 (1963).

27. A. W. Norman, J. Lund, and H. F. DeLuca, *Arch. Biochem. Biophys.*, *108*:12 (1964).

28. J. W. Blunt, H. F. DeLuca, and H. Schnoes, *Chem. Commun.*, p. 801 (1968).

29. J. W. Blunt, H. F. DeLuca, and H. K. Schnoes, *Biochemistry, 7*:3317 (1968).

30. D. E. M. Lawson (Ed.), *Vitamin D*. Academic Press, New York, 1978.

31. M. R. Haussler, J. F. Myrtle, and A. W. Norman, *J. Biol. Chem.*, *243*:4055 (1968).

32. D. E. M. Lawson, D. R. Fraser, E. Kodicek, H. R. Morris, and D. H. Williams, *Nature 230*:228 (1971).

33. A. W. Norman, J. F. Myrtle, R. J. Midgett, H. F. Nowicki, V. Williams, and G. Popjak, *Science, 173*:51 (1971).

34. M. F. Holick, H. K. Schnoes, H. F. DeLuca, T. Suda, and R. J. Cousins, *Biochemistry, 10*:2799 (1971).

35. D. R. Fraser and E. Kodicek, *Nature, 288*:764 (1970).

36. A. W. Norman, *Biol. Rev.*, *43*:97–137 (1968).

37. A. R. Baker, D. P. McDonnell, M. Hughes, T. M. Crisp, D. J. Manglesdorf, M. R. Haussler, J. W. Pike, J. Shine, and B. W. O'Malley, *Proc. Natl. Acad. Sci. USA, 85*:3294–3298 (1988).

38. P. P. Minghetti and A. W. Norman, *FASEB J.*, (in press).

39. D. Crowfoot and J. D. Dunitz, *Nature, 162*:608 (1948).

40. D. C. Hodgkin, B. M. Rimmer, J. D. Dunitz, and K. W. Trueblood, *J. Chem. Soc.*, *947*:4945 (1963).

41. W. H. Okamura, A. W. Norman, and R. M. Wing, *Proc. Natl. Acad. Sci. USA, 71*:4194 (1974).

42. E. G. Bligh and W. J. Dyer, *Can. J. Biochem. Physiol.*, *37*:911 (1959).

43. T. B. Woodward, F. Sondheimer, D. Taub, K. Heusler, and W. U. McLamore, *J. Am. Chem. Soc.*, *74*:4223 (1952).

44. H. M. E. Cardwell, J. W. Cornforth, S. R. Duff, H. Holterman, and R. J. Robinson, *Chem. Soc.*: 361 (1953).

45. P. Bruck, R. D. Clark, R. S. Davidson, W. H. H. Gunther, P. S. Littlewood, and B. Lythgoe, *J. Chem. Soc. C:* 2529 (1967).

46. M. F. Holick, H. K. Schnoes, H. F. DeLuca, T. Suda, and R. J. Cousins, *Biochemistry, 10*:2799 (1971).

47. R. G. Wong, A. W. Norman, C. R. Reddy, and J. W. Coburn, *J. Clin. Invest.*, *51*:1287 (1972).

48. R. A. Gibbs and W. H. Okamura, *Tetrahedr. Letters, 28*:6021 (1987).

49. W. H. Okamura, M. N. Mitra, D. A. Procsal, and A. W. Norman, *Biochem. Biophys. Res. Commun.*, *65*:24 (1975).

50. M. F. Holick, M. Garabedian, H. K. Schnoes, and H. F. DeLuca, *J. Biol. Chem.*, *250*:226 (1975).

51. R. L. Johnson, W. H. Okamura, and A. W. Norman, *Biochem. Biophys. Res. Commun.*, *67*:797 (1975).

52. M. R. Haussler, J. E. Zerwekh, R. H. Hesse, E. Rizzardo, and M. M. Pechet, *Proc. Natl. Acad. Sci. USA, 70*:2248 (1973).

53. M. F. Holick, P. Kasten-Schraufrogel, T. Tavela, and H. F. DeLuca, *Arch. Biochem. Biophys.*, *166*:63 (1975).

54. J. L. Napoli, M. A. Fivizzani, H. K. Schnoes, and H. F. DeLuca, *Biochemistry, 17*:2387 (1978).

55. A. W. M. Hay and G. Watson, *Nature, 256*:150 (1975).

56. J. D. Greaves and C. L. A. Schmidt, *J. Biol. Chem.*, *102*:101 (1983).

57. W. Heymann, *J. Biol. Chem.*, *118*:371 (1937).

58. W. Heymann, *J. Biol. Chem.*, *122*:256 (1937).

59. D. E. M. Lawson, in *Vitamin D: Molecular Biology and Clinical Nutrition*, A. W. Norman (Ed.). Marcel Dekker, New York, 1980.

60. M. F. Holick, *J. Invest. Dermatol., 76*:107–114 (1981).

61. H. F. DeLuca, *Vitam. Horm., 25*:315 (1967).

62. H. Rikkers and H. F. DeLuca, *J. Physiol., 213*:380 (1967).

63. H. G. Morgan, W. C. Thomas, L. Haddock, and J. Eager, *Trans. Assoc. Am. Physicians, 71*:93 (1958).

64. W. C. Thomas, H. G. Morgan, T. B. Connor, L. Haddock, C. E. Bills, and J. E. J. Howard, *Clin. Invest., 38*:1078 (1959).

65. P. DeCrousaz, B. Blanc, and I. Antener, *Helo. Odondol. Acta, 9*:151 (1965).

66. P. H. Bordier, L. Miravet, P. Marie, J. Gueris, F. Rousselet, A. W. Norman, H. Rasmussen and A. Ryckewaert, Revue du Rhumatisme, 45:241 (1978).

67. N. E. Cooke and E. V. David, *J. Clin. Invest., 76*:2420 (1985).

68. R. Bouillon, F. A. Van Assche, H. Van Baelen, W. Heyns, and P. De Moor, *J. Clin. Invest., 67*:589 (1981).

69. D. D. Bikle, P. K. Siiteri, E. Ryzen, J. G. Haddad, and E. Gee, *J. Clin. Endocrinol. Metab., 61*:969 (1985).

70. A. W. M. Hay and G. Watson, *Comp. Biochem. Physiol. B, 56*:131 (1977).

71. W. Heyman, *J. Biol. Chem., 118*:371–376 (1937).

72. J. Quaterman, A. C. Dalgarno, A. Adams, B. F. Fell, and R. Boyne, *Br. J. Nutr., 18*:65–77 (1964).

73. S. J. Rosenstreich, C. Rich, and W. Wolwiler, *J. Clin. Invest., 50*:679–687 (1971).

74. E. G. Mawer, J. Backhouse, C. A. Holman, G. A. Lumb, and S. W. Stanbury, *Clin. Sci., 43*:413 (1972).

75. A. W. Norman, J. Roth, and L. Orci, *Endocrinol. Rev., 3*:331–366 (1982).

76. D. T. Baran and M. L. Milne, *J. Clin. Invest. 77*:1622–1626 (19xx).

77. K. W. Colston, I. M. A. Evans, T. C. Spelsberg, and I. MacIntyre, Biochem. J., 164:83–89 (1977).

78. H. L. Henry, A. N. Taylor, and A. W. Norman, *J. Nutr., 107*:1918 (1977).

79. J. M. Canterbury, G. Gavellas, J. J. Bourgoignie, and E. Reiss, *J. Clin. Invest., 65*:571 (1980).

80. H. L. Henry and A. W. Norman, *Science, 201*:835 (1978).

81. A. W. Norman, V. L. Leathers, J. E. Bishop, S. Kadowaki, and B. E. Miller, in *Vitamin D: Chemical, Biochemical and Clinical Endocrinology of Calcium Metabolism*, A. W. Norman (Ed.). Walter deGruyter, Berlin, 1982.

82. S. Ishizuka, T. Ohba, and A. W. Norman, in *Vitamin D: Molecular, Cellular and Clinical Endocrinology*, A. W. Norman (Ed.). Walter deGruyter, Berlin, 1988.

83. R. Kumar, *Kidney International, 30*:793–803 (1984).

84. C. Perret, C. Desplan, A. Brehier, and M. Thomasset, *Eur. J. Biochem., 148*:61–66 (1985).

85. R. A. Corradino and R. H. Wasserman, *Arch. Biochem. Biophys., 219*:286–296 (1968).

86. H. C. Tsai and A. W. Norman, *Biochem. Biophys. Res. Commun., 54*:622–627 (1985).

87. P. D. Seibert, W. Hunziker, and A. W. Norman, *Arch. Biochem. Biophys., 219*:286–296 (1982).

88. G. Theofan, A. P. Nguyen, and A. W. Norman, *J. Biol. Chem., 261*:16943–16947 (1986).

89. P. P. Minghetti, L. Cancela, Y. Fujisawa, G. Theofan, and A. W. Norman, *Mol. Endocrinol., 2*:355–367 (1988).

90. I. Nemere and A. W. Norman, *J. Bone Mineral Res., 2*:99–107 (1987).

91. M. R. Haussler and T. A. McCain, *N. Engl. J. Med. 297*:974–983 (1977).

92. H. F. DeLuca and H. K. Schnoes, *Ann. Rev. Biochem., 52*:411–439 (1983).

93. J. T. McCarthy, S. S. Barham, and R. Kumar, *J. Steroid Biochem., 21*:253–265 (1984).

94. M. R. Clements, L. Johnson, and D. R. Fraser, *Nature, 325*:62–65, (1987).

95. H. L. Henry and A. W. Norman, *Ann. Rev. Nutr., 4*:493–520 (1984).

96. J. L. Underwood and H. F. DeLuca, Am. J. Physiol., 246:E493–498 (1984).

97. C. Cade and A. W. Norman, *Endocrinology, 119*:84–90 (1986).

98. O. Gedik and S. Akalin, *Diabetologia 29*:142–145 (1986).

99. J. Sonnenberg, V. N. Luine, L. C. Krey, and Christakos, S., *Endocrinology, 118*:1433–1439 (1985).

100. M. Thomasset, C. O. Parkes, and P. Cuisinier-Gleizes, *Am. J. Physiol., 243*:E483–488 (1982).

101. F. Glisson, De Rachitide. Sadler, London, 1660.

102. M. R. Walters, *Biochem. Biophys. Res. Commun., 103*:721–726 (1981).

103. J. Hosomi, J. Hosoi, E. Abe, T. Suda, T., and T. Kuroki, *Endocrinology, 113*:1950–1957 (1983).

104. E. L. Smith and M. F. Holick, in *Vitamin D: A Chemical, Biochemical and Clinical Update*, A. W. Norman (Ed.). Walter de Gruyter, Berlin, 1985, p. 255.

105. D. D. Bikle, M. K. Nemanic, J. O. Whitney, and P. W. Elias, *Biochemistry, 25*:1545–1548 (1986).

106. E. Abe, C. Miyaura, H. Sakagami, M. Takeda, K. Konno, T. Yamazaki, S. Yoshiki, and T. Suda, *Proc. Natl. Acad. Sci. USA, 78*:4990–4994 (1981).

107. H. P. Koeffler, T. Armatruda, N. Ikekawa, Y. Kobayashi, H. F. DeLuca, *Cancer Res., 44*:5624–5628 (1984).

108. H. Reichel, H. P. Koeffler, and A. W. Norman, *J. Biol. Chem., 262*:10931–10937 (1987).

109. S. Iho, T. Takahashi, F. Kura, H. Sugiyama, and T. Hoshino, *J. Immunol., 236*:4427–4431 (1986).

110. C. D. Tsoukas, D. M. Provvedini, and S. C. Manolagas, *Science, 224*:1438–1440 (1984).

111. W. F. C. Rigby, T. Stacy, and M. W. Fanger, *J. Clin. Invest., 74*:1451–1455 (1984).

112. R. Belsey, H. F. DeLuca, and J. T. Potts, *J. Clin. Endocrinol. Metab., 33*:554 (1971).

113. B. E. Miller and A. W. Norman, *Meth. in Enzym., 102*:291 (1983).

114. P. S. Chen and H. B. Bosmann, *J. Nutr., 83*:133 (1964).

115. A. J. Passannante and L. V. Avioli, *Anal. Biochem., 15*:287 (1966).

116. R. D. Coldwell, C. E. Porteous, D. J. H. Trafford, and H. L. J. Makin, *Steroids, 49*:155–196 (1987).

117. K. A. Tartivita, J. P. Sciarello, and B. C. Rudy, *J. Pharm. Sci., 65*:1024 (1976).

118. G. Jones and H. F. DeLuca, *J. Lipid Res. 16*:448 (1975).

119. P. F. Brumbaugh and M. R. Haussler, *Life Sci., 13*:1737 (1973).

120. D. A. Procsal, W. H. Okamura, and A. W. Norman, *J. Biol. Chem., 250*:8382 (1975).

121. T. A. Reinhardt, R. L. Horst, J. W. Orf, and B. W. Hollis, *J. Clin. Endocrinol. Metab., 58*:91–98 (1984).

122. B. W. Hollis and T. Kilbo, in *Vitamin D: Molecular, Cellular and Clinical Endocrinology*, A. W. Norman (Ed.). Walter deGruyter, Berlin, 1988.

123. T. A. Reinhardt and R. L. Horst, in *Vitamin D: Molecular, Cellular and Clinical Endocrinology*, A. W. Norman (Ed.). Walter deGruyter, Berlin, 1988.

124. L. E. Booher, E. R. Hartzler, and E. M. Hewston, U.S. Department of Agriculture Circular 638, 1942.

125. F. Bayard, P. Bec, and J. P. Louvet, *Eur. J. Clin. Invest., 2*:195 (1972).

126. T. Suda, H. F. DeLuca, H. K. Schnoes, G. Ponchon, Y. Tanaka, and M. F. Holick, *Biochemistry, 9*:2917 (1970).

126a. J. N. Hathcock, *Pharmacy Times*, May 1985, p. 104.

127. M. R. Hughes, D. J. Baylink, P. G. Jones, and M. R. Haussler, *J. Clin. Invest., 58*:61 (1976).

128. J. W. Coburn and N. Brautbar, in *Vitamin D: Molecular Biology and Clinical Nutrition*, A. W. Norman (Ed.). Marcel Dekker, New York, 1980.

129. G. L. Klein, C. M. Targoff, M. E. Ament, D. J. Sherrard, R. Bluestone, J. H. Young, A. W. Norman, and J. W. Coburn, *Lancet, 15*:1041 (1980).

130. J. K. Maesaka, V. Batuman, N. C. Pablo, and S. Shakamuri, *Arch. Int. Med., 142*:1206–1207 (1982).

131. J. S. Adams, F. R. Singer, M. A. Gacad, O. P. Sharma, M. J. Hayes, P. Vouros, and M. F. Holick, *J. Clin. Endocrinol. Metab., 60*:960–966 (1985).

132. S. Epstein, P. H. Stern, N. H. Bell, I. Dowdeswell, and R. T. Turner, *Calcif. Tissue Int.,*

36:541–544 (1984).

133. V. N. Hoffman and O. M. Korzseniowski, *Ann. Int. Med.*, 74:721–724 (1986).

134. A. H. Mudde, H. van den Berg, P. G. Boshuis, F. C. Breedveld, H. M. Markusse, P. M. Kluin, O. L. Bijvoet, and S. E. Papapoulos, *Cancer*, 59:1543–1546 (1987).

135. L. V. Avioli, S. W. Lee, J. E. McDonald, J. Lund, and H. F. DeLuca, *J. Clin. Invest.*, 46:983 (1967).

136. J. G. Haddad and K. Y. Chuy, *J. Clin. Endocrinol. Metab.*, 33:992 (1955).

137. M. R. Haussler, M. R. Hughes, J. W. Pike, and T. A. McCain, in *Vitamin D: Biochemical, Chemical and Clinical Aspects Related to Calcium Metabolism*, A. W. Norman (Ed.). Walter de Gruyter, Berlin, 1977, p. 473.

138. A. S. Brickman, J. W. Coburn, A. W. Norman, and S. G. Massry, *Am. J. Med.*, 57:28 (1974.

139. M. R. Haussler, D. J. Baylink, M. R. Hughes, P. F. Brumbaugh, J. E. Wergedal, F. H. Schen, R. L. Nielsen, S. J. Counts, K. M. Bursac, and T. A. McCain, *Clin. Endocrinol.* 5:15 (1976).

140. A. S. Brickman, J. Jowsey, D. J. Sherrard, G. Friedman, F. R. Singer, D. J. Baylink, N. Maloney, S. G. Massry, A. W. Norman, and J. W. Coburn, in *Vitamin D and Problems Related to Uremic Bone Disease*, A. W. Norman (Ed.). Walter de Gruyter, Berlin, 1975, p. 241.

141. B. J. Lund, O. H. Sorensen, B. I. Lund, J. E. Bishop, and A. W. Norman, *J. Clin. Endocrinol. Metab.*, 51:606 (1980).

142. H. Reichel and A. W. Norman, *Ann. Rev. of Med.* (in press).

143. H. Reichel, H. P. Koeffler, and A. W. Norman, *New Engl. J. Med.*, (submitted).

144. R. W. Winters, J. B. Graham, J. F. Williams, V. W. McFalls, and C. H. Burnett, *Medicine*, 37:97 (1958).

145. A. S. Brickman, J. W. Coburn, K. Kurokawa, J. E. Bethune, and A. W. Norman, *N. Engl. J. Med.*, 289:495 (1973).

146. S. Balsan and M. Garabedian, Endocrinology, *Proc. Int. Symp. 4th*, 1973, p. 147.

146. C. D. Arnaud, R. Maijer, T. Reade, C. R. Scrivner, and D. T. Whelan, *Pediatrics*, 46:871 (1970).

148. U. A. Liberman, in *Vitamin D: Molecular, Cellular and Clinical Endocrinology*, A. W. Norman (Ed.). Walter de Gruyter, Berlin, 1988.

149. T. J. Hahn, B. A. Hendin, C. R. Scharp, and J. G. Haddad, *New Engl. J. Med.*, 287:900 (1972).

150. A. W. Norman, J. D. Bayless, and H. C. Tsai, *Biochem. Pharmacol.*, 25:163 (1976).

151. W. Jubez, M. R. Haussler, T. A. McCain, and K. G. Tolman, *J. Clin. Endocrinol. Metab.*, 44:617 (1977).

152. R. A. Corradino, *Biochem. Pharmacol.*, 25:863 (1976).

153. M. V. Jenkins, M. Harris, and M. R. Wills, *Calcif. Tissue Res.*, 16:163 (1974).

154. M. R. Haussler, Vitamin D: Metabolism, Drug Interactions and Therapeutic Applications in Humans, in *Nutrition and Drug Inter-relations*, J. N. Hathcock, and J. Coon (Eds.). Academic Press, New York, 1978, pp. 718–750.

155. B. Garcia-Pascual, A. Donath, and B. Courvoisier, in *Vitamin D: Biochemical, Chemical and Clinical Aspects Related to Calcium Metabolism*, A. W. Norman (Eds.). Walter de Gruyter, Berlin, 1977, p. 819.

156. J. R. Bullamore, J. C. Gallagher, R. Wilkinson, and B. E. C. Nordin, *Lancet*, 2:535 (1970).

157. R. D. Lindeman, J. Tobin, N. W. Shock, *J. Am. Geriatr. Soc.*, 33:278–285 (1985).

158. R. W. Gray, D. R. Wilz, A. E. Caldas, and J. Lemann, *J. Clin. Endocrinol. Metab.*, 45:299 (1977).

159. S. W. Stanbury, and G. A. Lumb, *Medicine*, 41:1 (1962).

160. A. W. Ireland, J. S. Clubb, F. C. Neale, S. Posen, and T. S. Reeve, *Ann. Intern. Med.*, 69:81 (1968).

161. L. Binderup and E. Bramm, *Biochem. Pharmacol.*, 37:889 (1988).

162. J. Y. Zhou, A. W. Norman, E. D. Collins, M. Lubbert, M. R. Uskokovic, and H. P. Koeffler, (submitted).

3
Vitamin E

Lawrence J. Machlin
Hoffmann-La Roche, Inc.
Nutley, New Jersey

I. HISTORY AND INTRODUCTION

In the early 1920s, a young scientist named Herbert Evans started a series of investigations on the influence of nutrition on reproduction in the rat (1). He and his colleague, Katherine Bishop, discovered that rats failed to reproduce when fed a rancid lard diet unless lettuce or whole wheat were added to the diet. Subsequently, it was found that the wheat germ oil contained all the "vitamin" properties of the wheat. In 1925, Evans suggested adopting the letter E to designate the factor following the then recognized vitamin D. Emerson had purified the factor, and it was given the name tocopherol from the Greek *tokos*, meaning childbirth, and the verb *pherein*, to bring forth. The *ol* was added to indicate the alcohol nature of the material. Vitamin E is now accepted as the generic term for a group of tocol and tocotrienol derivatives possessing some degree of vitamin activity. The most active compound is α-tocopherol.

In 1938, Fernholz established the structure for α-tocopherol, and shortly after that, Karrer provided the first synthesis (2). During the two decades during which the vitamin was identified, purified, structured, and synthesized, considerable progress in determining its biological properties was also made. Mason found that male rats on deficient diets developed testis degeneration. Card not only showed embryonic failure in the chicken egg, but demonstrated that the cause of the failure resulted from damage to the circulatory system. Pappenheimer, Olcott, and others found that muscle degeneration was also a common deficiency symptom. In the 1940s and 1950s, other symptoms of vitamin E deficiency were identified, for example, exudative diathesis and encephalomalacia in chickens; liver necrosis and enamel depigmentation in rats; anemia in monkeys; and steatitis or "yellow fat" disease in a number of animals.

The antioxidant properties of vitamin E were recognized by many of the early investigators. The findings by Dam (3–5) of peroxides in adipose tissue of animals fed diets deficient in vitamin E and the demonstration by his group and others that a variety of synthetic antioxidants prevent vitamin E deficiency signs in animals provided the basis for an "antioxidant" theory of vitamin E function.

Although many additional theories have been proposed to explain vitamin E's function, the most accepted explanation for its activity is that it acts in concert with a number of small molecules, such as reduced glutathione and ascorbic acid, as well as with several enzymes, such as glutathione peroxidase, superoxide dismutase, and catalase, to defend the cell against the damaging effects of oxygen radicals. In this role the vitamin aids the body in maintaining its normal defenses against disease and environmental insults. In its absence there is damage to many cells, particularly the red blood cell, muscle, and nerve cells.

Until recently, no deficiency disease in humans had been established, in contrast to the bewildering array of vitamin E deficiency signs that manifest themselves in animals. However, studies in the last 10 years have now clearly demonstrated that there is indeed a vitamin E deficiency pathology in humans, namely a debilitating neuropathy occurring in children and adults with severe fat malabsorption.

The legacy of myth and misinformation from the past history of extravagant claims has given way in recent years to the development of a solid body of scientific evidence that vitamin E is indeed an essential vitamin in both animals and man, playing a unique role against free-radical injury. The vitamin not only prevents neuropathy but plays an important role in maintaining the health of the premature infant. In addition, the accumulation of evidence that vitamin E enhances the immune response and may play a role in the prevention of cancer, cardiovascular disease, cataracts, and Parkinson's disease continues to stimulate a huge amount of interest, as demonstrated by publication of a number of international conferences (7–13) and comprehensive reviews (14–16).

II. CHEMISTRY

A. Structure-Activity

At least eight compounds have been isolated from plant sources that have vitamin E activity (Fig. 1). All have a 6-chromanol ring structure and a side chain. The tocols have a phytol side chain, and the trienols have a similar structure, with double bonds at $3'$, $7'$, and $11'$ positions of the side chain. Both tocols and trienols occur as a variety of isomers that differ by the number and location of methyl groups on the chromanol ring. α-Tocopherol is the most active form of vitamin E (Table 1). The tocols contain three asymmetric carbons, specifically at the 2 position in the ring and in the $4'$ and $8'$ positions of the side chain, thus making possible a total of eight possible optical isomers. The epimeric configuration at the 2 position is apparently dominant in determining biological activity.

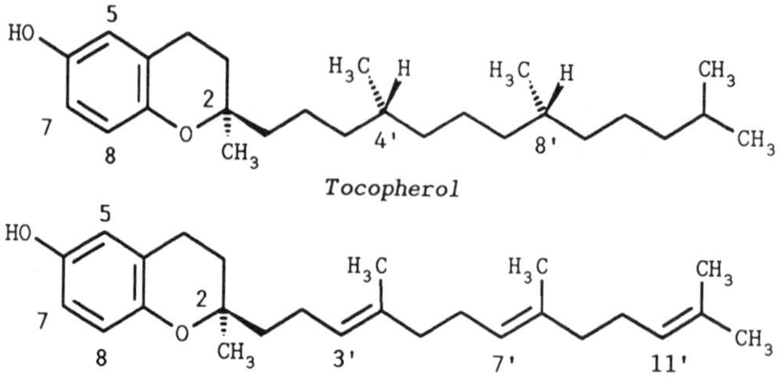

Tocopherol

Tocotrienol

Position of Methyl Groups	Trivial Names (Abbreviations)	
	Tocopherols	Tocotrienols
5, 7, 8	α-tocopherol (α-T)	α-tocotrienol (α-T-3)
5, 8	β-tocopherol (β-T)	β-tocotrienol (β-T-3)
7, 8	γ-tocopherol (γ-T)	γ-tocotrienol (γ-T-3)
8	δ-tocopherol (δ-T)	δ-tocotrienol (δ-T-3)

Figure 1 Formulas of eight members of tocopherol and tocotrienol series with vitamin E activity.

B. Nomenclature

Tentative recommendations on the nomenclature of tocopherol-related compounds have been made by the Commission on Biochemical Nomenclature (CBN) of the International Union of Pure and Applied Chemists (IUPAC) (17). Pending final adoption of this proposal, the American Institute of Nutrition has proposed the following nomenclature consistent with IUPAC-CBN proposals:

The term vitamin E should be used as the generic description for all tocol and tocotrienol derivatives qualitatively exhibiting the biological activity of α-tocopherol. Thus, phrases

Table 1 Biopotency of Tocopherols

		Fetal resorption (rat) (%)	Hemolysis (rat) (%)	Muscular Dystrophy	
				Preventive (chicken) (%)	Curative (rat) (%)
Abbreviation	Structure				
α-T	5,7,8-Trimethyl tocol	100	100	100	100
β-T	5,8-Dimethyl tocol	25–40	15–27	12	—
γ-T	7,8-Dimethyl tocol	1–11	3–20	5	11
δ-T	8-Methyl tocol	1	0.3–2	—	—
α-T-3	5,7,8-Trimethyl tocotrienol	27–29	17–25	—	28
β-T-3	5,8-Dimethyl tocotrienol	5	1–5	—	—

such as "vitamin E activity," "vitamin E deficiency," and "vitamin E in the form of ..." represent preferred usage.

The term tocol is the trivial designation of 2-methyl-2 (4′, 8′, 12′-trimethyl-tridecyl) chroman-6-ol.

The term tocopherols should be used as the generic description for all mono, di, and trimethyl tocols irrespective of biological activity. The term "tocopherols" is not synonymous with the term "vitamin E."

The only naturally occurring stereoisomers of α-tocopherol, formerly known as d-α-tocopherol or α-tocopherol should be designated RRR-α-tocopherol. The totally synthetic α-tocopherol, formerly known as *dl-α*-tocopherol should, be designated all-*rac*-α-tocopherol. Esters of tocopherols should be designated tocopheryl esters (e.g., α-tocopheryl acetate).

C. Analogs and Commercial Forms

Two principal sources of vitamin E in commercial use are RRR-α-tocopherol and all-*rac*-α-tocopherol, which are usually marketed as the acetate esters. The succinate ester has also been available. The esters are not found in most foods. The international unit which is equivalent to 1 mg all-*rac*-α-tocopheryl acetate is the accepted measure of biological activity (18) (Table 2). The all-*rac*-α-tocopherol is synthetic. The RRR-α-tocopherol is obtained from natural sources by molecular distillation and by methylation of the mixture of α-, β-, γ-, and δ-tocopherols, or by hydrogenation of α-tocotrienol. Since it is not isolated without extensive chemical processing, it cannot legally be called "natural" but only "derived from natural sources."

Vitamin E is also sold in a water-miscible form, which apparently is more readily absorbed. Vitamin E solution in oil for injection has been prepared, but the bioavailability is extremely poor. A water-miscible injectable vitamin E preparation has been developed (19). This contains free all-*rac*-α-tocopherol in a water-miscible form. In this form, α-tocopherol is more efficiently absorbed from intramuscular injection sites than a water-miscible preparation containing α-tocopheryl acetate or either form dissolved in an oil base. Injectable preparations have not received FDA approval and should only be used under an NDA. Tocopheryl nicotinate is available in Japan for medical use.

Generally, any significant changes in structures from α-tocopherol results in a loss of biological activity (20). For example, adding a double bond to the side chain, shortening or lengthening the side chain, or oxidation of the chromanol ring all result in major loss of biological activity. When the hydroxy group is masked as an ether, complete

Table 2 Commercially Available Forms of α-Tocopherol

Form	IU/mg
dl-α-Tocopheryl acetate (all-*rac*)	1.00
dl-α-Tocopherol (all-*rac*)	1.10
d,α-Tocopheryl acetate (RRR)	1.36
d,α-Tocopherol (RRR)	1.49
dl-α-Tocopheryl acid succinate (all-*rac*)	0.89
d,α-Tocopheryl acid succinate (RRR)	1.21

loss of activity occurs. Loss of any methyl group also results in significant loss of activity (Table 1). The only two modifications that have resulted in no loss and even an increase in activity are the substitution of an amine or *N*-methylamine group for the hydroxyl group of the chromanol ring and substitution of a dihydro benzofuran for the chromanol ring (21).

D. Synthesis

All-*rac*-α-tocopherol is usually synthesized by the condensation of trimethyl hydroquinone with isophytol (20). Earlier approaches employed natural phytol, which resulted in the synthesis of 2RS,4'R,8'R-α-tocopherol or "2-ambo-α-tocopherol." Enantiospecific total syntheses of RRR-α-tocopherol and its seven stereoisomers have also been reported (22).

E. Chemical Properties

α-Tocopherol is practically insoluble in water but is almost completely soluble in oils, fats, acetone, alcohol, chloroform, ether, benzene, and other fat solvents. Some physicochemical properties are given in Table 3.

Tocopherols are stable to heat and alkali in the absence of oxygen and are unaffected by acids at temperatures up to $100\,°C$. However, they are slowly oxidized by atmospheric oxygen. Oxidation is accelerated by exposure to light, heat, and alkali and the presence of iron and copper salts. Oxidation products include tocopheroxide, tocopheryl quinone, and tocopheryl hydroquinone (Fig. 2), as well as dimers and trimers. Since the esters of the free phenolic hydroxyl group are much more stable in the presence of oxygen, tocopherol is usually provided commercially as the acetate ester. The esters, however, cannot function as antioxidants.

III. ANALYTICAL PROCEDURES

A. Sample Preparation

Low-lipid samples, such as blood plasma and some other tissues, can be extracted directly with conventional lipid solvents, such as chloroform-methanol, hexane-ethanol, or acetone. Otherwise, samples are saponified first and then extracted with lipid solvents. Since tocopherol oxidizes readily, it is important that antioxidants such as ascorbic acid, pyrogallol, or *p*-hydroxyacetanilid be present during saponification. Following extraction further purification can be obtained by chromatographic procedures (23).

B. Emmerie–Engel Reaction

This spectrophotometric procedure is based on the generation of a red (or purple) complex between ferrous ions and αα'-dipyridyl or bathophenanthroline following the reduction of ferric ion to ferrous ion by tocopherol.

C. Spectrofluorometry

Free tocopherols have a strong natural fluorescence that has provided the basis for sensitive methods of analysis for tocopherol in serum and other tissues. The fluorometric procedures are simpler than the colorimeteric and in plasma are free from interference by carotene, a problem with the Emmerie–Engel procedure.

Table 3 Chemical Properties

Item	dl-α-Tocopherol	$d,$-α-Tocopherol	$dl,$α-Tocopheryl acetate	$d,$-α-Tocopheryl acetate
Color	Colorless to pale yellow, viscous oil	Colorless to pale yellow, viscous oil	Colorless to pale yellow, viscous oil	Colorless to pale yellow, viscous oil
Boiling point (°C)	200–220 (0.1 mm)	—	224 (0.3 mm)	—
Molecular weight	430.69	430.69	472.73	472.73
Spectrophometric data				
Absorption maxima (nm)	292–294	292–294	285.5	285.5
$E_{1cm}^{1\%}$ (ethanol)	71–76	72–76	40–44	40–44

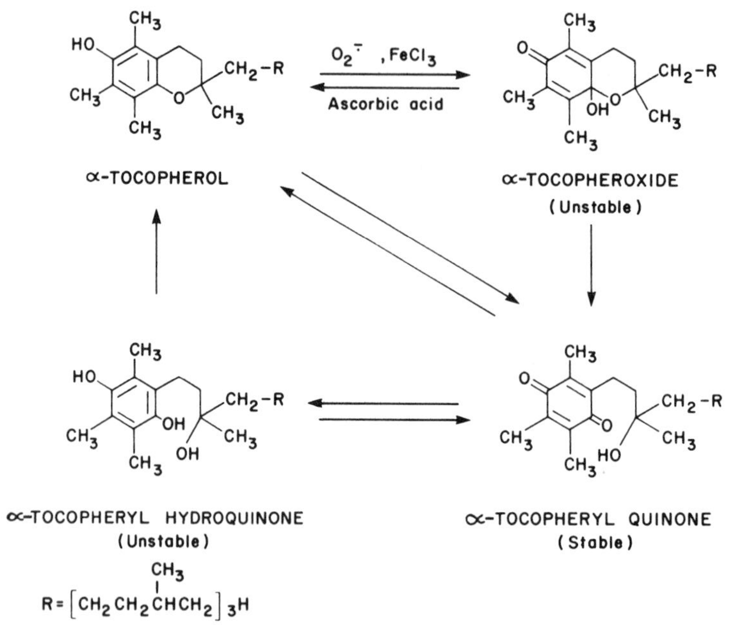

Figure 2 Oxidation products of tocopherols. (From Nesheim et al., *Nutrition of the Chicken*, M. Scott Pub., Ithaca, NY 1977.)

D. Chromatography

1. Thin-Layer

This procedure provides excellent separation of the tocopherols and requires little instrumentation. However, caution must be taken to avoid oxidative losses during separations (23).

2. Gas-Liquid

Tocopherols are first converted to more volatile derivatives, such as the trimethylsilyl ethers, as well as the acetate, propionate, and trifluoroacetate esters prior to chromatography (23). Methods are quite sensitive, with microgram quantities of tocopherols detectable. Recently, procedures were developed that permit the separation and quantitation of the four racemates present in all-*rac*-α-tocopherol (24).

3. High-Performance Liquid Chromatography (HPLC)

Procedures for the analysis of plasma (25), blood cells (26), tissues, foods (27), and animals feeds (28) are now available. Either reverse-phase or normal-phase procedures are used, coupled with either fluorometric or ultraviolet detectors. Although this necessitates sophisticated equipment, no derivatives are required and often saponification is not a necessity. The procedures, therefore, are specific, rapid, simple, and very sensitive. With fluorometric detection, nanogram quantities can be detected. Many procedures permit separation and quantitation of the α, β, and γ isomers of tocopherol and of α-tocopherol from α-tocopheryl quinone and the tocopherol dimer.

IV. BIOASSAY PROCEDURES

The true biological activity of vitamin E is determined by its ability to prevent or reverse specific vitamin E deficiency symptoms in animals in vivo (e.g., fetal resorption, muscular dystrophy, and encephalomalacia). Other tests, such as the erythrocyte hemolysis test, liver storage, and elevation of plasma tocopherol, have also been used. These latter methods are not a direct measure of biological activity in vivo, but they do reflect the relative absorption of the test compounds as well as their turnover in the liver or red blood cells. In general, the erythrocyte hemolysis and tissue storage tests correlate well with the in vivo procedures and may be correlated with alterations in red blood cell half-life observed in vitamin E–deficient humans. Therefore, although caution should be used in interpreting results with these methods, they are convenient and may have some utility.

A. Fetal Resorption

The antisterility assay based on fetal resorption in female rats is a classic method for testing the biopotency of various tocopherols (23). Vitamin E–depleted virgin female rats are mated with normal males. After successful mating, various levels of vitamin E are given by mouth to the female, in several divided doses. The rats are killed 20–21 days after mating, and the number of living, dead, and resorbed fetuses are counted and percentage of live young determined. The procedure is quite tedious and time consuming.

B. Muscular Degeneration Tests

In the chicken, muscular degeneration is evaluated directly after 3–4 weeks on deficient or supplemented diets, and the breast muscle is scored for severity of the lesion. Indirect measures of muscular degeneration, such as creatinuria, plasma aspartate aminotransferase, and lactic dehydrogenase, have also been used in ducks and rabbits. A method based on the reversal of muscular degeneration in the rat, using plasma pyruvate kinase levels as an index, is quite reliable, rapid, and sensitive (29).

C. Erythrocyte Hemolysis Test

This test is based on the protection by vitamin E against dialuric acid or hydrogen peroxide-induced hemolysis. Rats are depleted of vitamin E and are then given oral test doses selected to give a range of 20–80% hemolysis. The method is simple and agrees with the fetal resorption and chick liver-storage bioassays.

D. Other Methods

Biological assays based on liver storage, growth, encephalomalacia, and testicular degeneration have also been used in a limited number of studies.

V. VITAMIN E CONTENT IN FOOD

All eight isomers of the tocol and trienol series (Fig. 1) are widely distributed in nature. α-Tocopherol has the highest biological activity (Table 1). In foods of animal origin, it accounts for almost all vitamin E activity (Table 4). In vegetable seed oils, other isomers occur in substantial quantities (Table 5). In soybean oil, α-tocopherol represents only 8–10% of the total tocopherols but still represents the major portion of the biological activity.

Table 4 α-Tocopherol Content of Foods of Animal Origin

Food	Mean (range) (μg/g)		Percentage of total
Beef	6	(5–8)	> 75
Pork	5	(4–6)	> 89
Chicken	3	(2–4)	> 84
Fish			
Halibut	9	(4–13)	> 90
Cod	2	(15–33)	> 90
Shrimp	9	(6–19)	14
Milk			
Spring	0.2		> 90
Fall	1.1		> 90
Butter	24	(10–33)	> 90
Lard	12	(2–30)	> 90
Eggs	11	(8–12)	58–85

Source: Adapted from Ref. 30.

The α-tocopherol content of plant foods is given in Table 6. As more data on isomer distribution are obtained, a more precise assessment of the vitamin E content of foods based on the biological activities of all active isomers may be possible.

Unfortunately, there will always be serious limitations to the usefulness of tabular data in estimating vitamin E intakes of individuals or of a population. There is no correlation between intake estimated by direct analysis and that estimated by calculation from tabular data (30). The reason for this disparity is that a large number of factors influence the vitamin E content of foods (30) and result in a wide variation in vitamin content of

Table 5 Tocopherol Content (μg/g) of Vegetable Oils[a]

	α-T	β-T	γ-T	δ-T	α-T-3	β-T-3	δ-T-3
Coconut	11	—	—	6	5	1	19
Corn	159	50	602	—	—	—	—
Cottonseed	440	—	387	—	—	—	—
Olive	100	—	—	—	—	—	—
Peanut	189	—	214	21	—	—	—
Rapeseed	236	—	380	12	—	—	—
Safflower	396	—	174	—	—	—	—
Soybean	79	—	593	264	—	—	—
Sunflower	487	—	51	8	—	—	—
Wheat germ	1194	710	260	271	26	181	—
Palm	211	—	316	—	143	32	286
Margarine							
Soft	139	—	252	63	—	—	—
Hard	108	—	272	32	—	—	—

[a]All refined.
Source: Adapted from Ref. 30.

Table 6 α-Tocopherol Content (μg/g) of Foods of Plant Origin

Nut		Fruit	
Almond	270	Apple	3
Brazil	65	Banana	2
Filbert	210	Grapefruit	3
Peanut	72	Orange	2
Pecan	11	Peach	13
Walnut	5	Pear	5
Seeds and grains		Strawberry	12
Corn grain	10	Vegetables	
Milo grain	12	Asparagus	16
Oatmeal	17	Bean (fresh)	< 1
Poppyseed	18	Bean (navy, dry)	5
Rice (brown)	7	Brussels sprout	10
Rice (white)	1	Broccoli	20
Rye grain	10	Carrot	4
Wheat grain	11	Lettuce	3
Wheat germ	117	Potato (white)	< 1
Wheat bread (white)	0.9	Pea	< 1
Whole wheat bread	5	Turnip greens	22
		Spinach	25

Source: Adapted from Ref. 30.

a particular foodstuff. For many foods there is a three- to tenfold range in reported α-tocopherol values. For example, there can be a fivefold seasonal difference in the α-tocopherol content of milk.

The natural tocopherols are not very stable, and often significant losses from food occur during storage and during cooking. For example, there is a 48% loss of tocopherol in potato chips after storage for 2 weeks at room temperature. Losses of natural tocopherol during storage of vegetable oils are usually minimal but during cooking can be appreciable. Losses also occur during the processing of foods, particularly if there is any significant exposure to heat and oxygen. Anyone interested in precise values for vitamin E intake of individuals must currently resort to analytical assay of all foods just prior to ingestion. The α-tocopheryl acetate added to foods is very stable.

VI. METABOLISM

A. Absorption

Absorption of tocopherols takes place principally through the lymphatic system where they are transported as a lipoprotein complex (31). In man and other species, absorption of tocopherol is incomplete. For example, only 21–29% of labeled tocopherol was recovered in the thoracic duct lymph. In another study based on recovery in the feces, 36–50% was absorbed. As the dose increases, the percentage of absorption decreases (32). The efficiency of absorption is enhanced by the simultaneous digestion and absorption of dietary lipids. Medium-chain triglycerides particularly enhance absorption, whereas polyunsaturated fatty acids are inhibitory.

In animals, vitamin E was absorbed twice as readily from an aqueous-miscible emulsion as from an oil solution following oral administration (33). Water-miscible α-tocopheryl acetate was superior to the fat-soluble preparation in oral treatment of children with cystic fibrosis (34).

Tocopheryl acetate is almost completely hydrolyzed prior to absorption, probably by a duodenal mucosal esterase (35). When larger doses are administered, higher blood levels are attained with tocopherol than with tocopheryl acetate administration (36) (Fig. 3), suggesting some limitation in hydrolysis of the ester with high intakes.

Both bile and pancreatic juice are necessary for maximal absorption of vitamin E. Thus, patients with biliary obstruction or pancreatic insufficiencies have very limited ability to absorb the vitamin. Vitamin E is apparently absorbed as a lipid-bile micelle, together with free fatty acids, monoglycerides, and other fat-soluble vitamins, by penetrating the epithelial cells through the apical plasma membrane of the absorptive cells in the brush

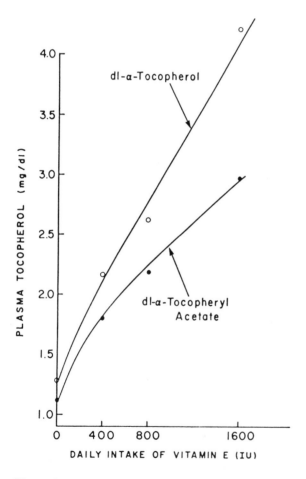

Figure 3 Relationship of intake of all-*rac*-α-tocopherol or all-*rac*-α-tocopheryl acetate to plasma levels of tocopherol in adult humans after 21 days of administration.(Based on Ref. 36.)

border (Fig. 4). The transfer of the vitamin across the epithelial cell may require several stages, most of them poorly understood, although they may involve diffusion processes. Absorption of vitamin E is maximal in the median portion of the small intestine. None is absorbed in the large intestine. In mammals, vitamin E is transported from the intestine to lymphatic capillaries. In contrast, in birds, tocopherol is transported via the portal vein directly to the liver. Unlike cholesterol or vitamin A, α-tocopherol is not reesterified during the absorption process.

B. Transport of Lymph and Blood

Vitamin E circulates in the lymph and blood bound to all of the lipoproteins, and it is generally distributed according to the fat composition of each fraction (37). Most is transported in the LDL fraction. There is some evidence that its distribution in the various lipoproteins is different in males and females (28). There is no evidence for the existence of a specific transport protein although there is some evidence of specific binding to HDL (38,39). There is a very high correlation between the total lipid or cholesterol in the serum and the tocopherol level. Thus, in disorders such as hypothyroidism, diabetes mellitus, and hypercholesterolemia, plasma vitamin E levels are higher than normal, whereas in conditions associated with low serum lipids, low tocopherol levels have been found. These conditions include certain liver diseases, abeta-lipoproteinemia, protein malnutrition, cystic fibrosis, and other malabsorption disorders.

Vitamin E is also transported in erythrocytes (39a). The concentration of vitamin E in the red blood cell is about 20% that in plasma, with all the vitamin E found in the membrane (40). Erythrocyte and platelet vitamin E concentrations usually reflect changes in plasma levels of the vitamin (Fig. 5).

C. Tissue Deposition, Storage, and Mobilization

The uptake of tocopherol by tissues varies directly with the logarithm of the tocopherol intake (37,41). This is illustrated by data on the tocopherol content of lung in rats and

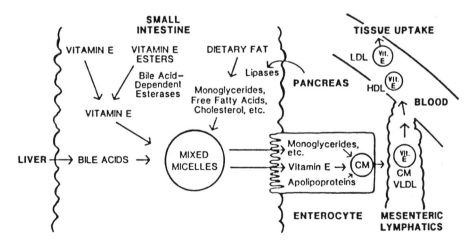

Figure 4 Schema of absorption and transport in man. (Reproduced with permission from *Clinical and Nutritional Aspects of Vitamin E*, Elsevier, Amsterdam, 1987, pp. 169–181.)

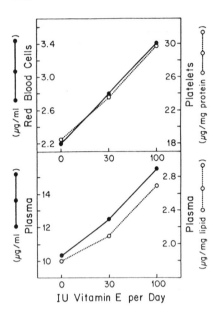

Figure 5 Effect of vitamin E supplements of α-tocopherol concentration in human blood. (Based on Ref. 116)

in the muscle of chickens (Fig. 6). This relationship represents a departure from what occurs with most other vitamins, which usually have distinct deposition thresholds in tissues other than the liver and may provide an explanation for the pharmacological effects of vitamin E. Tissues vary considerably in their vitamin E levels (Table 7) with no consistent relationship to lipid parameters. The adrenal and pituitary glands, testis, and platelets have the highest vitamin E concentrations. The vitamin is most concentrated in cell fractions rich in membrane, such as the mitochondria and microsomes (Table 8). Recent reports have demonstrated the existence of proteins in the cytosol that specifically bind α-tocopherol. The cytosolic binding proteins apparently facilitate the transport of tocopherol into mitochondrial (42) and microsomal membranes (43).

Although γ-tocopherol is absorbed and deposited in tissues readily, it is retained only to a limited degree compared with α-tocopherol. Thus, the differences of one methyl group on the chromanol ring has a profound effect on tissue retention. Lucy (44) has proposed that the phytyl side chain of α-tocopherol may interact with the fatty acyl chain of polyunsaturated phospholipids, particularly arachidonate. Alterations of the side chain of α-tocopherol drastically alter biological activity (20). Thus, the structure of both the ring and side chain may be important in determining the specific locus of the vitamin in the cell membrane. It is generally assumed that in membranes, α-tocopherol is oriented with the chromanol "head" group towards the surface of the membrane near the phosphate region of the phospholipid and with the hydrophobic phytyl "tail" buried within the hydrocarbon region. Tocopherol is probably not completely fixed in the membrane, but may "bob up and down" or laterally around its average position (45).

Preliminary reports suggests that specific binding proteins for tocopherol occur not only in the cytosol but also in the nucleus (46), in tumor cells (47), and in the membrane

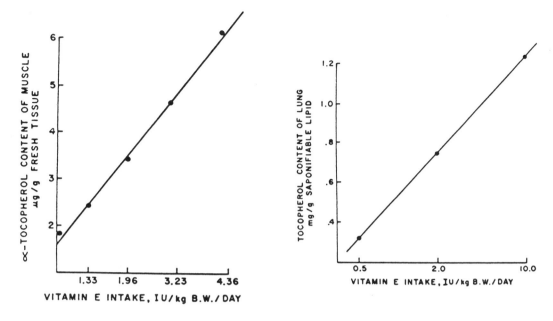

Figure 6 Relationship of vitamin E intake to tocopherol content of lungs (rat) and muscle (chickens).

of the red blood cell (48) and adrenals (49). The exact nature of the binding of α-tocopherol in the cell is an elusive problem awaiting resolution.

Adipose tissue, liver, and muscle represent the major storage deposits of the vitamin. The rate of depletion of tocopherol upon its withdrawal from the diet varies considerably, being relatively rapid in plasma and liver, slower from skeletal and heart muscle, and

Table 7 α-Tocopherol Content of Human Tissues

| | Normal | | Cystic fibrosis |
Tissue	μg/g	mg/g Lipid	(μg/g)
Plasma	9.5	1.4	2.4
Erythrocytes	2.3	0.5	0.5
Platelets	30.0	1.3	—
Adipose tissue	150.0	0.2	—
Kidney	7.0	0.3	—
Liver	13.0	0.3	3.5
Muscle	19.0	0.4	2.6
Ovary	11.0	0.6	—
Uterus	9.0	0.7	—
Heart	20.0	0.7	—
Adrenal	132.0	0.7	—
Testis	40.0	1.0	—
Pituitary	40.0	1.2	—

Table 8 Subcellular Distribution of Tocopherol in Rat Tissue

Cell fraction	Tocopherol in liver		Tocopherol in heart	
	μg/mg Protein	%[a]	μg/mg Protein	%[a]
Soluble	0.002	0.4	0.02	1.7
Heavy mitochondrial	0.27	53.8	0.26	21.8
Light mitochondrial	0.12	23.9	0.29	24.4
Microsomal	0.08	15.9	0.37	31.1
Nuclear	0.03	6.0	0.25	21.0

[a]Percentage of total recovered in five fractions.

very slow from adipose tissue (50). In the guinea pig, plasma levels decreased very rapidly to deficient levels in spite of negligible losses from adipose and muscle tissue.

When high levels of vitamin E are added to diets containing nutritionally adequate levels, the vitamin accumulates with time in all tissues studied (50). When the high supplementation levels are withdrawn, tissue levels rapidly return to their normal levels. There appear to be two different pools of vitamin E in most tissues, one at high tissue levels that is rapidly mobilized and one at low tissue levels that decreases very slowly.

D. Metabolism and Excretion

Vitamin E undergoes very little metabolism (37). Usually less than 1% of orally ingested vitamin E is excreted in the urine. The major route of excretion is fecal elimination. The absorbed α-tocopherol is largely deposited unmodified in its unesterified form in tissues. There is some evidence for the existence, in trace amounts, of tocopheryl quinone, tocopheryl hyroquinone, dimers, trimers, and more polar metabolites in tissues. However, it is still not clear whether these represent true metabolites or artifacts resulting from oxidation during their isolation. Compounds (Fig. 7) often referred to as Simon's metabolites (51,52) are found in the urine. The major portion of these are present as conjugates with glucuronic acid. They have no vitamin E activity and are considered to be simply detoxification products.

VII. BIOCHEMICAL FUNCTION

A. Membrane Antioxidant Hypothesis

Many early investigators recognized that α-tocopherol could function as an antioxidant in vivo (53,54). The commonly accepted theory (55) for initiation and propagation of free-radical–mediated oxidations and their inhibition by antioxidants is outlined in Table 9 (steps 1–4). Polyunsaturated fatty acids (PUFA) are particularly sensitive to autoxidation: the more double bonds the greater the susceptibility to such oxidation. The association of dietary PUFA with exacerbation of vitamin E–deficiency symptoms was recognized early in the history of the vitamin (5). It was first thought that dietary vitamin E was destroyed when PUFA were undergoing peroxidation in the diet. However, even when oxidation was prevented or tocopherol given separately from the dietary PUFA, the PUFA brought on symptoms of vitamin E deficiency. Furthermore, peroxides were detected in the adipose tissues of rats and chicks fed diets deficient in vitamin E and rich in PUFA (4). Finally,

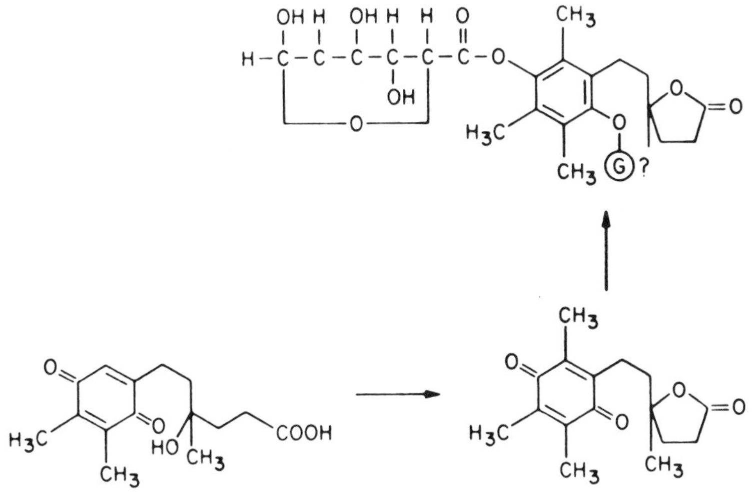

α – Tocopheronic Acid α – Tocopheronolactone

Figure 7 Simon's metabolites of vitamin E. G indicates possible second glucuronate.

Table 9 Autoxidation and Antioxidant Reactions Involving Vitamin E

1. Initiation (formation of a free radical)

$$LH \xrightarrow{\text{Initiators}} L\bullet$$

2. Reaction of radical with oxygen

$$L\bullet + O_2 \longrightarrow LO_2\bullet$$

3. Propagation

$$L0_2\bullet + LH \longrightarrow L\bullet + ROOH$$

4. Antioxidant reaction

$$LO_2\bullet + E \longrightarrow E + LOOH$$

5. Regeneration

$$E\bullet + C \longrightarrow E + C\bullet$$

$$C\bullet + NADPH \xrightarrow[\text{Semidehydro ascorbate reductase}]{} C + NADP$$

$$E\bullet + 2GSH \xrightarrow[\text{Enzyme?}]{} E\bullet + GSSG$$

$$GSSG + NADPH \xrightarrow[\text{Glutathione reductase}]{} 2GSH + NADP$$

6. Termination

$$E\bullet + E\bullet \longrightarrow \text{E-E (dimer)}$$

$$E\bullet + LO_2\bullet \longrightarrow \text{EOOL (?)}$$

Abbreviations: LH, fatty acid; L•, fatty acid radical; LO_2•, peroxy radical; E, tocopherol; E•, tocopheroxy radical; LOOH, hydroperoxide; C, ascorbic acid; C•, ascorbyl radical; GSH, reduced glutathione; GSSG, oxidized glutathione.

it has been observed that a variety of synthetic antioxidants, such as ethoxyquin and diphenyl-*p*-phenylenediamine (DPPD), with structures quite unrelated to tocopherol, were found to prevent many symptoms of vitamin E deficiency (54,56). This effect was not a result of the sparing of vitamin E in tissues, since rats that had insufficient tissue reserves to maintain normal reproduction responded to administration of DPPD (57). These observations led to the proposal by Tappel (58) that vitamin E functions as in vivo antioxidant that protects tissue lipids from free radical attack. Some of the evidence for the role of vitamin E is summarized in Table 10 (59).

It is now understood that:

- Tocopherol is located primarily in the membrane portion of the cell.
- Free radicals are generated by a number of enzymatic and nonenzymatic reactions occurring in cells.
- Tocopherol is part of the cell's defense against oxygen-containing radicals. The enzymes superoxide dismutase, catalase, glutathione peroxidase, and glutathione reductase also play a protective role. Small molecules, such as reduced glutathione, ascorbic acid, bilirubin, and uric acid, can also function as antioxidants.

Molenaar et al. (60) proposed that the chromanol ring of tocopherol is located at the polar surface of membranes and that the phytyl side chain interacts with PUFA of the phospholipids (44) in the nonpolar interior of the membrane.

Although the antioxidant role of vitamin E has not been accepted by all investigators (60a,61), many of the biochemical and pathological effects of vitamin E inadequacy may be explained by an alteration of membrane structure by free-radical attack. For example, almost all of the enzymes affected by vitamin E status are either membrane bound or are concerned with the glutathione peroxidase system (62).

One criticism (60a) of the antioxidant hypothesis is that one should expect to detect peroxides in tissues that have pathology resulting from a vitamin E deficiency (e.g., liver, testis, and muscle). Unequivocal evidence for the existence of peroxides in these tissues has been difficult to obtain. Peroxidized fatty acids are preferentially hydrolyzed by phospholipase A_2 and are then rapidly destroyed by glutathione peroxidase so that there is little opportunity for fatty peroxides to accumulate. Breakdown products of lipid peroxidation, however, have been observed. For example, aldehydes are found in tissues of

Table 10   Evidence for the Antioxidant Role of Vitamin E

In vitro:
  Prevents lipid peroxidation
  Reacts directly with:
    peroxy radical
    superoxide radical
    singlet oxygen
In vivo (in vitamin E–deficient animals):
  Increased peroxides found in fat tissue
  Increased aldehydes found in many tissues
  Increased exhalation of ethane and pentane
  Synthetic antioxidants prevent deficiency symptoms
  More severe deficiency symptoms when dietary PUFA increased
  Lipofuscin accumulates in some tissues

E-deficient animals (63), and pentane (64) and ethane (65) are exhaled in E-deficient animals and humans (66). In addition, a decrease in tocopherol and appearance of tocopheryl quinone has been observed (67) in the alveolar fluid of heavy smokers.

If vitamin E is merely an in vivo antioxidant, what is special about the vitamin compared with synthetic antioxidants? Vitamin E is unique in its more specific localization in membranes and in the tenacity with which it remains in most tissues. Thus, even small changes in the ring structure or in the phytol side chain result in altered pharmacokinetics and a large difference in biological activity. In order to be effective, most synthetic antioxidants have to be administered continuously in relatively large amounts compared with vitamin E.

Another aspect of α-tocopherol that makes it unique as an in vivo antioxidant is its ability to be regenerated from the tocopheroxy radical by vitamin C and by reduced glutathione (Table 9, Fig. 8). Ascorbate reduces the tocopheroxy radical with concurrent formation of an ascorbate radical (68,69). The ascorbate radical can be enzymatically reduced back to ascorbate by an NADH-dependent system. Thus, a mechanism exists for continuously regenerating tocopherol. Ascorbate can be effective even though it is in the cytosol and tocopherol is in the membrane by acting at the interface of the aqueous and

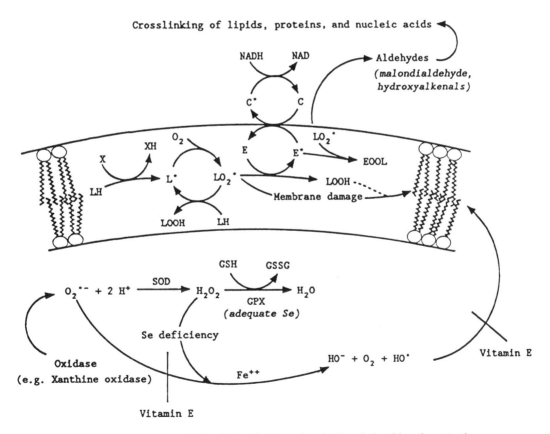

Figure 8 Interrelationships of vitamin E, selenium, vitamin C, and glutathione in protecting membranes. Abbreviations see Table 9. $O_2 \div$, superoxide anion; HO•, hydroxyl radical.

lipid phases (Fig. 8). Reduced glutathione also reduces tocopheroxy radical, perhaps by an enzymatically mediated process (70).

It is now clear that α-tocopherol plays a unique role as the major lipid-soluble antioxidant protecting all membranes from injury from free radicals and aldehydes resulting from lipid peroxidation.

B. Arachidonic Acid and Prostaglandin Metabolism

Both the lipoxygenase and the cycloxygenase pathways of arachidonic acid metabolism involve free-radical–mediated reactions. As an in vivo antioxidant, vitamin E might therefore inhibit some of the reactions leading to the formation of hydroxy eicosatetraenoic acid (HETE), thromboxane (TXA_2), or prostaglandins (71). Thromboxane is considered the most potent platelet-aggregating factor, and indeed, many studies have demonstrated that vitamin E inhibits platelet aggregation (72). There is evidence for enhanced prostaglandin synthesis in platelets (73), spleen, and bursa (74) of vitamin E deficient animals. On the other hand, synthesis of prostaglandin F (PGF) is depressed in testes (75) and muscle of deficient animals (76). There is some evidence that vitamin E suppresses thromboxane synthesis and enhances prostacyclin formation (77,78) and may inhibit lipoxygenase (79) and phospholipase activity (80). The inhibition of phospholipase activity may be a secondary effect of vitamin E decreasing formation of lipid peroxides which in turn activate phospholipase A_2. Administration of 800 IU per day of vitamin E had no effect on the indices of thromboxane and prostacyclin production (81). In view of the potential significance of these pathways in thrombotic diseases and inflammation, it will be important to establish the specific role of vitamin E in modulating these processes.

C. Nucleic Acid, Protein, and Lipid Metabolism

Increased rates of DNA synthesis were observed in muscles in vitamin E–deficient rabbits and in bone marrow of deficient monkeys. It is unlikely that this reflects a direct participation of vitamin E in DNA synthesis. Rather, it may reflect increased erythropoiesis in response to decreased erythrocyte survival time and increased muscle cell turnover resulting from the necrotizing myopathy produced by vitamin E deficiency. Similarly, it has been difficult to define a direct role of vitamin E in RNA or protein synthesis (62).

Many enzyme levels are altered in vitamin E–deficient animals. There is good evidence that, for xanthine oxidase and creatine kinase, elevated levels in deficient animals represent true increases in apoenzyme synthesis and not merely changes in enzyme activity. Based on these observations, it has been proposed (82) that the vitamin may serve as a repressor for the synthesis of certain enzymes.

In protozoans (83,84), addition of tocopherol to the food supply results in a morphogenic transformation. Specifically, protozoans, which are small and predominantly bactivorous, become enlarged and carnivorous. It has been proposed that α-tocopherol may either protect the cell membrane, allowing continued growth and gigantism, or that the compound might act as a transcriptional control agent. Vitamin E treatment enhances the morphological differentiation of neuroblastoma cells in culture (85) and also influences differentiation of myeloid leukemia cells (86). Whether these are indirect effects of its antioxidant role or whether vitamin E plays a more direct role in cell differentiation remains to be established.

It has also been proposed that vitamin E plays a specific role in the synthesis of heme proteins (87), but this suggestion has not been verified by other investigators (88). An enzymatic function in the desaturation of fatty acids has also been proposed (61).

D. Mitochondrial Function

Mitochondria contain high levels of tocopherol (Table 8), most of which is in the inner membranes. Electron microscope examination of muscle and heart tissue indicates that disruption of mitochondria is one of the earliest pathological events observed in vitamin E–deficient animals.

There is a decline in oxidation of α-ketoglutarate and succinate in livers from deficient rats (89). The effect of vitamin E seems to involve the early part of the eletron-transport chain, perhaps close to the dehydrogenases themselves. α-Tocopherol may protect dehydrogenase sulfhydryl groups from oxidation or reaction with metal ions because of its location close to the sulfhydryl groups in the cell. The role of tocopherol as an electron acceptor in the electron-transport system has been suggested. However, no clear evidence for this speculation is at present available.

The mitochondria from liver and muscle of vitamin E–deficient rats are very susceptible to damage induced by visibile light or steady-state respiration with substrate (90).

E. Relationship to Hormones

Although spermatogenesis is drastically inhibited in the testes of vitamin E–deficient animals, production of male sex hormones appears unimpaired. Similarly, although deficient females fail to reproduce, female sex hormones are produced normally.

In vitro, steroidogenesis is inhibited in adrenals of E–deficient rats. However, no clear evidence for in vivo alterations of adrenal function is available. When subjects with mammary dysplasia are treated with vitamin E, the abnormal ratio of progesterone to estradiol in the serum is normalized (91). There is some evidence that thyroid activity is diminished in vitamin E–deficient rats (92).

VIII. DEFICIENCY SIGNS

A. Animals

A large number of tissues can be affected by vitamin E deficiency (Table 11). The specific tissue affected appears to depend on the particular species and the effects of other nutrients, such as polyunsaturated fatty acids and selenium. The most common deficiency sign is necrotizing myopathy. This occurs in almost all species in the skeletal muscles but is also observed in the heart and some smooth muscles. In lambs and calves, myopathy results primarily from a selenium deficiency, whereas in other species vitamin E status is the main determinant. Some species, such as the guinea pig and rabbit, develop a severe debilitating myopathy when fed diets low in vitamin E. In contrast, rats manifest a relatively benign myopathy on diets that are free of vitamin E, and chickens develop no myopathy unless the diet is simultaneously deficient in sulfur amino acids and vitamin E.

In the chicken, the interrelationships between PUFA and selenium have been clearly established. When a vitamin E–deficient diet high in PUFA of the linoleate series is fed, chickens develop encephalomalacia, a disorder characterized by localized hemorrhage and necrosis in the cerebellum. Selenium does not prevent this disorder. When selenium is

Table 11   Effects of Vitamin E Deficiency in Animals

Tissue	Observation	Species
Muscles		
Skeletal	Necrotizing myopathy	Monkey, pig, rat, dog, rabbit, guinea pig, horse, calf,[a] lamb,[a] kid,[a] mink, chicken,[b] duck, salmon,[a] catfish, antelope
Heart	Necrotizing myopathy	Pig, rat, dog, rabbit, guinea pig, calf, cow, sheep, goat, baboon, antelope, elephant, deer
Gizzard	Necrotizing myopathy	Turkey
Reproductive		
Placental blood vessels	Fetal death and resorption	Pig, rat,mouse, guinea pig, cow,[a] ewe[a], chicken
Uterus	Lipofuscin accumulation	Rat
Testis	Degeneration of epithelium	Monkey, pig, rat, rabbit, guinea pig, hamster, dog, chicken
Gastrointestinal		
Intestine	Lipofuscin accumulation	Dog
Stomach	Gastric ulceration	Pig
Adipose tissue	Lipofuscin accumulation	Pig, rat, mouse, hamster, cat, mink
Vascular		
Blood vessels	Exudative diathesis[c]	Chicken, turkey, salmon, catfish
Erythrocytes	Anemia	Monkey, pig, rat, salmon, catfish
	Hemolysis (in vitro)	Monkey, rat, chicken
Platelets	Increased number	Rat
	Increased ability to aggregate (in vitro)	Rat
Eyes	Cataracts	Turkey embryo, rabbit
	Retinal degeneration	Dog, monkey, rat
Nervous system		
Brain (cerebellum)	Encephalomalacia[d]	Chicken
Nerves	Axonal dystrophy	Monkey, rat, dog, duck, mouse, guinea pig
	Lipofuscin accumulation	Rat, mouse
Liver	Necrosis[c]	Pig, rat, mouse

[a]Vitamin E not effective if diets are severely deficient in selenium; both nutrients are required.
[b]Preventable by sulfur amino acids.
[c]Preventable by selenium.
[d]Neural changes may be secondary to vascular pathology.

almost absent from the diet, as well as vitamin E, chickens develop exudative diathesis, a disorder characterized by increased capillary permeability resulting in subcutaneous edema. Addition of either nutrient will prevent the disorder. With even lower selenium diets, chickens develop a pancreatic necrosis which can be prevented by low levels of selenium or extremely high levels of vitamin E.

What accounts for the wide species difference, the variety of symptoms, and the observation that selenium and/or PUFA may, or may not, affect the manifestation of vitamin E deficiency signs? There are species differences in the efficiency with which dietary vitamin E is deposited in tissues. For example, turkeys deposit much less tocopherol than chickens in their tissues. Selenium functions as a constituent of GSH peroxidases. This enzyme occurs in different concentrations in various tissues and in different species. Also, the concentration of a non–selenium-dependent reduced glutathione (GSH) peroxidase can vary as well. The level of labile PUFA, such as 20:4, 22:5, and 22:6, can very considerably from tissue to tissue and from one species to another. Also, the efficiency with which dietary PUFA are deposited in the lipid structure of the cell varies with species, tissue, and stage of growth. Finally, endogenous radical-generating systems may be still another variable. It will take considerably more research to define which specific variables are the main determinants of the manifestations of a particular deficiency sign in a particular species.

Excellent descriptions of the pathology of vitamin E deficiency are available (93,94).

B. Humans

1. Blood Tocopherol

When human plasma levels of tocopherol are less than 0.5 mg/dl, the red blood cells (RBC) are increasingly subject to oxidative hemolysis in vitro and have a shorter life span in vivo than normal RBC. Based on these observations and considerable information from animal experiments, it is generally accepted that people with plasma levels of less than 0.5 mg/dl are vitamin E deficient. According to this guideline, several groups of human subjects fall into this category (Table 12). Some of the clinical consequences of vitamin E deficiency in humans are given in Table 13.

2. Infants

The infant is born in a state of relative tocopherol deficiency (Table 12). The smaller the infant, the greater the degree of deficiency. Term infants who are breast-fed quickly attain adult blood tocopherol values. The vitamin E deficiency state of premature infants over the first few weeks of life can be attributed to limited tissue storage at birth, relative dietary deficiency, intestinal malabsorption, and rapid growth (95,96). After development of a mature digestive system, tocopherol absorption improves and blood vitamin E levels rise. Most infants become sufficient in vitamin E by several weeks after birth (97).

Extremely low blood levels of tocopherol have been associated with a hemolytic anemia. The typical syndrome generally manifests itself at approximately 4–6 weeks of age in premature infants with birth weights less than 1500 g. Hemoglobin levels are in the range of 7–9 g/dl, and the anemia is accompanied by reticulocytosis and hyperbilirubinemia (98). In these infants, thrombocytosis is generally present and the platelets are hyperaggregable (72). Occasionally, infants display some edema. Administration of iron may exacerbate the red blood cell destruction unless vitamin E is also administered. The anemia has been associated with ingestion of formulae that are high in polyunsaturated fatty acids and not adequately fortified with vitamin E. Manufacturers have generally increased the vitamin E concentration and decreased the PUFA in infant formulae, so that a hemolytic anemia resulting from a vitamin E deficiency is now unlikely.

Administration of intramuscular vitamin E appears to reduce but not to eliminate the accelerated red cell destruction in the preterm infant.

Table 12 Blood Tocopherol Levels[a] in Humans

Subjects	Total tocopherol[b] (mg/dl)
Adults	0.95
Young adults	0.86
Elderly adults	1.20
Children (2–12 years)	0.76
Term infants	0.40
Premature infants	0.26
Infants and children with protein–calorie malnutrition	0.45
Kwashiorkor	0.30
Enteropathies	
Cholestatic liver disease	< .1
Abetalipoproteinemia	< .1
Celiac disease	0.32
Nontropical sprue	0.25
Tropical sprue	0.28
Chronic pancreatitis	0.40
Ulcerative colitis	0.24
Gastrectomy	0.42
Cystic fibrosis	0.23
Hemolytic anemias	
β-Thalassemia major	0.42
Thalassemia intermedia	0.21
Sickle-cell anemia	0.62
Glucose-6-phosphate dehydrogenase deficiency	0.53
Hereditary spherocytosis	0.52
Miscellaneous	
Total parenteral nutrition	0.55
Gaucher's disease	
(severe)	0.08
(chronic)	0.35

[a]Average values for plasma or serum. Based mostly on Ref. 95 and 173–175.
[b]Mostly α-tocopherol.

3. Oxygen Toxicity

Low-birth-weight infants are often exposed to high oxygen levels to relieve the respiratory distress that frequently occurs in premature infants. Apparently their low vitamin E status contributes to the risks of oxygen toxicity, such as retinopathy of prematurity (ROP), which involves damage to the retina and can result in blindness. Administration of vitamin E has reduced the severity of the retinopathy in some studies, although a review of all studies indicated that there was no conclusive evidence of benefit (or harm) from vitamin E administration (97).

Bronchopulmonary dysplasia (BPD) is a form of chronic pulmonary insufficiency in infants that has also been partially attributed to exposure to high oxygen levels. Preliminary experiments indicating that administration of vitamin E to premature infants ameliorated BPD were not confirmed, although the authors still support the role for vitamin E in the defense against oxygen-induced lung injury. The BPD in the second study was less severe.

Table 13 Clinical Consequences of Vitamin E Deficiency in Humans

---

I. Low-birth weight infants (< 1500 g)
   A. Hemolytic anemia
      Hemoglobin levels 7–9 g/dl
      Reticulocytosis
      Hyperbilirubinemia
   B. Thrombocytosis (elevated platelet count)
   C. Hyperaggregability of platelets
   D. Greater risk of intraventricular hemorrhage
   E. Increased severity of retinopathy of prematurity (ROP)
II. Children with severe malabsorption (i.e., cholestatic liver disease, cystic fibrosis, abetalipoproteinemia)
   A. Reduced red blood cell half-life
   B. Axonal dystrophy
   C. Neuromuscular deficits
III. Adults (malabsorption, total TPN, familial deficiency, or experimental deficiency)
   A. Reduced red blood cell half-life
   B. Lipofuscinosis (ceroid in smooth muscle)
   C. Neuromuscular deficit

A survey (100) has shown that blood tocopherol levels of premature infants have risen dramatically in recent years, presumably as a result of higher intakes of vitamin E by the mothers while they are pregnant. Thus, some problems caused by vitamin E deficiency have been substantially reduced.

Premature infants who have been treated with high levels of vitamin E had a reduced incidence of intraventricular hemorrhage (IVH) compared with nontreated controls (101,102). Since IVH is a common cause of death in premature infants, it will be important to confirm this observation.

Since absorption of vitamin E by the premature infant is limited, in many of the studies with ROP, BPD, and IVH, the infants were injected intramuscularly or intravenously with a preparation of tocopherol as a water-miscible emulsion (103). This preparation has not yet been approved by the Food and Drug Administration, so that investigators must obtain an IND or administer vitamin E orally. Some investigations indicate that absorption of tocopherol, even in infants weighing less than 1500 g, is sufficient to increase blood levels to a more normal range.

The Committee on Nutrition of the American Academy of Pediatrics recommends that formula fed to premature infants should provide 0.7 IU vitamin E per 100 kcal and at least 1.0 IU vitamin E per gram of linoleic acid. In addition, the multivitamin supplement given to the low-birth-weight infants should provide 5 IU of vitamin E, preferably as a water-miscible emulsion.

4. Children

Children generally have lower blood tocopherol levels than adult (Table 11). This lower level can be partially explained by the lower lipid levels in children. However, even when values are expressed on a lipid basis, they are low (104).

5. Protein-Calorie Malnutrition (PCM); Kwashiorkor

Vitamin E status appears much more critical in kwashiorkor where plasma tocopherol levels were found to be extremely low (Table 11). Free-radical tissue injury has been proposed to be important in the pathogenesis of this disease (105).

6. Malabsorption and Neuromuscular Disorders

The only children who show clinical signs of vitamin E deficiency are those with severe malabsorption (Tables 11 and 12). Over the past decade, it has become established that vitamin E deficiency occurs in 49-77% of children with chronic cholestasis. Persistent vitamin E deficiency causes a well-characterized progressive neurologic disorder beginning with hyporeflexia at about 18 months of age, followed by truncal and limb ataxia, depressed vibratory and position sensation, ophthalmoplegia, muscle weakness, ptosis, and scoliosis within the first decade. The following neuromuscular lesions in children with chronic cholestasis resemble those described in animal models of vitamin E deficiency: degeneration of the posterior columns of the spinal cord and nuclei gracilis and cuneatus, degeneration and loss of large-caliber myelinated fibers in peripheral nerve, and neuropathic and myopathic muscle lesions. Administration of vitamin E results in improved neurological (106) and hepatic (107) function particularly if given at an early age before symptoms develop significantly. Neurological disorders apparently related to low vitamin E states are also observed in children with cystic fibrosis (108) and abetalipoproteinemia (109).

7. Adults

Experimental dietary deprivation.   One study was carried out by Horwitt and his associates in which adult subjects were fed diets containing 2-3 mg tocopherol per day (95). After 1-2 years on the diet, blood levels of tocopherol were below 0.5 mg/dl. Erythrocytes from these subjects had increased susceptibility to peroxidative hemolysis and a decreased half-life compared with those of control subjects fed 15 mg tocopherol per day. No other symptoms were observed in the deficient group. Increasing the polyunsaturated fatty acid (linoleic acid) intake accelerated the decline of blood tocopherol.

Malabsorption.   Adults with malabsorption often have low tocopherol levels (95) (Table 11). The erythrocytes from subjects with low levels of tocopherol are associated with an increased susceptibility to peroxidative hemolysis and a shortening of the mean red cell survival time (110). Abnormal ceroid deposition in smooth muscle, such as the intestine, often accompanies low vitamin E status. Increased creatinuria or abnormalities in other indices of muscular dysfunction have not been well established. Neuropathy has also been observed in adults with prolonged and severe malabsorption (111). Neurological dysfunction in vitamin E-deficient adults generally requires 10-20 years of malabsorption whereas symptoms develop within 18-24 months in children with the vitamin deficiency. Most affected adults have responded to large oral doses of vitamin E.

Isolated vitamin E deficiency (familial deficiency).   Patients have been reported who developed the neuromuscular features of vitamin E deficiency but had no fat malabsorption, ate a normal diet and yet were vitamin E deficient (106,112). Absorption of pharmacological doses of vitamin E were normal or near normal, and all patients responded to 800-1000 IU per day. This disorder appears to be an inborn error of vitamin E metabolism.

IX. METHODS OF NUTRITIONAL ASSESSMENT

Serum (or plasma) tocopherol levels have been the most convenient and useful index of vitamin E status (95,113). A hydrogen peroxide hemolysis test has also been used, although this requires vigorous standardization of experimental conditions and is less precise than blood tocopherol levels. In groups of individuals with widely varying plasma lipid there is a correlation between plasma tocopherol level and plasma total lipid. Therefore, subjects with hypolipidemia may have low vitamin E levels as a direct consequence of the low lipid levels and may not be truly vitamin E deficient. In contrast, hyperlipidemic persons may have falsely high plasma vitamin E levels. However, for individuals with normal lipid levels, this relationship is much weaker. Nevertheless, the ratio of plasma tocopherol to lipid is usually a more reliable criterion of adequacy (Table 14) than tocopherol alone (114). The ratio of tocopherol to cholesterol is often a more convenient index than total lipid. Release of malondialdehyde (MDA) from erythrocytes has also been used to monitor vitamin E status (Table 14,115).

Platelet tocopherol has been suggested (116) as an index of status, since it is highly correlated with tocopherol content of other tissues, but it presents technical difficulties, and its utility in humans has not been established. Analysis of red blood cells has also been suggested (117). The increase in the tocopherol content of red blood cells and platelets following supplementation closely parallels the increase in plasma tocopherol (Fig. 5). However, plasma may not reflect the level of tocopherol in tissues with very slow turnover such as adipose and brain.

Recently, a reliable procedure (118) for analysis of adipose tissue in a biopsy sample has been developed. Since α-tocopherol turnover in adipose tissue is very slow (50), this technique may provide a tool for evaluating long-term intake of the vitamin. Breath pentane analysis, an index of in vivo lipid peroxidation, has also been suggested as a functional test of vitamin E status (127a).

Table 14 Tentative Guidelines for Interpreting Vitamin E Status

Age group	Category		
	Deficient	Low	Acceptable
All ages—serum or plasma vitamin E (mg/dl)[a]	< 0.5	0.5– 0.7	> 0.7
All ages—erythrocyte H_2O_2 hemolysis (%)[a]	>20	10–20	<10
All ages—erythrocyte MDA release (%)[b]	> 6.0	—	< 6.0
Serum or plasma vitamin E			
Adults mg/g lipid[c]	< 0.8	—	> 0.8
Adults mg/g cholesterol	< 2.5	—	> 2.5
Children mg/g lipid[d]	< 0.6	—	> 0.6

[a]*Source*: Ref. 113.
[b]*Source*: Ref. 115.
[c]*Source*: Ref. 114.
[d]*Source:* Refs. 104 and 116.

X. NUTRITIONAL REQUIREMENTS

A. Animal

It is difficult to define the requirement for vitamin E since polyunsaturated fatty acids, selenium, and, occasionally, sulfur amino acids can influence the need for the vitamin. Dietary PUFA have a particularly large influence on the requirement (120).

All animals studied, as well as fish, have been shown to require vitamin E (Table 10 and 14). The estimated dietary requirement varies from 3 to 70 IU/kg of diet (Table 15) (121).

There are some species, such as the Rotnest Quokka, that are extraordinary sensitive to vitamin E deficiency (122). Within a species there can also be large strain differences. For example, the spontaneously hypertensive rat is more sensitive to a deficiency than the Wistar-Kyoto or Sprague-Dawley strains (123).

Table 15   Minimum Vitamin E Requirement for Animals

Animal	Requirements[a] (IU/kg diet)
Chickens	
Starting and breeding	30
Growing and laying	10
Turkeys	
Starting and growing	30
Breeding	40
Swine	
Baby piglets	20
Growing pigs	10
Breeding gilts, sows, and boars	20
Cattle: young and breeding	20
Horses: young and breeding	20
Dogs	40
Cats	70
Minks and foxes	40
Fish	
Salmon	30
Catfish	25[b]
Rat	30[c]
Mouse	30[c]
Guinea pig	50[c]
Hamster	3[c]

[a]These levels are estimated to be adequate in complete diets (1) containing at least 0.1 ppm Se, (2) adequate in sulfur amino acids, and (3) containing no more than 1.5% linoleic acid. Vitamin E requirement increases in direct proportion to increased dietary intake of PUFA.
[b]In the presence of 125 mg ethoxyquin per kilogram diet; requirement in the absence of ethoxyquin was 100 IU/kg diet.
[c]Based on recommendations of the National Research Council of the National Academy of Sciences.
Source: Based on Ref. 121.

Requirements are often higher when dietary selenium levels are low and linoleic acid levels are high. Generally, requirements have been established by determining the level necessary to prevent vitamin E deficiency symptoms. When optimum immune response is the criterion, the requirement might be higher (124).

B. Humans

Studies on the vitamin E requirement of infants established that the amount necessary to prevent peroxidative hemolysis was 2–10 IU/day (95). These observations, plus estimates of normal intakes when fed human milk, provided a basis for establishment of the requirement for infants (the 1989 RDA is 4.5 IU/day).

The 1968 RDA of 30 IU for an adult was based on experiments with human subjects who were fed high levels of PUFA (125). Reassessment of the normal range of PUFA intakes and of the vitamin E content of U.S. diets as consumed led in 1974 to a revised, reduced recommendation of 15 IU (126). Analysis of typical U.S. daily diets as consumed averaged 7.4–9.0 mg α-tocopherol. Thus, there remains an unexplained discrepancy between the estimate of the vitamin E requirement based on epidemiological and dietary evidence and that derived from human experiments by Horwitt (127), who considers that 15 IU is at the lower end of a range of requirements that extends to 45 IU/day.

In the 1980 RDA (128), an effort was made to take into account the dietary contribution of β- and γ-tocopherol, as well as α-tocotrienol. The requirement was expressed as tocopherol equivalents (TE); 1 TE is equal to 1 mg RRR-α-tocopherol. The other isomers were converted to TE by multiplying the mg of each isomer by the appropriate relative activity factor:

Isomer	Factor
β-Tocopherol	0.5
γ-Tocopherol	0.1
α-Tocotrienol	0.3

In practice, TE from β- and γ-tocopherol rarely account for more than 20% of the total dietary intake of vitamin E.

The 1989 RDA expressed both in TE and IU is given in Table 16.

XI. INTERACTIONS

A. Nutritional

1. Polyunsaturated Fatty Acids

In animals, the dietary requirement for vitamin E increases when the intake of PUFA increases (5,120). For example, diets high in linoleate increase the requirement for prevention of encephalomalacia in the chicken. High levels of fish oils, such as cod-liver oil, often exacerbate skeletal and cardiac myopathy in many animals. In the only experimental study in humans (129), doubling the PUFA intake with a fixed amount of dietary vitamin E resulted in a gradual decrease in plasma α-tocopherol. The significance of the relationship between dietary α-tocopherol and PUFA in human diets is not clear. The primary dietary sources of PUFA, vegetable oils and soft margarines, are generally rich sources

Table 16 Recommended Dietary Allowances of the Food and Nutrition Board

Category	Age (yr)	Weight		Vitamin E	
		kg	lb	mg α-TE[a]/day	IU/day[b]
Infants	0.0–0.5	6	13	3	4.5
	0.5–1.0	9	20	4	6.0
Children	1–3	13	29	6	9.0
	4–6	20	44	7	10.5
	7–10	28	62	7	10.5
Males	11–14	45	99	10	15.0
	15–18	66	145	10	15.0
	18+	70	154	10	15.0
Females	11–14	4	101	8	12.0
	15+	55	120	8	12.0
Pregnant				10	15.0
Lactating (1st 6 mo)				12	18.0

[a]α-TE = α-tocopherol equivalents. 1 mg d-α-tocopherol = 1 TE.
[b]IU = International Unit. Based on 1 α TE = 1.49 IU.
Source: From *Recommended Dietary Allowances*, National Academy of Sciences, Washington, DC, 1989.

of vitamin E. However, it has been very difficult to define the adequacy of human diets in terms of E/PUFA ratios. When plasma vitamin E levels are used as the criterion, a ratio of 0.4 has been sufficient in children (120,128).

On the other hand, consumption of soybean oil has increased considerably in the last 20 years, and the ratio of vitamin E to PUFA (mg vitamin E per g PUFA) in soybean oil is only 0.2, much lower than in most other foods or fats. In addition, there is now increased interest in the use of fish oils to reduce cardiovascular disease risk. Highly purified fish oils have low E/PUFA ratios. With the continued increase in consumption of a variety of sources of PUFA, reevaluation of the E/PUFA relationship is warranted.

2. Selenium

The selenium-containing enzyme glutathione peroxidase is primarily a cytosolic enzyme that reduces H_2O_2 to H_2O and which also can reduce fatty acid hydroperoxides to fatty alcohols (130). This latter activity is speculated to facilitate the action of vitamin E in reducing peroxy radicals. Figure 8 summarizes some of these events and provides a bicohemical basis for a vitamin E–selenium interaction.

In animals, such symptoms as liver necrosis in rats or exudative diathesis and pancreatic atrophy in chickens can be prevented by either selenium or vitamin E. Vitamin E absorption, at least in chickens, is impaired by a severe selenium deficiency. In the chicken, selenium alleviates such vitamin E deficiencies, both by permitting higher levels of vitamin E to be absorbed and by serving as a precursor of glutathione peroxidase. In other animals there is little evidence that selenium spares vitamin E by enhancing absorption.

In selenium-deficient areas, such as New Zealand, selenium levels are quite low but there is no evidence of exacerbated vitamin E deficiency. Blood levels of tocopherol in human subjects in New Zealand are similar to those in selenium-replete areas. In China, children develop a cardiomyopathy (Keshan's disease) in selenium-deficient areas, but there is no clear evidence that vitamin E status is low or that vitamin E deficiency contributes to the pathology observed.

3. Amino Acids

Necrotic liver degeneration in the rat can be prevented with either vitamin E, cystine, or selenium. Induction of muscular dystrophy in the chicken requires a vitamin E–deficient diet containing a low level of sulfur amino acids (121). Although the activity of sulfur amino acids in vitamin E deficiency is still not completely understood, it presumably is derived from the reducing properties of the sulfhydryl groups of cysteine in proteins and in peptides, such as glutathione.

Simultaneous restriction of tryptophan and vitamin E (but not of either alone) in the maternal diet of rats led to a high incidence of lenticular opacities in the eyes of the progeny (131). The biochemical explanation of this relationship is unknown.

4. Vitamin B_{12}

Urinary excretion of methylmalonic acid, an indicator of vitamin B_{12} deficiency, was observed in a limited number of premature infants and in a few cystic fibrosis patients. Administration of vitamin E to these subjects was followed by a disappearance or decrease in urinary methylmalonate (132). A possible explanation of these findings is that vitamin E deficiency may interfere with the conversion of vitamin B_{12} to its coenzyme, 5'-deoxyadenosyl cobalamin (133). This coenzyme is part of methylmalonyl CoA-mutase, necessary for the conversion of methylmalonyl CoA to succinyl CoA.

5. Zinc

There is considerable evidence that, in addition to its role as a component of many enzymes, zinc can function as a stabilizer of biomembranes (134). RBC from vitamin E–and zinc-deficient animals are very susceptible to peroxidative hemolysis (132). Supplementation of these diets with either zinc or vitamin E results in greater stability of the RBC. When chickens are fed zinc-deficient diets containing 30 IU vitamin E per kilogram, they develop skin and joint abnormalities. These abnormalities are completely alleviated by addition of 500 IU/kg of vitamin E to the diet (135).

Zinc deficiency in rats resulted in lowered plasma tocopherol levels (136). Maximum plasma tocopherol levels were not observed in sickle-cell anemia subjects until supplements containing zinc were administered (137). These studies suggest that poor zinc status could result in reduced absorption of vitamin E.

6. Vitamin A

Vitamin A is very susceptible to peroxidation. As an effective in vivo antioxidant, vitamin E can protect vitamin A. Indeed, vitamin E–deficient animals absorb and store vitamin A more poorly and deplete existing liver reserves of vitamin A more rapidly than do normal animals (138,139). Very high levels of dietary vitamin A increase the vitamin E requirement (140). Many effects of vitamin A toxicity can be counteracted by vitamin E administration in animals (139,141–143).

Only a limited amount of data with humans is available. The addition of vitamin E to an oral preparation of vitamin A did not significantly improve the retention of vitamin A in malnourished children (144). However, most data indicate that vitamin E is needed for efficient vitamin A utilization and liver storage and suggest that it may also alleviate hypervitaminosis A. Based on these observations, it has been recommended (139,145) that vitamin E be included in the high-potency, prophylactic oral preparations of vitamin A used in intervention programs.

7. Iron

Vitamin E protects against the skeletal and cardiac myopathies that can occur following administration of iron to piglets (146). Vitamin E also reduces hemolysis in mice (147) and epileptiform discharges in rats when these animals are injected with iron-dextran (148). Vitamin E reduced the iron-dextran–induced elevation in ethane exhalation in rats (149). This suggests that vitamin E prevents iron-induced lipid peroxidation in vivo presumably due to its antioxidant properties.

In thalassemia major and other severe forms of congenital hemolytic anemias, iron overload is associated with peroxidation of erythrocyte lipids and reduced serum vitamin E levels. In low-birth-weight infants, iron administration may lead to the development of vitamin E–deficiency anemia (150–152), particularly in infants fed a high PUFA formula.

8. Vitamin C

Vitamin E and C are synergistic in their antioxidant properties in vitro. Ascorbate can reduce the tocopheroxy radical in vitro with the concurrent formation of an ascorbate radical (68,69), which can be enzymatically reduced back to ascorbate by an NADH-dependent system. Thus a mechanism exists for continuously regenerating tocopherol (Fig. 8).

The sparing effect of ascorbate can be demonstrated even when the tocopherol is in a lipid phase, and the ascorbate is in the aqueous phase. Presumably they can interact at the interface of the lipid and aqueous phases. When vitamin C–deficient diets are fed to guinea pigs, decreased levels of vitamin E are observed in the lung and adrenals suggesting that vitamin C can spare vitamin E in vivo.

9. Vitamin K

In animals, extremely large doses of vitamin E will cause bleeding if diets are low or marginal in vitamin K. This can be explained by the inhibition of the vitamin K–dependent gamma carboxylase by both α-tocopherol and α-tocopheryl quinone.

B. Environmental

1. Drugs

Oral contraceptives: Women using oral contraceptives had reduced plasma vitamin E levels and increased platelet clotting. Supplementation with 200 IU/day of vitamin E markedly reduced platelet activity (153).

Anthracyclines (Adriamycin):   Anthracyclines are known to generate free radicals in vitro. Vitamin E, therefore, has been proposed as an agent that might alleviate their toxicity. Vitamin E has been shown to be effective in reducing acute adriamycin toxicity in several animal models. In one clinical trial (154) vitamin E therapy may have allowed administration of an additional 100 mg/m² of adriamycin, however, this increase was not considered sufficient to be clinically useful. Anthracyclines are mutagenic and carcinogenic and are thought to generate secondary cancers in humans. It is of interest that administering vitamin E reduced the occurrence and development of daunorubicin-induced mammary tumors in rats (155).

Nitrofurantoin: This urinary tract antibacterial commonly causes pulmonary damage in rats and humans. In rats, toxicity is exacerbated by feeding a vitamin E–deficient diet (156).

Whether administration of vitamins E to humans can affect nitrofurantoin toxicity has not been established.

Carbon tetrachloride: There is now ample evidence that hepatotoxicity from carbon tetrachloride is mediated by the production of free radicals and that, at least in animals, administration of vitamin E reduces the toxicity (157).

Acetaminophen: This analgesic also causes liver toxicity at high levels. In rats the hepatotoxicity is alleviated by vitamin E administration (158).

Nitrosamines: Secondary and tertiary amines react with nitrate at low pH (i.e., comparable with that present in the stomach) to produce nitrosamines that are often both hepatotoxic and carcinogenic (159). α-Tocopherol has been found to prevent nitrosamine formation by causing destruction of nitrosating agents. γ-Tocopherol is much less effective than α-tocopherol. When α-tocopherol is added to bacon, nitrosamine formation during frying is drastically reduced. Vitamin E also prevents nitrosamine formation in vivo in experimental animals. Oral administration of vitamin E to humans greatly reduced the level of fecal mutagens (160). However, whether this effect is directly related to lowering the intestinal or fecal content of nitrosamine has not been established.

Anticonvulsants: Epileptic children treated with anticonvulsants (phenobarbital, phenytoin, carbamazepine) had significantly lower plasma tocopherol levels than normal children or epileptics not on anticonvulsants (160a).

2. Heavy Metals

Lead: Vitamin E treatment reduced the coproporphyrinemia and anemia in rabbits with subacute lead poisoning. Increased splenomegaly and anemia is found in vitamin E–deficient lead-poisoned rats. Although there is strong evidence that vitamin E deficiency exacerbates lead damage to red cells, it is still not known if vitamin E status is of any significance in lead-induced encephalopathies in humans (161).

Mercury: High levels of vitamin E reduced methyl mercury toxicity in rats and quail compared to control animals fed diets with nutritionally adequate levels of vitamin E and selenium. Similar protection by vitamin E was also reported in respect to inorganic mercury with quail. Furthermore, the neurotoxicity of methyl mercury in hamsters was prevented by vitamin E. These findings have not yet been extended to humans (161).

Copper: Administration of high levels of copper to ducklings (162) and sheep (163) results in muscle lesions characteristic of a vitamin E deficiency. Furthermore, when vitamin E- and selenium-deficient rats were given copper, there was an increase in ethane exhalation (an increased in vivo peroxidation), concomitant with increased mortality. Administration of vitamin E prevented both the increase in ethane and mortality (164).

3. Ozone and Nitrogen Dioxide

Ozone (O_3) and nitrogen dioxide (NO_2) are common environmental pollutants that are powerful oxidizing agents that can cause lung damage. Many studies in animals (161,165,166) have demonstrated that vitamin E–deficient animals are unusually susceptible to toxicity by these agents. This suggests that individuals with poor vitamin E status (e.g., premature infants, malabsorption patients, and hemolytic anemia subjects) may be at noticeably increased risks of O_3 or NO_2 toxicity. Administration of vitamin E to normal, well-nourished subjects did not enhance ozone-inhibited lung functions (167). On the other hand, shock lung syndrome, a form of respiratory distress thought to be caused by such oxidizing agents as O_2, O_3, or NO_2, seems to respond to vitamin E administration (168). In rats, poor vitamin E status predisposed the animals to an ozone-related increase in respiratory infection (169). The significance of this observation to human conditions remains to be investigated.

4. Smoking

There is no effect of smoking on plasma tocopherol levels (170). However, in the lung alveolar fluid, tocopherol levels are depressed and an increase in tocopheryl quinone is apparent (67). Furthermore, administration of vitamin E reduced the elevated levels of pentane in the exhaled air of chain smokers (171). Whether vitamin E has any effect on the harmful sequelae of smoking (e.g., emphysema, lung cancer) remains to be established. An increased risk of lung cancer has been reported in persons with lower serum vitamin E levels (171a).

C. Genetic

There are extremely wide species differences in susceptibility of animals to vitamin E deficiency. For example, rabbits and guinea pigs readily develop a debilitating myopathy when fed diets low in vitamin E, whereas rats and chickens are relatively resistant. Spontaneous myopathy is observed in Nyala and the Rottnest Quokka eating diets with moderate amounts of vitamin E. Large doses of vitamin E prevent myopathy in these species.

Within a species there are also notable strain differences. Some strains of owl monkeys develop a hemolytic anemia even when fed diets with nutritionally adequate levels of vitamin E (172). High levels of vitamin E prevent the disorder. Strain differences are also observed in rats. For example, spontaneously hypertensive rats (SHR) are more susceptible to a vitamin E deficiency than are the genetically related normotensive Wistar-Kyoto strain and Sprague-Dawley rats (123). Although people with inherited hemolytic anemias such as sickle-cell anemia (173), G-6-P-D deficiency (174), and thalassemia (175) usually have low vitamin E levels in their blood, this effect is likely to be secondary to the pathology involved in the hemolytic anemia. An inborn error of vitamin E metabolism has been reported (112) in humans.

XII. MISCELLANEOUS EFFECTS

A. Aging and Life Span

Many age-related alterations in tissues are mimicked in vitamin E–deficient animals. Specifically, lipofuscin accumulation in a variety of tissues, neuroaxonal dystrophy, loss of muscle function with increased creatinuria, and decreased immune function are all observed in aged or vitamin E–deficient animals and humans. These parallel changes have suggested that vitamin E may prolong the life span. Harman (176) and others (177,177a) have proposed a "free radical" explanation for aging.

Addition of vitamin E to the diet has enhanced the life span of small mammals in some studies (178) but not in others (179), and many gerontologists remain skeptical of any true effect. The life span of nematodes (180), drosophila (177), and rotifers (181) is prolonged when vitamin E is added to the diet early in life. Supplementation with vitamin E has reduced the number of spontaneously occurring tumors later in life in rats (177). Whether this latter observation is related to an enhancement of the immune response in aged animals by the vitamin remains to be determined. There is limited epidemiological evidence that populations consuming high levels of vitamin E have reduced mortality rates

(182), although it is impossible to conclude that vitamin E per se was responsible for this beneficial effect.

Rather than any expectation of increased life span, vitamin E is more liable to play a role in slowing the onset of age-related health problems such as cataracts, cancer, cardiovascular disease, and decreased immune function.

B. Cancer

Free radicals and lipid peroxides have been postulated to be directly involved in the etiology of cancer (183). Animal models and in vitro experiments suggest that vitamin E could play some role in the prevention of cancer by blocking the formation of carcinogens, inhibiting carcinogens from reaching target sites, suppressing the expression of neoplasia, and enhancing the immune system (184).

Eight prospective studies have shown that higher serum levels of vitamin E are associated with a lower risk of cancer (Table 17). Five other studies have failed to find much relationship, although the direction of the changes was similar. Six cancer prevention trials involving intervention with vitamin E are now underway.

Generally, tumor tissues peroxidize less readily than their normal counterparts (177). This resistance to peroxidation could be partially attributed to the greater concentration of tocopherol in the tumor tissue than in normal tissue (185). The physiological significance of these observations is not clear at present.

Vitamin E inhibits both in vitro and in vivo formation of nitrosamines, compounds that are generally carcinogenic (184). α-Tocopherol prevents nitrosamine formation by irreversibly reacting with nitrosating agents to form α-tocopheryl quinone.

Table 17 Summary of Epidemiological Studies of Serum Vitamin E and Cancer

Site of cancer	Mean difference in serum vitamin E (μg/ml) cases minus controls	Relative risk lowered vs. highest quintile	Ref.
Prospective studies			
Breast	−1.3**	5	242
All	−1.0	—	244
Lung	−1.4***	25	238
All	−0.1	—	245
5 sites	0.0	—	240
All	−0.9	—	241
All	−0.2	—	243
Lung	−0.8	—	237
All	−1.3**	4.4	237
All	−0.3*	1.56	236
Retrospective studies			
Gastric dysplasia	−1.2*	—	234
Ovary	−1.1	—	235
Lung	−3.1***	—	239
Offspring of lung cancer patients	−1.2*	—	239

*P < 0.05; ** P < 0.025; *** P < 0.001.

C. Exercise

Physical exertion increases the severity of myopathy induced by vitamin E–selenium deficiency (186), induces free radical reactions in muscle tissue (187) and results in a decrease
in muscle tocopherol (188). In humans, vitamin E is mobilized during heavy exercise (189).
Administration of vitamin E reduced pentane exhalation in exercisers (190) and high altitude
mountain climbers (191) suggesting an inhibition of exercise-induced lipid peroxidation.
Generally, vitamin E supplementation has failed to result in any improvement in athletic
performance (i.e., speed of running, swimming), but whether it can improve endurance
or protect against exercise induced muscle damage requires further investigation.

D. Wound Healing/Skin

1. Healing of Wounds and Burns

Animal studies have suggested that administration of vitamin E might help reduce scar
formation (192) and accelerate healing of wounds (193) and burns (194). Well-controlled
human studies, however, are not available.

2. Skin, Cosmetic Applications

Topically applied α-tocopherol or α-tocopheryl acetate can be absorbed into the skin and
is useful as a moisturizer since, unlike petrolatum which has an occlusive effect, vitamin
E can moisturize from within. α-Tocopherol is also useful in cosmetics in extending their
shelf life and inhibiting nitrosamine formation. Whether the vitamin provides protection
against ultraviolet damage or "aging" of skin remains to be established (195).

XIII. EFFICACY OF PHARMACOLOGICAL DOSES

When large amounts of water-soluble vitamins are consumed, tissue levels are not increased
appreciably. In contrast, when large amounts of vitamin E are administered to animals,
the tissue content generally increases proportionally to the logarithm of the dose administered. When high levels of α-tocopheryl acetate are given to humans, serum and
blood cell levels increase proportionately to the dose (Figs. 3 and 5). Thus, if higher tissue
levels afford some advantage, there is at least a potential for benefit from administration
of high levels of the vitamin.

   A large number of diseases have been reported to be responsive to administration
of high levels of vitamin E. These claims are generally difficult to evaluate since they
are often anecdotal or poorly controlled or are carried out for only limited amounts of
time. Marks (196) and Farrel (95) have critically reviewed much of this literature. They
concluded that, with the exception of intermittent claudication, there was little evidence
for efficacy of vitamin E. More recent studies have tended to confirm the possible benefit
of vitamin E for treatment of intermittent claudication (197) and have suggested that vitamin
E may be a useful in the alleviation of the symptoms of a number of diseases and more
importantly for the prevention of some infectious and chronic diseases in animals and man.

A. Immune Function (Infectious Diseases)

Lymphocytes and mononuclear cells have the highest concentration of vitamin E of any
cells in the body. It is therefore not surprising that vitamin E has a profound effect on
the immune system. Many parameters of the immune system are depressed in vitamin
E–deficient animals. This includes T- and B-lymphocyte stimulation, mixed lymphocyte

response, plaque-forming cell activities, interleukin-2 levels, and neutrophil and macrophage chemotaxis and adhesion (198). The requirement for optimum immune response in the rat is higher than for the prevention of classical vitamin E–deficiency symptoms (124). This may partially explain why addition of vitamin E to diets nutritionally adequate in the vitamin not only enhanced antibody formation, but reduced morbidity and mortality in response to infection with *E. coli* in chickens, *Mycoplasma pulmonaris* in rats, histomoniasis in turkeys, and *Chlamydia* in lambs. Moreover, neutrophil-induced damage to lung tissue following burn injury is reduced when rats are preinjected with vitamin E (199).

Possible explanations for the immune-enhancing properties of vitamin E are alterations in eicosanoid metabolism and alterations in membrane fluidity of immune cells. Moreover, antioxidant properties may explain the reduction in self-destruction of neutrophils during the oxidative burst.

Administration of vitamin E to children with respiratory tract infection improved their clinical status and normalized the ratio of OKT_4^+ to OKT_8^+ cells in their peripheral blood (200). Administration of 1600 IU/day of vitamin E to adults improved phagocytosis, presumably as a result of reduced autotoxicosis by reducing the H_2O_2 produced (201). At this level of intake, in vitro bacterial killing was reduced, although the reduction was not considered clinically relevant.

Two studies indicate that vitamin E may be of considerable importance in maintaining or enhancing the immune system in the elderly. In a prospective epidemiological study, it was found that 66% of subjects over 60 years of age, with plasma tocopherol levels of less than 1.35 mg/dl, experienced at least three infections over a 3-year period. In contrast, only 37% of subjects with plasma tocopherol over 1.35 mg/dl had at least three infections (202). Based on the dose-response (Fig. 5), an intake of 40–60 IU of vitamin E per day would be necessary to attain blood levels this high. In a double-blind study in healthy elderly (60–85 years), those given 800 IU vitamin E per day had enhanced delayed-type hypersensitivity and lymphocyte mitogen responses compared to placebo controls (203).

Clearly the immune-enhancing effect of vitamin E on man could have considerable public health implications and warrants continued investigation.

B. Genetic Hemolytic Anemias

Although blood levels of tocopherol are low in β-thalassemia (Table 11), administration of vitamin E resulted in only minimal benefit in reducing transfusion requirements or increasing hemoglobin levels (204). Blood tocopherol levels are also low in sickle-cell anemia (SCA) patients. Administration of vitamin E to SCA patients results in a lowered proportion of irreversibly sickled cell (205), but there is still no clear evidence of a therapeutic benefit from vitamin E. In contrast, there is a definite improvement in hemoglobin levels, reticulocyte counts, and RBC half-lives in patients with glucose-6-phosphate dehydrogenase deficiency or glutathione synthetase deficiency following administration of 800–1000 IU/day of vitamin E (206).

C. Malabsorption Defects

It is now clear that the neurological problems associated with abetalipoproteinemia, cholestatic liver disease, and cystic fibrosis can be ameliorated or even prevented by the administration of high levels of vitamin E early in the disease process (206).

D. Cardiovascular Disease

Early claims that vitamin E was effective in treatment of angina or heart failure have not been confirmed. However, there is increasing evidence that vitamin E status may be an important factor in a number of aspects of cardiovascular disease:

1. Intermittent Claudication

Administration of 300–600 IU vitamin E per day for at least 6 months to subjects with intermittent claudication appears to enhance blood flow and permit longer walking periods without pain (197).

2. Platelet Function

In normal adults administration of 800 IU/day or less has little or no effect on platelet aggregation (208,209). However, the adhesion of platelets to collagen is significantly decreased by as little as 400 IU/day of vitamin E (210). Inhibition of platelet adhesion could help prevent thrombus formation. Furthermore, in hyperlipemic subjects (211), women on oral contraceptives (153), and in insulin-dependent diabetics (212), administration of 200–1000 IU/per day of vitamin E suppressed abnormal levels of platelet aggregation.

3. Lipoproteins

One current theory suggests that LDL becomes atherogenic only after peroxidation (213), and recent evidence suggests that vitamin E can help prevent this critical lipoperoxidative step (214,215). Administration of vitamin E does not alter serum LDL cholesterol or triglyceride levels. Reports of an increase in HDL levels following vitamin E administration have not been reproducible.

4. Ischemia-Reperfusion Injury

Ischemia-reperfusion injury is thought to result from a burst of free-radical production following restriction of blood flow to the heart and subsequent reperfusion. This occurs during bypass surgery, angioplasty, or fibrinolysis treatment. Preadministration of vitamin E has been found to protect against such injury in many animal models and in man during cardiopulmonary bypass surgery (216,217).

5. Mortality from Cardiovascular Disease

Epidemological studies have been equivocal. One carefully controlled study failed to show any relationship between plasma tocopherol and risk of death from coronary heart disease (CHD), whereas a multinational study of over 11 countries showed a clear inverse correlation of plasma tocopherol and mortality from CHD (218).

6. Stroke

Thrombosis or hemorrhage in the brain can lead to free-radical injury from the resulting ischemia and reperfusion (220). Vitamin E has been shown to ameliorate brain edema and injury in animal models. Markedly reduced serum vitamin E levels and elevated MDA is observed in stroke cases within 48 hours of the acute event (221). Daily administration of 100 mg of α-tocopherol via a drainage tube or spinal tap significantly reduced the evidence of symptomatic vasospasms in patients with subarachnoid hemorrhages (222). Further studies in the preventive and therapeutic role of vitamin E in stroke are warranted.

7. Disseminated Intravascular Coagulation (DIC)

Pigs on high-PUFA, low-vitamin E diets die with symptoms of DIC being characterized by multiple microthrombi in small vessels. Administration of vitamin E inhibits endotoxin-induced experimental DIC in rats (219).

E. Parkinsonism

There is some evidence that Parkinsonism is caused by damage to the substantia nigra of the brain resulting from autoxidation and metabolism of dopamine (223). Epidemiological studies (224,225) suggest that consumption of higher intake of vitamin E is associated with lower risk of the disease. One study has suggested that 3200 IU per day of vitamin E (with vitamin C) to persons with early Parkinsonism delayed the time before dopaminergic drugs were required (226). Another reported that the progression of the severity of symptoms was slower in subjects taking vitamin E supplements (227). Based on this background a large-scale, multicentered study is underway to evaluate the effect of 2000 IU per day on the progression of this disease (228)

F. Cataracts

There is considerable evidence that cataracts are a result of cumulative damage resulting from light-induced free-radical damage (229). Cataracts have been observed in vitamin E–deficient turkey embryos and rats with a combined deficiency with tryptophan. Furthermore, vitamin E delayed onset of cataracts in a variety of in vitro and in vivo animal models. Epidemiological studies have shown that persons low in vitamin E in combination with low vitamin C or β-carotene have a higher risk of cataracts (230) and that persons consuming vitamin E supplements (average 400 IU) had a lower risk of cataracts (231).

XIV. SAFETY

Both acute and chronic studies with animals have shown that vitamin E is relatively nontoxic (232).For example, the LD_{50} for all-*rac*-α-tocopherol or all-*rac*-α-tocopheryl acetate is in excess of 2000 mg/kg body weight for rats, mice, and rabbits. The vitamin is not mutagenic, carcinogenic, or teratogenic. In those instances in which deleterious effects were observed, the doses used were in the range of 1 g/kg body weight.

In human studies with double-blind protocols and other large studies of oral vitamin E supplementation, few side effects have been reported, even at doses as high as 3200 mg/day (3200 IU/day) (233). The majority of side effects were reported in letters to the editor as individual case reports or uncontrolled studies. Most of these side effects have not been observed in the larger well-controlled studies. There are no consistent effects of vitamin E supplementation on serum lipid and lipoprotein levels.

Oral intake of vitamin E can exacerbate the coagulation defect produced by vitamin K deficiency caused by either malabsorption or anticoagulant therapy. Therefore, high levels of supplemental vitamin E may be contraindicated in such conditions. Vitamin E has not been found to produce coagulation abnormalities in individuals who are not vitamin K deficient.

REFERENCES

1. H. E. Evans, *Vitam. Horm.*, 20:379 (1963).
2. K. Mason, in *Vitamin E, A Comprehensive Treatise*, L. J. Machlin (Ed.), Marcel Dekker, New York, 1980, pp. 1–8.
3. H. Dam, *Pharmacol. Rev.*, 9:1 (1957).
4. H. Dam and H. Granados, *Acta Physiol. Scand.*, 10:162 (1945).
5. H. Dam, *Vitam. Horm.*, 20:527 (1962).

6. H. J. Kayden and P. P. Nair (Eds.), International Conference on Vitamin E and its role in cellular metabolism, *Ann. N.Y. Acad. Sci.*, *203*:1–247 (1972).

7. J Moustgaard and J. Hyldgaard-Jensen (Eds.), Viamin E animal nutrition, *Acta Agric. Scand. (Suppl.)*, *19*:11–230 (1971).

8. M. K. Horwitt (Eds.), International symposium on vitamin E, *Am. J. Clin. Nutr.*, *27*:939–1194 (1974).

9. E. deDuve and O. Hayaishi (Eds.), *Tocopherol, Oxygen, and Bio-membranes*. Elsevier/North Holland Biomedical Press, New York, 1978.

10. B. Lubin and L. J. Machlin (Eds.), Conference on vitamin E: Biochemical, hematological, and clinical aspects, *Ann. N.Y. Acad. Sci.*, *393* (1982).

11. O. Hayaishi and M. Mino (Eds.), *Clinical and Nutritional Aspects of Vitamin E*. Elsevier Science Pub., New York 1987.

12. A. T. Diplock, L. J. Machlin, L. Packer, and W. A. Pryor, Vitamin E: Biochemistry and health implications, *Ann. N.Y. Acad. Sci.*, *570* (1989).

13. Anon, *Biology of Vitamin E*, Ciba Foundations Symposium 101. Pitman, London, 1983.

14. J. Bieri and P. M. Farrell, *Vitam. Hormon.*, *34*:31 (1976).

15. L. J. Machlin (Ed.), *Vitamin E, A Comprehensive Treatise*. Marcel Dekker, New York, 1980.

16. A. T. Diplock, in *Fat Soluble Vitamins Their Biochemistry and Applications*, A. T. Diplock (Ed.). Technomic Pub. Co., Lancaster, PA, 1985, pp. 154–224.

17. Anon., *Eur. J. Biochem.*, *46*:217 (1974).

18. *U. S. Pharmacopaea*, XX, 846 (1980).

19. H. L. Newmark, W. Pool, J. C. Bauernfeind, and E. DeRitter, *J. Pharmacol. Sci.*, *64*:655 (1975).

20. S. Kasparek, in *Vitamin E, A Comprehensive Treatise*, L. J. Machlin (Ed.). Marcel Dekker, New York, 1980, p. 7.

21. K.C. Ingold, G. W. Burton, D. O. Foster, M. Zuler, L. Hughes, S. Lacolle, E. Lusztyk, and M. Slaby, *FEBS*, *205*:117 (1986).

22. N. Cohen, C. G. Scott, C. Neukom, R. J. Lopresti, G. Weber, and G. Saucy, *Helv. Chim. Acta*, *64*:1158 (1981).

23. I. D. Desai and L. J. Machlin, in *Methods of Vitamin Assay 4/E*, J. Augustin and B. P. Klein (Eds.). J. Wiley and Sons, Inc., New York, 1985, p. 255.

24. C. G. Scott, N. Cohen, P. P. Riggio, and G. Weber, *Lipids*, *17*:97 (1982).

25. J. G. Bieri, T. J. Tolliver, and G. L. Catignani, *Am. J. Clin. Nutr.*, *32*:2143 (1979).

26. L. J. Hatam and H. J. Kayden, *J. Lipid Res.*, *20*:639 (1979).

27. J. M. Thompson and G. Hatina, *J. Liquid Chromatogr.*, *2*:327 (1979).

28. H. Cohen and M. R. Lapointe, *J. Assoc. Off. Anal. Chem.*, *63*:1254 (1980).

29. L. J. Machlin, E. Gabriel, and M. Brin, *J. Nutr.*, *112*:1437 (1982).

30. J. C. Bauernfeind, in *Vitamin E, A Comprehensive Treatise*, L. J. Machlin (Ed.). Marcel Dekker, New York, 1980, p. 99.

31. H. E. Gallo-Torres, in *Vitamin E, A Comprehensive Treatise*, L. J. Machlin (Ed.). Marcel Dekker, New York, 1980, p. 170.

32. H. Schmandke, C. Sima, and R. Manne, *Int. Z. Vitam. Forsch.*, *39*:796 (1969).

33. H. Schmandke and G. Schmidt, *Int. Z. Vitam. Forsch.*, *35*:128 (1965).

34. S. Gross and K. K. Melhorn, *J. Pediatr.*, *85*:753 (1974).

35. P. M. Mathias, J. T. Harres, T. J. Petern, and D. P. R. Muller, *J. Lipid Res.*, *22*:829 (1981).

36. H. Baker, O. Frank, B. DeAngelis, and S. Feingold, *Nutr. Rep. Int.*, *21*:531 (1980).

37. H. E. Gallo-Torres, in *Vitamin E, A Comprehensive Treatise*, L. J. Machlin, (Ed.). Marcel Dekker, New York, 1980, p. 193.

38. W. A. Behrens, J. N. Thompson, and R. Madere, *Am. J. Clin. Nutr.*, *35*:691 (1982).

39. H. J. Kayden, C-K Chow, and L. K. Bjornson, *J. Lipid Res.*, *14*:533 (1973).

39a. B. A. Clevidence and J. Lehman, *Lipids*, *24*:137 (1989).

40. C. K. Chow, *Am. J. Clin. Nutr.*, *28*:756 (1975).

41. J. G. Bieri, *Ann. N.Y. Acad. Sci.*, *203*:181 (1972).
42. H. Mowri, Y. Nakagawa, K. Inoue, and S. Nojima, *Eur. J. Biochem.*, *117*:537 (1981).
43. D. J. Murphy and R. D. Mavis, *J. Biol. Chem.*, *256*:10464 (1981).
44. J. A. Lucy, in *Tocopherol, Oxygen, and Biomembranes*, E. deDuve, and O. Hayaishi (Eds.). Elsevier/North Holland Biomedical Press, New York, 1978, p. 109.
45. G. W. Burton and K. V. Ingold, *Accounts of Chem. Res.*, *19*:194 (1986).
46. R. Patnaik, *Int. J. Biochem.*, *13*:1087 (1981).
47. K. N. Prasad, D. Gaudreau, and J. Brown, *Proc. Soc. Exp. Biol. Med.*, *166*:167 (1981).
48. A. E. Kitabchi, *Ann. N. Y. Acad. Sci.*, *393*:300 (1982).
49. A. E. Kitabchi, J. Winnalasena, and J. Barker, *Biochem. Biophys. Res. Commun.*, *96*:1739 (1980).
50. L. J. Machlin and E. Gabriel, *Ann. N.Y. Acad. Sci.*, *393*:48 (1982).
51. E. J. Simon, L. S. Gross, and A. T. Milhorat, *J. Biol. Chem.*, *221*:797 (1956).
52. E. J. Simon, A. Eisengart, L. Sundheim, and A. T. Milhorat, *J. Biol. Chem.*, *221*:807 (1956).
53. H. S. Olcott and H. A. Matill, *Chem. Rev.*, *29*:257 (1941).
54. H. Dam, *Pharmacol. Rev.*, *9*:1 (1957).
55. J. F. Mead, Free radical mechanisms of lipid damage and consequences for cellular membranes, in *Free Radicals*, Vol. I, W. A. Pryor (Ed.). Academic Press, New York, 1976, pp. 51–68.
56. L. J. Machlin, *J. Am. Oil Chem. Soc.*, *40*:368 (1963).
57. H. H. Draper, J. G. Bergan, M. Chin. A. Csallany, and A. V. Boara, *J. Nutr.*, *84*:395 (1964).
58. A. L. Tappel, *Vitam. Horm.*, *20*:493 (1962).
59. L. J. Machlin, *Nutrition*, pp. 51–54 (1987).
60. I. Molenaar, C. E. Hulstaert, and M. J. Hadonk, in *Vitamin E, A Comprehensive Treatise*, L. J. Machlin (Ed.). Marcel Dekker, New York, 1980, pp. 372–389.
60a. J. Green and J. Bunyan, *Nutr. Abstr. Rev.*, *39*:321 (1969).
61. J. P. Infante, *Molecular & Cellular Biochem.*, *69*:93 (1986).
62. G. L. Catigani, in *Vitamin E, A Comprehensive Treatise*, L. J. Machlin (Ed.). Marcel Dekker, New York, 1980, pp. 318–332.
63. H. S. Lee and A. S. Csallany, *Lipids*, *22*:104 (1987).
64. C. E. Dillard, E. E. Dumelin, and A. L. Tappel, *Lipids*, *12*:109 (1977).
65. G. Lawrence, G. Cohen, and L. J. Machlin, *Ann. N.Y. Acad. Sci.*, *393*:227 (1982).
66. M. Lemoyne, A. VanGossum, R. Kurian, M. Ostro, J. Axler, and K. N. Jeejeeboy, *Am. J. Clin. Nutr.*, *46*:267 (1987).
67. E. R. Pacht, H. Kaseki, J. R. Mohammed, D. G. Cornwell, and W. B. Davis, *J. Clin. Invest.*, *77*:789 (1986).
68. A. Bendich, L. J. Machlin, O. Scandurra, G. W. Burton, and D. D. M. Waynes, *Adv. Free Radical Biology & Medicine* *2*:419 (1986).
69. E. Niki, *Chem. & Physics of Lipids*, *44*:227 (1987).
70. P. B. McCay, *Ann. N.Y. Acad. Sci.*, *570*:32 (1989).
71. R. V. Panganamala and D. G. Cornwell *Ann. N.Y. Acad. Sci.*, *393*:376 (1982).
72. M. Stuart, *Ann. N.Y. Acad. Sci.*, *393*:277 (1982).
73. W. C. Hope, L. J. Machlin, R. J. Filipski, and F. M. Vane, *Prostaglandins*, *10*:557 (1975).
74. R. O. L. Koff, D. R. Guptill, L. M. Lawrence, C. C. McKan, M. M. Mathias, C. F. Nockels, and R. P. Tengerdy, *Am. J. Clin. Nutr.*, *34*:245 (1981).
75. M. P. Carpenter, *Fed. Proc.*, *40*:189 (1981).
76. A. C. Chan, C. E. Allen, and P. V. J. Hegarty, *J. Nutr.*, *110*:66 (1980).
77. A. C. Chan and M. K. Leith, *Am. J. Clin. Nutr.*, *34*:2341 (1981).
78. C. W. Karpen, A. J. Merola, R. W. Trewyn, D. G. Cornwell, and R. V. Panganamala, *Prostaglandins*, *22*:651 (1981).
79. E. J. Goetzl, *Nature*, *288*:183 (1980).
80. Y-Z Cao, O. Karmin, P. C. Choy, and A. C. Chan., *Biochem. J.*, *247*:135 (1987).

81. M. J. Stampfer, J. A. Jakubowski, D. Faigel, R. Vaillancourt, and D. Deykin, *Am. J. Clin. Nutr.*, *47*:700 (1988).

82. R. O. Olson, *Am. J. Clin. Nutr.*, *27*:1117 (1974).

83. J. J. Gilbert, *Am. J. Clin. Nutr.*, *27*:1005 (1974).

84. D. C. Lennartz and E. C. Bovee, *Trans. Am. Micros. Soc.*, *99*:310 (1980).

85. K. Prasad, S. Ramanujam, and P. Gaudreau, *Proc. Soc. Exp. Biol. Med.*, *161*:570 (1979).

86. H. Sakagami, K. Asaka, E. Abe, C. Miyaura, T. Suda, and K. Konna, *J. Nutr. Sci. Vitaminol.*, *27*:291 (1981).

87. P. I. Caasi, J. W. Hauswirth, and P. P. Nair, *Ann. N. Y. Acad. Sci.*, *203*:93 (1972).

88. L. R. Horn, L. J. Machlin, M. O. Barker, and M. Brin, *Arch. Biochem. Biophys.*, *172*:270 (1976).

89. L. M. Corwin, in *Vitamin E, A Comprehensive Treatise*, L. J. Machlin, (Ed.). Marcel Dekker, New York, 1980, pp. 332–347.

90. A. T. Quintanhila, L. Packer, J. M. S. Davies, T. L. Racanelli, and K. J. Davies, *Ann. N.Y. Acad. Sci.*, *393*:32 (1982).

91. R. S. London, G. S. Sundarem, M. Schultz, P. P. Nair, and P. J. Goldstein, *Cancer Res.*, *41*:3811 (1981).

92. H. Weiser, V. Actervalh, and W. Boguth, *Acta. Agric. Scand. (Suppl)*, 19:208 (1973).

93. K. E. Mason, in *The Vitamins*, Vol. 3, Part VII, W. H. Sebrell and R. S. Harris (Eds.). Academic Press, New York, 1954, pp. 514–562.

94. J. S. Nelson, in *Vitamin E, A Comprehensive Treatise*, L. J. Machlin (Ed.). Marcel Dekker, New York, 1980, pp. 397–428.

95. P. Farrel, in *Vitamin E, A Comprehensive Treatise*, L. J. Machlin (Ed.). Marcel Dekker, New York, 1980, pp. 520–620.

96. F. Oski, in *Textbook of Pediatric Nutrition*, R. M. Suskind (Ed.). Raven Press, New York, 1981, pp. 145–151.

97. Institute of Medicine. Report of a Study, "Vitamin E and Retinopathy of Prematurity." National Academy Press, Washington, DC, June 1986.

98. S. J. Gross and S. A. Landaw, *Ann. N.Y. Acad. Sci.*, *393*:316 (1982).

99. R. A. Ehrenkranz, R. C. Ablow, and J. B. Warshaw, *Ann. N.Y. Acad. Sci.*, *393*:452 (1982).

100. L. J. Johnson (unpublished).

101. M. L. Chiswick, M. Johnson, C. Woodhall, M. Gowland, J. Davies, N. Toner, and D. G. Sims, *Br. Med. J.* *287*:81–84 (1983).

102. M. E. Speer, C. Blifeld, A. J. Rudolph, P. Chadda, B. Holbein, and H. M. Hittner, *Pediatrics*, *74*:1107–1112 (1984).

103. H. L. Newmark, W. Pool, J. C. Bauernfeind, and E. DeRitter, *J. Pharm. Sci.*, *64*:655 (1975).

104. P. M. Farrell, S. L. Levine, M. D. Murphy, and A. J. Adams, *Am. J. Clin. Nutr.*, *31*:1720 (1978).

105. M. H. M. Golden and D. Ramdath, *Proc. Nutr. Soc.*, *46*:53–68 (1987).

106. R. J. Sokol, *Ann. Rev. Nutr.*, *8*:351 (1988).

107. R. J. Sokol, J. E. Heubi, C. McGraw, and W. F. Balistreri, *Hepatology*, *6*:1263–1269 (1986).

108. E. Elias, D. P. R. Muller, and J. Scott, *Lancet*, *2*:1319 (1981).

109. D. P. R. Muller and J. K. Lloyd, *Ann. N.Y. Acad. Sci.*, *393*:133 (1982).

110. P. J. Leonard and M. S. Losowsky, *Am. J. Clin. Nutr.*, *24*:388 (1981).

111. R. E. Knight, A. J. Bourne, and M. Newton, *Gastroenterol.*, *91*:209–211 (1986).

112. R. J. Sokol, H. J. Kayden, D. B. Davis, M. G. Traber, H. Neville, S. Ringel, W. B. Wilson, and D. A. Stumpf, *J. Lab. Clin. Med.*, *11*:548 (1988).

113. H. E. Sauberlich, R. P. Dowdy, and J. H. Skala, Laboratory test for the assessment of nutritional status, *CRC Crit. Rev. Clin. Lab. Sci.*, 288 (1973).

114. M. K. Horwitt, C. C. Harvey, D. H. Dahm, and M. T. Searcy, *Ann. N.Y. Acad. Sci.*, *203*:233 (1972).

115. H. Cynamon, *J. Pediatr. Gastroenterol. Nutr.*, *6*:46–50 (1987).

116. J. Lehman, D. D. Rao, J. J. Canary, and J. T. Judd, *Am. J. Clin. Nutr., 47*:470 (1988).

117. M. Mino, M. Kitagawa, and S. Nakagawa, *Am. J. Clin. Nutr., 41*:631–638 (1988).

118. G. J. Handelman, W. L. Epstein, L. J. Machlin, F. J. VanKuijk, and E. A. Dratz, *Lipids, 23*:598–604 (1988).

119. M. Lemoyne, A. VanGossum, R. Kurian, M. Ostro, J. Axler, and K. N. Jeejeeboy, *Am. J. Clin. Nutr., 46*:267 (1987).

120. H. Draper, In *Vitamin E, A Comprehensive Treatise*, L. J. Machlin (Ed.). Marcel Dekker, New York, 1980, pp. 272–288.

121. M. L. Scott, in *Handbook of Lipid Research*, Vol. 2, H. F. DeLuca (Ed.). Plenum Press, New York, (1978), p. 133.

122. B. A. Kakulas and R. D. Adams, *Ann. N.Y. Acad. Sci., 138*:90 (1966).

123. E. Gabriel, A. Bendich, and L. J. Machlin, *Proc. Soc. Exptl. Biol. Med., 176*:378 (1984).

124. A. Bendich, E. Gabriel and L. J. Machlin, *J. Nutr., 116*:675 (1986).

125. Food and Nutrition Board, *Recommended Dietary Allowance* (7th ed.). U. S. National Academy of Sciences Publication, Washington, DC, 1964, 1968.

126. Food and Nutrition Board, *Recommended Dietary Allowance* (8th ed.). U.S. National Academy of Sciences Publication, Washington DC, 1974.

127. M. K. Horwitt, *Am. J. Clin. Nutr., 27*:1182 (1974).

128. Food and Nutritional Board, *Recommended Dietary Allowance* (9th ed.). U.S. National Academy of Sciences Publication, Washington, DC, 1980.

129. M. K. Horwitt, *Vitam. Horm., 20*:541 (1962).

130. F. Ursini and A. Bindoli, *Chem. and Physics of Lipids, 44*:255 (1987).

131. G. E. Bunce and J. L. Hess, *J. Nutr., 106*:222 (1976).

132. L. J. Machlin and E. Gabriel, *Ann. N.Y. Acad. Sci., 335*:98 (1980).

133. A. S. Pappu, P. Fatterpaker, and R. Sreenvasan, *Biochem. J., 172*:115 (1978).

134. M. S. Chvapil, S. L. Elias, J. M. Ryan, and C. F. Zukoski, *Int. Rev. Neurobiol., 1*:105 (1972).

135. W. J. Bettger, P. G. Reeves, J. E. Savage, and B. L. O'Dell, *Proc. Soc. Exp. Biol. Med., 163*:432 (1980).

136. M. J. Bunk, A. Dnistrian, M. K. Schwarz, and R. S. Rivlin, *Am. J. Clin. Nutri., 45*:865 (1987).

137. L. Sindel, S. Banga, V. Mankad, and A. Bendich, *Fed. Proc., 46*:1163 (1987).

138. S. Gerger, *Bibl. Nutr. Diet, 15*:85 (1969).

139. J. C. Bauernfeind, H. Newmark, and M. Brin, *Am. J. Clin. Nutr., 27*:234 (1974).

140. W. J. Pudelkiewicz, L. Webster, and L. D. Matterson, *J. Nutr. 84*:113 (1964).

141. L. W. McCuaig and I. Motzok. *Poultry Sci., 49*:1090 (1970).

142. M. K. Soliman, *Int. J. Vitaminol. Nutr. Res., 42*:389 (1972).

143. M. Y. Jenkins and G. V. Mitchell, *J. Nutr., 105*:1600 (1975).

144. J. A. Kusin, V. Reddy, and B. Sivakumar, *Am. J. Clin. Nutr., 27*:774 (1974).

145. L. M. DeLuca, J. Glover, J. Heller, J. A. Olson, and B. Underwood, Vol. VI, *Guidelines for the Eradication of Vitamin A Deficiency and Xerophthalmia*—A Report of IVAGG, Nutrition Foundation, New York, 1978.

146. G. Tollerz, *Acta Agric. Scand. (Suppl). 19*:184 (1973).

147. K. A. Smith and C. E. Mengel, *J. Lab. Clin. Med., 72*:505 (1968).

148. J. J. Rubin and L. J. Willmore, *Exp. Neurol., 67*:472 (1980).

149. A. L. Tappel and C. J. Dillard, *Fed. Proc., 40*:174 (1981).

150. M. L. Willmore, R. J. Schott, P. L. O'Neal, and F. A. Oski, *N. Engl. J. Med., 292*:887 (1974).

151. P. R. Dallam, *J. Pediatr., 85*:742 (1974).

152. D. K. Melhorn and S. Gross, *J. Pediatr., 79*:569 (1971).

153. S. Renaud, M. Ciavatti, L. Perrot, F. Berthezene, D. Dargent, and P. Condamin, *Contraception 36*:347 (1987).

154. S. S. Legha, Y-M. Wang, B. MacKay, M. Ewer, G. N. Hortobagyi, R. S. Benjamin, and M. K. Ali, *Ann. N.Y. Acad. Sci., 393*:411 (1982).

155. Y-M. Wang and S. K. Howell, *Ann. N.Y. Acad. Sci., 393*:186 (1982).

156. M. R. Boyd, G. L. Catignani, H. A. Sasame, J. R. Mitchell, and A. W. Stiko, *Am. Rev. Respir. Dis., 120*:93 (1967).

157. R. O. Recknagel, *Pharmacol. Rev., 19*:145 (1967).

158. J. Kelleher, N. P. Keaney, B. E. Walker, M. S. Losowsky, and M. F. Dixon, *J. Int. Med. Res., 4(Suppl. Y)*:138 (1977).

159. H. L. Newmark and W. J. Mergens, in *Gastrointestinal Cancer*, W. R. Bruce, P. Correa, M. Lopkin, S. R. Tannenbaum, T. D. Wilkins (Eds.). Banbury Report 7, Cold Spring Harbor Laboratory, Cold Spring Harbor, NY, 1981, pp. 285-303.

160. W. R. Bruce, A. J. Varghese, S. Wang, and P. Dion, in *Naturally Occurring Carcinogens—Mutagens and Modulators of Carcinogenesis*, E. C. Miller, J. A. Miller, I. Hiron, T. Sugimura, and S. Takayama (Eds.). University Park Press, Baltimore, 1979, pp. 221-228.

160a. A. O. Ogunmekan, *Trop. Geogr. Med., 37*:175 (1985).

161. E. J. Calabrese, in *Nutrition and Environmental Health*, Vol. 1. John Wiley & Sons, New York, 1980, pp. 491-571.

162. J. F. VanVleet, G. D. Boon, and V. J. Ferrans, *Am. J. Vet. Res., 42*:1206 (1981).

163. S. R. Gooneratne and J. McHowell, *Res. Vet. Sci., 28*:351 (1980).

164. J. J. Dougherty and W. G. Hoekstra, *Proc. Soc. Exptl. Biol. Med., 169*:201 (1982).

165. B. L. Fletcher and A. L. Tappel, *Environ. Res., 6*:165 (1973).

166. D. B. Menzel, in *Vitamin E, A Comprehensive Treatise*, L. J. Machlin (Ed.). Marcel Dekker, New York, 1980, pp. 474-494.

167. J. P. Hackney, W. S. Linn, R. D. Buckley, M. P. Jones, L. H. Wightman, and S. K. Karuza, *J. Toxicol. Environ. Health, 7*:383 (1981).

168. H. R. D. Wolf and H. W. Seeger, *Ann. N.Y. Acad. Sci., 393*:392 (1982).

169. D. Warshauer, E. Goldstein, P. D. Hoepride, and W. Lippert, *J. Lab. Clin. Med.,83*:228 (1974).

170. W. C. Stryker, L. A. Kaplan, E. A. Stein, M. J. Stampfer, A. Sober, and W. C. Willet, *Am. J. Epidem., 127*:283 (1988).

171. R. Shariff, E. Hosino, J. Allard, C. Pichard, R. Kurian, and K. M. Jeejeebhoy, *Am. J. Clin. Nutr., 47*:758 (1988).

172. P. K. Seghal, R. T. Bronson, P. S. Brady, K. McIntyre, and M. W. Elliot, *Lab. Anim. Sci., 30*:92 (1980).

173. C. Natta and L. J. Machlin, *Am. J. Clin. Nutr., 32*:1359 (1979).

174. L. M. Corash, M. Shultz, J. G. Bieri, C. Bartsocas, S. Moses, N. Barban, and J. D. Schulman, *Ann. N.Y. Acad. Sci., 393*:348 (1982).

175. E. A. Rachmilewitz, A. Kornberg, and M. Acker, *Ann. N.Y. Acad. Sci., 393*:336 (1982).

176. D. Harman, *Age, 1*:143 (1978).

177. J. R. Walton and L. Packer, in *Vitamin E, A Comprehensive Treatise*, L. J. Machlin (Ed.). Marcel Dekker, New York, 1980, p. 495.

177a. J. B. Blumberg and S. N. Meydani, in *Nutrition and Aging*, M. L. Hutchinson and H. N. Munro (Eds.). Academic Press, Orlando, FL, 1986, p. 85.

178. D. Harman, *Age, 3*:64 (1980).

179. A. Blackett and D. A. Hall, *Gerontology, 27*:133 (1981).

180. M. Kahn and H. E. Enesco, *Age, 4*:109 (1981).

181. H. E. Enesco and C. Verdone-Smith, *Exp. Gerontol, 15*:335 (1980).

182. J.E. Enstrom and L. Pauling, *Proc. Natl. Acad. Sci. USA, 79*:6023 (1982).

183. D. C. H. McBrien and T. F. Slater (Eds.), *Free Radicals, Lipid Peroxidation and Cancer*. Academic Press, New York, 1982.

184. W. J. Mergens and H. N. Bhagavan, in *Nutrition and Cancer Prevention: The Role of Micronutrients*, T. E. Moon and M. Micozzi (Eds.). Marcel Dekker, New York, 1989, p. 305.

185. R. W. Swick and C. A. Bauman, *Cancer Res., 11*:948 (1951).

186. P. S. Brady, L. J. Brady, and D. E. Ullrey, *J. Nutr., 109*:1103 (1979).

187. K. J. Davies, A. T. Quintanilha, G. A. Brooks, and L. Packer, *Biochem. Biophys. Res. Commun., 107*:1198 (1982).

188. K. M. Aikawa, A. T. Quintanilha, B. O. deLumen, G. A. Brooks, and L. Packer, *Bioscience Reports, 4*:253 (1984).

189. J. Pincemail, C. Deby, G. Camus, F. Pirnay, R. Bouchez, L. Massaux, and R. Goutier, *Eur. J. Appl. Physiol., 57*:189 (1988).

190. C. J. Dillard, R. E. Litov, W. M. Savin, E. E. Dumelin, and A. L. Tappel, *J. Appl. Physiol., 45*:927 (1978).

191. I. Simon-Schnass, H. Pabst, and K. M. Hengkoffer, *Deutsche Zeit. für Sportmedizin, 38*:200 (1987).

192. H. P. Ehrlich, H. Tarver, and T. K. Hunt, *Ann. Surg., 175*:235 (1972).

193. J. E. Kim and G. Shklar, *J. Periodontal, 54*:305 (1983).

194. A. S. Melkumian, E. L. Tumanian, and M. I. Aghajamov, *Zhurnal. Eksperimental Klinicheskoi Meditsing, 18*:52 (1978).

195. D. Djerassi, L. J. Machlin, and C. Nocka, *Drug and Cosmetic Industry*, January:29–34 (1986).

196. J. Marks, *Vitam. Horm., 20*:573 (1962).

197. K. Haeger, *Ann. N.Y. Acad. Sci., 393*:369 (1982).

198. A. Bendich, in *Nutrition and Immunology*, R. K. Chandra (Ed.). Alan Liss, New York, 1988, pp. 125–147.

199. G. O. Till, J. R. Hatherhill, W. W. Tourtellotte, M. J. Lutz, and P. A. Ward, *Am. J. Pathol, 119*:376 (1985).

200. E. Skopinska-Rozewska, A. Blaim, B. Wlodarska, M. Olszewski, B. Galazka, *Arch. Immunol. et Therap. Exp., 35*:207 (1987).

201. R. L. Baehner, L. A. Boxer, J. M. Allen, and J. Davies, *Blood, 50*:327 (1977).

202. M. Chavance, B. Hecketh, J. Mikstacki, C. Fournier, G. Vernher, and C. Janot, *Brit. Med. J., 291*:1348 (1985).

203. S. Meydani, *Ann. N.Y. Acad. Sci., 570*:283 (1989).

204. E. A. Rachmilewitz, A. Shifter, and I. Kahane, *Am. J. Clin. Nutr., 32*:1850 (1979).

205. C. Natta and L. J. Machlin, *Am. J. Clin. Nutr., 33*:968 (1980).

206. L. M. Corash, M. Sheetz, J. G. Bieri, C. Bartsocas, S. Moses, N. Barban, and J. D. Schulman, *Ann. N.Y. Acad. Sci., 393*:348.

207. R. S. London, G. S. Sundarem, L. Murphy, and P. J. Goldstein, *J. Am. Coll. Nutrition, 2*:115 (1983).

208. M. J. Stampfer, J. A. Jakobowski, D. Faigel, R. Vallancourt, and D. Deykin, *Am. J. Clin. Nutr., 47*:700 (1988).

209. P. C. Huijgens, A. M. VanDenBerg, L. M. Imandt, and M. M. Langenhuijsen, *Acta. Haemot., 65*:217 (1981).

210. J. Jandak, M. Steiner, and P. D. Richardson, *Thrombosis Res., 49*:393 (1988).

211. A. Szczeklik, R. J. Gryglewski, D. Domagala, D. Dworski, and M. Basista, *Thrombosis and Haemostosis, 54*:425 (1985).

212. L. Colette, N. Pares-Herbute, L. H. Monnier, and E. Cartry, *Am. J. Clin. Nutr., 47*:256 (1988).

213. D. Steinberg, S. Parthasarathy, T. E. Carew, J. C. Khoo, and J. L. Witzum, *New Engl. J. Med., 320*:915 (1989).

214. G. Bittolo-Bon, G. Cazzolato, M. Saccardi, P. Avogaro, in *Clinical and Nutritional Aspects of Vitamin E*, O. Hayaishi and M. Mino (Eds.). Elsevier Science Pub. P.V., Amsterdam, 1987, pp. 109–120.

215. H. Esterbauer, *Ann. N.Y. Acad. Sci., 570*:254 (1989).

216. N. C. Cavarocchi, M. D. England, J. F. O'Brien, E. Solis, P. Russo, H. Schaff, T. A. Orszulak, J. R. Pluth, and M. P. Kane, *J. Surg. Res., 40*:419 (1986).

217. J. Pincemail, *Ann. N.Y. Acad. Sci., 570*:501 (1989).

218. F. Gey and P. Puska, *Ann. N.Y. Acad. Sci., 570*:268 (1989).

219. T. Yoshikawa, Y. Furukawa, M. Murakami, K. Watanabe, and M. Kondo, *Thromb. Haemostas.*, *48*:235 (1982).
220. P. H. Chan, in *Cellular Antioxidant Defense Mechanisms*, Vol. III, C. K. Chow (Ed.). CRC Press Inc, Boca Raton, FL, 1988, pp. 89–110.
221. M. Kibata, Y. Shimizu, K. Miyake, K. Shoji, K. Miyahara, Y. Masu, and I. Kimura, in *Tocopherol, Oxygen and Biomembranes*, C. deDuve and O. Haiyaishi (Eds.). Elsevier, North Holland Biomedical Press, New York, 1978, pp. 283–295.
222. Y. Kato, H. Sano, V. K. Jain, K. Katada, Y. Kamei, T. Asai, M. Abe, and T. Kanno, in *Clinical and Nutritional Aspects of Vitamin E*, O. Haiyaishi and M. Mino (Eds.). Elsevier Science Pub, New York, 1987, pp. 363–366.
223. J. D. Grimes, M. N. Hassan, and J. H. Thaker, *Prog. Neuro-Psychopharmacol. and Biol. Psychiat.*, *12*:165 (1988).
224. L. I. Golbe, T. M. Farrell, and P. H. Davis, *Arch. Neurol.*, *45*:1350, (1988).
225. C. M. Tanner, J. A. Cohen, B. C. Summerville, and C. G. Goetz, *Ann. Neurol.*, *23*:224 (1988).
226. S. Fahn, *Arch. Neurol.*, *45*:810 (1988).
227. S. Factor and W. S. Weiner, *Ann. N.Y. Acad. Sci.*, *570*:441 (1989).
228. S. Fahn, *Ann. N.Y. Acad. Sci.*, *570*:186 (1989).
229. L. J. Machlin, *Nutrition*, pp. 51–54 (1987).
230. P. F. Jacques, L. T. Chylack, R. B. McGandy, and S. C. Hartz, *Arch. Opthalmol.*, *106*:337 (1988).
231. J. M. D. Robertson and J.R. Trevithick, *Ann. N.Y. Acad. Sci.*, in press, 1989.
232. Anon., Evaluations of the health aspects of tocopherols and α-tocopheryl acetate as food ingredients. Report No. PB 262 653 prepared for the FDA by the Federation of American Societies for Experimental Biology, Bethesda, MD, 1975.
233. A. Bendich and L. Machlin, *Am. J. Clin. Nutr.*, *48*:612 (1988).
234. W. Haenzel, et al., *Int. J. Cancer Res.*, *36*:43 (1985).
235. P. K. Heinonen et al., Arch. Gynecol., 237:37 (1985).
236. P. Knekt, et al., *Am. J. Epidemiol.*, *127*:28 (1988).
237. F. J. Kok, et al., *N. Engl. J. Med.*, *316*:1416 (1987).
238. M. S. Menkes, et al., *N. Engl. J. Med.*, *315*:1250 (1986).
239. H. Miyamoto, et al., *Cancer*, *60*:1159 (1987).
240. A. M. Y. Nomura, et al., *Cancer Res.*, *45*:2369 (1985).
241. H. B. Staehlin, et al., *J. Natl. Cancer Inst.*, *73*:1463 (1984).
242. N. J. Wald, et al., *Br. J. Cancer*, *49*:321 (1984).
243. N. J. Wald, et al., *Br. J. Cancer*, *56*:69 (1987).
244. W. Willett, et al., *N. Engl. J. Med.*, *310*:430 (1984).
245. J. T. Salonen, et al., *Br. Med. J.* *290*:417–420 (1985).

4
Vitamin K

J. W. Suttie

College of Agricultural and Life Sciences
University of Wisconsin at Madison
Madison, Wisconsin

I. HISTORY

The discovery of vitamin K was the result of a series of experiments by Henrik Dam on the possible essential role of cholesterol in the diet of the chick. Dam (1) noted that chicks ingesting diets that had been extracted with nonpolar solvents to remove the sterols developed subdural or muscular hemorrhages and that blood taken from these animals clotted slowly. The disease was subsequently observed by McFarlene et al. (2), who described a clotting defect seen when chicks were fed ether-extracted fish or meat meal, and also by Holst and Halbrook (3). Studies in a number of laboratories soon demonstrated that this disease could not be cured by the administration of any of the known vitamins or other known physiologically active lipids. Dam continued to study the distribution and lipid solubility of the active component in vegetable and animal sources and in 1935 proposed (4,5) that the antihermorrhagic vitamin of the chick was a new fat-soluble vitamin, which he called vitamin K. Not only was K the first letter of the alphabet that was not used to described an existing or postulated vitamin activity at that time, but it was also the first letter of the German word *Koagulation*. Dam's reported discovery of a new vitamin was followed by an independent report of Almquist and Stokstad (6,7), describing their success in curing the hemorrhagic disease with ether extracts of alfalfa and clearly pointing out that microbial action in fish meal and bran preparations could lead to the development of antihemorrhagic activity.

The only plasma proteins involved in blood coagulation that were clearly defined at that time were prothrombin and fibrinogen, and Dam et al. (8) succeeded in preparing a crude plasma prothrombin fraction and demonstrating that its activity was decreased when it was obtained from vitamin K–deficient chick plasma. At about the same period of time, the hemorrhagic condition resulting from obstructive jaundice or biliary problems was shown to be due to poor utilization of vitamin K by these patients, and the bleeding episodes were attributed to a lack of plasma prothrombin. The prothrombin assays used at that time were not specific for prothrombin, and it was widely believed that the defect in the plasma of animals fed vitamin K–deficient diets was due solely to a lack of prothrombin. A real understanding of the various factors involved in regulating the generation of thrombin from prothrombin did not begin until the mid-1950s, and during the next 10 years, factors VII, IX, and X were discovered and shown to be dependent on vitamin K for their synthesis.

A number of groups were involved in the attempts to isolate and characterize this new vitamin, and Dam's collaboration with Karrer of the University of Zurich resulted in the isolation of the vitamin from alfalfa as a yellow oil. Subsequent studies soon established that the active principle was a quinone and vitamin K_1 was characterized as 2-methyl-3-phytyl-1,4-naphthoquinone (9) and synthesized by Doisy's group in St. Louis. Their identification was confirmed by independent synthesis of this compound by Karrer et al. (10), Almquist and Klose (11), and Fieser (12). The Doisy group also isolated a form of the vitamin from putrified fish meal, which in contrast to the oil isolated from alfalfa was a crystalline product. Subsequent studies demonstrated that this compound, called vitamin K_2, contained an unsaturated side chain at the 3 position of the naphthoquinone ring. Early investigators recognized that sources of the vitamin, such as putrified fish meal, contained a number of different vitamins of the K_2 series with differing cabin-length polyprenyl groups at the 3 position. Early observations suggested that the alkylated forms of vitamin K could be formed in animal tissues from the parent compound, menadione. This was not definitely established until Martius and Esser (13) demonstrated that they could isolate a radioactive polyprenylated form of the vitamin from tissues of rats fed radioactive menadione. Much of the early history of the discovery of vitamin K has been reviewed by Almquist (14), and Almquist (15), Dam (16), and Doisy et al. (17) reviewed the literature in this field shortly after the discovery of the vitamin.

II. CHEMISTRY

A. Isolation

Vitamin K can be isolated from biological material by standard methods used to obtain physiologically active lipids. The isolation is always complicated by the small amount of desired product in the initial extracts. Initial extractions are usually made with the use of some type of dehydrating conditions, such as the chloroform-methanol, or by first grinding the wet tissue with anhydrous sodium sulfate and then extracting it with acetone followed by hexane or ether. Large samples (kilogram quantities) of tissues can be extracted with acetone alone, and this extract is partitioned between water and hexane to obtain the crude vitamin. Small samples, such as in vitro incubation mixtures or buffered subcellular fractions, can be effectively extracted by shaking the aqueous suspension with a mixture of isopropanol and hexane. The phases can be separated by centrifugation and the upper layer analyzed directly. Matschiner (18) has also reported that extraction with Claisen's alkali will effectively recover both phylloquinone and the long-chain menaquinones from tissues. This procedure has been very useful in separating and concentrating vitamin K from the bulk lipids during preliminary column fractionation.

Crude nonpolar solvent extracts of tissues contain large amounts of contaminating lipid in addition to the desired vitamin. Further purification and identification of vitamin K in this extract can be facilitated by a preliminary fractionation of the crude lipid extract on hydrated silicic acid (19). A number of the forms of the vitamin can be separated from each other and form other lipids by reversed-phase partition chromatography, as described by Matschiner and Taggart (20). These general procedures appear to extract the majority of vitamin K from tissues. Following separation of the total vitamin K fraction from much of the contaminated lipid, the various forms of the vitamin can be separated by the procedures described in Section III.

B. Structure and Nomenclature

The nomenclature of compounds possessing vitamin K activity has been modified a number of times since the discovery of the vitamin. The nomenclature in general use at the present time is that most recently adopted by the IUPAC-IUB Subcommittee on Nomenclature of Quinones (21). The term *vitamin K* is used as a generic descriptor of 2-methyl-1,4-naphthoquinone (I) and all derivatives of this compound that exhibit an antihemorrhagic activity in animals fed a vitamin K–deficient diet. The compound 2-methyl-3-phytyl-1,4-naphthoquinone (II) is generally called vitamin K_1, or phylloquinone. The USP nomenclature for phylloquinone is phytonadione. The compound first isolated from putrified fish meal and called at that time vitamin K_2 is one of a series of vitamin K compounds with unsaturated side chains, called multiprenylmenaquinones, which are found in animal tissues and bacteria. This particular menaquinone had seven isoprenoid units or 35 carbons in the side chain and was once named vitamin $K_2(35)$ but now is called menaquinone-7 (MK-7) (III). Vitamins of the menaquinone series with up to 13 prenyl groups have been identified, as well as several partially saturated members of this series.

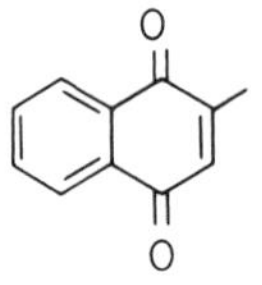

I 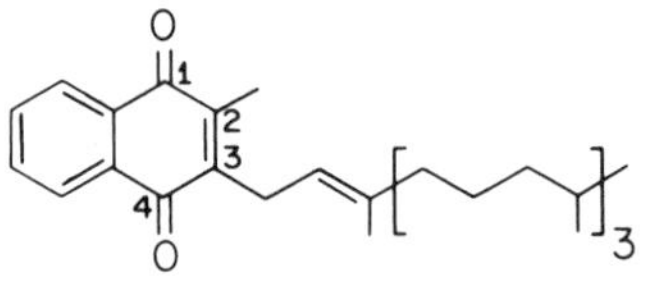   II

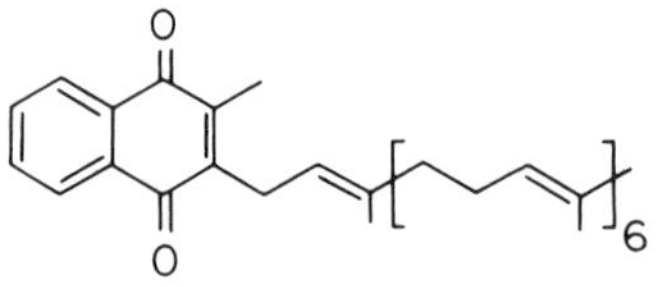

III

The parent compound of the vitamin K series, 2-methyl-1,4-naphthoquinone, has often been called vitamin K_3 but is more commonly and correctly designated as menadione. This nomenclature is summarized in Table 1. Nomenclature in this field has been completed by an attempt of the International Union of Nutrition Sciences (IUNS) to promote the IUNS nomenclature shown in Table 1. These differences have not been resolved, but at the present time most workers in the field see little advantage in a change from the IUPAC nomenclature.

C. Structures of Important Analogs, Commercial Forms, and Antagonists

1. Analogs and Their Biological Activity

Following the discovery of vitamin K, a number of related compounds were synthesized in various laboratories and their biological activity compared with that of the isolated forms. A large number of compounds were synthesized by the Fieser group (22), and data on the biological activity of these and other compounds have been reviewed and summarized elsewhere (23,24). The data from some of the early studies are somewhat difficult to compare because of variations in methods of assay, but a number of generalities were apparent rather early. Although there were early suggestions that menadione (I) might be functioning as a vitamin, it is now usually assumed that the compound is alkylated to a biologically active menaquinone either by intestinal microorganisms or by tissue

Table 1 Comparison of Vitamin K Nomenclature

Chemical name	IUPAC (abbreviation)[a]	IUNS (abbreviation)	Old
2-Methyl-1,4-naphthoquinone (I)	Menadione	Menaquinone	K_3
2-Methyl-3-phytyl-1,4-naphthoquinone (II)	Phylloquinone (K)	Phytylmenaquinone (PMQ)	K_1
2-Methyl-3-multiprenyl-1,4-naphthoquionone (class)	Menaquinone-n (MK-n)	Prenylmenaquinonone-n (MQ)	$K_{2(n)}$
2-Methyl-3-farnesylgeranylgeranyl-1,4-naphthoquinone (III)	Menaquinone-7 (MK-7)	Prenylmenaquinone-7 (MQ-7)	$K_{2(35)}$

[a]The IUPAC nomenclature should be used at the present time.

alkylating enzymes. The range of compounds that can be utilized by animals (or intestinal bacteria) is wide, and compounds such as 2-methyl-4-amino-1-naphthol or 2-methyl-1-naphthol have biological activity similar to that of menadione when fed to animals. Compounds such as the diphosphate, the disulfate, the diacetate, and the dibenzoate of reduced vitamin K series have been prepared, and they have been shown to have full biological activity. Most early studies compared the activities of various compounds with that of menadione. The 2-methyl group is usually considered essential for activity, and alterations at this position, such as the 2-ethyl derivative (IV), result in inactive compounds. This is not due to the inability of the 2-ethyl derivative to be alkylated, as 2-ethyl-3-phytyl-1,4-naphthoquionone is also inactive. There is some evidence from feeding experiments that the methyl group may not be absolutely essential. 2-Phytyl-1,4-naphthoquionone (V) has biological activity, but the available data do not establish that V functions as a biologically active desmethyl phylloquinone rather than being methylated to form phylloquinone.

Studies with substituted 2-methyl-1,4-naphthoquinones have revealed that polyisoprenoid side chains are the most effective substituents at the 3 position. The biological activity of phylloquinone, 2-methyl-3-phytyl-1,4-naphthoquinone (II), is reduced by saturation of the double bond to form 2-methyl-3-(β, γ-dihydrophytyl)-1,4-naphthoquinone (VI). This compound is, however, considerably more active than 2-methyl-3-octadecyl-1,4-naphthoquinone (VII), which has an unbranched alkyl side chain of similar size. Natural phylloquinone is the *trans* isomer, and although there has been some confusion in the past, Matschiner and Bell (25) have shown that the *cis* isomer of phylloquionone (VIII) is essentially inactive. The naphthoquinone nucleus cannot be altered appreciably, as methylation to form 2,6-dimethyl-3-phytyl-1,4-naphthoquinone (IX) results in loss of activity, and the

IV   V

VI   VII

VIII   IX

benzoquinone most closely corresponding to phylloquinone, 2,3,5-trimethyl-6-phytyl-1, 4-benzoquinone, has been reported (22) to have no activity. Much of the data on biological activity of these compounds was obtained by the use of an 18-hr oral dose curative test utilizing vitamin K–deficient chickens. This type of assay allows sufficient time for metabolic alterations of the administered form to an active form of the vitamin, and the observations of an antihemorrhage activity of a compound by this assay do not mean that it was in fact substituting for the vitamin at its active site. Activity varies with length of the isoprenoid side chain, and isoprenalogs with three to five isoprenoid groups in either a menaquinone or a phylloquinone-type compound have maximum activity (24) when administered orally. The lack of effectiveness of higher isoprenalogs in this type of assay may be due to the relatively poor absorptions of these compounds. Matschiner and Taggart (26) have shown that when the intracardial injection of vitamin K to deficient rats is used as a criterion, the very high molecular weight isoprenalogs of the menaquinone series are the most active; maximum activity was observed with MK-9 (Table 2).

The activity of various structural analogs of vitamin K in whole-animal assay systems is, of course, a summation of the relative absorption, transport, metabolism, and effectiveness of this compound at the active site as compared with that of the reference compound. In vitro systems to study the action of vitamin K are now available (see Section VII), and these have been used (27–30) to determine the structural requirements for vitamin K activity. The available data suggest that much of the structure-function relationships that have been seen in intact animals are a function of the interaction of the substituent on the 3 position of the vitamin with the microsomal membrane, and that the critical molecualr requirement is for a 2-methyl-3-substituted 1,4-naphthoquinone ring that can be reduced to the hydroquinone. A wide range of hydrophobic residues can be substituted at the 3 position with retention of activity. Both the 3-thioethers and 3-O-ethers of menadione are active compounds if the group attached is hydrophobic, and a number of nonisoprenoid substituents have appreciable activity. The des-methyl or *cis* analogs of vitamin K have little or no activity in these in vitro systems, and the shorter chain homologs have relatively higher activity than they do in the intact animal.

Table 2 Effect of Route of Administration on Biological Activity[a]

Number of C atoms in side chain	Relative biological activity		
	Phylloquinone series	Menaquinone series	
	Oral (chick)	Oral (chick)	Intracardial (rat)
10	10	15	<2
15	30	40	—
20	100	100	13
25	80	>120	15
30	50	100	170
35	—	70	1700
40	—	68	—
45	—	60	2500
50	—	25	1700

[a]Data are expressed on a molar basis with phylloquinone assigned a value of 100.
Source: From Refs. 24 and 26.

2. Commercial Form of Vitamin K

Only a few forms of the vitamin are commercially important. The major use of vitamin K in the animal industry is in poultry diets. Chicks are very sensitive to vitamin K restriction, and antibiotics that decrease intestinal vitamin synthesis are often added to poultry diets. Supplementation is therefore required to ensure an adequate supply. Phylloquinone is too expensive for this purpose, and different forms of menadione have been used. Menadione itself possesses high biological activity in a deficient chick, but its effectiveness depends on the presence of lipids in the diet to promote absorption. There are also problems of its stability in feed products, and because of this, water-soluble forms are used. Menadione forms a water-soluble sodium bisulfite addition product, menadione sodium bisulfite (MSB) (X), which has been used commercially but which is also somewhat unstable in mixed feeds. In the presence of excess sodium bisulfite, MSB crystallizes as a complex with an additional mole of sodium bisulfite; this complex, known as menadione sodium bisulfite complex (MSBC) (XI), has increased stability and it is widely used in the poultry industry. A third water-soluble compound is a salt formed by the addition of dimethylpyridionol to MSB; it is called menadione pyridionol bisulfite (MPB) (XII). Comparisons of the relative biopotency of these compounds have often been made on the basis

of the weight of the salts rather than on the basis of menadione content, and this has caused some confusion in assessing their value in animal feeds. A number of studies (35–37), however, have indicated that MPB is somewhat more effective in chick rations than in MSBC. This form of the vitamin has also been demonstrated to be effective in swine rations (38).

The clinical use of vitamin K is largely limited to two forms. A water-soluble form of menadione, menadiol sodium diphosphate, which is sold as Kappadione or Synkayvite, is still used in some circumstances, but the danger of hyperbilirubinemia associated with menadione usage (see Section XI) had led to the use of phylloquinone as the desired form of the vitamin. Phylloquinone (USP phytonadione) is sold as AquaMEPHYTON, Konakion, Mephyton, and Mono-Kay.

3. Antagonists of Vitamin Action

The history of the discovery of the first antagonists of vitamin K, the coumarin derivatives, has been documented and discussed by Link (39). A hemorrhagic disease of cattle, traced to the consumption of improperly cured sweet clover hay, was described in Canada and the American Midwest in the 1920s. If serious hemorrhages did not develop, animals could be aided by transfusion with whole blood from healthy animals, and by the early 1930s, it was established that the cause of the prolonged clotting times was a decrease in the concentration of prothrombin in the blood. The compound present in spoiled sweet clover that was responsible for this disease had been studied by a number of investigators but was finally isolated and characterized as 3,3′-methyl-bis-(4-hydroxycoumarin) by Link's group (40,41) during the period from 1933 to 1941 and was called dicumarol (XIII). Dicumarol was successfully used as a clinical agent for anticoagulant therapy in some early studies, and a large number of substituted 4-hydroxycoumarins were synthesized both in Link's laboratory and elsewhere. The most successful of the both clinically for long-term lowering of the vitamin K–dependent clotting factors and subsequently as a rodenticide, have been warfarin, 3-(α-acetonylbenzyl)-4-hydroxycoumarin (XIV), or its sodium salt; Marcumar, 3-(1-phenylpropyl)-4-hydroxycoumarin (XV); and Tromexan, 3,3′-carboxymethylene-bis-(4-hydroxycoumarin) ethyl ester (XVI). The various drugs that have

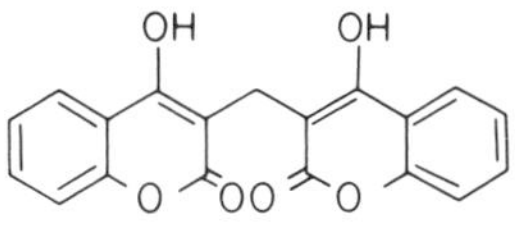

XIII

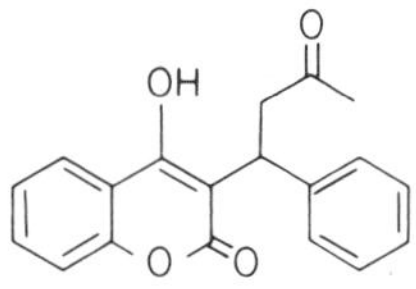

XIV

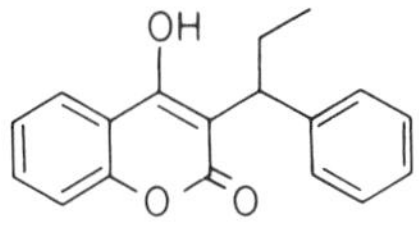

XV

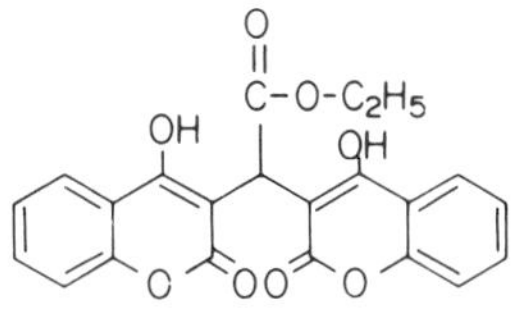

XVI

been used differ in the degree to which they are absorbed from the intestine, in their plasma half-life, and presumably in their effectiveness as a vitamin K antagonist in the active site. Because of this, their clinical use differs. Much of the information on the structure-activity relationships of the 4-hydroxycoumarins has been reviewed by Renk and Stoll (37). These drugs are synthetic compounds, and although the clinically used compound is the racemic mixture, studies of the two optical isomers of warfarin have shown that they differ both in their effectiveness as anticoagulants and in the influence of other drugs on their metabolism. The clinical use of these compounds and many of their pharmacodynamic interactions have recently been reviewed by O'Reilly (38).

Warfarin is widely used as a rodenticide, and concern has been expressed in recent years because of the identification of anticoagulant-resistant rat populations. These were first observed in northern Europe (39) and subsequently in the United States (40). Resistance is now a significant problem in both North America (41) and Europe (42), and concern over the spread of resistance has led to the synthesis of new, more effective, coumarin derivatives. Two of the most promising appear to be 3-(3-p-diphenyl-1,2,3,4-tetrahydronaphth-1-yl)-4-hydroxycoumarin, Difenacoum (XVII) and 3-(3-[4′-bromobiphenyl-4-yl]-1,2,3,4-tetrahydronaphth-1-yl)-4 hydroxycoumarin, Bromodifenacoum (XVIII). The genetics

XVII   XVIII

of resistance and the differences between various resistant strains are now better understood (43), and it appears that the problems can be brought under control.

A second class of chemical compounds having anticoagulant activity that can be reversed by vitamin K administration (44) are the 2-substituted 1,3-indandiones. Many of these compounds also have been synthesized, and two of the more commonly used members of the series have been 2-phenyl-1,3-indandione (XIX) and 2-pivalyl-1,3-indandione (XX).

XIX   XX

These compounds have had some commercial use as rodenticides, but because of the potential for hepatic toxicity (38), they are no longer used clinically. Studies on the mechanism of action of these compounds have not been as extensive as those on the 4-hydroxycoumarins, but the observations that warfarin-resistant rats are also resistant to the indandiones and their effects on vitamin K metabolism (45) suggest that the mechanism of action of the indandiones is similar to that of the 4-hydroxycoumarins.

During the course of a series of investigations into the structural requirements for vitamin K activity, it was shown (46) that replacement of the 2-methyl group of phylloquinones by a chlorine atom to form 2-chloro-3-phytyl-1,4-naphthoquinone (XXI) or by

XXI

a bromine atom to form 2-bromo-3-phytyl-1,4-naphthoquinone resulted in compounds that were potent antagonists of vitamin K. The most active of these two compounds is the chloro derivative (commonly called (chloro-K). Lowenthal (47) has shown that, in contrast to the coumarin and indandione derivatives, Chloro-K acts as if it were a true competitive inhibitor of the vitamin at its active site(s). Because its mechanism of action is distinctly different from that of the commonly used anticoagulants, Chloro-K has been used to probe the mechanism of action of vitamin K, and, as it is an effective anticoagulant in coumarin anticoagulant-resistant rats (48), it has been suggested as a possible rodenticide. Lowenthal's studies of possible agonists and antagonists of vitamin K indicated (49) that, in contrast to earlier reports (22), some of the *para*-benzoquinones do have biological activity. The benzoquinone analog of vitamin K_1, 2,5,6,-trimethyl-3-phytyl-1,4-benzoquinone, was found to have weak vitamin K activity, and 2-chloro-5,6-dimethyl-3-phytyl-1,4-benzoquinone (XXII) is an antagonist of the vitamin. When these compounds were modified to contain shorter isoprenoid side chains at the 3 position, they were neither agonists nor antagonists.

Two compounds that appear to be rather unrelated to either vitamin K or the coumarins and that have anticoagulant activity have recently been described. Marshall (50) has shown that 2,3,5,6-tetrachloro-4-pyridinol (XXIII) has anticoagulant activity, and on the basis of its action in warfarin-resistant rats (45), it would appear that it is functioning as a direct antagonist of the vitamin, as does Chloro-K. A second series of compounds even less structurally related to the vitamin are the 6-substituted imidazole-[4-5-*b*]-pyrimidines. These compounds were described by Bang et al. (51) as antagonists of the vitamin, and the action of 6-chloro-2-trifluoromethylimidazo-[4,5-*b*]-pyrimidine (XXIV) in warfarin-resistant rats (51,52) suggest that they function in the same way as a coumarin or indandione type of compound.

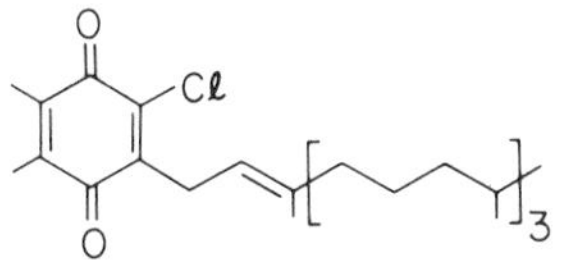

XXII

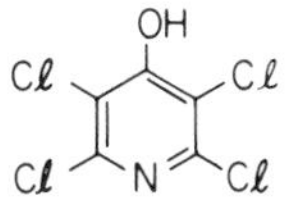

XXIII

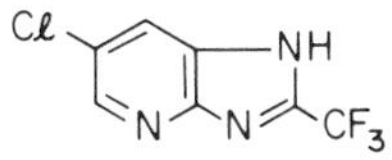

XXIV

A hypoprothrombinemia can also be produced in some species by feeding animals sulfa drugs and antibiotics. There is little evidence that these compounds are doing anything other than decreasing intestinal synthesis of the vitamin by altering the intestinal flora. They should, therefore, not be considered antagonists of the vitamin.

D. Synthesis of Vitamin K

The methods used in the synthesis of vitamin K have remained essentially those originally described by Doisy's group (53), Almquist and Klose (11,54), and Fieser (12,55) in 1939. Those procedures involved the condensation of phytol or its bromide with menadiol or its salt to form the reduced addition compound, which is then oxidized to the quinone. Purification of the desired product from unreacted reagents and side products occurred either at the quinol stage or after oxidation. These reactions have been reviewed in considerable detail, as have methods to produce the specific menaquinones rather than phylloquinonone (56,57). The major side reactions in this general scheme is the formation of the *cis* rather than the *trans* isomer at the Δ^2 position and alkylation at the 2 rather than the 3 position to form the 2-methyl-2-phytyl derivative. The use of monoesters of menadiol and newer acid catalysts for the condensation step (58) is the basis for the general method of industrial preparation used at the present time. More recently, Naruta and Maruyama (59) have described a new method for the synthesis of compounds of the vitamin K series based on the coupling of polyprenyltrimethyltins to menadione. This method is a regio- and stereocontrolled synthesis that gives a high yield of the desired product. It is likely that this method may have particular utility in the synthesis of radiolabeled vitamin K for metabolic studies, as the purification of the desired product appears to be somewhat simpler than with the synthesis currently used.

E. Physical and Chemical Properties

Compounds with vitamin K activity are substituted 1,4-naphthoquinones and, therefore, have the general chemical properties expected of all quinones. The chemistry of quinoids has been reviewed in a book edited by Patai (60), and much of the data on the spectral and other physical characteristics of phylloquinone and the menaquinones have been summarized by Sommer and Kofler (61) and Dunphy and Brodie (62). The oxidized form of the K vitamins exhibits an ultraviolet spectrum that is characteristic of the naphthoquinone nucleus, with four distinct peaks between 240 and 280 nm and a less sharp absorption at around 320–330 nm. The extinction coefficient ($E_{1cm}^{1\%}$) decreases with chain length and has been used as a means of determining the length of the side chain. The molar extinction value ϵ for both phylloquinone and the various menaquinones is about 19,000. The absorption spectrum changes drastically upon reduction to the hydroquinone, with an enhancement of the 245 nm peak and disappearance of the 270 nm peak. These compounds also exhibit characteristic infrared and nuclear magnetic resonance absorption spectra that are again largely those of the naphthoquinone ring. Nuclear magnetic resonance analysis of phylloquinone has been used to establish firmly that natural phylloquinone is the *trans* isomer and can be used to establish the *cis-trans* ratio in synthetic mixtures of the vitamin. Mass spectroscopy has been useful in determining the length of the side chain and the degree of saturation of vitamins of the menaquinone series isolated from natural sources. The ultraviolet, infrared, nuclear magnetic resonance, and mass fragmentation spectra of phylloquinone are shown in Figure 1. Phylloquinone is an oil at room temperature; the various menaquinones can easily be crystallized from organic solvents and have melting points from 35 to 60 °C, depending on the length of the isoprenoid chain.

III. ANALYTICAL PROCEDURES

Vitamin K can be analyzed by a variety of color reactions or by direct spectroscopy (61,62). The chemical reactivity is a function of the naphthoquinone nucleus, and other quinones, as would be expected, also react with many of the colorimetric assays that have been described. The number of interfering substances present in crude extracts is such that a significant amount of separation is often required before ultraviolet absorption spectra can be used during isolation of vitamin K. It is possible to overcome many problems caused by this interference by measuring the difference between the oxidized and reduced form of the vitamin (63). Spectrographic methods are useful for extracts containing large amounts of the vitamin, such as those obtained from bacterial cultures, but are of little value in the determination of the small amount of vitamin present in most natural sources. These determinations have depended on a biological assay, and only recently have attempts been made to develop analytical methods suitable for the small amounts of vitamin K present in most food sources.

Although plant material contains vitamin K in the form of phylloquinone, animal and bacterial sources often contain an extensive mixture of various isoprenalogs of the menaquinone series. Separation of these forms has been accomplished on thin-layer silica gel plates impregnated with either silver nitrate or paraffin (64). A large number of other thin-layer and paper chromatographic systems are available (56,61,62). Some progress has also been made in the separation of various forms of the vitamin by countercurrent distribution and by vapor phase chromatography. All separations involving concentrated extracts of vitamin K should be carried out in subdued light to minimize ultraviolet decomposition of the vitamin. Compounds with vitamin K activity are also sensitive to alkali, but are relatively stable to an oxidizing atmosphere and heat and can be vacuum distilled with little decomposition.

Interest in the metabolism of vitamin K in animal tissues and, in particular, the interconversion of the vitamin and its 2,3-epoxide (see Section VI.D) has led to an increasing emphasis on the use of high-performance liquid chromatography (HPLC) as an analytical tool to investigate vitamin K metabolism. This method was first demonstrated to be applicable to the separation of vitamin K by Williams et al. (65). The general development of HPLC techniques for the quantitation of phylloquinone and menaquinones in biological materials has been reviewed (66), and specific methods will be discussed in sections V and VI.

IV. BIOASSAY PROCEDURES

The classical assay for the vitamin K content of an unknown source was based on determination of the whole blood clotting time of the chick (67). A small amount of material to be assayed was placed in the crop of vitamin K–deficient chicks and the response at 20 hr compared to that of known amounts of vitamin K. When larger amounts of material were available, they were fed for 2 weeks and the degree of vitamin sufficiency compared to known amounts of the vitamin. This assay was improved by utilizing more sensitive plasma clotting factor assays (68,69), and the factors influencing the sensitivity have been discussed (70). The sensitivity of this bioassay can be improved by better standardization of the degree of deficiency (71), and the degree of hypoprothrombinemia of the test chicks has been modified by anticoagulant administration (33,68,69). This modification makes the assay rather insensitive to menadione and other unalkylated forms of the vitamin.

Because of the ease in producing a vitamin K deficiency in this species, chicks have most often been used in biological assays. Intracardial injection of relatively pure forms of the vitamin into vitamin K–deficient rats has also been used (26). All oral bioassay procedures are complicated by the effects of different rates and extents of absorption of the desired nutrients from the various products being assayed. It is likely that they will be largely superseded by HPLC techniques and used in the future only to compare the biological activity of different forms of the vitamin or to investigate nutrient interactions that modify biological activity.

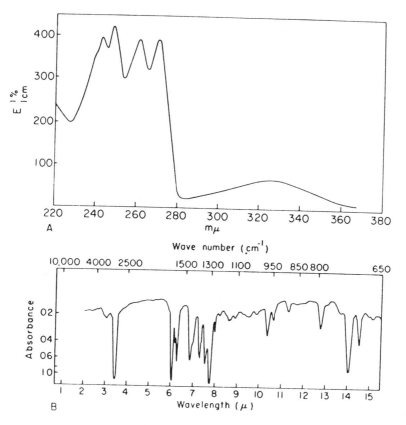

Figure 1 Physical properties of phylloquinone. (A) Ultraviolet absorption specta in petroleum ether. (B) infrared absorption spectra. (C) Nuclear magnetic resonance spectra in CDCl₃ at 60 Mc. (D) Mass fragmentation spectrum of the parent molecular ion is seen at m/e 450.

V. CONTENT IN FOOD

Satisfactory tables of the vitamin K content of various commonly consumed foods are not yet available. Many of the values commonly quoted have apparently been recalculated in an unspecified way from data originally published by Dam's group (72,73) utilizing a chick bioassay that was not intended to be more than qualitative and should not in any sense be used to give absolute values. Another table that is widely quoted (74) also apparently contains data from this source, as well as considerable amounts of unpublished data. A major problem has been the lack of suitable bioassays or chemical assays for the vitamin. Interest in the effects of irradiation for food preservation on nutrient quality has yielded some values for the vitamin K content of meat (69,75,76) and vegetable (77) products Doisy (78), utilizing a chick bioassay, and Shearer et al. (79) and Kodaka et al. (80), utilizing chromatographic procedures, have assayed the vitamin K content of a number of vegetables.

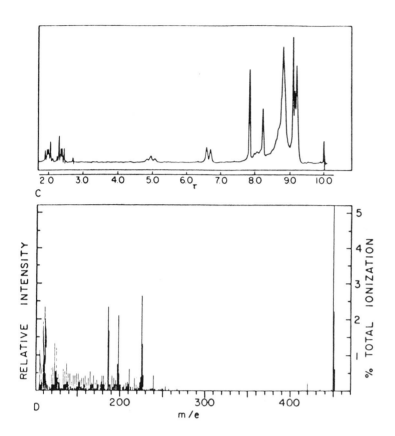

The range of values that has been reported for the same foods is illustrated by the data shown in Table 3. The significant variation observed suggests that reporting a single value for the vitamin K content of different foods gives an erroneous impression of the confidence that should be given such a value. The data in Table 4 have therefore been compiled to give a general indication of the vitamin K content of common foods and to point out relatively good sources of the vitamin. Where possible, values from a number of sources have been considered in compiling Table 4. In general, green and/or leafy vegetables are the best source of the vitamin. Due to the low dietary requirement for vitamin K, most foods contribute a significant amount toward satisfying this requirement, and an uncomplicated deficiency is unlikely.

There are undoubtedly significant changes in the vitamin K content of plants during growth and maturity, but these have not been extensively investigated. The effect of food processing and cooking on vitamin K content has not been carefully considered. Richardson et al. (77) have investigated the effect of heat processing (canning) or of sterilization by ionizing radiation on the vitamin K content of six vegetables. The vitamin K content of these foods, as determined by chick bioassay, did not differ consistently from that of the fresh frozen food, nor did storage of any of the products for 15 months have a significant effect. These data suggest that a general assumption, that vitamin K in food is relatively stable, is warranted, but only limited data are available.

Table 3 Determination of Vitamin K by Bioassay and Chemical Methods

Food	Vitamin K (μg per 100 g fresh)			
	Bioassay		Chemical assay	
	I[a]	II[b]	III[c]	IV[d]
Beans, green	14	22	46	—
Broccoli	200	65	147	—
Cabbage	95	37	110	61
Cauliflower	136	<10	27	—
Carrots	20	—	5	—
Peas	19	—	39	—
Potatoes, white	4	—	<1	—
Spinach	177	130	415	231
Tomato, ripe	11	—	6	—

[a]Doisy (78), chick bioassay of fresh food with phylloquinone as a standard.
[b]Richardson et al. (77) chick bioassay of frozen food with menadione as a standard.
[c]Shearer et al. (79), HPLC assay for phylloquinone.
[d]Seifert (81), gas chromatography assay of phylloquinone; data have been recalculated from dry weight basis.

Interest in the hemorrhagic disease of the newborn has led to a determination of phylloquinone in cow and human milk (83) and in infant formula foods (82–84). Human milk contains only 1–2 ng of phylloquinone/ml (83,85,86), which is somewhat less than that found in cows' milk (83). Infant formulas are currently supplemented with vitamin K, providing a much higher intake than that provided by breastmilk.

VI. METABOLISM

A. Absorption

Vitamin K is absorbed from the intestine into the lymphatic system (87). The absorption of nonpolar lipids, such as vitamin K, depends on their incorporation into mixed micelles, and optimal formation of these micellar structures requires the presence of both bile and pancreatic juice. Shearer et al. (88) have studied the absorption of radioactive phylloquinone in normal subjects and in patients with impaired fat absorption caused by obstructve jaundice, pancreatic insufficiency, or adult celiac disease. Normal subjects were found to excrete less than 20% of a 1 mg dose of phylloquinone in the feces, but as much as 70–80% of the ingested phylloquinone was excreted unaltered in the feces of the diseased patients. Treatment of the disease state was shown to drastically improve phylloquinone absorption. The total amount of radioactivity in the feces of normal subjects was about 50% of that ingested, but most of the activity was due to polar biliary excretion products.

The absorption of various forms of vitamin K has been studied and found to differ significantly. Hollander (89) utilized the inverted rat gut sac to demonstrate uptake of phylloquinone in proximal gut segments but relatively poor uptake from distal segments. This uptake was saturable and inhibited by incubation under N_2 or in the presence of 2,4-dinitrophenol. It was concluded from these studies that ingested phylloquinone was absorbed by an energy-dependent process from the proximal portion of the small intestine.

Table 4 Vitamin K Content of Ordinary Foods[a]

Foods	Vitamin K (μg per 100 g)			
	< 10	10–50	50–100	< 100
Dairy and protein				
Fluid milk	X			
Cheese		X		
Butter		X		
Skeletal meats	X			
Beef liver			X	
Other liver		X		
Eggs		X		
Cereals and cereal products				
Whole corn	X			
Corn oil		X		
Oats		X		
Whole wheat	X			
Bread	X			
Vegetables				
Potatoes	X			
Carrots	X			
Tomatoes	X			
Green beans		X		
Peas		X		
Cabbage			X	
Cauliflower			X	
Broccoli				X
Spinach				X
Lettuce				X
Brussel sprouts				X
Fruits				
Oranges	X			
Peaches	X			
Applesauce	X			
Bananas	X			
Beverages				
Coffee		X		
Green tea				X

[a]Values considered in assigning vitamin K content was taken from Refs. 69,74–79,81,82. Many of the values in Ref. 98 are from unpublished sources, or may be from Dam and Glavind (73) and have therefore been recalculated in a manner not clearly defined.

Subsequent investigations (90,91) utilizing a recirculating perfusion of an isolated gut segment in vivo confirmed these observations and demonstrated that addition of menaquinones or menadione had no influence on phylloquinone absorption. The addition of short- or medium-chain fatty acids to the bile salt micellar perfusate decreased phylloquinone appearance in the lymph, but long-chain unsaturated fatty acids enhanced this process.

In contrast to the active transport of phylloquinone observed in inverted gut sacs, menaquinone-9 was absorbed from the small intestine by a passive noncarrier-mediated process (92). In the colon, where menaquinone concentrations are higher, uptake was also by a passive, nonsaturable process (93). Additional studies of in vivo absorption utilizing isolated ileal or colonic segments have been interpreted as evidence that bacterial mena- quinones can be a significant source of vitamin K for the human (94), although there is some question as to the availability of a sufficient concentration of bile salts for this proc- ess (88). Menadione can be absorbed from both the small intestine and the colon by a passive process (95,96) and can be alkylated to a biologically active form.

B. Transport

The lymphatic system has been demonstrated to be the major route of transport of ab- sorbed phylloquinone from the intestine. There is no evidence that the vitamin in the lymph is in any way modified, and it has been shown (87) that it is associated with chylomicrons. Shearer et al. (97) have demonstrated the association of phylloquinone with serum lipopro- teins, but little is known of the existence of specific carrier proteins. The clearance of an injected dose of radioactive phylloquinone from plasma has been investigated in humans (98,99) and shown to consist of a two-phase exponential decline in radioacitivity. The first phase had a half-life of from 20 to 30 min and the second a half-life of from 120 to 165 min. Although the body pool of vitamin K cannot be calculated from such data, it can be calculated (98) that the total body pool of vitamin K is replaced approximately every 2.5 hr.

C. Plasma Concentrations

The resolution provided by the development of HPLC systems (66) and the increased sen- sitivity provided by newer methods of detection have made it possible to obtain a quan- titative measure of the amount of vitamin K in serum or plasma. The clinical significance of these measurements is not yet fully established, and little information on the relation- ship between dietary intake and serum levels is available. Measurements of endogenous serum phylloquinone concentrations (0.5–2 ng/ml) require a preliminary semi-preparative column to rid the sample of contaminating lipids followed by an analytical column. The chief alterations and improvement in methodology in recent years have been associated with the use of different methods of detection. Early methods (100–102) utilized UV detec- tors which are stable but are relatively insensitive and subject to interference from a number of plasma lipids. Electrochemical detection (103–105) offers increased sensitivity but is unstable and difficult to use in a reductive mode. The reduced form of vitamin K, the naphthohydroquinone, is fluorescent, and increased sensitivity has been achieved by either postcolumn chemical reduction of the vitamin (106–107) or by electrochemical reduction (108). In all cases, the reduced vitamin was detected by fluorescence. Detection of vitamin K with a dual electrode system has also been reported (109).

Methodology is still improving, and the reported mean values from a number of small populations have ranged from 0.3 ng/ml (102) to 2.6 ng/ml (101) for two groups utilizing an electrochemical detector in a reductive mode. In a more extensive study (110), the me- dian serum phylloquinone concentration for 95 subjects was 1.1 ng/ml with a mean value of 1.3 ± 0.64 (SD). More recent studies (111,112) have found fasting levels more in the range of 0.5 ng/ml. From the available data, it is not possible to determine whether or not there have been real differences in the vitamin K intakes of the groups studied or if analytical problems still exist. The lowest values reported have been obtained from subjects following an overnight fast, but little information on the diurenal variation of serum vitamin K or the effect of recent meal ingestion is available.

D. Tissue Deposition and Storage

Early studies of the distribution of dietary vitamin K in tissues were hampered by the low specific radioactivity of the vitamin available. These studies utilized milligram quantities of vitamin K injected into rats and indicated that phylloquinone was specifically concentrated and retained in the liver but that menadione was poorly retained in this organ. Menadione was found to be widely distributed in all tissues and to be very rapidly excreted. The metabolism of more physiological doses of the vitamin has also been studied, and even at low doses (113,114), there are significant differences in the tissue distribution of phylloquinone and a water-soluble form of menadione. Almost 50% of a 10-μg dose of phylloquinone was found in the liver at 3 hr, but only 2% of a 2-μg dose of menadiol diphosphate was localized in this tissue. The major lipophilic product of menadione metabolism formed when low doses of menadione were administered was menaquinone-4 (115,116). Phylloquinone is rapidly concentrated in liver, but after a rapid drop during the first few hours following injection, radioactive phylloquinone was shown (116) to be removed from rat liver with a half-life of about 17 hr. The inability to rapidly develop a vitamin K deficiency in most species is, therefore, not the result of significant storage of the vitamin, Konishi et al. (117) studied vitamin K distribution by the technique of whole-body radiography following administration of radioactive menadione, phylloquinone, or menaquinone-4. They found essentially equal body distribution of phylloquinone and menaquinone-4 at 24 hr following intravenous injection. Radioactive menadione was spread over the whole body much faster than the other two compounds, but the amount retained in the tissues was low. Whole-body radiography also conformed that vitamin K is concentrated by organs other than liver and the highest activity was seen in the adrenal glands, lungs, bone marrow, kidneys, and lymph nodes.

The distribution of vitamin K within the liver has also been determined. Early studies (118) depended on bioassay of isolated fractions of normal liver and indicated that the vitamin was distributed in all subcellular organelles. Bell and Matschiner (119) injected 0.02 or 3 μg of phylloquinone into vitamin K–deficient rats and found that over 50% of the liver radioactivity was recovered in the microsomal fraction and that substantial amounts were found in the mitochondria and cellular debris fractions. Thierry and Suttie (114) studied the specific activity (picomoles vitamin K per milligram protein) of injected radioactive phylloquinone and found that only the mitochondrial and microsomal fractions had a specific activity that was enriched over that of the entire homogenate and that the highest specific activity was in the mitochondrial fraction. A subsequent study (25), utilizing the less biologically active *cis* isomer of phylloquinone, indicated that the largest fraction of liver radioactivity was in the microsomal fraction, but that the mitochondrial fraction had the highest specific activity. Nyquist et al. (120) found the highest specific activity (dpm/mg protein) of radioactive phylloquinone to be in the Golgi and smooth microsomal membrane fractions. Factors influencing intracellular distribution of the vitamin are not well understood, but it is known that the *cis* and *trans* forms of phylloquinone are not handled the same (121) and that the inhibitor chloro-K can influence subcellular distribution (114,122). The vitamin does appear to be lost more rapidly from the cytosol than from membrane fractions as a deficiency develops (123).

Because of the small amounts of vitamin K in animal tissues, it has been difficult to determine which of the vitamers are present in tissue from different species. Martius and his co-workers (124) utilized radioactive menadione to establish that it could be converted to a more lipophilic compound that, on the basis of their limited characterization, appeared to be menaquinone-4. Their data also suggested that intestinal flora or animal tissues can dealkylate lipophilic forms of the vitamin and utilize the menadione released. Because of the limited data available and the demonstration that liver tissue can form menaquinone-4 from menadione, it has often been assumed that this derivative was the major form of the vitamin in animal tissues. The available data, largely from Matschiner's laboratory, have been reviewed by Matschiner (18,125), and they indicate that phylloquinone is found in the liver of those species ingesting plant material and that, in addition to this, menaquinones containing from 6 to 13 prenyl units in the alkyl chain are found in the liver of most species. Some of these long-chain vitamers appear to be partially saturated. It is of interest that menaquinone-4, which is the major metabolite formed when menadione is ingested, has not been identified as a normal liver form of the vitamin. The data in Table 5, therefore, suggest that, in addition to some dietary phylloquinone, the liver of most species contains a number of menaquinones that are presumably of bacterial origin.

E. Metabolism

1. Alkylation of Menadione

Animals cannot synthesize the naphthoquinone ring, and this portion of the vitamin must be furnished in the diet. Bacteria and plants synthesize this aromatic ring system from shikimic acid, and these pathways have recently been reviewed (126,127). It appears that

Table 5   Various Forms of Vitamin K in Liver[a]

| | Species of liver studied | | | | | | |
Vitamin	Beef	Rabbit	Chicken	Pig	Dog	Horse	Human
Total K_1 equivalent							
(μg)	1.2	—	—	0.4	0.6	0.1	0.06
Number of forms found	4	2	2	13	19	1	10
Form identified							
Phylloquinone	X	X	X	X		X	X
MK-4 (H_4)[b]		X	X	X			
MK-6					X[c]		
MK-7				X[c]	X[c]		X
MK-8				X[c]	X[c]		X[c]
MK-9				X[c]	X[c]		X[c]
MK-10	X			X[c]	X[c]		X[c]
MK-11	X				X		X
MK-12	X				X		
MK-13					X		

[a]Adapted from Matschiner (18) and specific references to studies of each species can be found there. The presence of a particular form (indicated by X) does not mean that it represents a significant amount of the total activity, and the original data should be consulted.
[b]2-Methyl-3-δ^6-dehydrophytyl-1,4-naphthoquinone.
[c]Partially saturated forms of these menaquinones were also identified.

bacterial synthesis of menaquinones does not usually proceed through free menadione as an intermediate, but rather 1,4-dihydroxy-2-naphthoic acid is prenylated, decarboxylated, and then methylated to form the menaquinones. The transformation of menadione to menaquinone-4 in animal tissues was first observed by Martius and Esser (13), and Martius subsequently presented evidence that administered phylloquinone or other alkylated forms could be converted to menaquinone-4 (128). It was originally believed that the dealkylation and subsequent realkylation with a geranylgeranyl side chain occurred in the liver, but it was subsequently shown (129) that phylloquinone was not converted to menaquinone-4 unless it was administered orally. This suggested that intestinal bacterial action was required for the dealkylation step. It is, however, probable (124) that some dealkylation does occur in animal tissue and that some interconversion of phylloquinone and menaquinones can occur without bacterial action.

The alkylation of menadione has also been demonstrated in systems in vitro. Martius (130) demonstrated that menadione could be converted to menaquinone-4 by an in vitro incubation of rat or chick liver homogenates with geranylgeranyl pyrophosphate. The activity in chick liver was much higher than that in the rat. Dialameh extended these studies (131,132) and demonstrated that other isoprenoid pyrophosphates could serve as alkyl donors for menaquinone synthesis. There is no evidence that menadione can function as an active form of the vitamin without alkylation, and menaquinone-4 is the major product of menadione alkylation.

2. Metabolic Degradation and Excretion

Menadione metabolism has been studied in both whole animals (133,134) and isolated perfused livers (135). The phosphate, sulfate, and glucuronide of menadiol have been identified in urine and bile, and studies with hepatectomized rats (136) have suggested that extrahepatic metabolism is significant. Early studies of phylloquinone metabolism (137) demonstrated that the major route of excretion was in the feces and that very little unmetabolized phylloquinone was present. Wiss and Gloor (112) observed that the side chains of phylloquinone and menaquinone-4 were shortened by the rat to seven carbon atoms, yielding a carboxylic acid group at the end that cyclized to form a γ-lactone. This lactone was excreted in the urine, presumably as a glucuronic acid conjugate. The metabolism of radioactive phylloquinone has now been studied in humans by Shearer's group (97,99,138). They found that about 20% of an injected dose of either 1 mg or 45 μg of vitamin K was excreted in the urine in 3 days, and that 40–50% was excreted in the feces via the bile. Two different aglycones of phylloquinone were tentatively identified as the 5 and 7 carbon side-chain carboxylic acid derivatives, respectively. It was concluded that the γ-lactone previously identified was an artifact formed by the acidic extraction conditions used in previous studies.

More recent studies of vitamin K metabolism have been conducted after the significance of the 2,3-epoxide of the vitamin (XXV) was discovered. This metabolite, commonly called vitamin K-oxide, was discovered by Matschiner et al. (139), who were investigating an

XXV

observation (119) that warfarin treatment caused a buildup of liver phylloquinone. This increase in radioactive vitamin was shown to be due to the presence of a significant amount of a metabolite more polar than phylloquinone that was isolated and characterized as phylloquinone 2,3-epoxide. Further studies of this compound (140) revealed that abut 10% of the vitamin K in the liver of a normal rat is present as the epoxide and that this can become the predominant form of the vitamin following treatment with coumarin anticoagulants.

As might be expected from the effects of coumarin anticoagulants on tissue metabolism of vitamin K, anticoagulant treatment has a profound effect on vitamin K excretion. A series of investigations (98,99,141–143) has established that the rate of disappearance of radiolabeled vitamin K from the plasma is not significantly altered by coumarin anticoagulant administration. The ratio of plasma vitamin K epoxide to vitamin K does, however, increase drastically under these conditions. Warfarin administration also greatly increases urinary excretion and decreases fecal excretion of phylloquinone (142). The distribution of the various urinary metabolites of phylloquinone is also substantially altered by warfarin administration. The amounts of the two major urinary glucuronides that have tentatively been identified as the conjugates of 2-methyl-3-(5′-carboxy-3′-methyl-2′pentenl)-1,4-naphthoquinone (XXVI) and 2-methyl-3-(3′-carboxy-3′-methylpropyl)-1,4-naphthoquinone (XXVII) are substantially decreased, and three new metabolites appear (141).

XXVI   XXVII

It is likely that there are a number of excretion products of vitamin K that have not yet been identified. Matschiner (125) has fed doubly labeled phylloquinone—a mixture of [6,7-^{3}H]phylloquinone and [^{14}C]phylloquinone-(phytyl-U) with a ^{3}H:^{14}C ratio of 66 to vitamin K–deficient rats and recovered radioactivity in the urine with a ^{3}H:^{14}C ratio of 264. This ratio is higher than would be expected for the excretion of a metabolite with seven carbons remaining in the side chain and is more nearly that expected from the excretion of the metabolite with five carbons remaining in the side chain (138). These data suggest that some more extensively degraded metabolites of phylloquinone are also formed. An exchange of the phytyl side chain of phylloquinone for the tetraisoprenoid chain of menaquinone-4 before degradative metabolism would also be expected to contribute to an increase in the ^{3}H:^{14}C ratio, and current data suggest that this exchange may occur. It is doubtful, however, that this exchange is extensive enough to account for the increased ratio of naphthoquinone ring atoms to side-chain atoms that was observed in this study.

The available data relating to vitamin K metabolism therefore suggest that menadione is rapidly metabolized and excreted and that only a relatively minor portion of this synthetic form of the vitamin gets converted to biologically active menaquinone-4. The degradative metabolism of phylloquinone and the menaquinones is much slower. The major products appear to have been identified, but there may be a number of urinary and biliary products not yet characterized. The ratio of the various metabolites formed is drastically altered by anticoagulant administration. There is, however, no evidence to indicate that the isoprenoid forms of the vitamin must be subjected to any metabolic transformation before they serve as a cofactor for the vitamin K–dependent carboxylases.

VII. BIOCHEMICAL FUNCTION

A. The Vitamin K–Dependent Clotting Factors

Soon after Dam's discovery of a hemorrhagic condition in chicks that could be cured by certain plant extracts, it was demonstrated that the plasma of these chicks contained a decreased concentration of prothrombin. At this time, the complex series of reactions involved in the conversion of circulating fibrinogen to a fibrin clot were poorly understood. A basis for a clear understanding of the role of the multitude of factors involved in coagulation came with the realization (144,145) that many of the proteins involved could be looked at as zymogens that could be activated by a specific protease and that these modified proteins cold in turn activate still other zymogens. This led to the development of a generalized "cascade" or "waterfall" theory of blood coagulation, which has now been shown to be an oversimplification. As shown in Figure 2, the key step is the activation of

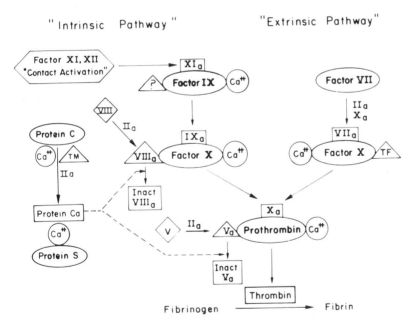

Figure 2 Involvement of vitamin K–dependent clotting factors in coagulation. The vitamin K–dependent proteins (ellipses) circulate as inactive forms of serine proteases until converted to their active (subscript a) forms. These conversions occur in stages where an active protease, a substrate, and a protein cofactor (triangles) form a Ca^{2+}-mediated association with a phospholipid surface. The protein cofactors V and VII are activated by thrombin (II_a) to achieve their full activity. The clotting system is traditionally divided into two pathways: the extrinsic pathway, which involves a tissue factor (TF) in addition to blood components, and an intrinsic pathway, which involves components present in the blood. Protein C is activated by II_a in the presence of an endothelial cell protein called thrombomodulin (TM). Protein C is not a procoagulant but rather functions in a complex with protein S to inactivate V_a and VIII_a.

prothrombin (factor II) to thrombin by the activated form of factor X (factor Xa). Factor X can be activated by two pathways involving the vitamin K–dependent proteins, factor VII, and factor IX. These activations are carried out in a Ca^{2+}/phospholipid dependent manner, and the enzymology of these conversions is now well understood. The four proteins involved in thrombin generation were collectively called the "vitamin K–dependent clotting factors" for 25 years before protein C (146) and protein S (147) were discovered. These two proteins have an anticoagulant role as they are able to inactivate the accessory proteins, factor Va, and factor VIIIa (148). A seventh vitamin K–dependent protein called protein Z has been described, but its function is not known.

A number of incorrect theories to explain the role of vitamin K in prothrombin synthesis have been proposed during the last 50 years. Proposals that the vitamin, or at least a portion of it, was a part of the prothrombin molecule could never be confirmed. Martius postulated (149) that the vitamin had a function in mammalian electron transport, as it does in some bacteria, and that a deficiency would lead to a defect in oxidative phosphorylation and a low cellular ATP level. This would then result in a decrease in the concentration of proteins with a rapid turnover rate, such as prothrombin. This theory could not be substantiated, nor could the postulate (150) that the rate of prothrombin production is regulated by an effect of vitamin K on DNA transcription. Beginning in the middle to late 1960s, investigators centered around two alternative hypotheses: (1) that the vitamin acts at a ribosomal site to regulate the de novo rate of prothrombin synthesis or (2) that it functions postribosomally in a metabolic step that converts a precursor protein that can be produced in the absence of the vitamin to active prothrombin.

The possibility that a precursor protein was involved in the formation of prothrombin was probably first clearly stated by Hemker et al. (151), who noted an abnormal clotting time in plasma from patients receiving anticoagulant therapy and postulated that it was due to the presence of an inactive form of plasma prothrombin in these patients. The rate of appearance of prothrombin in the plasma when vitamin K was administered to severely hypoprothrombinemic rats also suggested the presence of a significant pool of a precursor protein that could be converted to prothrombin following vitamin administration. The lack of sensitivity of this initial prothrombin response to the protein synthesis inhibitor, cycloheximide, strongly suggested that protein synthesis was not involved in the vitamin K–dependent step of prothrombin synthesis. Direct evidence of the presence of a liver precursor protein was obtained when Shah and Suttie (152) demonstrated that the prothrombin produced when hypoprothrombinemic rats were given vitamin K and cycloheximide was not radiolabeled if radioactive amino acids were administered at the same time as the vitamin. These observations were consistent with the presence of a precursor protein pool in the hypopothrombinemic rat that was rapidly being synthesized and that could be converted to prothrombin in a step that did not require protein synthesis. This hypothesis was strengthened by direct observations (153) that the plasma of patients treated with coumarin anticoagulants contained a protein that was antigenically similar to prothrombin but lacked biologial activity. A similar protein was first demonstrated in bovine plasma by Stenflo (154) but it appears (155) to be absent in the plasma of other species that were given anticoagulants.

The identification of this abnormal prothrombin in the plasma of anticoagulant-treated animals led to investigations of the bovine plasma protein that culminated in an understanding of the chemical nature of the postribosomal modification of prothrombin. The initial studies of this protein (156–159) demonstrated that it contained normal thrombin, had the same molecular weight and amino acid composition as normal prothrombin, but did not absorb to insoluble barium salts as did normal prothrombin. This difference, and its altered calcium-dependent electrophoretic and immunochemical properites, suggested a difference in calcium-binding properties of these two proteins that was subsequently demonstrated by direct calcium-binding measurements. The critical difference in the two proteins was the inability of the abnormal protein to bind to calcium ions, which are needed for the phospholipid-stimulated activation by factor X_a (160). These studies of the abnormal prothrombin clearly implicated the calcium-binding region of prothrombin as the vitamin K–dependent region but provided no evidence of the chemical nature of this region. Nelsestuen and Suttie (161) and Stenflo (162) both isolated acidic, Ca^{2+}-binding peptides from a tryptic digest of the fragment 1 region of normal bovine prothrombin. The peptides isolated by these two groups could not be obtained when similar isolation procedures were applied to preparations of abnormal prothrombin. The nature of the vitamin K–dependent modification was elucidated when Stenflo et al. (163) succeeded in isolating an acidic tetrapeptide (residues 6–9 of prothrombin) and demonstrating that the glutamic acid residues of this peptide were modified so that they were present as γ-carboxyglutamic acid (3-amino-1,1,3-propanetricarboxylic acid) residues (Fig. 3). Nelsestuen et al. (164) independently characterized γ-carboxyglutamic acid (Gla) from a dipeptide (residues 33 and 34 of prothrombin), and these characterizations of the modified glutamic acid residues in prothrombin were confirmed by Magnusson et al. (165), who demonstrated that all 10 Glu residues in the first 33 residues of prothrombin are modified in this fashion.

B. Vitamin K–Dependent Carboxylase

After the vitamin K–dependent step in prothrombin synthesis was shown to be the formation of γ-carboxyglutamic acid residues, Esmon et al. (166) demonstrated that the addition of vitamin K and $H^{14}CO_3$ to vitamin K–deficient rat liver microsomal preparations resulted in the fixation of CO_2 into microsomal proteins. It was possible to isolate radioactive prothrombin from this incubation mixture and show that essentially all the incorporated radioactivity was present as γ-carboxyglutamic acid residues in the fragment 1 region of prothrombin. These observations would appear to offer final proof of the biochemical role

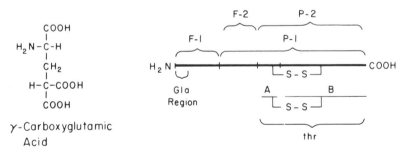

Figure 3   Structure of γ-carboxyglutamic acid (Gla) and a diagramatic representation of the prothrombin molecule. Specific proteolysis of prothrombin by factor X_a and thrombin will cleave prothrombin into the specific large peptides shown: fragment 1 (F-1), fragment 2 (F-2), prethrombin 1 (P-1), prethrombin 2 (P-2), and thrombin (thr). For details of the activation of prothrombin to thrombin and for sequences of vitamin K–dependent proteins, see Ref. 146. The Gla residues in bovine prothrombin are located at residues 7, 8, 15, 17, 20, 21, 26, 27, 30, and 33, and they occupy homologous positions in the other vitamin K–dependent plasma proteins.

of vitamin K as a cofactor for this microsomal glutamyl carboxylase (Fig. 4). Initial studies of the vitamin K–dependent carboxylase (27,28,167,168) were carried out in washed microsomes, where the activity was shown to require the presence of endogenous precursor proteins, O_2, vitamin K, and HCO_3^-. The activity was stimulated by an energy source and factor(s) present in the postmicrosomal supernatant. This supernatant contains pyridine nucleotides and a protein(s) acting as a NAD^+ ($NADP^+$) reductase, and the supernatant requirement can be replaced by the reduced form of vitamin K. The vitamin K–dependent carboxylase activity was soon solubilized (167,169,170) and the solubilized preparation was found to retain the basic requirement for reduced vitamin K and O_2 of the membrane-associated system. The absence of ATP and the presence of an ATP inhibitor did not inhibit the solubilized system, suggesting that the energy to drive the carboxylation comes only from the reoxidation of the reduced vitamin in the system. The available data (171) also indicate that the active species in the carboxylation reaction is CO_2 rather than HCO_3^-.

Early studies of this enzyme system utilized the endogenous microsomal precursors of the vitamin K–dependent proteins as substrates for the reaction. Studies of the mechanism of action of this carboxylase were facilitated by the observation (172) that the pentapeptide Phe-Leu-Gluc-Glu-Val would serve as a substrate for the enzyme, and most recent studies of the system have utilized soluble peptide substrates. The general properties of this system are presented in Table 6. The general properties of this enzyme system are now understood in some detail and have been described in recent reviews (173–176).

Studies of the microsomal vitamin K–dependent carboxylase have not yet led to a clear definition of the molecular role of the vitamin in this reaction. The same microsomal preparations catalyze the conversion of the reduced form of the vitamin to its 2,3-epoxide. Willingham and Matschiner (177) postulated that the formation of the epoxide ("epoxidase" activity) is an obligatory step in the action of the vitamin in promoting prothrombin biosynthesis. The properties of the epoxidase are known in some detail (178), and the relationship between these two reactions has been reviewed (179,180). The reactions are both localized in the rough endoplasmic reticulum (181) and have the same oxygen dependence (182). Epoxidase activity can be stimulated by the presence of a Glu site substrate of the carboxylase (183), but recent evidence (184) has demonstrated that some epoxide formation can occur in the absence of carboxylation.

A critical observation in assessing the role of vitamin K in this reaction was the demonstration by Friedman et al. (185) that removal of a hydrogen from the γ-position of the Glu substrate was vitamin K– and O_2-dependent, but not CO_2-dependent. The stereochemistry of this abstraction has now been determined (186). It is not possible to unequivocally determine if hydrogen abstraction is a radical or ion forming event, but current evidence favors the formation of a carbanion at the γ-position (187,188). Current evidence favors a mechanism for the carboxylation reaction similar to that shown in

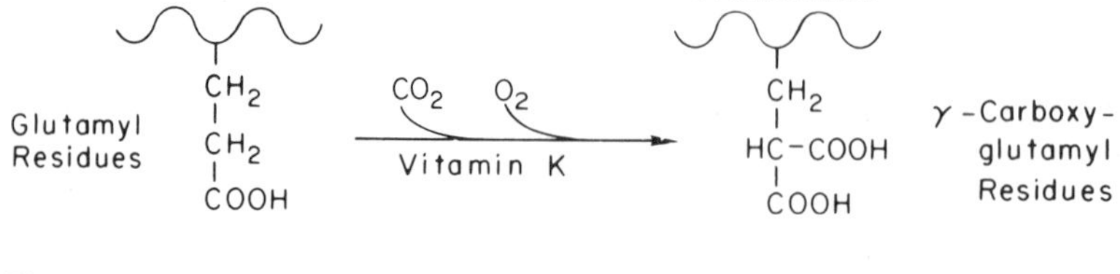

Figure 4 The vitamin K-dependent carboxylation reaction.

Table 6 Properties of the Microsomal Vitamin K–Dependent Carboxylase[a]

Required	Reported inhibitors
Vitamin KH_2 or	Chloro-K
[Vitamin K + NADH]	Tetrachlorphyridinol
O_2	Sulfhydryl poisons
CO_2	Free-radical traps
Stimulatory conditions	Warfarin
Dithiothreitol	KCN
High salt concentrations	Chelating agents
Pyridoxal-P	t-Butyl-OOH
Mn^{2+} salts	GSH-px
	Superoxide dismutase

[a]Stimulation and inhibition of the caboxylase appear to depend on the system and conditions of incubation. There is considerable disagreement as to the effects of some inhibitors (173–176).

Figure 5. Although the available data is consistent with this mechanism, no direct evidence for an oxygenated form of the vitamin is available, and it is likely that an unambiguous role for the vitamin will not be determined until the membrane protein has been purified.

C. Vitamin K–Dependent Proteins in Skeletal Tissues

Hauschka et al. (189) first reported the presence of Gla in the EDTA-soluble proteins of chick bone and demonstrated that it was located in an abundant low molecular weight protein which would bind tightly to $BaSO_4$. Price et al. (190) independently discovered a low molecular weight Gla-containing protein in bovine bone which bound tightly to hydroxyapatite and which inhibited hydroxyapatite formation from saturated solutions of calcium phosphate. This protein was soon sequenced (191) and shown to contain three Gla residues in a 49-residue sequence (MW 5700) that shows no apparent homology to the vitamin K–dependent plasma proteins. These initial reports have led to extensive investigations of the properties and function of this protein, and reviews are available (192,193). This protein has been called either "osteocalcin" or bone Gla protein (BGP), and the terms are used interchangeably by most investigators.

Osteocalcin from various species is very homologous (193), and much of the structure appears to have been conserved during evolution. Calcium ions binds weakly to osteocalcin, but it has been shown (194) that the secondary structure is strongly influenced by calcium concentrations in the physiological range. Microsomal preparations obtained from chick embryo bones carry out the vitamin K–dependent carboxylation reaction (195), and evidence from primary bone cultures (196) indicates that osteocalcin is synthesized in bone rather than accumulating in bone after synthesis in a different organ.

Clear evidence for the physiological role of osteocalcin has been difficult to obtain. Early reports tended to assume some role of the protein in bone mineralization, but evidence to support this type of role has been difficult to obtain. Price and Williamson (197) developed a vitamin K–deficient rat model where animals were maintained by administration of a ratio of Warfarin to vitamin K that prevent hemorrhagic problems but resulted in bone osteocalcin levels only 2% of normal. No defect in bone size, morphology, or mineralization was observed in these animals, and calcium homeostasis was not impaired. Subsequent

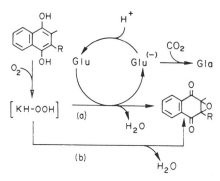

Figure 5 Proposed mechanism for the vitamin K–dependent carboxylase/epoxidase system. The available data strongly support the vitamin K–dependent formation of a carbanion at the γ-position of the Glu residue in a reaction coupled to epoxide formation. This event is followed by carboxylation in a step not involving the vitamin (pathway a). Neither the chemical nature of the proposed oxygenated intermediate nor the mechanism by which hydrogen abstraction is linked to epoxide formation can be determined from the available data. In the absence of a Glu substrate, the enzyme will also carry out an epoxidation reaction not linked to the hydrogen abstraction (pathway b).

studies demonstrated that when rats were maintained on this protocol for 8 rather than 2 months, a mineralization disorder characterized by complete fusion of proximal tibia growth plate and cessation of longitudinal growth was observed. Whether this response is due to a defect in osteocalcin synthesis or the synthesis of a second closely related protein, matrix Gla protein (MGP) (200), is not yet known. These data do suggest that these skeletal vitamin K–dependent proteins are in some manner regulating crystallization of bone mineral.

The active vitamin D metabolite 1,25-dihydroxyvitamin D_3 has been shown (201) to stimulate the formation of osteocalcin by cultured osteosarcoma cells, and the vitamin D metabolites will also increase the level of circulation of osteocalcin in the rat (202). Some relationships between the action of these two fat-soluble vitamins appears to be present, and warfarin administration (203) will influence the degree to which 1,25-dihydroxyvitamin D_3 will mobilize bone from the tibia metaphysis. Osteocalcin has also been shown to evoke a chemotactic response to osteoclast precursors (204), and this response (205) might be related to the ability to mobilize bone.

The discovery that circulating levels of osteocalcin can be measured by a radioimmunoassay has led to investigations of the level of this protein under various physiological conditions. Circulating osteocalcin is four- to fivefold higher in young children than adults and reaches the adult level of 5–7 ng/ml at puberty. Levels are probably slightly higher in males, and a slight but constant increased in circulating osteocalcin in females from the 30–39-year age group up to 90–94-year age group has been found (207). It has been shown that plasma osteocalcin increases in Paget's disease, bone metastasis, renal osteodystrophy, hyperparathyroidism, and osteopenia (208). In general, plasma osteocalcin was increased by diseases characterized by increased resorption and increased bone formation and was highly elevated in Paget's disease.

D. Other Vitamin K–Dependent Proteins

Proteins containing Gla residues have been found in mineralized tissues other than bone (209) and in pathologically calcified tissues (210–212). These proteins have not been extensively characterized, and their relationship to osteocalcin has not always been clarified. A Gla-containing protein has been purified from kidney (213) and shown to be distinct from osteocalcin, but its function has not been established. Proteins of unknown function reported to contain Gla have also been purified from liver mitochondria (214), spermatozoa (215), and urine (216). The presence of Gla in a calcium-binding protein purified from the chick chorioallantoic membrane (217) has not been confirmed (210). Gla-containing proteins are found in the calcified cartilage of elasmobranch species (219) and have been identified in snake venoms (218) and in marine gastropods (219).

These reports of purified or nearly purified proteins containing Gla residues makes it abundantly clear that the action of vitamin K–dependent carboxylase is not limited to the hepatic modification of a few mammalian plasma proteins. The presence of vitamin K–dependent carboxylase activity in various tissues and cultured cells has also been assessed. These efforts have been reviewed (220–222), and they indicate that with the exception of muscle, most mammalian tissues and organs contain significant levels of carboxylase activity. In considering the physiological role of these newly discovered vitamin K–dependent proteins, the widespread use of vitamin K antagonists as clinical anticoagulants should be considered. Large numbers of patients are routinely given sufficient amounts of coumarin anticoagulants to depress vitamin K–dependent clotting factor levels of from 15–35% of normal. It might, therefore, have been expected that a number of problems unrelated to clotting factor synthesis would have been observed in these patients. A number of factors may have contributed to a failure to observe widespread clinical problems associated with an effect on synthesis of other vitamin K–dependent proteins during routine anticoagulant therapy. Vitamin K metabolism in these other tissues may not be as sensitive to coumarin anticoagulants as is that in the liver, or the normal level of these proteins may be in excess of that needed for their physiological function. It may also be that these proteins do not serve an important physiological function at this time and are merely an evolutionary vestige of a once-important functional system.

E. Metabolic Effects of 4-Hydroxycoumarins

Because of their use as clinical anticoagulants, investigations of the mechanism of action of the 4-hydroxycoumarins have been of interest to researchers in the vitamin K field. Although other theories have been proposed (223) and found inadequate to explain the available data, recent investigations have centered on the interconversion of vitamin K and its 2,3-epoxide as the site of coumarin action. Matschiner et al. (139) noted that the ratio of liver vitamin K-oxide to vitamin K increased when rats were given warfarin. They postulated that the epoxide acted as a competitive inhibitor of vitamin K at its site of action and that warfarin was an inhibitor of vitamin K action only to the extent that it increased the cellular ratio of oxide to vitamin through an inhibition of the liver epoxide to reductase activity (224,225). This theory rested on the observation that prothrombin production was blocked when the oxide to vitamin K ratio in the liver was high and observations (45,226–228) that rats with a genetic resistance to warfarin did not respond to warfarin administration by increasing the concentration of the epoxide. Warfarin was always administered to keep this ratio high, and it was difficult to determine if the high epoxide level was responsible for the block in prothrombin production, or if it was merely occurring at the same time. Subsequent studies (229–231), which demonstrated that prothrombin synthesis could occur in the presence of a high epoxide to vitamin K ration, appeared to rule out a role of the epoxide as a direct inhibitor of vitamin K action. They did not, however, invalidate the hypothesis that the inhibition of the epoxide reductase (Figure 6) might be involved in the anticoagulant action of warfarin.

If the liver pool of vitamin K is continually cycling between the epoxide and free vitamin form, a block in the reduction of the epoxide would result in a concentration of vitamin inadequate to drive the carboxylase. The development of in vitro systems to study the action of vitamin K provided additional tools to study the mechanism of action of the coumarins. The activity of the vitamin K–dependent carboxylase in intact microsomes can be influenced by varying ratios of vitamin K and warfarin (168), but the carboxylase activity in microsomes solubilized with detergent Triton X-100 loses much of its warfarin sensitivity (169). This observation was followed up by Whitlon et al. (232), who demonstrated that vitamin K epoxide can serve as a source of vitamin K for the carboxylase activity in intact microsomes if dithiothreitol (DTT) is used as a reductant rather than NAD(P)H. This DTT-stimulated activity is strongly inhibited by warfarin, as is the DTT-dependent epoxide reductase in these preparations. It was shown that the epoxide reductase activity of liver microsomes prepared from rats genetically resistant to warfarin was relatively insensitive to warfarin inhibition. The epoxide reductase activity in these preparations was, however, inhibited by Difenacoum, a coumarin anticoagulant shown to be an effective rodenticide in this strain of rats. These data, and other studies that have recently been reviewed (180) are consistent with the hypothesis that the metabolic effects of these componds are the consequence of their inhibition of the microsomal epoxide reductase and subsequent decreases in vitamin K concentration.

The sensitivity of the other vitamin K–dependent enzymes that might be involved in the anticoagulant response has also been investigated. A survey of these enzymes (233) indicated that the epoxide reductase was the most sensitive site and the most likely site of action of these drugs. The DTT-dependent vitamin K quinone reductase was not assayed in that survey, and its sensitivity to warfarin (234) and its decreased response to warfarin in the warfarin-resistant rat (235) was subsequently demonstrated. It is, therefore, likely as shown in Figure 6 that the effects of 4-hydroxycoumarins involve not only the reduction of vitamin K epoxide to the quinone but also the reduction of the quinone to the hydroquinone. The NADH-dependent quinone reductases are less sensitive to warfarin inhibition and constitute a pathway for vitamin K quinone reduction in the anticoagulant-treated animal (236). The presence of this pathway explains the ability of administered vitamin K to counteract the hemorrhagic condition resulting from a massive dose of warfarin.

VIII. DEFICIENCY SIGNS AND METHODS OF NUTRITIONAL ASSESSMENT

The only currently available method to measure an inadequate intake of vitamin K is to measure the plasma concentration of one of the vitamin K–dependent clotting factors,

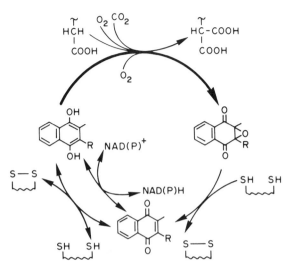

Figure 6 Vitamin K–related activities in rat liver microsomes. Vitamin K epoxide formed in the carboxylation reaction is reduced by a warfarin-sensitive pathway "vitamin K epoxide reductase" that is driven by dithiothreitol (DTT) as a reducing agent in in vitro studies. The quinone form of the vitamin can be reduced to the hydroquinone either by a warfarin-sensitive DTT-driven quinone reductase or by one or more nicotinamide nucleotide-linked quinone reductases which are less sensitive to warfarin. Warfarin and other coumarin anticoagulants do not have a significant effect on the carboxylase/epoxidase activity.

prothrombin (factor II), factor VII, factor IX, or factor X. The various tests of clotting function used in clinical practice have been summarized by Denson and Biggs (237), and the application of some of these as a measure of vitamin K status has been reviewed (238).

Whole-blood clotting times, which were used in early work, are notoriously inaccurate, variable, and insensitive and should not be used. Tests used at present measure the time it takes recalcified citrated or oxalated plasma to form a fibrin clot. The standard "one-stage prothrobin time" assay measures clotting time after the addition of calcium and a lung or brain extract (thromboplastin) preparation to furnish phospholipids and tissue factor. Variations of this assay have been developed, and commercial reagent kits are available. Because of the presence of tissue extract, factor IX is bypassed, and the assay responds to the level of prothrombin and factors VII and X. Of these, factors VII has the shortest half-life, and its concentration decreases earliest when vitamin K action is impaired. It is likely, therefore, that these one-stage prothrombin assays often measure the level of factor VII rather than prothrombin. Specific assays for factors VII and X are also available, but one seldom used in studies of vitamin K sufficiency. The classic assay for prothrombin is a "two-stage" assay in which thrombin is generated from prothrombin in one tube and a sample of this added to fibrinogen in a second tube to measure thrombin concentration. This is a much more tedious procedure, although capable of giving an accurate measurement of the amount of prothrombin in a plasma sample, it has seldom been used for routine assay of vitamin K status. A number of snake venom preparations liberate thrombin from prothromin and have been used (155,239,240) to develop one-stage clotting assays for prothrombin. The enzymes in these preparations do not require that prothrombin be present in a calcium-dependent phospholipid complex for activation, and they will therefore activate the descarboxyprothrombin formed in vitamin K deficient animals. For this reason they cannot be used to monitor a vitamin K deficiency.

All these methods depend on the observation of the formation of a fibrin clot as an end point to assay and are not amenable to automation. The vitamin K–dependent clotting factors are serine proteases, and in recent years, there has been a considerable interest in the development of chromogenic substrates for the assay of these proteins, particularly factor X and prothrombin. These assays, when utilized to assay prothrombin activity, actually measure the concentration of thrombin that has been generated from prothrombin by various methods (239). Because they can be readily adapted to an automated analysis, these substrates are receiving a great deal of attention as clinical tools to follow anticoagulant therapy but have not yet been utilized in any attempt to monitor vitamin K adequacy.

Human vitamin K deficiency results in the secretion into the plasma of partially carboxylated prothrombin molecules. Because these species lack the full complement of γ-carboxyglutamic acid residues, their calcium-binding affinity is altered and they can be separated from normal prothrombin by crossed immuno-electrophoresis (153). This technique has been used to follow the development of vitamin K deficiency. Direct (241) and indirect (242) methods for measuring this species of prothrombin have been described, and antibodies which are specific for these "abnormal" prothrombins have been developed. These can also be used to detect a vitamin K deficiency (243). This method appears to be more sensitive to alterations in vitamin K sufficiency than alterations of prothrombin time and will probably be the method of choice in future investigations. It is likely that vitamin K status is reflected in alterations of circulating levels of the vitamin. The extremely low concentration of vitamin K in plasma has made these measurements very difficult, but HPLC methods for the determination of plasma or serum phylloquinone have recently been developed (see Sect. VI.C). The amount of vitamin K found in "normal" plasma appears to be between 0.5 and 1.0 ng/ml (113), and only a limited amount of information on the response of circulating vitamin K to changes in dietary vitamin K is currently available. No assessment of the concentration of circulating menaquinones has yet been made, but it is likely that further development of this methodology will be of importance in monitoring the human vitamin K requirement.

IX. NUTRITIONAL REQUIREMENT

A. Animals

The establishment of a dietary viatmin K requirement for various species has been difficult. The difficulties involved in demonstrating dietary requirement in many species presumably comes from the varying degrees to which they utilize the large amount of vitamin K synthesized by intestinal bacteria and the degree to which different species practice coprophagy. A spontaneous deficiency of vitamin K was first noted in chicks, and poultry are much more likely to develop symptoms of a dietary deficiency than any other species. It is usually assumed that the site of vitamin K synthesis in the chick is too close to the distal end of the tract to permit absorption, although it is also possible that the rapid rate of passage of material through the chick intestine and the relatively short length of large intestine in this species contribute to the problem.

Ruminal microorganisms synthesize large amounts of vitamin K, and ruminants do not appear to need a source of vitamin in the diet. Deficiencies have, however, been produced in most monogastric species. Estimations of vitamin K requirements by different workers are difficult to compare because of the different forms of the vitamin that were used and different methods that were employed to establish the requirement. Some studies have utilized a curative assay in which animals were first made hypoprothrombinemic by feeding a vitamin K–deficient diet. They were then either injected with the vitamin and prothrombin levels assayed after a few hours or a day, or they were fed diets containing various amounts of the vitamin for a number of days and the response in clotting factor synthesis noted. Preventive or prophylatic assays have also been used, and an attempt made to determine the minimum concentration of the vitamin that must be present in a diet to maintain normal clotting factor levels.

Phylloquinone has often been used in experimental nutrition studies, whereas other forms of vitamin K are usually used in practical rations. Menadione is usually considered to be from 20 to 40% as effective as phylloquinone on a molar basis, but this depends a great deal on the type of assay which is used. It is rather ineffective in a curative assay, where the rate of its alkylation to a menaquinone is probably the rate-limiting factor, but often shows activity nearly equal to phylloquinone in a long-term preventive assay. Practical nutritionists have often preferred to utilize a water-soluble form of menadione, such as menadione sodium bisulfite complex (MSBC). This compound appears to be about as active on a molar basis as phylloquinone in poultry rations, and at least in this species, the activity of menadione, MSBC, and phylloquinone are roughly equal on a weight basis.

Detailed discussions of the vitamin K requirements of various species are available in articles by Scott (244,245), Doisy and Matschiner (115), Griminger (90). The data indicate that the requirement for most species falls in a range of 2–200 μg vitamin K per kilogram body weight per day. The data in Table 7, which have been adopted from a table presented by Griminger (90), give an indication of the magnitude of the requirement for various species. It should be remembered that this requirement can be altered by age, sex, or strain, and that any condition influencing lipid absorption or conditions altering intestinal flora will have an influence of these values (see Sect. X). A considerably higher level of dietary vitamin K has been recommended for most laboratory animals by the National Research Council (246). Recommendations for most species are in the range of 3000 μg/kg of diet, but the rat requirement has been set at 50 μg/kg. This is the level recommended by the American Institute of Nutrition (247) in their purified diet for rats and mice. Subsequent observations (248,249) have indicated that this level is not always adequate and that to ensure sufficient dietary vitamin K for rats the recommended level of vitamin K should be increased to 500 μg menadione per kilogram diet.

B. Humans

The requirement of the adult human for vitamin K is extremely low, and there seems little possibility of a simple dietary deficiency developing in the absence of complicating factors. The low requirement and the relatively high levels of vitamin K found in most diets prevented an accurate assessment of the requirement until recent years. Frick et al. (250) studied the vitamin K requirement of starved intravenously fed debilitated patients given

Table 7 Vitamin K Requirements of Various Species[a]

Species	Daily intake (μg/kg per day)	Dietary concentration (μg/kg diet)
Dog	1.25	60
Pig	5	50
Rhesus monkey	2	60
Rat, male	11–16	100–150
Chicken	80–120	530
Turkey poult	180–270	1200

[a]Data have been summarized from a more extensive table (Ref. 90) and are presented as the amount of vitamin needed to prevent the development of a deficiency. No correction for differences in potency of equal weights of different forms of the vitamin has been made.

antibiotics to decrease intestinal vitamin K synthesis. They determined that 0.1 μg/kg per day was not sufficient to maintain normal prothrombin levels and that 1.5 μg/kg per day was sufficient to prevent any decreases in clotting factor synthesis. Their data indicate that the requirement was of the order of 1 μg/kg per day. Doisy (78) fed a chemically defined diet providing less than 10 μg of vitamin K per day to two normal subjects and was able to deplete prothrobmin concentrations to less than 50% by about 20 weeks. Mineral oil and antibiotics were administered during a portion of this period to decrease vitamin absorption and synthesis. These patients responded to the administration of about 0.5 μg vitamin K per kilogram per day by rapidly restoring clotting activity to normal. It was concluded from this study that about 1 μg vitamin K per kilogram per day was sufficient to maintain normal clotting factor synthesis in the normal adult human. O'Reilly (251) maintained four normal volunteers on a diet containing about 25 μg vitamin K per day and administered antibiotics to decrease intestinal synthesis. Prothrombin activity was maintained in a normal range of from 70 to 100% of normal during a 5-week period, with lower values observed near the end of the study. These data suggest that prothrombin concentrations can be maintained near the low end of the normal range on a diet containing about 0.5 μg vitamin K per kilogram per day. The limited studies available therefore suggest that the vitamin requirement of the human is in the range of 0.5–1.0 μg vitamin K per kilogram per day. A recent study modifying the vitamin K intake of young adults by restriction of foods with a high phylloquinone content (252) has resulted in mild deficiency symptoms and alterations of circulating phylloquinone concentrations. These responses were reversed by additional dietary vitamin, and the data obtained are consistent with a requirement in the range previously suggested.

X. FACTORS INFLUENCING VITAMIN K STATUS AND POSSIBLE GROUPS AT RISK

A. Adult Human Considerations

The human population normally consumes a diet containing a great excess of vitamin K, but a vitamin K–responsible hypoprothrombinemia can sometimes be a clinically significant human problem. O'Reilly (38) has reviewed the potential problem areas and has pointed out the basic fators needed to prevent a vitamin K deficiency: (1) a normal diet containing the vitamin (2) the presence of bile in the intestine, (3) a normal absorptive surface in the small intestine, and (4) a normal liver. Cases of an acquired vitamin K deficiency do, therefore, occur in the adult population, and although relatively rare, they do present a significant problem for some individuals. It has usually been assumed that a general deficiency is not possible, but Hazell and Bloch (253) have observed that a relatively high percentage of an older adult hospital-admitted population has a hypoprothrombinemia that responds to administration of oral vitamin K. The basis for this apparent increase in vitamin K requirement was not determined and was probably multicausal. It has, however, been shown (254) that it is much easier to develop a vitamin K deficiency in older than in young rats. Whether this is related to anything other than an increased intake of nutrients/unit of body weight in the younger animals has not been determined.

B. Hemorrhagic Disease of the Newborn

A hemorrhagic disease of the human newborn has been a long-recognized syndrome (255) and one that appears to be at least in part responsive in vitamin K therapy. The newborn infant has low prothrombin levels, and these normally increase with time. The gut of the newborn is relatively sterile and provides little vitamin K, and many infant formulas, as is human breast milk, are low in vitamin K. The condition is at its worst a few days after birth, and serious problems appear to be associated almost exclusively with breast-fed infants (256). Because of the possibility of hemorrhagic episodes, the American Academy of Pediatrics has recommended (257) that milk-substitute formulas be supplemented with vitamin K or that the infant be supplemented. Current recommendations for breast-fed infants or for infants fed low vitamin K milk substitutes are 1 mg phylloquinone intramuscularly per month (258).

Improvement in methodology has led to a renewed interest in vitamin K nutrition in the infant, and the importance of the low vitamin K intake of breast fed infants to the development of signs of deficiency is now more clearly understood (86,259). Assessment of vitamin K status in infants is complicated by a general hypoprothrombinemia that is not vitamin responsive, which is seen in many infants. This condition is probably due to a general lack of maturity of the liver and an inability of immature liver to synthesize normal levels of clotting factors (260) but has also been ascribed to a heparin-like inhibitor in plasma (261).

C. Effects of Drugs

Early studies (see Ref. 254) of vitamin K action and requirement established the need to prevent coprophagy to produce a vitamin K deficiency in the rat. It is easily demonstrated that the vitamin K requirement of the rat is greatly increased under germ-free conditions (263) and that feeding sulfa drugs increases the vitamin K requirement of the chick (264). The effect of decreased intestinal flora on the vitamin K status of noncoprophagenic animals will depend on the ability of different species to absorb bacterially synthesized vitamin K from the lower intestinal tract. It was assumed at one time that the human absorbed little bacterially synthesized vitamin K and that oral antimicrobial therapy was not a hazard. It is now clear that the most common condition known to result in vitamin K–responsive hemorrhagic events is the patient who has a low dietary intake of vitamin K and is also receiving antibiotics. These cases are numerous and have been reviewed by Savage and Lindenbaum (264). The prevalence of this condition suggests that patients with restricted food intake or on total parenteral nutrition who are also receiving antibiotics should be closely observed for signs of vitamin K deficiency. The second- and third-generation cephalosporins have been implicated in a large number of hypothrombinemic episodes; although it has been suggested that these drugs have a direct effect on the vitamin K–dependent carboxylase (265), it is more likely that they are exerting a weak coumarin-like response (266,267).

A series of recent reports have demonstrated (268,269) that dietary butylated hydroxytoluene causes a hemorrhagic condition in rats that can be cured by vitamin K supplementation. The mechanism by which the effect is mediated has not yet been clarified. Phenobarbital and diphenylhydantoin administration to mothers has been reported (270) to produce a vitamin K–responsive hemorrhage in the newborn, and clofibrate appears to alter coumarin responsiveness (271) through an effect on vitamin K utilization of availability. The nature of these effects has not been extensively investigated.

The widely used coumarin anticoagulants (see Sections II.C and VII.E) effectively antagonize the action of vitamin K and also influence metabolism of the vitamin. Clinically, the effect of this vitamin K antagonism has been thought to be limited to their effect on clotting factor synthesis. The discovery of a vitamin K–dependent bone protein has raised the possibility that the lack of synthesis of this protein is responsible for the "fetal warfarin syndrome," which can develop from coumarin administration during pregnancy (272). Whether this effect is related to the drug antagonisms of vitamin K or if it an unrelated drug effect has not yet been established.

D. Influence of Hormones

Early studies of vitamin K requirements indicated that female rats had higher plasma prothrombin concentrations and a lower vitamin K requirement. Plasma prothrombin levels are also higher in pregnant rats, and this increased concentration of prothrombin in female and pregnant rats results from an effect on rate of synthesis rather than rate of prothrombin degradation (273). Castration of both sexes unifies that vitamin K response, and in the castrated rat, prothrombin concentrations can be increased with estrogens and decreased with androgens (274). There are some indications (123) from studies utilizing [H³] vitamin K_1 that the estrogen effects are related to the amount of vitamin needed in the liver to maintain normal levels of prothrombin. The available evidence suggests that the influence of estrogens on rate of synthesis is reflected in a higher rate of synthesis and accumulation of prothrombin precursors in the microsomes (275,276).

The effect of other hormones on vitamin K metabolism or action is less clear. Nishino (277) has shown that hypophysectomy prevents the estrogen stimulation of prothrombin synthesis in castrated females, and that prolactin injections protect intact males from the development of hypoprothrombinemia. It has also been shown that hypothyroidism in humans results in a decrease in both the rate of synthesis and destruction of the vitamin K–dependent clotting factors (278). It is likely that the effects of these hormones are related to rates of synthesis of the proteins involved rather than to any effect on vitamin K metabolism. But is is possible that there are also effects on the vitamin itself.

E. Other Dietary and Disease State Factors

Early studies of vitamin K functions (279) established that the inclusion of mineral oil in diets prevented its absorption, and mineral oil has often been used in vitamin K–deficient diets. High dietary vitamin A has also been recognized for some time to adversely influence vitamin K action (245). Whether this is a general effect on nonpolar lipid absorption or a specific vitamin K antagonism is not clear, but it can be observed at relatively low dietary levels of retinol acetate and retinoic acid (254). Dietary oxidized squalene also has a potent hemorrhagic effect (254), and a d-α-tocopherol hydroquinone administration has been shown to produce a vitamin K–responsive hemorrhagic syndrome in the pregnant rat (280). High vitamin E consumption may be of some clinical significance, as the addition of vitamin K to the diet of a patient on coumarin anticoagulant therapy has been shown to result in a hemorrhagic episode (281). It is therefore possible that a borderline deficiency of vitamin K might be exacerbated by high vitamin E intakes.

Insufficient assimilation of vitamin K can occur in adults on protracted antibiotic treatment or those receiving long-term parenteral hyperaliminentation without vitamin K supplementation. Malabsorption of vitamin K has also occurred as a result of obstructive jaundice, biliary fistula, pancreatic insufficiency, steatorrhea, or chronic diarrhea. Specific references to observations of vitamin K–responsive hemorrhagic conditions in these various diseases states can be found in Refs. 38 and 264.

XI EFFICACY AND HAZARDS OF PHARMACOLOGICAL DOSES OF VITAMIN K

No hazards attribute to the long-term ingestion of elevated amounts of the natural forms of vitamin K have been reported (282). For treatment of prolonged clotting times when hemorrhage is not a problem, vitamin K can be given orally or parenterally. If given orally to patients with impaired biliary function, bile salts should also be administered. Vitamin K_1 is available as the pure compound or as an aqueous colloidal solution that can be given intramuscularly or intravenously. Some adverse reactions have been noted following intervenous administration (258), and unless a severe hemorrhagic episode is present, intramuscular infection is the recommended route of therapy. Effective therapy requires synthesis of normal clotting factors, and a couple of hours may be necessary before a substantial decrease in clotting times is apparent.

The relative safety of phylloquinone and, presumably, menaquinone does not hold for menadione or its water-soluble derivatives. These compounds can be safely used at low levels to prevent the development of a deficiency but should not be used as a pharmacological treatment for a hemorrhagic condition. Although once prescribed for treatment of the hemorrhagic disease of the newborn, these compounds are known to react with free sulfhydryl groups of various tissues and to cause hemolytic anemia, hyperbilirubinemia, and kernicterus. This marked increase in conjugated bilirubin is extremely toxic to the neonatal brain and has caused death in some instances (282).

REFERENCES

1. H. Dam, Cholesterinstoffwechsel in Hühnereiern and Hünchen. *Biochem. Z. 215*:475–492 (1929).
2. W. D. McFarlane, W. R. Graham, and F. Richardson, The fat-soluble vitamin requirements of the chick. I. The vitamin A and vitamin D content of fish meal and meat meal. *Biochem. J. 25*:358–366 (1931).
3. W. F. Holst and E. R. Halbrook, A "scurvy-like" disease in chicks. *Science 77*:354 (1933).
4. H. Dam. The antihaemorrhagic vitamin of the chick. *Biochem. J. 29*:1273–1285 (1935).
5. H. Dam. The antihaemorrhagic vitamin of the chick. Occurrence and chemical nature. *Nature 135*:652–653 (1935).

6. H. J. Almquist and E. L. R. Stokstad, Dietary haemorrhagic disease in chicks. *Nature* *136*:31(1935).

7. H. J. Almquist and E. L. R. Stokstad, Hemorrhagic chick disease of dietary origin. *J. Biol. Chem. 111*:105–113 (1935).

8. H. Dam, F. Schønheyder, and E. Tage-Hansen, Studies on the mode of action of vitamin K. *Biochem. J. 30*:1075–1079 (1936).

9. D. W. MacCorquodale, L. C. Cheney, S. B. Binkley, W. F. Holcomb, R. W. McKee, S. A. Thayer, and E. A. Doisy, The constitution and synthesis of vitamin K. *J. Biol. Chem. 131*:357–70 (1939).

10. P. Karrer, A. Geiger, R. Legler, R. Rüegger, and H. Salomon, Über die isolierung des α-Phyllochinones (Vitamin K aus Alfalfa) sowie über dessen Entdeckungsgeschechter. *Helv. Chim. Acta 22*:1464–1470 (1939).

11. H. J. Almquist and A. A. Klose, Synthetic and natural antihemorrhagic compounds. *J. Am. Chem. Soc. 61*:2557–2558 (1939).

12. L. F. Fieser, Synthesis of 2-methyl-3-phytyl-1,4-naphthoquinone. *J. Am. Chem. Soc. 61*:2559–2561 (1939).

13. C. Maritous and H. O. Esser. Über die Konstitution des im Tierkorper aus Methyl Naphthochinongelbildenten K-Vitamines. *Biochem Z. 331*:1–9 (1958).

14. H. J. Almquist, The early history of vitamin K. *Am. J. Clin. Nutr. 28*:656–659 (1975).

15. H. J. Almquist, Vitamin K. *Physiol. Rev. 21*:194–216 (1941).

16. H. Dam, Vitamin K, its chemistry and physiology. *Adv. Enzymol. 2*:285–324 (1942).

17. E. A. Doisy, S. B. Binkley, and S. A. Thayer, Vitamin K. *Chem. Rev. 28*:477–517 (1941).

18. J. T. Matschiner, Isolation and identification of vitamin K from animal tissue. In *Symposium Proceedings on the Biochemistry, Assay, and Nutritional Value of Vitamin K and Related Compounds*. Assn. Vitamin Chem., Chicago, 1971, pp. 21–37.

19. J. T. Matschiner, W. V. Taggart, and J. M. Amelotti. The vitamin K content of beef liver, detection of a new form of vitamin K. *Biochemistry 6*:1243–1248 (1967).

20. J. T. Matschiner and W. V. Taggart, Separation of vitamin K and associated lipids by reversed-phase partition column chromatography. *Anal. Biochem. 18*:88–93 (1967).

21. IUPAC-IUB, Commission on Biochemical Nomenclature. Nomenclature of quinones with isoprenoid side chains. *Eur. J. Biochem. 53*:15–18 (1975).

22. L. F. Fieser, M. Tishler, and W. L. Sampson, Vitamin K activity and structure. *J. Biol. Chem. 137*:659–692 (1941).

23. P. Griminger, Biological activity of the various vitamin K forms. *Vitamins and Hormones 24*:605–618 (1966).

24. F. Weber and O. Wiss, Vitamin K group: active compounds and antagonists. In *The Vitamins*, vol. III (W. H. Sebrell and R. S. Harris, eds.). Academic Press, New York, 1971, pp. 457–466.

25. J. T. Matschiner and R. G. Bell, Metabolism and vitamin K activity of *cis* phylloquinone in rats. *J. Nutr. 102*:625–630 (1972).

26. J. T. Matschiner and W. V. Taggart, Bioassay of vitamin K by intracardial injection in deficient adult male rats. *J. Nutr. 94*:57–59 (1968).

27. P. A. Friedman and M. Shia, Some characteristics of a vitamin K-dependent carboxylating system from rat liver microsomes. *Biochem. Biophys. Res. Commun. 70*:647–654 (1976).

28. J. P. Jones, A. Fausto, R. M. Houser, E. J. Cardner, and R. E. Olson, Effect of vitamin K homologues on the conversion of preprothrombin to prothrombin in rat liver microsomes. *Biochem. Biophys. Res. Commun. 72*:589–597 (1976).

29. D. O. Mack, M. Wolfensberger, J-M. Girardot, J. A. Miller, and B. C. Johnson, The carboxylation activity of vitamin K analogs with substitutions at position 2, 3, or 5. *J. Biol. Chem. 254*:2656–2664 (1979).

30. B. C. Johnson, D. O. Mack, R. Delaney, M. R. Wolfensberger, C. Esmon, J. A. Price, E. Suen, and J-M. Girardot, Vitamin K analogs in the study of vitamin K-dependent carboxylation. In *Vitamin K Metabolism and Vitamin K-dependent Proteins* (J. W. Suttie, ed.).

University Park Press, Baltimore, 1980, pp. 455–466.

31. P. Griminger, Relative vitamin K potency of two water-soluble menadione analogues. *Poultry Sci. 44*:211–213 (1965).

32. P. N. Dua and E. J. Day, Vitamin K activity of menadione dimethylpyrimidinol bisulfite in chicks. *Poultry Sci. 45*:94–96 (1966).

33. O. W. Charles, B. C. Dilworth, and E. J. Day, Chick bioassay of vitamin K compounds using dicumarol and pivalyl as anticoagulants. *Poultry Sci. 47*:754–760 (1968).

34. K. P. Link, The discovery of dicumarol and its sequels. *Circulation 19*:97–107 (1959).

35. H. A. Campbell and K. P. Link, Studies on the hemorrhagic sweet clover disease. IV. The isolation and crystallization of the hemorrhagic agent. *J. Biol. Chem. 138*:21–33 (1941).

36. M. A. Stahmann, C. F. Huebner, and K. P. Link, Studies on the hemorrhagic sweet clover disease. V. Identification and synthesis of the hemorrhagic agent. *J. Biol. Chem. 138*:513–527 (1941).

37. E. Renk and W. G. Stoll, Orale Antikoagulantien. *Prog. Drug. Res. 11*:226–355 (1968).

38. R. A. O'Reilly, Vitamin K and the oral anticoagulant drugs. *Ann. Rev. Med. 27*:245–261 (1976).

39. C. M. Boyle, Case of apparent resistance of *Rattus norvegicus* Berkenhout to anticoagulant poisons. *Nature 188*:517 (1960).

40. W. B. Jackson and D. Kaukeinen, Resistance of wild norway rats in North Carolina to warfarin rodenticide. *Science 176*:1343–1344 (1972).

41. W. B. Jackson, A. D. Ashton, and K. Delventhal, Overview of anticoagulant rodenticide usage and resistance. In *Current Advances in Vitamin K Research* (J. W. Suttie, ed.). Elsevier Science Publishers, New York, 1988, pp. 381–388.

42. M. Lund, Detection and monitoring of resistance to anticoagulant rodenticies in populations of brown rats (*Rattus norvegicus*) in Denmark. In *Current Advances in Vitamin K Research* (J. W. Suttie, ed.). Elsevier Science Publishers, New York, 1988, pp. 399–405.

43. J. H. Greaves and P. B. Cullen-Ayres, Genetics of Difenacoum resistance in the rat. In *Current Advances in Vitamin K Research* (J. W. Suttie, ed.). Elsevier Science Publishers, New York, 1988, pp. 389–397.

44. H. Kabat, E. F. Stohlman, and M. I. Smith, Hypoprothrombinemia induced by administration of indandione derivatives. *J. Pharmacol. Exp. Ther. 80*:160–170 (1944).

45. P. Ren, R. E. Laliberte, and R. G. Bell, Effects of warfarin, phenylindanedione, tetrachloropyridinol, and chloro-vitamin K_1 on prothrombin synthesis and vitamin K metabolism in normal and warfarin-resistant rats. *Mol. Pharmacol. 10*:373–380 (1974).

46. J. Lowenthal, J. A. MacFarlene, and K. M. McDonald, The inhibition of the antidotal activity of vitamin K_1 against coumarin anticoagulant drugs by its chloro analogue. *Experentia 16*:428–429 (1960).

47. J. Lowenthal, Vitamin K analogs and mechanisms of action of vitamin K in *The Fat-Soluble Vitamins* (H. F. DeLuca and J. W. Suttie, eds.). University of Wisconsin Press, Madison, 1970, pp. 431–446.

48. J. W. Suttie, Anticoagulant-resistant rats: Possible control by the use of the chloro analog of vitamin K. *Science 180*:741–743 (1973).

49. J. Lowenthal and J. A. MacFarlene, Vitamin K-like and antivitamin K activity of substituted *para*-benzoquinones. *J. Pharmacol. Exp. Therap. 147*:130–138 (1965).

50. F. N. Marshall, Potency and coagulation factor effects of 2,3,5,6-tetrachloropyridinol compared to warfarin and its antagonism by vitamin K. *Proc. Soc. Exp. Biol. Med. 139*:806–810 (1972).

51. N. U. Bang, G. O. P. O'Doherty, and R. D. Barton, Selective suppression of vitamin K-dependent procoagulant synthesis by compounds structurally unrelated to vitamin K. *Clin. Res. 23*:521A (1975).

52. P. A. Friedman and A. E. Griep, *In vitro* inhibition of vitamin K-dependent carboxylation by tetrachloropyridinol and the imidazopyridines. *Biochemistry 19*:3381–3386 (1980).

53. S. B. Binkley, L. C. Cheney, W. F. Holcomb, R. W. McKee, S. A. Thayer, D. W. Mac-Corquodale, and E. A. Doisy, The constitution and synthesis of vitamin K_1. *J. Am. Chem. Soc. 61*:2558–2559 (1939).

54. H. J. Almquist, Vitamin K: Discovery, identification, synthesis, functions. *Fed. Proc. 28*:2687–2689 (1979).

55. L. F. Fieser, Identity of synthetic 2-methyl-3-phytyl-1,4-naphthoquinone and vitamin K_1. *J. Am. Chem. Soc. 61*:2561 (1939).

56. H. Mayer and O. Isler, Vitamin K group—chemistry. In *The Vitamins*, 2nd ed., vol. III (W. H. Sebrell and R. S. Harris, eds.). Academic Press, New York, 1971, pp. 418–443.

57. H. Mayer and O. Isler, Synthesis of vitamins K. In *Methods in Enzymology*, vol. XVIII-C (D. B. McCormick and L. D. Wright, eds.). Academic Press, New York, 1971, pp. 491–547.

58. H. Mayer and O. Isler, Vitamin K group—industrial preparation. In *The Vitamins*, 2nd ed., vol. III (W. H. Sebrell and R. S. Harris, eds.) Academic Press, New York, 1971, pp. 444–445.

59. Y. Naruta and K. Maruyama, Regio- and stereocontrolled polyprenylation of quinones. A new synthetic method of vitamin K series. *Chem. Lett.*:991–884 (1979).

60. S. Patai, The chemistry of the quinoid compounds, Parts 1 and 2. John Wiley and Sons, New York, 1974.

61. P. Sommer and M. Kofler, Physiochemical properties and methods of analysis of phylloquinones, menaquinones, ubiquinones, phostoquinones, menadione, and related compounds. *Vitamins and Hormones 24*:349–399 (1966).

62. P. J. Dunphy and A. F. Brodie, The structure and function of quinones in respiratory metabolism. In *Methods in Enzymology*, vol. XVIII-C (D. B. McCormick and L. D. Wright, eds.). Academic Press, New York, 1971, pp. 407–461.

63. H. Mayer and O. Isler, Isolation of vitamin K. In *Methods in Enzymology*, vol. XVIII-C (D. B. McCormick and L. D. Wright, eds.). Academic Press, New York, 1971, pp. 469–491.

64. J. T. Matschiner and J. M. Amelotti. Characterization of vitamin K from bovine liver *J. Liver Res. 9*:176–179 (1968).

65. R. C. Williams, J. A. Schmidt, and R. A. Henry, Quantitative analysis of fat-soluble vitamins by high-speed liquid chromatography. *J. Chromatog. Sci. 10*:494–501 (1972).

66. M. J. Shearer, High-performance liquid chromatography of K vitamins and their antagonists. In *Advances in Chromatography*, vol. 21 (J. C. Giddings, E. Grushka, J. Cazes, and P. R. Brown, eds.). Marcel Dekker, Inc., New York, 1983, pp. 243–301.

67. H. Dam and E. Søndergaard, The determination of vitamin K. In *The Vitamins*, 2nd ed., vol. VI (P. Gyorgy and W. N. Pearson, eds.). Academic Press, New York, 1967, pp. 245–260.

68. P. Griminger and O. Donis, Potency of vitamin K_1 and two analogs in counteracting the effects of dicumarol and sulfaquinoxaline in the chick. *J. Nutr. 70*:361–368 (1960).

69. J. T. Matschiner and E. A. Doisy, Jr., Bioassay of vitamin K in chicks. *J. Nutr. 90*:97–100 (1966).

70. P. Griminger, Nutritional requirements for vitamin K-animal studies. In *Symposium Proceedings on the Biochemistry, Assay, and Nutritional Value of Vitamin K and Related Compounds*. Assn. Vitamin Chemists, Chicago, 1971, pp. 39–59.

71. H. Weiser and A. W. Kormann, Biopotency of vitamin K. *Int. J. Vitamin Nutr. Res. 53*:143–155 (1983).

72. H. Dam and F. Schønheyder, The occurrence and chemical nature of vitamin K. *Biochem. J. 30*:897–901 (1936).

73. H. Dam and J. Glavind. Vitamin K in the plant. *Biochem. J. 32*:485–487 (1938).

74. R. E. Olson, Vitamin K. In *Modern Nutrition in Health and Disease* (R. S. Goodhart and M. E. Shils, eds.). Lea & Febiger, Philadelphia, 1980, pp. 170–180.

75. M. S. Mameesh, V. C. Metta, P. B. Rama Rao, and B. C. Johnson, On the cause of vitamin K deficiency in male rats fed irradiated beef and the production of vitamin K deficiency using an amino acid synthetic diet. *J. Nutr. 90*:165–170 (1962).

76. J. T. Matschiner and E. A. Doisy, Jr., Vitamin K content of ground beef. *J. Nutr. 90*:331–334 (1966).

77. L. R. Richardson, S. Wilkes, and S. J. Ritchey, Comparative vitamin K activity of frozen, irradiated and heat-processed foods. *J. Nutr. 73*:369–373 (1961).

78. E. A. Doisy, Vitamin K in human nutrition. In *Symposium Proceedings on the Biochemistry, Assay and Nutritional Value of Vitamin K and Related Compounds*. Assn. Vitamin Chemists, Chicago, 1971, pp. 79–92.

79. M. J. Shearer, V. Allan, Y. Haroon, and P. Barkhan, Nutritional aspects of vitamin K in the human. In *Vitamin K Metabolism and Vitamin K-Dependent Proteins* (J. W. Suttie, ed.). University Park Press, Baltimore, 1980, pp. 317–327.

80. K. Kodaka, T. Ujiie, T. Ueno, and M. Saito, Contents of vitamin K_1 and chlorophyll in green vegetables. *J. Jap. Soc. Nutr. Food Sci. 39*:124–126 (1986).

81. R. M. Seifert, Analysis of vitamin K_1 in some green leafy vegetables by gas chromatography. *J. Agric. Food Chem. 27*:1301–1304 (1979)).

82. D. L. Schneider, H. B. Fluckiger, and J. D. Manes, Vitamin K_1 content of infant formula products. *Pediatrics 53*:273–275 (1974).

83. Y. Haroon, M. J. Shearer. S. Rahim. W. G. Gunn, G. McEnery, and P. Barkhan, The content of phylloquinone (vitamin K_1) in human milk, cows' milk and infant formula foods determined by high-perforamnce liquid chromatography. *J. Nutr. 112*:1105–1117 (1982).

84. J. D. Manes, H. B. Fluckiger, and D. L. Schneider, Chromatographic analysis of vitamin K_1; application to infant formula products. *J. Agric. Food Chem. 20*:1130–1132 (1972).

85. L. M. Canfield, G. S. Martin, and K. Sugimoto, Vitamin K in human milk. In *Current Advances in Vitamin K Research* (J. W. Suttie, ed.). Elsevier Science Publishers, New York, 1988, pp. 499–504.

86. R. V. Kries, M. J. Shearer, M. Haug, G. Harzer, and U. Gobel, Vitamin K deficiency and vitamin K intake in infants. In *Current Advances in Vitamin K Research* (J. W. Suttie ed.) Elsevier Science Publishers, New York, 1988, pp. 515–523.

87. R. Blomstrand and L. Forsgren, Vitamin K_1-^{3}H in man. Its intestinal absorption and transport in the thoracic duct lymph. *Int. Z. Vitamin Forschung 38*:46–64 (1968).

88. M. J. Shearer, A. McBurney, and P. Barkhan, Studies on the absorption and metabolism of phylloquinone (vitamin K_1) in man. *Vitamins and Hormones 32*:513–542 (1974).

89. D. Hollander, Vitamin K_1 absorption by everted intestinal sacs of the rat. *Am. J. Physiol. 225*:360–364 (1973).

90. D. Hollander, E. Rim, and K. S. Muralidhara, Vitamin K_1 intestinl absorption in vivo: Influence of luminal contents on transport. *Am. J. Physiol. 232*:E69–E74 (1977).

91. D. Hollander and E. Rim, Effect of luminal constituents on Vitamin K_1 absorption into thoracic duct lymph. *Am. J. Physiol. 234*:E54–E59 (1978).

92. D. Hollander and E. Rim, Vitamin K_2 absorption by rat everted small intestinal sacs. *Am. J. Physiol. 231*:415–419 (1976).

93. D. Hollander, K. S. Muralidhara, and E. Rim, Colonic absorption of bacterially synthesized vitamin K_2 in the rat. *Am. J. Physiol. 230*:251–255 (1976).

94. D. Hollander, E. Rim, and P. E. Ruble, Jr., Vitamin K_2 colonic and ileal *in vivo* absorption: Bile, fatty acids, and pH effects on transport. *Am. J. Physiol. 233*:E124–E129 (1977).

95. D. Hollander and T. C. Truscott, Colonic absorption of vitamin K-3. *J. Lab. Clin. Med. 83*:648–656 (1974).

96. D. Hollander and T. C. Truscott, Mechanism and site of vitamin K-3 small intestinal transport. *Am. J. Physiol. 226*:1526–1522 (1974).

97. M. J. Shearer, P. Barkhan, and G. R. Webster, Absorption and excretion of an oral dose of tritiated vitamin K_1 in man. *Brit. J. Haematol. 18*:297–308 (1970).

98. T. D. Bjornsson, P. J. Meffin, S. E. Swezey, and T. F. Blaschke, Disposition and turnover of vitamin K_1 in man. In *Vitamin K Metabolism and Vitamin K-Dependent Proteins* (J. W. Suttie, ed.). University Park Press, Baltimore, 1980, pp. 328–332.

99. M. J. Shearer, C. N. Mallinson, G. R. Webster, and P. Barkhan, Clearance from plasma and excretion in urine, faeces and bile of an intravenous dose of tritiated vitamin K_1 in man. *Brit. J. Haematol. 22*:579–588 (1972).

100. M. F. LeFevere, A. P. DeLeenheer, and A. E. Claeys, High-performance liquid chromatographic assay of vitamin K in human serum. *J. Chromatog. 186*:749–762 (1979).

101. M. F. LeFevere, A. P. DeLeenheer, A. E. Claeys, I. V. Claeys, and H. Steyaert, Multidimensional liquid chromatography: A breakthrough in the assessment of physiological vitamin K levels. *J. Lipid Res. 23*:1068–1072 (1982).

102. M. J. Shearer, S. Rahim, P. Barkhan, and L. Stimmler, Plasma vitamin K_1 in mothers and their newborn babies. *Lancet 2*:460–463 (1982).

103. S. Ikenoya, K. Abe, T. Tsuda, Y. Yamano, O. Hiroshima, M. Ohmae, and K. Kawabe, Electrochemical detector for high-performance liquid chromatography II. Determination of tocopherols, ubiquinones, and phylloquinone in blood. *Chem. Pharm. Bull. 27*:1237–1244 (1979).

104. T. Ueno and J. W. Suttie, High-pressure liquid chromatographic-electrochemical detection analysis of serum trans-phylloquinone. *Analyt. Biochem. 133*:62–67 (1983).

105. J. P. Hart, M. J. Shearer, P. T. McCarthy, and S. Rahim, Voltammetric behavior of phylloquinone (vitamin K_1) at a glassy-carbon electrode and determination of the vitamin in plasma using high-performance liquid chromatography with electrochemical detection. *Analyst 109*:477–481 (1984).

106. J. P. Langenberg and U. R. Tjaden, Determination of (endogenous) vitamin K_1 in human plasma by reversed-phase high-performance liquid chromatography using fluorometric detection after post-column electrochemical reduction. Comparison with ultraviolet, single and dual electrochemical detection. *J. Chromatog. 305*:61–72 (1984).

107. Y. Haroon, D. S. Bacon, and J. A. Sadowski, Liquid-chromatographic determination of vitamin K_1 in plasma, with fluorometric detection. *Clin. Chem. 32*:1925–1929 (1986).

108. J. P. Langenberg and U. R. Tjaden, Improved method for the determination of vitamin K_1 epoxide in human plasma with electrofluorimetric reaction detection. *J. Chromatog. 289*:377–385 (1984).

109. Y. Haroon, C. A. W. Schubert, and P. V. Hauschka, Liquid chromatographic dual electrode detection system for vitamin K compounds. *J. Chromatog. Sci. 22*:89–93 (1984).

110. L. L. Mummah-Schendel and J. W. Suttie, Serum phylloquinone concentrations in a normal adult population. *Am. J. Clin. Nutr. 44*:686–689 (1986).

111. J. A. Sadowski, D. S. Bacon, S. Hood, K. W. Davidson, C. M. Ganter, Y. Haroon, and D. C. Shepard, The application of methods used for the evolution of vitamin K nutritional status in human and animal studies. In *Current Advances in Vitamin K Research* (J. W. Suttie, ed.). Elsevier Science Publishers, New York, 1988, pp. 453–463.

112. M. J. Shearer, P. T. McCarthy, O. E. Crampton, and M. B. Mattock, The assessment of human vitamin K status for tissue measurements. In *Current Advances in Vitamin K Research* (J. W. Suttie, ed.). Elsevier Science Publishers, New York, 1988, pp. 437–452.

113. M. J. Thierry and J. W. Suttie, Distribution and metabolism of menadiol diphosphate in the rat. *J. Nutr. 97*:512–516 (1969).

114. M. J. Thierry and J. W. Suttie, Effect of warfarin and the chloro analog of vitamin K on phylloquinone metabolism. *Arch. Biochem. Biophys. 147*:430–435 (1971).

115. W. V. Taggart and J. T. Matschiner, Metabolism of menadione-6,7-^{3}H in the rat. *Biochemistry 8*:1141–1146 (1969).

116. M. J. Thierry, M. A. Hermodson, and J. W. Suttie, Vitamin K and warfarin distribution and metabolism in the warfarin-resistant rat. *Am. J. Physiol. 219*:854–859 (1970).

117. T. Konishi, S. Baba, and H. Sone, Whole-body autoradiographic study of vitamin K distribution in rat. *Chem. Pharm. Bull. 21*:220–224 (1973).

118. J. P. Green, E. Søndergaard, and H. Dam, Intracellular distribution of vitamin K in beef liver. *Biochim. Biophys. Acta. 19*:182–183 (1956).

119. R. G. Bell and J. T. Matschiner, Intracellular distribution of vitamin K in the rat. *Biochim. Acta 184*:597–603 (1969).

120. S. E. Nyquist, J. T. Matschiner, and D. J. James Morre, Distribution of vitamin K among rat liver cell fractions. *Biochim. Biophys. Acta 244*:645–649 (1971).

121. T. E. Knauer, C. Siegfried, A. K. Willingham, and J. T. Matschiner, Metabolism and biological activity of *cis*- and *trans*-phylloquinone in the rat. *J. Nutr. 105*:1519–1524 (1975).

122. M. J. Thierry-Palmer, M. S. Stern, C. A. Kost, and J. C. Montgomery, Effect of the chloro analog of vitamin K on phylloquinone metabolism in liver mitochondria. In *Vitamin K Metabolism and Vitamin K–Dependent Proteins* (J. W. Suttie, ed.). University Park Press, Baltimore 1980, pp. 333–336.

123. T. E. Knauer, C. M. Siegfried, and J. T. Matschiner, Vitamin K requirement and the concentration of vitamin K in rat liver. *J. Nutr. 106*:1747–1756 (1976).

124. C. Martius, Chemistry and function of vitamin K. In *Blood Clotting Enzymology* (W. H. Seegers, ed.). Academic Press, New York, 1967, pp. 551–575.

125. J. T. Matschiner, Occurrence and biopotency of various forms of vitamin K. In *The Fat-Soluble Vitamins* (H. F. DeLuca and J. W. Suttie, eds.). University of Wisconsin Press, Madison, 1970, pp. 377–397.

126. R. Bentley, Biosynthesis of vitamin K and other natural naphthoquinones. *Pure Appl. Chem. 41*:47–68 (1975).

127. R. Meganathan, T. Folger, and R. Bentley, Enzymes involved in vitamin K biosynthesis. In *Vitamin K Metabolism and Vitamin K–Dependent Proteins* (J. W. Suttie, ed.). University Park Press, Baltimore, 1980, pp. 188–192.

128. C. Martius, Recent investigations on the chemistry and function of vitamin K. In *Ciba Fdn. Symposium on Quinones in Electron Transport* (G. E. W. Wolstenholme and C. M. O'Connor, eds.). Little, Brown, Boston, 1961, pp. 312–326.

129. M. Billeter, W. Bollinger, and C. Martius, Untersuchungen über die Umwandlung von verfutterten K-Vitaminen durch Austausch der Seitenkette und die Rolle der Darmbakterien hierbei. *Biochem. Z. 340*:290–303 (1964).

130. C. Martius, The metabolic relationships between the different K vitamins and the synthesis of the ubiquinones. *Am. J. Clin. Nutr. 9*:97–103 (1961).

131. G. H. Dialameh, W. V. Taggart, J. T. Matschiner, and R. E. Olson, Isolation and characterization of menaquinone-4 as a product of menadione metabolism in chicks and rats. *Int. J. Vit. Nutr. Res. 41*:391–400 (1971).

132. G. H. Dialameh, Stereobiochemical aspects of warfarin isomers for inhibition of enzymatic alkylation of menaquinone-0 to menaquinone-4 in chick liver. *Int. J. Vit. Nutr. Res. 48*:131–135 (1978).

133. F. C. G. Hoskin, J. W. T. Spinks, and L. B. Jaques, Urinary excretion products of menadione (vitamin K_3). *Can. J. Biochem. Physiol. 32*:240–250 (1954).

134. K. T. Hart, Study of hydrolysis of urinary metabolites of 2-methyl-1,4-naphthoquinone. *Proc. Soc. Exp. Biol. Med. 97*:848–851 (1958).

135. R. Losito, C. A. Owen, Jr., and E. V. Flock, Metabolism of [C^{14}] menadione. *Biochemistry 6*:62–68 (1967).

136. R. Losito, C. A. Owen, Jr., and E. V. Flock, Metabolic studies of vitamin K_1-^{14}C and menadione-^{14}C in the normal and hepatectomized rats. *Thromb. Diath. Haemorrhag. 19*:383–388 (1968).

137. J. D. Taylor, G. J. Miller, L. B. Jaques, and J. W. T. Spinks, The distribution of administered vitamin K_1-^{14}C in rats. *Can. J. Biochem. Physiol. 34*:1143–1152 (1956).

138. M. J. Shearer and P. Barkhan, Studies on the metabolites of phylloquinone (vitamin K_1) in the urine of man. *Biochim. Biophys. Acta 297*:300–312 (1973).

139. J. T. Matschiner, R. G. Bell, J. M. Amelotti, and T. E. Knauer, Isolation and characterization of a new metabolite of phylloquinone in the rat. *Biochim. Biophys. Acta 201*:309–315 (1970).

140. R. G. Bell, J. A. Sadowski, and J. T. Matschiner, Mechanism of action of warfarin. Warfarin and metabolism of vitamin K$_1$. *Biochemistry 11*:1959–1961 (1972).

141. M. J. Shearer, A. McBurney, A. M. Breckenridge, and P. Barkhan, Effect of warfarin on the metabolism of phylloquinone (vitamin K$_1$):Dose-response relationships in man. *Clin. Sci. Mol. Med. 52*:621–630 (1977).

142. M. J. Shearer, A. McBurney, and P. Barkhan, Effect of warfarin anticoagulation on vitamin-K$_1$ metabolism in man. *Brit. J. Haematol. 24*:471–479 (1973).

143. B. K. Park, J. B. Leck, A. C. Wilson, M. J. Serlin, and A. M. Breckenridge, A study of the effect of anticoagulants on [^{3}H] vitamin K$_1$ metabolism and prothrombin complex activity in the rabbit. *Biochem. Pharmacol. 28*:1323–1329 (1979).

144. E. W. Davie and O. D. Ratnoff, Waterfall sequence for intrinsic blood clotting. *Science 145*:1310–1312 (1964).

145. R. G. Macfarlane, Haematology an enzyme cascade in the blood clotting mechanism, and its function as a biochemical amplifier. *Nature 202*:498–499 (1964).

146. J. Stenflo, A new vitamin K-dependent protein. Purification from bovine plasma and preliminary characterization. *J. Biol. Chem. 251*:355–363 (1976).

147. R. G. Di Scipio, M. A. Hermodson, S. G. Yates, and E. W. Davie, A comparison of human prothrombin, factor IX (Christmas Factor), factor X (Stuart Factor), and protein S. *Biochemistry 16*:698–706 (1977).

148. L. H. Clouse and P. C. Comp, The regulation of hemostasis: The protein C system. *New Engl. J. Med. 314*:1298–1304 (1986).

149. C. Martius and D. Nitz-Litzow, Oxydative phosphorylierung und Vitamin K Mangel. *Biochim. Biophys. Acta 13*:152–153 (1954).

150. R. E. Olson, Vitamin K induced prothrombin formation: Antagonism by actinomycin D. *Science 145*:926–928 (1964).

151. H. C. Hemker, J. J. Veltkamp, A. Hensen, and E. A. Loeliger, Nature of prothrombin biosynthesis: Preprothrombinaemia in vitamin K-deficiency. *Nature 200*:589–590 (1963).

152. D. V. Shah and J. W. Suttie, Mechanism of action of vitamin K: Evidence for the conversion of a precursor protein to prothrombin in the rat. *Proc. Natl. Acad. Sci. USA 68*:1653–1657 (1971).

153. P. O. Ganrot and J. E. Nilehn, Plasma Prothrombin during treatment with dicumarol. II. Demonstration of an abnormal prothrombin fraction. *Scand. J. Clin Lab. Invest. 22*:23–28 (1968).

154. J. Stenflo, Dicumarol-induced prothrombin in bovine plasma. *Acta Chem. Scand. 24*:3762–3763 (1970).

155. T. L. Carlisle, D. V. Shah, R. Schlegel, and J. W. Suttie, Plasma abnormal prothrombin and microsomal prothrombin precursor in various species. *Proc. Soc. Exp. Biol. Med. 148*:140–144 (1975).

156. J. Stenflo, Vitamin K and the biosynthesis of prothrombin II. Structural comparison of normal and dicoumarol-induced bovine prothrombin. *J. Biol. Chem. 247*:8167–8175 (1972).

157. J. Stenflo and P. O. Ganrot, Vitamin K and the biosynthesis of prothrombin. I Identification and purification of a dicoumarol-induced abnormal prothrombin for bovine plasma. *J. Biol. Chem. 247*:8160–8166 (1972).

158. G. L. Nelsestuen and J. W. Suttie, Mode of action of vitamin K. Calcium binding properties of bovine prothrombin. *Biochemistry 11*:4961–4964 (1972).

159. G. L. Nelsestuen and J. W. Suttie, The purification and properties of an abnormal prothrombin protein produced by dicoumarol-treated cows. A comparison to normal prothrombin. *J. Biol. Chem. 247*:8176–8182 (1972).

160. C. T. Esmon, J. W. Suttie, and C. M. Jackson, The functional significance of vitamin K action. Difference in phospholipid binding between normal and abnormal prothrombin. *J. Biol. Chem. 250*:4095–4099 (1975).

161. G. L. Nelsestuen and J. W. Suttie, The mode of action of vitamin K. Isolation of a peptide

containing the vitamin K-dependent portion of prothrombin. *Proc. Natl. Acad. Sci. USA* *70*:3366–3370 (1973).

162. J. Stenflo, Vitamin K and the biosynthesis of prothrombin. IV. Isolation of peptides containing prosthetic groups from normal prothrombin and the corresponding peptides from dicoumarol-induced prothrombin. *J. Biol. Chem. 249*:5527–5535 (1974).

163. J. Stenflo, P. Fernlund, W. Egan, and P. Roepstorff, Vitamin K dependent modificatiaons of glutamic acid residues in prothrombin. *Proc. Natl. Acad. Sci. USA 71*:2730–2733 (1974).

164. G. L. Nelsestuen, T. H. Zytkovicz, and J. B. Howard, The mode of action of vitamin K. Identification of γ-carboxyglutamic acid as a component of prothrombin. *J. Biol. Chem. 249*:6347–6350 (1974).

165. S. Magnusson, L. Sottrup-Jensen, T. E. Petersen, H. R. Morris, and A. Dell, Primary structure of the vitamin K-dependent part of prothrombin. *FEBS Lett. 44*:189–193 (1974).

166. C. T. Esmon, J. A. Sadowski, and J. W. Suttie, A new carboxylation reaction. The vitamin K-dependent incorporation of $H^{14}CO_3^-$ into prothrombin. *J. Biol. Chem. 250*:4744–4748 (1975).

167. J-M. Girardot, D. O. Mack, R. A. Floyd, and B. C. Johnson, Evidence for vitamin K semi-quinone as the functional form of vitamin K in the liver vitamin K-dependent protein carboxylation reaction. *Biochem. Biophys. Res. Commun. 70*:655–662 (1976).

168. J. A. Sadowski, C. T. Esmon, and J. W. Suttie, Vitamin K-dependent carboxylase. Requirements of the rat liver microsomal enzyme system. *J. Biol. Chem. 251*:2770–2775 (1976).

169. C. T. Esmon and J. W. Suttie, Vitamin K-dependent carboxylase: Solubilization and Properties. *J. Biol. Chem. 251*:6238–6243 (1976).

170. D. O. Mack, E. T. Suen, J-M. Girardot, J. A. Miller, R. Delaney, and B. C. Johnson, Soluble enzyme system for vitamin K-dependent carboxylation. *J. Biol. Chem. 251*:3269–3276 (1976).

171. J. P. Jones, E. J. Gardner, T. G. Cooper, and R. E. Olson, Vitamin K-dependent carboxylation of peptide-bound glutamate. The active species of "CO_2" utilized by the membrane-bound preprothrombin carboxylase. *J. Biol. Chem. 252*:7738–7742 (1977).

172. J. W. Suttie, J. M. Hageman, S. R. Lehrman, and D. H. Rich, Vitamin K-dependent carboxylase: Development of a peptide substrate. *J. Biol. Chem. 251*:5827–5830 (1976).

173. B. C. Johnson, Post-translational carboxylation of preprothrombin. *Mol. Cell. Biochem. 38*:77–121 (1981).

174. C. Vermeer, The vitamin K-dependent carboxylation reaction. *Mol. Cell. Biochem. 61*:17–35 (1984).

175. R. E. Olson, The function and metabolism of vitamin K. *Ann. Rev. Nutr. 4*:281–337 (1984).

176. J. W. Suttie, Vitamin K-dependent carboxylase. *Ann. Rev. Biochem. 54*:459–477 (1985).

177. A. K. Willingham and J. T. Matschiner, Changes in phylloquinone epoxidase activity related to prothrombin synthesis and microsomal clotting activity in the rat. *Biochem. J. 140*:435–441 (1974).

178. J. A. Sadowski, H. K. Schnoes, and J. W. Suttie, Vitamin K epoxidase: Properties and relationship to prothrombin synthesis. *Biochemistry 16*:3856–3863 (1977).

179. J. W. Suttie, A. E. Larson, L. M. Canfield, and T. L. Carlisle, Relationship between vitamin K-dependent carboxylation and vitamin K epoxidation. *Fed. Pro. 37*:2605–2609 (1978).

180. R. G. Bell, Metabolism of vitamin K and prothrombin synthesis: Anticoagulants and the vitamin K-epoxide cycle. *Fed. Proc. 37*:2599–2604 (1978).

181. T. L. Carlisle and J. W. Suttie, Vitamin K dependent carboxylase: Subcellular location of the carboxylase and enzymes involved in vitamin K metabolism in rat liver. *Biochemistry 19*:1161–1167 (1980).

182. J. J. McTigue and J. W. Suttie, Oxygen dependence of vitamin K-dependent carboxylase and vitamin K epoxidase. *FEBS Lett. 200*:71–75 (1986).

183. J. W. Suttie, L. O. Geweke, S. L. Martin, and A. K. Willingham, Vitamin K epoxidase: Dependence of epoxidase activity on substrates of the vitamin K-dependent carboxylation

reaction. *FEBS Lett.* *109*:267–270 (1980).

184. A. Y. Cheung, G. M. Wood, S. Funakawa, C. P. Grossman, and J. W. Suttie, Vitamin K dependent carboxylase: substrates, products, and inhibitors. In *Current Advances in Vitamin K Research* (J. W. Suttie, ed.). Elsevier Science Publishers, New York, 1988, pp. 3–16.

185. P. A. Friedman, M. A. Shia, P. M. Gallop, and A. E. Griep, Vitamin K-dependent γ-carbon-hydrogen bond cleavage and the non-mandatory concurrent carboxylation of peptide bound glutamic acid residues. *Proc. Natl. Acad. Sci. USA* *76*:3126–3129 (1979).

186. R. Azerad, P. Decottignies-Le Marechal, C. Ducrocq, A. Righini-Tapie, A. Vidal-Cros, S. Bory, J. Dubois, M. Gaudry, and A. Marquet, The vitamin K-dependent carboxylation of peptide substrates: Stereochemical features and mechanistic studies with substrate analogues. In *Current Advances in Vitamin K Research* (J. W. Suttie, ed.). Elsevier Science Publishers, New York, 1988, pp. 17–23.

187. J. J. McTigue and J. W. Suttie, Vitamin K-dependent carboxylase: Demonstration of a vitamin K- and O_2-dependent exchange of ^{3}H from ^{3}H$_2$O into glutamic acid residues. *J. Biol. Chem.* *258*:12129–12131 (1983).

188. D. L. Anton and P. A. Friedman, Fate of the activated γ-carbon-hydrogen bond in the un-coupled vitamin K-dependent γ-glutamyl carboxylation reaction. *J. Biol. Chem.* *258*:14084–14087 (1983).

189. P. V. Hauschka, J. B. Lian, and P. M. Gallop, Direct identification of the calcium-binding amino acid γ-carboxyglutamate, in mineralized tissue. *Proc. Natl. Acad. Sci. USA* *72*:3925–3929 (1975).

190. P. A. Price, A. S. Otsuka, J. W. Poser, J. Kristaponis, and N. Raman, Characterization of a γ-carboxyglutamic acid-containing protein from bone. *Proc. Natl. Acad. Sci. USA* *73*:1447–1451 (1976).

191. P. A Price, J. W. Poser, and N. Raman, Primary structure of the γ-carboxyglutamic acid-containing protein from bovine bone. *Proc. Natl. Acad. Sci. USA* *73*:3374–3375 (1976).

192. J. B. Lian, P. V. Hauschka, and P. M. Gallop, Properties and biosynthesis of a vitamin K-dependent calcium binding protein in bone. *Fed. Proc. 37*:2615–2620 (1978).

193. P. A. Price, Vitamin K-dependent formation of bone Gla protein (osteocalcin) and its func-tion. *Vitamins and Hormones 42*:65–108 (1985).

194. P. V. Hauschka and S. A. Carr, Calcium-dependent α-helical structure in osteocalcin. *Biochemistry 21*:2538–2547 (1982).

195. J. B. Lian and P. A. Friedman, The vitamin K-dependent synthesis of γ-carboxyglutamic acid by bone microsomes. *J. Biol. Chem. 253*:6623–6626 (1978).

196. S. K. Nishimoto and P. A. Price, Proof that the γ-carboxyglutamic acid-containing bone protein is synthesized in calf bone. Comparative synthesis rate and effect of coumarin on synthesis. *J. Biol. Chem. 254*:437–441 (1979).

197. P. A. Price and M. K. Williamson, Effects of warfarin on bone. Studies on the vitamin K-dependent protein of rat bone. *J. Biol. Chem. 256*:12754–12759 (1981).

198. P. A. Price, M. K. Williamson, T. Haba, R. B. Dell, and W. S. S. Jee, Excessive mineraliza-tion with growth plate closure in rats on chronic warfarin treatment. *Proc. Natl. Acad. Sci. USA 79*:7734–7738 (1982).

199. P. A. Price, Bone Gla protein and matrix Gla protein: Identification of the probable struc-tures involved in substrate recognition by the γ-carboxylase and discovery of tissue differences in vitamin K metabolism. In *Current Advances in Vitamin K Research* (J. W. Suttie, ed.). Elsevier Science Publishers, New York, 1988, pp. 259–273.

200. P. A. Price and M. K. Williamson, Primary structure of bovine matrix Gla protein, a new vitamin K-dependent bone protein. *J. Biol. Chem. 260*:14971–14975 (1985).

201. P. A Price and S. A. Baukol, 1,25-Dihydroxyvitamin D$_3$ increases synthesis of the vitamin K-dependent bone protein by osteosarcoma cells. *J. Biol. Chem. 255*:11660–11663 (1980).

202. P. A. Price and S. A. Baukol, 1,25-Dihydroxyvitamin D$_3$ increases serum levels of the vitamin K-dependent bone protein. *Biochem. Biophys. Res. Commun. 99*:928–935 (1981).

203. P. A. Price and S. A. Sloper, Concurrent warfarin treatment further reduces bone mineral levels in 1,25-dihydroxyvitamin D_3-treated rats *J. Biol. Chem. 258*:6004–6007 (1983).

204. J. D. Malone, S. L. Teitelbaum, G. L. Griffin, R. M. Senior, and A. J. Kahn, Recruitment of osteoclast precursors by purified bone matrix constituents. *J. Cell Biol. 92*:227–230 (1982).

205. J. B. Lian, Osteocalcin: Functional studies and postulated role in bone resorption. In *Current Advances in Vitamin K Research* (J. W. Suttie, ed.). Elsevier Science Publishers, New York, 1988, pp. 245–257.

206. C. M. Gundberg, D. E. C. Cole, J. B. Lian, T. M. Reade, and P. M. Gallop, Serum osteocalcin in the treatment of inherited rickets with 1,25-dihydroxyvitamin D_3. *J. Clin. Endocrinol. Metab. 56*:1063–1067 (1983).

207. P. D. Delmas, D. Stenner, H. W. Wahner, K. G. Mann, and B. L. Riggs, Increase in serum bone γ-caboxyglutamic acid protein with aging in women. Implications for the mechanism of age-related bone loss. *J. Clin. Invest. 71*:1316–1321 (1983).

208. P. A. Price, J. G. Parthemore, and L. J. Deftos, New biochemical marker for bone metabolism. Measurement by radioimmunoassay of bone Gla protein in the plasma of normal subjects and patients with bone disease. *J. Clin. Invest. 66*:878–883 (1980).

209. M. J. Glimcher, B. Lefteriou, and D. Kossiva, Identification of O-phosphoserine, O-phosphothreonine and γ-carboxyglutamic acid in the non-collagenous proteins of bovine cementum; comparison with dentin, enamel and bone. *Calc. Tiss. Intl. 28*:83–86 (1979).

210. J. B. Lian, R. J. Levy, J. T. Levy, and P. A. Friedman, Other vitamin K dependent proteins. In *Calcium-Binding Proteins: Structure and Function* (F. L. Siegel, E. Carafoli, R. H. Kretsinger, D. H. MacLennan, and R. H. Wasserman, eds.). Elsevier North-Holland, New York, 1980, pp. 449–460.

211. R. J. Levy, C. Gundberg, and R. Scheinman, The identification of the vitamin K-dependent bone protein osteocalcin as one of the γ-carboxyglutamic acid containing proteins present in calcified atherosclerotic plaque and mineralized heart valves. *Atherosclerosis 46*:49–56 (1983).

212. J. A. Helpern, S. J. McGee, and J. M. Riddle, Observations suggesting a possible link between gamma-carboxyglutamic acid and porcine bioprosthetic valve calcification. *Henry Ford Hosp. Med. J. 30*:152–155 (1982).

213. A. E. Griep and P. A. Friedman, Purification of a protein containing γ-carboxyglutamic acid from bovine kidney. In *Vitamin K Metabolism and Vitamin K-Dependent Proteins* (J. W. Suttie, ed.). University Park Press, Baltimore, 1980, pp. 307–310.

214. A. Gardemann and G. F. Domagk, The occurrence of γ-carboxyglutamate in a protein isolated from ox liver mitochondria. *Arch. Biochem. Biophys. 220*:347–353 (1983).

215. B. A. M. Soute, W. Muller-Ester, M. A. G. de Boer-van den Berg, M. Ulrich, and C. Vermeer, Discovery of a γ-carboxyglutamic acid-containing protein in human spermatozoa. *FEBS Lett. 190*:137–141 (1985).

216. Nakagawa, Y., V. Abram, F. J. Kezdy, E. T. Kaiser, and F. L. Coe, Purification and characterization of the principal inhibitor of calcium oxalate monohydrate crystal growth in human urine. *J. Biol. Chem. 258*:12594–12600 (1983).

217. R. S. Tuan, W. A. Scott, and Z. A. Cohn, Purification and characterization of calcium-binding protein from chick chorioallantoic membrane. *J. Biol. Chem. 253*:1011–1016 (1978).

218. G. Tans, J. W. P. Govers-Riemslag, J. L. M. L. van Rijn, and J. Rosing, Purification and properties of a prothrombin activator from the venom of *Notechis scutatus scutatus*. *J. Biol. Chem. 260*:9366–9370 (1985).

219. P. V. Hauschka, E. A. Mullen, G. Hintsch, and S. Jazwinski, Abundant occurrence of γ-carboxyglutamic acid (Gla)-containing peptides in the marine gastropod family *Conidae*. In *Current Advances in Vitamin K Research* (J. W. Suttie, ed.). Elsevier Science Publishers, New York, 1988, pp. 237–243.

220. J. W. Suttie, Vitamin K. In *The Fat-Soluble Vitamins* (A. T. Diplock, ed.). William Heinemann Ltd., London, 1985, pp. 225–311.

221. C. Vermeer, Comparison between hepatic and nonhepatic vitamin K-dependent carboxylase. *Haemostasis 16*:239–245 (986).

222. M. C. Roncaglioni, A. P. B. Dalessandro, B. Casali, C. Vermeer, and M. B. Donati, γ-Glutamyl carboxylase activity in experimental tumor tissues: A biochemical basis for vitamin K dependence of cancer procoagulant. *Haemostasis 16*:295–299 (1986).

223. J. W. Suttie, Vitamin K. In *Handbook of Lipid Research,* vol. 2, *The Fat-Soluble Vitamins* (H. F. DeLuca, ed.). Plenum Press, New York, 1978, pp. 211–277.

224. R. G. Bell and J. T. Matschiner, Vitamin K activity of phylloquinone oxide. *Arch. Biochem. Biophys. 141*:473–476 (1970).

225. R. G. Bell and J. T. Matschiner, Warfarin and the inhibition of vitamin K activity by an oxide metabolite. *Nature 237*:32–33 (1972).

226. A. Zimmerman and J. T. Matschiner, Biochemical basis of hereditary resistance to warfarin in the rat. *Biochem. Pharmacol. 23*:1033–1040 (1974).

227. J. T. Matschiner, A. Zimmerman, and R. G. Bell, The influence of warfarin on vitamin K epoxide reductase. *Thrombos. Diathes. Haemorrh.* (suppl 57):45–52 (1974).

228. R. G. Bell and P. T. Caldwell, The mechanism of warfarin resistance. Warfarin and the metabolism of vitamin K_1. *Biochemistry 12*:1759–1762 (1973).

229. J. A. Sadowski and J. W. Suttie, Mechanism of action of coumarins. Significance of vitamin K epoxide. *Biochemistry 13*:3696–3699 (1974).

230. S. R. Goodman, R. M. Houser, and R. E. Olson, Ineffectiveness of phylloquinone epoxide as an inhibitor of prothrombin synthesis in the rat. *Biochem. Biophys. Res. Commun. 61*:250–257 (1974).

231. P. T. Caldwell, P. Ren, and R. G. Bell, Warfarin and metabolism of vitamin K. *Biochem. Pharmacol. 25*:3353–3362 (1974).

232. D. S. Whitlon, J. A. Sadowski, and J. W. Suttie, Mechanism of coumarin action: Significance of vitamin K epoxide reductase inhibition. *Biochemistry 17*:1371–1377 (1978).

233. E. F. Hildebrandt and J. W. Suttie, Mechanisms of coumarin action: sensitivity of vitamin K metabolizing enzymes of normal and warfarin-resistant rat liver. *Biochemistry 21*:2406–2411 (1982).

234. M. J. Fasco and L. M. Principe, R- and S-warfarin inhibition of vitamin K and vitamin K 2,3-epoxide reductase activities in the rat. *J. Biol. Chem. 257*:4894–4901 (1982).

235. M. J. Fasco, E. F. Hildebrandt, and J. W. Suttie, Evidence that warfarin anticoagulant action involves two distinct reductase activities. *J. Biol. Chem. 257*:11210–11212 (1982).

236. R. Wallin, S. D. Patrick, and J. O. Ballard, Vitamin K antagonism of coumarin intoxication in the rat. *Thromb. Haemostas.* (Stuttg.) *55*:235–239 (1986).

237. K. W. E. Denson and R. Biggs, Laboratory diagnosis, tests of clotting function and their standardization. In *Human Blood Coagulation, Haemostasis and Thrombosis* (R. Biggs, ed.). Blackwell Scientific Publishers, 1972, pp. 278–332.

238 H. E. Sauberlich, R. P. Dowdy, and J. H. Skala, CRC laboratory tests for the assessment of nutritional status. CRC Press:83–88 (1974).

239. B. R. J. Kirchhof, C. Vermeer, and H. C. Hemker, The determination of prothrombin using synthetic chromogenic substrates; choice of a suitable activator. *Thromb. Res. 13*:219–232 (1978).

240. K. W. E. Denson, R. Borrett, and R. Biggs, The specific assay of prothrombin using the Taipan snake venom *Brit. J. Haematol. 21*:219–226 (1971).

241. R. M. Bertina, W. van der Marel-van Nieuwkoop, J. Dubbeldam, R. J. Boekhout-Mussert, and J. J. Veltkamp, New Method for the Rapid Detection of Vitamin K Deficiency. *Clin. Chim. Acta 105*:83–98 (1980).

242. P. M. Allison, L. L. Mummah-Schendel, C. G. Kindberg, C. S. Harms, N. U. Bang, and J. W. Suttie, Effects of a vitamin K-deficient diet and antibiotics and normal human volunteers. *J. Lab. Clin. Med. 110*:180–188 (1987).

243. R. A. Blanchard, B. C. Furie, M. Jorgensen, S. F. Kruger, and B. Furie, Acquired vitamin

dependent carboxylation deficiency in liver disease. *New Engl. J. Med. 305*:242–248 (1981).

244. M. L. Scott, Vitamin K in animal nutrition. *Vitamins and Hormones 24*:633–647 (1966).

245. E. A. Doisy and J. T. Matschiner, Biochemistry of vitamin K. In *Fat-Soluble Vitamins* (R. A. Morton, ed.). Pergamon Press, Oxford, 1970, pp. 293–331.

246. National Academy of Sciences. *Nutritional Requirements of Laboratory Animals*, 3rd ed., Washington, D. C. (1978).

247. J. G. Bieri, G. S. Stoewsand, G. M. Briggs, R. W. Phillips, J. C. Woodard and J. J. Knapka, Report of the American Institute of Nutrition, Ad Hoc Committee on Standards for Nutritional Studies. *J. Nutr. 107*:1340–1348 (1977).

248. B. D. Roebuck, S. A. Wilpone, D. S. Fifield, and J. D. Yager, Letter to the editor. *J. Nutr. 109*:924–925 (1979).

249. J. G. Bieri, Letter to the editor. *J. Nutr. 109*:925–926 (1979).

250. P. G. Frick, G. Riedler, and H. Brogli, Dose response and minimal daily requirement for vitamin K in man. *J. Appl. Physiol. 23*:387–389 (1967).

251. R. A. O'Reilly, Vitamin K in hereditary resistance to oral anticoagulant drugs. *Am. J. Physiol. 221*:1327–1330 (1971).

252. J. W. Suttie, L. L. Mummah-Schendel, D. V. Shah, B. J. Lyle, and J. L. Greger, Development of human vitamin K deficiency by dietary vitamin K restriction. *Am. J. Clin. Nutr. 47*:475–480 (1988).

253. K. Hazell and K. H. Baloch, Vitamin K deficiency in the elderly. *Gerontol. Clin. 12*:10–17 (1970).

254. E. A. Doisy, Jr., Nutritional hypoprothrombinemia and metabolism of vitamin K. *Fed. Proc. 20*:989–994 (1961).

255. C. A. Owen, Jr., Vitamin K group: Deficiency effects in animals and human beings. In *The Vitamins*, vol. III, 2nd ed. (W. H. Sebrell and R. S. Harris, eds.). Academic Press, New York, 1971, pp. 470–491.

256. W. J. Keenan, T. Jewett, and H. I. Glueck, Role of feeding and vitamin K in hypoprothrombinemia of the newborn. *Am. J. Dis. Child. 121*:271–277 (1971).

247. American Academy of Pediatrics, Committee on Nutrition. Vitamin K supplementation for infants receiving mil substitute infant formulas and for those with fat malabsorption. *Pediatrics 48*:483–487 (1971).

258. American Hospital Formulary Service, Washington, D. C. Vitamin K activity. *Am. Soc. Hosp. Pharm. 88*:24 (1979).

259. F. Endo, K. Motohara, and I. Matsuda, Vitamin K deficiency in the newborn–milk intake and plasma PIVKA-II. In *Current Advances in Vitamin K Research* (J. W. Suttie, ed.). Elsevier Science Publishers, New York, 1988, pp. 505–507.

260. S. Suzuki, Studies on coagulation in newborn infants: LIver maturation and vitamin K procoagulant-inhibitor relations. *J. Perinat. Med. 7*:229 (1979).

261. J. M. van Doorm, A. D. Muller, and H. C. Hemker, Heparin-like inhibitor, not vitamin K deficiency, in the newborn. *Lancet 1*:852–853 (1977).

262. B. E. Gustafsson, F. S. Daft, E. G. McDaniel, and J. C. Smith, Effects of vitamin K-active compounds and intestinal microorganisms in vitamin K-deficient germfree rats. *J. Nutr. 78*:461–468 (1962).

263. T. S. Nelson and L. C. Norris, Studies on the vitamin K requirement of the chick. II. Effect of sulfaquinoxaline on the quantitative requirements of the chick for vitamin K_1, menadione and menadione sodium bisulfite. *J. Nutr. 73*:135–142 (1961).

264. D. Savage and J. Lindenbaum, Clinical and experimental human vitamin K deficiency. In *Nutrition in Hematology* (J. Lindenbaum, ed.). Churchill Livingstone, New York, 1983, pp. 271–320.

265. J. J. Lipsky, Mechanism of the inhibition of the γ-carboxylation of glutamic acid by *N*-methylthiotetrazole-containing antibiotics. *Proc. Natl. Acad. Sci. USA 81*:2893–2897 (1984).

266. H. Bechtold, K. Andrassy, E. Jahnchen, J. Koderisch, H. Koderisch, L. S. Weilemann,

H-G. Sonntag, and E. Ritz, Evidence for impaired hepatic vitamin K_1 metabolism in patients treated with N-methyl-thiotetrazole cephalosporins. *Thromb. Haemostas.* (Stuttg.) *51*:358–361 (1984).

267. K. A. Creedon and J. W. Suttie, Effect of N-methyl-thiotetrazole on vitamin K epoxide reductase. *Thromb. Res. 44*:147–153 (1986).

268. H. Suzuki, T. Nakao, and K, Hiraga, Vitamin K deficiency in male rats fed diets containing butylated hydroxytoluene (BHT). *Toxicol. Appl. Pharmacol. 50*:261–266 (1979).

269. O. Takahashi and K. Hiraga, Preventive effects of phylloquinone on hemorrhagic death induced by butylated hydroxytoluene in male rats. *J. Nutr. 109*:453–457 (1979).

270. K. R. Mountain, A. S. Gallus, and J. Hirsch, Neonatal coagulation defection due to anticonvulsant drug treatment in pregnancy. *Lancet*:1:265 (1970).

271. A. S. Rogen and J. C. Ferguson, Clinical observataion on patients treated with atronid and anticoagulants. *J. Atherscler Res. 3*:671–676 (1963).

272. J. T. Matschiner and R. G. Bell, Effect of sex and sex hormones on plasma prothrombin and vitamin K deficiency. *Proc. Soc. Exp. Biol. Med. 144*:316–320 (1973).

273. J. G. Hall, R. M. Pauli, and K. M. Wilson, Maternal and fetal sequelae on anticoagulation during pregnancy. *Am. J. Med. 68*:122–140 (1980).

274. J. T. Matschiner and A. K. Willingham, Influence of sex hormones on vitamin K deficiency and epoxidation of vitamin K in the rat. *J. Nutr. 104*:660–665 (1974).

275. D. W. Jolly, B. M. Kadis, and T. E. Nelson, Jr., Estrogen and prothrombin synthesis. The prothrombinogenic action of estrogen. *Biochem. Biophys. Res. Commun. 74*:41–49 (1977).

276. C. M. Siegfried, G. R. Knauer, and J. T. Matschiner, Evidence for increased formation of preprothrombin and the noninvolvement of Vitamin K-dependent reactions in sex-linked hyperprothrombinemia in the rat. *Arch. Biochem. Biophys. 194*:486–495 (1979).

277. Y. Nishino, Hormonal control of prothrombin synthesis in rat liver microsomes, with special reference to the role of estradiol, testosterone and prolactin. *Arch. Toxicol. Suppl. 2*:397–402 (1979).

278. A. T. van Oosterom, P. Kerkhoven, and J. J. Veltkamp, Metabolism of the coagulation factors of the prothrombin complex in hypothyroidism in man. *Thrombos. Haemostas.* (Stuttg.) *41*:273–285 (1979).

279. M. C. Elliott, B. Isaacs, and A. C. Ivy, Production of "prothrombin deficiency" and response to vitamins A, D and K. *Proc. Soc. Exp. Biol. Med. 43*:240–245 (1940).

280. G. H. Rao and K. E. Mason, Antisterility and antivitamin K activity of d-α-tocopheryl hydroquionone in the vitamin E-deficient female rat. *J. Nutr. 105*:495–498 (1975).

281. J. J. Corrigan, Jr., and F. I. Marcus, Coagulopathy associated with vitamin E ingestion. *J. Am. Med. Assn. 230*:1300–1301 (1974).

282. C. A. Owen, Vitamin K group. XI. Pharmacology and toxicology. In *The Vitamins*, vol. III, 2nd ed. (W. H. Sebrell and R. S. Harris, eds.). Academic Press, New York,1971, pp. 492–509.

5
Vitamin C

Ulrich Moser
F. Hoffmann-La Roche, Ltd.
Basel, Switzerland

Adrianne Bendich
Hoffmann-La Roche, Inc.,
Nutley, New Jersey

I. INTRODUCTION

Vitamin C was named ascorbic acid because it prevents and cures scurvy, one of the oldest diseases known to mankind. The word "scurvy" means "ulcerated, swollen mouth," which is a typical sign of the disease and can be traced back to the old Scandinavian forms skjoerbug, skörbjugg or the Icelandic *skyrbjûgr*; old English forms are *scarby* and *scorby* (1). Although this nutritional deficiency disease has been decribed throughout history, the cause of the illness was not recognized until 1753 when James Lind published his famous "Treatise of the Scurvy." Once discovered in 1928, ascorbic acid rapidly became a major area of research in many laboratories. Chemists as well as biochemists tried to unravel its secrets, and physicians looked for medical uses beyond curing scurvy. The number of publications, which increased from 364 in 1969 to over 1160 in 1986 (BIOSIS), documents the attention the scientific world pays to this compound. Although many functions have been described, the exact amount the human being needs is still a matter of discussion. Humans, other primates, guinea pigs, fruit-eating bats, some birds including the red-vented bulbul and related Passeriforme species, fish such as coho salmon, rainbow trout, and carp, are the only species that cannot synthesize ascorbic acid due to a lack of the enzyme L-gulono-gamma-lactone oxidase (2,3). One might speculate that nature gave up ascorbic acid synthesis in these animals in order to conserve glucose, the precursor of ascorbic acid. This would mean that a signfiicant amount of glucose, a major source of energy, would be conserved in the species that cannot synthesize ascorbic acid.

II. HISTORY

The book *The History of Scurvy and Vitamin C* by K. J. Carpenter deals extensively with the theories and problems of scurvy throughout history (4). Scurvy affected many people in ancient Egypt, Greece, and Rome and was probably already known to Hippocrates and the Roman naturalist Pliny. It influenced the course of history because the diet soldiers and sailors had eaten during military campaigns and during long ocean voyages very often did not contain adequate amounts of vitamin C (5). At the end of the Middle Ages, scurvy became epidemic in northern and central Europe. Between 1556 and 1857, 114 scurvy epidemics were reported in several countries, most occurring during the winter season, when fresh fruits and vegetables were not available.

Many observations were made that associated the eating of certain fresh foods with the cure of the disease and were rediscovered at various times during the fifteenth to the eighteenth centuries. In 1536, on the advice from New Foundland Indians, Jacques Carter gave his crew suffering from scurvy an extract from evergreen needles, probably from the white cedar *Thuja occidentalis*. Everybody who was willing to drink the extract recovered. Only 7 years later about 50 French people died of scurvy when a party of 200 wintered at almost the same place. Captain Sir James Lancaster, on route to East India in 1601, prevented an outbreak of scurvy by distributing three spoonfuls of lemon juice every morning to his men. Thousands of Austrian soldiers died of scurvy during the war against the Turks until the physician J. G. H. Kramer found in 1720 that fresh herbs and lemons cured the disease (6). Twenty-four years later in 1744, only 144 of 1000 sailors returned to England from Admiral Anson's voyage; the majority died of scurvy. Finally, James Lind, a surgeon of the Royal Navy, carried out his famous experiment in 1747, which was probably the first controlled clinical trial proving that lack of a component of the diet was responsible for scurvy and that oranges and lemons were the most effectual remedies against this disease. He published his results in a 400-page book in 1753 in Edinburgh as *A Treatise of the Scurvy. Containing an inquiry into the Nature, Causes and Cure of that Disease. Together with a Critical and Chronological View of what has been published on the subject* (7).

Captain James Cook maintained a healthy crew during his voyages around the world in 1772–1776 by adding sauerkraut, lemons and oranges to the provisions. It is not clear whether he was familiar with Lind's treatise. It wasn't until 1804 that the British Navy adopted the use of lime juice rations for all crews, which resulted in the nickname "limeys" for British sailors. Still, scurvy incidents continued to occur periodically, although prevention had been demonstrated. In the United States, when gold was found in California, thousands of settlers died from scurvy on the long voyages. During the Civil War, poor nutrition also claimed its tribute. Particularly, wars evoked scurvy epidemics, even among civilians, as seen during the siege of Paris 1870–71. Explorer Captain Scott and his team probably died of scurvy in 1912 while on their expedition to the South Pole. Their diet (pemmican, biscuits, butter, cocoa, sugar, and tea) lacked vitamin C (8). Today, incidents of scurvy can be observed occasionally in infants nourished exclusively with cow's milk, which is deficient in vitamin C, in aged persons on limited diets, and in adults with nutritional problems due to alcoholism, social affiliation, or strict, ill-balanced diets (9).

A breakthrough of scurvy research was the discovery by the Norwegian bacteriologist Axel Holst and the pediatrician Theodor Frölich in 1907 that guinea pigs were susceptible to scurvy and thus a valuable animal model for this disease (10). In earlier studies in the United States (11) and in Germany (12), signs of scurvy had been reported in guinea pigs, however, the importance of these observations have not been recognized. Between 1910 and 1921 researchers found that monkeys were also susceptible to scurvy, which gave more credence to the results obtained with guinea pigs (13). Zilva and his associates isolated the antiscorbutic activity as a crude fraction from lemons, which was easily destroyed by oxidation and protected by reducing agents like 2,6-dichloroindophenol (14). Because McCollum had already named the growth factors "A" and "B," Drummond's proposal was accepted to name the antiscorbutic factor "C," which later became "vitamin C" (15,16).

The isolation was first achieved by the Hungarian scientist Albert Szent-Györgyi, who was working on the nature of the oxidation of nutrients in relation to energy production. He isolated a reducing factor from adrenals in crystalline form, which he called "hexuronic acid" with the empirical formula $C_6H_8O_6$ (17,18). At the same time, King and Waugh found an identical compound in lemon juice (19). Shortly thereafter, Hirst and Haworth announced the structure of vitamin C (20) and suggested with Szent-Györgyi that the name be changed to L-ascorbic acid to convey its antiscorbutic properties. In the same year Reichstein reported the synthesis of D-ascorbic acid and L-ascorbic acid, which still forms the basis for large-scale industrial production (21). The synthetic product was proved to have the same biological activity as the substance isolated from natural tissues. In 1937, Haworth (chemistry) and Szent-Györgyi (medicine) were awarded the Nobel Prize for their work with vitamin C.

III. CHEMISTRY

A. Nomenclature and Structure

The designation of the compound 2-oxo-L-threo-hexono-1,4-lactone-2,3-ene-diol or vitamin C was changed to ascorbic acid or L-ascorbic acid in 1965 by the IUPAC-IUB Commission on Biochemical Nomenclature (22). Furthermore, the names L-xyloascorbic acid, 3-oxo-L-gulofuranolactone (enol form) and L-3-ketothreohexuronic acid lactone are listed in the Merck Index (23). The structure of ascorbic acid is given in Figure 1. The molecule has an almost planar five-membered ring. The two chiral centers at positions 4 and 5 determine the four stereoisomers (Fig. 1). Besides L-ascorbic acid, only erythorbic acid shows a limited level of vitamin C activity (Table 1). The stereochemical assignment of ascorbic acid to the L-series was confirmed by the synthesis from L-xylose (21).

Dehydroascorbic acid, the oxidized form of ascorbic acid which retains vitamin C activity, has a side chain that forms a hydrated hemiketal (Fig. 2) (24). Furthermore, the structure of crystalline dehydro-L-ascorbic acid was reported to be a dimer (25).

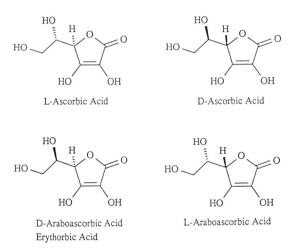

Figure 1 Isomers of ascorbic acid.

Table 1 Ascorbic Acid Isomers

Substance	M.P. (°C)	$[\alpha]_D(H_2O)(°)$	Activity
L-Ascorbic acid	192	+24	1
D-Ascorbic acid	192	−23	0
D-Araboascorbic acid	174	−18.5	0.025–0.05
L-Araboascorbic acid	170	+17	0

B. Physical and Chemical Properties

A selected number of physical properties of ascorbic acid are listed in Table 2. Besides the structure elucidation by X-ray crystallographic analysis (26,27), vitamin C has been intensively studied by [¹H] and [¹³C] NMR spectroscopy (28), IR-spectroscopy (29), mass spectra (30,31), and UV spectra (32,33). Due to the enediol substructure, the proton on O-3 is highly acidic ($pK_1 = 4.17$). The reversible oxidation to semidehydro-L-ascorbic acid and further to dehydro-L-ascorbic acid is the most important chemical property of ascorbic acid and is the basis for its known physiological activities.

Degradation reactions of L-ascorbic acid in aqueous solution depend on several factors, such as pH (the range with the highest stability being between 4 and 6), temperature, and the presence of oxygen or metals like copper. On standing, dehydro-L-ascorbic acid undergoes irreversible hydrolysis to 2,3-diketo-L-gulonic acid, which is oxidized to oxalic acid and L-threonic acid (Fig. 3). In acidic solutions, the degradation proceeds in forming L-(+)-tartaric acid, furfurol, and other furan derivatives, as well as some condensation products (34). Alkali-catalyzed degradation results in over 50 compounds, mainly mono-, di-, and tricarboxylic acids (35). Oxalic acid exerts an inhibitory effect on the oxidation of ascorbic acid, probably by chelating copper. The vitamin can also be stabilized in biological samples with trichloracetic acid or metaphosphoric acid (36).

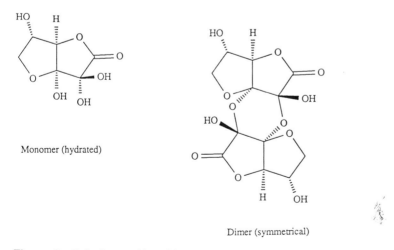

Monomer (hydrated)

Dimer (symmetrical)

Figure 2 Dehydroascorbic acid.

Table 2   Physical Properties of L-Ascorbic Acid

Property	Characteristics
Appearance	White, odorless, crystalline solid
Formula	$C_6H_8O_6$; MW 176.13
Crystal form	Monoclinic; usually plates, sometimes needles
Melting point	190–192 °C (decomposition)
Density	1.65
Optical rotation	$[\alpha]_D^{25} = +20.5°$ to $+21.5°$ (C = 1 in water)
	$[\alpha]_D^{23} = +48°$ (C = 1 in methanol)
pK_1	4.17
pK_2	11.57
Redox potential	First stage: $E_0 + 0.166$ V (pH 4)
Solubilities	1 g dissolves in 3 ml water, 30 ml 95% ethanol, 50 ml absolute ethanol, 100 ml glycerol USP, or 20 ml propylene glycol. Insoluble in ether, chloroform, benzene, petroleum ether, oils, fats, and other fat solvents

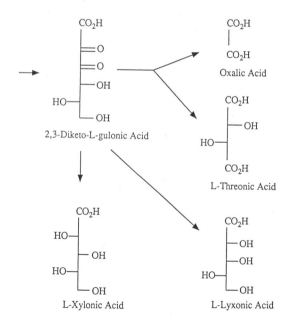

Figure 3   Degradation of ascorbic acid.

C. Isolation

The basis of the early isolation procedure of ascorbic acid from plants and fruits was the publication of Szent-Györgyi in 1928 (17). Cabbage, red pepper, and leaves of gladiolus were the sources of an industrial-scale isolation until the chemical synthesis proved to be superior to extraction. An efficient isolation method is also essential for the detection and measurement of vitamin C in foods, feeds, and pharmaceutical products (37). Aqueous solvents like 3–6% metaphosphoric acid containing acetic acid and EDTA, 0.5–2% oxalic acid, dilute trichloracetic acid with EDTA, dilute perchloric acid, or 0.5% 2,3-dimercaptopropanol are used for the extraction, which should be completed quickly in subdued light and inert atmosphere to avoid destruction from exposure of light and to oxygen, especially when small quantities of the vitamin are involved. Interfering substances can be removed by carbon decolorization, column chromatography, or solvent extraction with methylene chloride.

D. Synthesis

The approach to a synthesis of vitamin C depends on the purpose of the application of the product. Coupling of either a C-1 fragment with a C-5 fragment, or of a C-2 fragment with a C-4 fragment, or a conversion of a C-6 chain are suitable for the preparation of analogues and radiolabeled derivatives of L-ascorbic acid (38). The basis for industrial production is an efficient synthesis developed by Reichstein and Grüssner in 1934 starting from D-glucose (39). In a first step, D-glucose is reduced to D-sorbitol, which is then fermentatively oxidized to L-sorbose. The hydroxyl groups are protected by treatment with acetone and acid, and the formed diacetone-L-sorbose can then be oxidized to the corresponding acid, diacetone-2-keto-L-gulonic acid, which is easily converted to L-ascorbic acid by hydrolysis, lactonization, and enolization (Fig. 4).

Much time and effort has been devoted to finding other methods of vitamin C synthesis by fermentation (40). An important breakthrough was recently achieved using the recombinant DNA technology. It is possible to introduce the 2,5-diketo-D-gluconic acid reductase gene from *Corynebacterium* into *Erwinia herbicola*, which gives it the ability to produce 2-keto-L-gulonic acid directly from D-glucose (41). The use of this technology for the cost-effective production of L-ascorbic acid, however, requires further improvements of the process.

IV. ANALYTICAL PROCEDURES

A multitude of analytical procedures have been published since the discovery of ascorbic acid, because food products and biological and pharmaceutical samples require different extractions and because new analytical techniques allow a more specific determination of the vitamin. The methodology for determining ascorbic acid in biological samples, food products, and pharmaceuticals has been reviewed by L. A. Pachla and D. L. Reynolds (42); spectroscopic and chromatographic methods have been described in more detail by J. R. Cooke and R. E. D. Moxon (37). A selection of different methods is listed in Table 3.

Today, the biological test is only used in order to analyze derivatives of ascorbic acid for their vitamin C activity. Redox indicators like 2,6-dichloroindophenol or colorimetric reactions with metal ions are unspecific and subject to interference by a large number of substances contained in foods and natural products. These methods do not distinguish between the different stereoisomers, i.e. erythorbic acid gives the same results as ascorbic

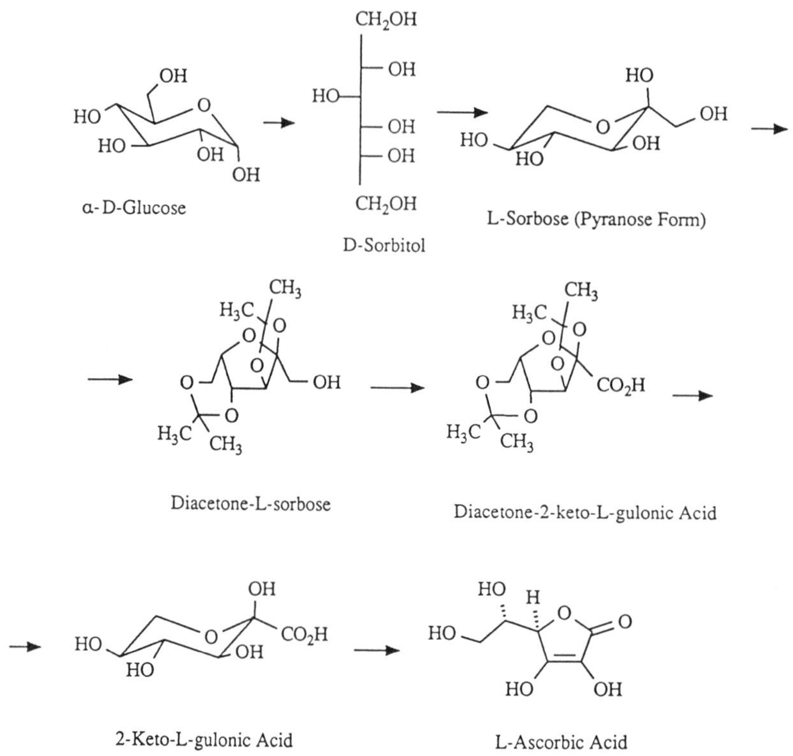

Figure 4   Chemical synthesis of L-ascorbic acid.

acid. Using ascorbate oxidase in a blank increases the specificity of these fast and simple methods (43).

The simultaneous determination of dehydroascorbic acid (DHA) and ascorbic acid is possible by calculating the difference between total ascorbate, obtained by reducing DHA with, for example, dithiothreitol, and the reduced form (44). Another colorimetric method involves oxidation of ascorbic acid with a suitable oxidizing agent and derivatization of the resulting dehydroascorbic acid with dinitrophenylhydrazine, yielding a colored product which can be measured at 520 nm. This classical method, commonly termed the Roe and Kuether method (45), has been modified with the purpose of measuring leukocyte ascorbate levels (46). Only 30–53% of the 2,4-dinitrophenylhydrazone is formed under optimal derivatization conditions (47).

Many electrochemical methods were used to determine ascorbic acid in fresh fruits, vegetables, beverages, and multivitamin tablets. The electro-oxidation at an electrode has the advantage of a higher selectivity, and metal ions do not interfere (48).

The introduction of the plant enzyme ascorbate oxidase (EC 1.10.3.3) caused an increase of the specificity of almost every method (49). One of a pair of replicate samples is pretreated with the enzyme, and the difference of the reading is proportional to ascorbate concentrations. The enzyme catalyzes the reduction of oxygen to O_2^-, which is coupled with the two protons of ascorbic acid to form water. Therefore, the consumption of oxygen is a direct measure for ascorbate concentrations. Immobilized ascorbate oxidase has been coated onto a Clark oxygen electrode and used for food analysis (50).

Table 3 Analytical Procedures

Method	Basic Principle; Reagents	Reference
Biological	Cure scurvy in guinea pigs	220
Spectroscopy	UV absorption	221
Redox Reactions	2,6-Dichlorphenolindophenol	222
	1,2-Naphthoquinone-1-sulfonic acid	223
	N-bromosuccinimide	224
	Methylene blue	225
	Chloramine	226
	3-(4,5-Trimethylthiazolyl-2)-2,5-diphenyl tetrazolium bromide	43
	Metal ions:	
	2,4,6-Tripyridyl-S-triazine	227
	Ferrozine	228
	K-ferricyanide	229
	α,α'-Dipyridine	230
	Ferricinium trichloroacetate	231
	Copper(I)-2,2 bisquinoline	232
Derivatization	2,4-Dinitrophenylhydrazine (DNPH)	45
	Diazotized 4-methoxy-2-nitroaniline	233
	o-Phenylene diamine	234
Electrochemical	Oxidation at an electrode	235
	Differential pulse voltametry	48
	Electron spin resonance	53
Enzymatic	Horseradish peroxidase	236
	Ascorbic acid oxidase	49
Chromatographic	Paper chromatography	237
	Gas-liquid chromatography	238
	Thin-layer chromatography	239
	Gas chromatography–mass spectroscopy	240
	Isotachophoresis	241
	HPLC: anion exchange, UV detection	242
	derivatization with DNPH	243
	reverse phase ion pair, amp. det.	244

Because spectroscopic and electrochemical methods do not distinguish between ascorbic acid and erythorbic acid, different separation methods have been developed to increase selectivity, such as paper, thin-layer, and gas chromatography. The high-performance liquid chromatography (HPLC) technology allows a rapid separation and detection of ascorbic acid as well as of erythorbic acid if appropriate conditions are chosen (51). However, many variations of columns and detectors are possible depending on the material to be analyzed. HPLC methods are fully automatizable and therefore suitable for routine assays (52). Besides ascorbic acid, dehydroascorbic acid, and erythorbic acid, the ascorbate free radical was observed and measured in human serum by electron spin resonance techniques (53).

V. SOURCES OF VITAMIN C

Ascorbic acid occurs in significant amounts in vegetables, fruits, and animal organs such as liver, kidney, and brain. Potatoes and cabbage are probably the most important sources of vitamin C for the majority of the Western population, at least during the winter season. Today, fresh fruits and vegetables are available all year. During storage and cooking, part of the ascorbic acid is lost due to oxidation (54). Only trace amounts of ascorbic acid are contained in milk, grains, and meat, whereas in the Australian fruit *Terminalia fernandiana*, over 3000 mg/100 g were found (55). Ascorbate values of up to 300 mg/100 g were measured in several tropical fruits (56). Neotropical plants eaten by primates and herbivorous bats accumulate ascorbic acid up to a concentration of 585 mg/100 g fresh weight with averages between 46.5 and 96.3 mg/100 g depending on the parts (fruits, foliages, or flowers), providing the monkeys with about 100 mg/kg body weight/day and the bat with 260 mg/kg body weight/day (57). The vitamin C content of some representative foods is listed in Table 4.

Table 4 Content of Ascorbic Acid in Selected Foods

Fruits and meat	Ascorbic acid (mg/100 g)	Vegetables	Ascorbic acid (mg/100 g)
Fruits of *Terminalia fernandiana*	3000	Peppers	125–200
Acerola	1300	Kale	120–180
Rose hips	1000	Parsley	170
Hawthorn berries	160–800	Turnip greens	139
Guava	300	Horseradish	120
Black currant	150–230	Collard greens	100–150
Lemons	50–80	Brussels sprouts	90–150
Strawberries	40–90	Broccoli	70–160
Oranges	40–60	Spinach	50–90
Grapefruit	35–45	Watercress	79
Red currant	40	Cauliflower	60–80
Tangerines	30	Kohlrabi	66
Pineapples	20–40	Cabbage	30–60
Raspberries	18–25	Turnips	15–40
Melons	13–33	Asparagus	15–30
Apples	10–30	Leek	15–30
Cherries	10	Potatoes	10–30
Peaches	7–14	Beans	10–30
Bananas	5–10	Peas	10–30
Liver, kidney	10–40	Onion	10–30
Fish	0–3	Tomatoes	10–30
Meat (beef, port)	0–2	Squash	8–25
Milk		Corn (sweet)	12
Human	3–6	Rhubarb	10
Cow	1–2	Celery	7–10
		Carrots	5–10
		Oat, rye, wheat	0
		Rice	0

Source: Refs. 55, 245–247.

VI. BIOCHEMISTRY

A. Plants

Ascorbic acid has not been detected in yeasts and prokaryotes, except cyanobacteria, and it is not clear whether it is produced by colorless forms of plants. It is present in all higher plants in growing and developing tissues; resting seeds, however, contain little if any (58).

Ascorbic acid is synthesized in plants from D-glucose by oxidation of the carbon atom C-2, epimerization of C-5 and finally oxidation of C-1. Thus, the carbon chain sequence of glucose is conserved. The first oxidation of D-glucose is catalyzed by pyranose-2-oxidase (EC 1.1.3.10) and yields D-glucosone. The epimerization of C-5 probably involves an oxidation-reduction linked to hydrogen carriers or a keto-enol rearrangement since the [³H] of D-[5-³H,6-¹⁴C]-glucose is not incorporated in ascorbic acid, but the [¹⁴C] appears in position 6 (59). So far, attempts to isolate an epimerase have been unsuccessful (58). A speculative scheme of ascorbic acid biosynthesis in plants based on tracer studies is given in Figure 5.

Little is known about the functions and metabolism of ascorbic acid in plants except that it is a precursor of oxalic acid and tartaric acid. Oxalate-accumulating plants cleave ascorbic acid between C-2 and C-3 to form oxalic acid and L-threonic acid. The latter undergoes either decarboxylation, resulting in a three-carbon acid which is recycled in the hexose phosphate metabolism, or oxidation to L-tartaric acid. Glycolic acid and glyoxylic acid are possible intermediates of oxalic acid generation (60). Cleavage between C-4 and C-5 in grape leaves leads to the formation of 2-keto-L-idonic acid, L-idonic acid, 5-keto-L-idonic acid, and finally to L-tartaric acid and glycolaldehyde (61). The oxidative reactions are interrupted in mature leaves at the level of L-idonic acid that accumulates (62). Ascorbic acid may function in protective mechanisms in chloroplasts (63) and contribute to plant growth, differentiation, and metabolism (64). Four enzymes are involved in the ascorbic acid metabolism in plants, of which monodehydroascorbate reductase (EC

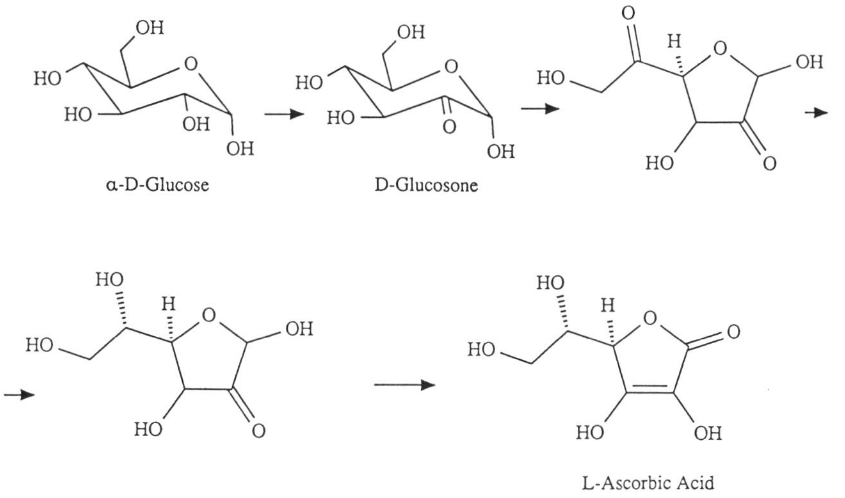

Figure 5 Biosynthesis of ascorbic acid in plants.

1.6.5.4) and dehydroascorbate reductase (EC 1.8.5.1) maintain ascorbic acid in the reduced form. Ascorbate peroxidase (EC 1.11.1.11) catalyzes the reaction:

$$H_2O_2 + 2 \text{ ascorbate} \Longrightarrow 2H_2O + 2 \text{ monodehydroascorbate}$$

and ascorbate oxidase (EC 1.10.3.3) catalyzes the oxidation as follows:

$$2 \text{ ascorbate} + O_2 \Longrightarrow 2 \text{ dehydroascorbate} + H_2O$$

Whereas peroxide-scavenging enzymes like ascorbate peroxidase fulfill a vital role in protecting the cells from oxidative damage, a specific function for the copper-containing ascorbate oxidase has yet to be found (65).

B. Animals

In the progress of evolution, the ability to synthesize ascorbic acid started in the kidney of amphibians. Insects, invertebrates, and fishes are unable to produce the vitamin and rely on a sufficient supply from the food. The key enzyme of the synthesis, L-gulonolactone oxidase (GLO, EC 1.1.3.8), still resides in the kidney of reptiles but has been transferred to the liver of mammals (66). The shift in organs containing the enzyme occurred in the marsupials; monotremes like the duckbill exhibit L-gulonolactone oxidase activity exclusively in the kidneys, most marsupials in the liver only. Bandicoots show similar activities in liver as well as in kidney, whereas some macropods have normal GLO values in the liver and about 10-fold lower levels in the kidneys (67). A similar transition in the biosynthesis of ascorbic acid was observed in birds (68). Finally, the enzyme disappeared in the guinea pig, fruit-eating bats, primates, and man. By administration of the missing enzyme, guinea pigs are able to live on an ascorbic acid–deficient diet (69).

In contrast to plants, the biosynthesis of ascorbic acid in animals is part of the glucuronic acid pathway. α-D-Glucose is first phosphorylated to α-D-glucose-6-phosphate, then isomerized to α-D-glucose-1-phosphate, which reacts with uridinetriphosphate (UTP) to form UDP-glucose, the precursor of glycogen synthesis. UDP-glucose is oxidized to UDP-D-glucuronate, which is also used for the synthesis of certain glycosaminoglycans and for conjugation with substances such as steroids, drugs, or bilirubin to be eliminated as glucuronides by the urinary tract. D-Glucuronic acid can further be reduced to L-gulonic acid, which lactonizes to form L-gulono-γ-lactone. Finally, the last oxidation is accomplished by the microsomal enzyme L-gulono-γ-lactone oxidase leading to the final product, ascorbic acid (70). D-Galactose may also serve as a precursor of vitamin C since it can be converted to D-glucose. Thus, in contrast to plants, the carbon chain of glucose is converted in ascorbic acid, where the C-1 of glucose becomes C-6 of ascorbic acid (Fig. 6).

Xenobiotics and drugs such as polychlorinated biphenyls, DDT, aminopyrine, barbital, and chloretone produce a marked increase in the biosynthesis of ascorbic acid in rats (71,72).

Ascorbic acid is carried in the bloodstream nonspecifically and is taken up by organs where specific transport mechanisms are responsible for its accumulation within the cells (Table 5). The stereoisomers, erythorbic acid and D-ascorbic acid, are poor substrates of the carrier; on the contrary, they inhibit the transport of L-ascorbic acid (72,73). The carrier does not exhibit the same reaction kinetics in all cell types; the uptake in adrenocortical cells is sodium and potassium dependent, whereas stimulation of granulocytes with N-formyl peptides, ionophore A23187, or with bacteria causes an increased uptake which is calcium dependent (74). The half-maximum velocity of the transport occurs within physiological limits of plasma concentrations, as can be seen from Table 5.

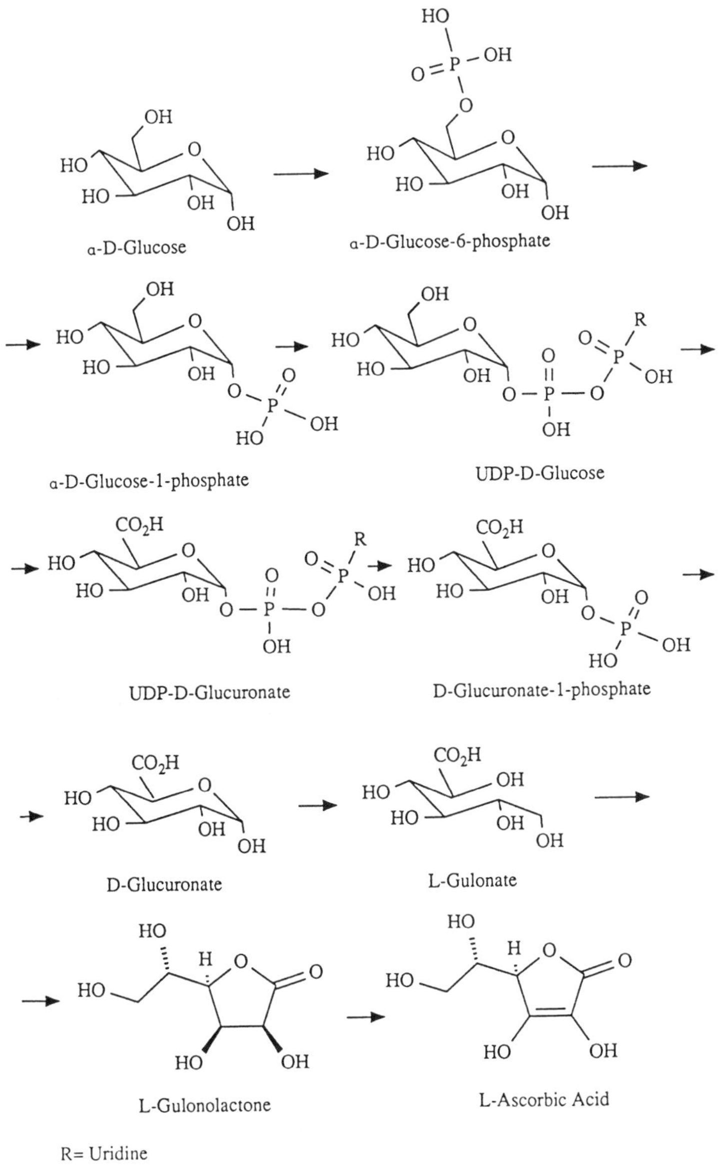

Figure 6 Biosynthesis of ascorbic acid in animals.

Ascorbic acid is kept in the reduced state by the enzymes semidehydroascorbate reductase (EC 1.6.5.4) and the glutathione-dependent dehydroascorbate resductase (EC 1.8.5.1). Only a limited quantity of ascorbic acid is metabolized yielding the primary oxidation products dehydroascorbic acid and 2,3-diketo-L-gulonic acid, which can be decarboxylated to CO_2 and products of the pentose phosphate cycle or oxalic acid plus threonic acid. In man, the formation of these urinary metabolites is limited to about 30–50 mg a day and even the intake of large doses of ascorbic acid up to 10 g per day does not result in an appreciable increase in urinary metabolites (75). In rats and guinea pigs, CO_2 is a

Table 5 Kinetic Data on Ascorbate Uptake

Cell type	Km (μmol/l)	V_{max} (amol/cell/m)	Reference
Porcine adrenocortical cells	20.5	73	73
Bovine adrenocortical cells	16.6	40[c]	248
Bovine adrenomedullary cells	29.0	68	249
Bovine retinal capillary pericytes	76	42[a]	250
Rat lung cells	160[b]	3[c]	251
Rat pituitary cells	9–18	7.3–38	252
Cat retinal pigment cells	42	117[a]	74
Human granulocytes	38.7	2.8	73
Human mononuclear leukocytes	100	3.1	73
Human skin fibroblasts	30.0	24	253

[a]pmol/μg DNA/m.
[b]Probably overestimated due to experimental design.
[c]Estimated from publication.

major metabolite of ascorbic acid degradation (76); in humans, however, CO_2 can be formed in the intestine upon ingestion of gram amounts of vitamin C (77). Furthermore, ascorbate-2-sulfate has been found in human urine as an excretory metabolite (78). In contrast to humans, fish are able to hydrolyze ascorbate-2-sulfate with the enzyme L-ascorbic acid-2-sulfate sulfohydrolase, which is similar to the human arylsulfatase A (79). It is proposed that ascorbate-2-sulfate is the storage form of the vitamin in fish (80).

VII. BIOCHEMICAL FUNCTIONS

A. Introduction

Ascorbic acid has a number of biochemical functions that are a consequence of the ability of this compound to donate one or two electrons. Ascorbic acid is required for the optimal activity of several enzymes involved in hydroxylation reactions (81) (Table 6) and in the metabolism of several nutrients and pharmacological agents in the body. Recent studies show that ascorbic acid is essential in the enzymatic amidation of neuropeptides leading to the formation of bioactive compounds in the brain and peripheral nervous system (82). Ascorbic acid also activates certain liver-detoxifying enzyme systems.

In addition to its importance in many enzymatic reactions, ascorbic acid can act directly as an antioxidant to inactivate highly reactive oxygen species. The ascorbate radical is less reactive than the oxy-radicals, and the ascorbate radical can be either oxidized further to form dehydroascorbic acid or reduced to ascorbate. The donation of the ascorbate electron to the tocopheryl radical restores the antioxidant potential to vitamin E (83).

The third major biochemical activity of ascorbic acid involves its capacity to compete with compounds for binding to substrates. This function is particularly important with regard to the inhibition of the formation of carcinogenic nitrosamines.

Table 6 Enzymes Dependent on Ascorbic Acid for Maximum Activity

Enzyme	Function
Proline hydroxylase (EC 1.14.11.2)	*trans*-4-Hydroxylation of proline in procollagen biosynthesis
Procollagen-proline 2-oxoglutarate 3-dioxygenase (EC 1.14.11.7)	*trans*-3-Hydroxylation of proline in procollagen biosynthesis
Lysine hydroxylase (EC 1.14.11.4)	5-Hydroxylation of lysine in procollagen biosynthesis
gamma-Butyrobetaine, 2-oxoglutarate 4-dioxygenase (EC 1.14.11.1)	Hydroxylation of a carnitine precursor
Trimethyllysine-2-oxoglutarate dioxygenase (EC 1.14.11.8)	Hydroxylation of a carnitine precursor
Dopamine β-monooxygenase (EC 1.14.17.1)	Dopamine β-hydroxylation in norepinephrine biosynthesis
Peptidyl glycine α-amidating monooxygenase activity	Carboxyterminal α-amidation of glycine-extended peptides in peptide hormone processing
4-Hydroxypenylpyruvate dioxygenase (EC 1.13.11.27)	Hydroxylation and decarboxylation of a tyrosine metabolite

Source: Ref. 82.

B. Electron Transport

The metabolism of ascorbic acid involves the reversible two-step oxidation-reduction resulting in the formation of the oxidized form of ascorbic acid, dehydroascorbic acid. Dehydroascrobic acid can also be metabolized to form 2,3-dioxo-L-gulconic acid via an irreversible opening of the lactone ring. The ratio of dehydroascorbic acid/ascorbic acid has been suggested as an indicator of the oxidation status of the cell (24). The ability of ascorbic acid to donate electrons is significant in the respiratory cycle of plants as well as in a number of chemical reactions in animals discussed below.

C. Enzymatic Reactions

Ascorbic acid is required for the optimal activity of several enzymes involved in the hydroxylation reactions associated with collagen formation as well as with carnitine and norepinephrine synthesis, tryptophan metabolism, and a number of other reactions. Ascorbic acid can donate electrons to the enzymes involved in the metabolism of tyrosine, histamine, and cholesterol (84). Recent studies show that ascorbic acid is essential in the enzymatic amidation of neuropeptides leading to the formation of bioactive compounds in the brain and peripheral nervous system (82). Ascorbic acid activates the liver-detoxifying enzyme systems, thus enhancing biotransformation of xenobiotics and natural metabolites (85).

D. Antioxidant

In contrast with oxidation/reduction reactions in which ascorbate donates two electrons, in the inactivation of highly reactive free radicals, ascorbic acid donates one electron. The products of this reaction are the quenched reactive species and the less reactive ascorbyl free radical. The ascorbyl free radical can be either reversibly reduced to ascorbic acid or oxidized to form dehydroascorbic acid (83) (Fig. 7).

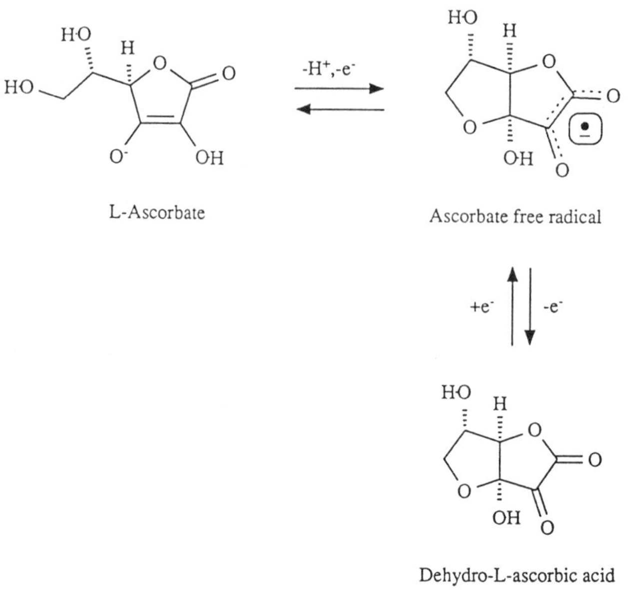

L-Ascorbate

Ascorbate free radical

Dehydro-L-ascorbic acid

Figure 7 Oxidation of ascorbic acid. (From Refs. 83,254.)

Ascorbic acid can react directly with aqueous free radicals such as the hydroxyl and peroxyl radicals and quench their reactivity. Since free-radical species have been associated with damaging effects to intracellular and extracellular structures, the antioxidant function of ascorbic acid is important in the protection of cellular functions. As an example, ascorbic acid has been shown to protect the rabbit cornea from free-radical–related damage by inhibiting the activity of corneal lipoxygenase (86).

In addition to reacting directly with aqueous free radicals, ascorbic acid indirectly affects the balance between oxidative products and antioxidant defense mechanisms. Vitamin E is the major fat-soluble antioxidant involved in protecting cellular membranes from free-radical–initiated oxidation. In the process of sparing fatty acid oxidation, tocopherol (vitamin E) is oxidized to the tocopheryl free radical. Ascorbic acid can donate an electron to the tocopheryl free radical, regenerating the reduced antioxidant form of tocopherol (83). Evidence for the in vivo importance of this sparing action of ascorbic acid is clearly demonstrated in an experiment in which guinea pigs were fed the same level of vitamin E and two levels of vitamin C. The guinea pigs fed the higher level of vitamin C had significantly more vitamin E in their lungs and plasma than the animals fed the low dose of vitamin C. It is concluded that the higher level of vitamin C protected tissue levels of vitamin E from oxidative degeneration (87).

The concentration of ascorbic acid in phagocytic cells found in the circulating blood is many times higher than in red blood cells and is approximately 150 times the concentration in plasma (88–90) (Table 7). These phagocytic cells use free radicals and other highly reactive oxygen containing molecules to help kill pathogens that invade the body. In the process, however, cells and tissues may be damaged by these reactive species. The antioxidant action of ascorbic acid helps to protect these cells from oxidative damage (91).

Table 7 Vitamin C Content of Human Blood Components

Component	Cell volume ($1/10^{15}$ cells)	Ascorbic acid Content (μmol/10^9 cells)	Ascorbic acid Concentration (μmol/l)
Granulocyte	450	0.53	1200
Mononuclear	360	1.37	3800
Platelet	16	0.030	1900
Erythrocyte	90	0.0039	43
Plasma			45

Source: Ref. 89.

E. Autooxidation

The in vitro addition of transition metals to a solution of ascorbic acid in the presence of oxygen results in the formation of free radicals. The formation of free radicals is further enhanced when hydrogen peroxide is added to the mixutre. The reactive chemical species formed can kill bacteria and inactivate viruses. None of the reactants alone can destroy these pathogens, however, the combination produces a potent antimicrobial agent (92–94). An example of the usefulness of the antimicrobial activity is the use of ascorbic acid solutions to retard the growth of bacteria on freshly cut up broiler chicken parts (95).

F. Inhibition of Nitrosamine Formation

Nitrosamines, a class of carcinogenic compounds, are formed when nitrite reacts with certain nitrogen-containing compounds, usually amines or amides. The anionic form of ascorbic acid, readily formed in aqueous solutions, can block the formation of *n*-nitroso compounds (including nitrosamines) by efficiently forming nitric oxide and dehydroascorbic acid (96).

The concentration of *n*-nitroso compounds formed in the body is dependent to some extent upon the intake of the nitrite precursor, nitrate, found in some drinking water and certain foods. Bacterial conversion of nitrate to nitrite occurs in the stomach. Nitrite is added as part of the preserving process for cured and pickled meats. High levels of nitrite are also present in cigarette smoke. Amines found in foods can combine with the nitrites to form nitrosamines in the digestive tract. Nitrosamines can also be directly consumed since these are found in foods (97).

In test tube experiments, ascorbic acid in molar ratios of 2–5:1 with nitrite completely blocked the formation of nitrosamines. Ascorbic acid has no direct effect on preformed nitrosamines (96).

The significance of the ability of ascorbic acid to interfere in nitrosamine formation is linked to the carcinogenicity of these nitroso compounds (88). Epidemiological studies have shown a strong association of digestive system cancers with high levels of nitrates in drinking water and nitrites in foods (97). In addition, individuals suffering from clinical conditions, such as partial gastrectomy and pernicious anemia, in which endogenous nitrosamine levels are increased, have significantly higher incidences of stomach cancer (99).

Epidemiological data have shown that populations with a high risk of stomach cancer have a prevalence of gastritis. Plasma ascorbic acid levels were significantly lower in individuals with gastritis than in those with no history of gastritis (100). When gastrec- tomy patients were given high doses of vitamin C, the concentration of *n*-nitroso com- pounds formed was significantly reduced, and the concentration of the nitrite precursor was reduced in all clinical conditions assessed (101).

Several epidemiological studies have also found an inverse relationship between the consumption of vitamin C–rich foods and stomach, esophageal, and lung cancers (102). The lower incidence of cancer in the populations consuming higher levels of vitamin C may be due to the ability of ascorbic acid to block the formation of mutagenic nitrosamines, as found in experiments with guinea pigs (103), rats (104,105), and, recently, in Chinese subjects with a high risk for developing esophageal cancer (106). In a preliminary study, a volunteer given the nonmutagenic precursors of the *n*-nitroso compound, nitrosoproline, and 1 g of ascorbic acid simultaneously, had complete inhibition of the nitrosation reac- tion, and no detectable level of nitrosoproline could be measured (107). Similarly, sup- plementation of patients with ascorbic acid significantly reduced intragastric mutagenic activity of the gastric juice without affecting the gastric pH (108).

Ascorbic acid is also added during the curing process used in the production of sausages and bacon to retard formation of nitrosamines (109).

G. Drug Interactions

Ascorbic acid is important for the optimal activity of certain of the intracellular drug- metabolizing systems including the hepatic cytochrome P-450 mixed-function oxidase (MFO) and flavin-containing monooxygenase systems (FMO). These systems are involved in the detoxification of nonprescription and prescription, legal and illicit drugs as well as environmental pollutants, which may actively or passively enter the body. The detox- ification process protects against the damaging effects of xenobiotics (85).

Ascorbic acid–deficient guinea pigs have significantly decreased ability to detoxify a number of foreign substances. Specifically, the activities as well as the concentration of the two enzyme systems were significantly reduced in ascorbic acid deficiency. Vitamin C deficiency causes the FMO to become highly unstable (85). Elderly patients with a long history of low vitamin C intakes had a decreased ability to eliminate drugs that are metabo- lized by these enzyme systems in the liver. Vitamin C supplementation restored the pa- tient's ability to metabolize the drugs (110).

In some instances, the intermediate formed as a result of drug metabolism is a toxic substance, which may bind to critical cellular components, causing damage. Ascorbic acid blocks the binding of benzene metabolites to guinea pig bone marrow, a target tissue for benzene toxicity (111). In addition, there is recent evidence that ascorbic acid accelerates the detoxification of alcohol by a catalase-mediated reaction which results, in guinea pigs, in a decrease in alcohol toxicity as measured by serum levels of liver enzymes (85).

Circulating ascorbic acid levels have been shown to be reduced during the prolonged administration of certain drugs including oral contraceptives containing estrogen, tetracycline, and aspirin (112). The decrease in ascorbic acid may be due to drug-induced impaired absorption or increased utilization of the vitamin for drug metabolism.

H. Influence on Mineral Metabolism

Dietary ascorbic acid can affect the gastrointestinal absorption of several essential minerals. The mechanism may be due to the reducing properties of ascorbic acid, or by chelation and subsequent enhancement of transport of the metal into the circulation. The result of ascorbic acid interaction with a specific element can be to either enhance or decrease its solubility.

1. Iron Absorption

The U.S. recommended dietary allowance (RDA) for iron for adults ranges from 10 mg in men to 18 mg in premenopausal women (9). The second National Health and Nutrition Examination survey indicated a prevalence of impaired iron status in adult women of 2.7–9% (113). The problem is more acute in less industrialized nations where iron deficiency anemia is a major health concern. The majority of dietary iron in these countries (as well as in poverty areas in the United States) is in the form of nonheme iron.

Ascorbic acid has been convincingly shown to enhance the absorption of nonheme iron. Iron deficiency anemia can exist even though there is ample nonheme iron in the diet because of its very limited absorption. Therefore, dietary vitamin C can be of considerable importance in the treatment of iron deficiency anemia (114,115). The mechanism of this effect may involve the ability of ascorbic acid to reduce the ferric iron found in foods to the more absorbable ferrous state. Ascorbic acid also forms soluble chelates with iron (116–119).

Ascorbic acid does not appear to significantly enhance iron absorption in individuals with an adequate iron status. In addition, ascorbic acid intake does not seem to affect the high level of iron absorption found in individuals with iron overload disorders (120).

2. Iron Metabolism and Excretion

In the presence of iron, ascorbic acid is oxidized, thus reducing the circulating ascorbic acid status at the expense of enhancement of iron absorption (117).

3. Zinc and Copper Absorption

Ascorbic acid does not affect zinc absorption in humans. Ascorbic acid does decrease copper absorption in rodent and chick models (117). However, in a controlled trial in which male volunteers were given 605 mg/day of ascorbic acid, no effect was found on the level of copper absorption, copper retention, total serum copper, or serum ceruloplasmin. In the same experiment, an intake of 5 mg/day of ascorbic acid also did not affect copper status (121). When subjects were given 1500 mg/day of ascorbic acid, there was a decrease in serum copper and ceruloplasmin levels over the 64-day supplementation period, however, these levels remained within the physiological range of normal values (122).

4. Heavy Metal Absorption

Ascorbic acid, alone or in combination with chelators, lowers the concentration of lead in the tissues of the body. The mechanism is thought to involve the formation of lead-ascorbate chelates, which results in enhancement of lead absorption from the intestine. Lead, in the chelated state, is more rapidly excreted by the kidney than unchelated lead (123) and thus more rapidly removed from the circulation (124).

Ascorbic acid supplementation effectively reduces the circulating levels of mercury, nickel, and vanadium in animal models (125,126). The enhancement of iron absorption by ascorbic acid was associated with decreased levels of cadmium in the tissues of laboratory animals (127).

VIII. PHYSIOLOGICAL EFFECTS

A. Antimutagenic Effects

Ascorbic acid has been shown to inhibit the formation of carcinogenic as well as mutagenic *n*-nitroso compounds in foods. However, several reports have appeared in the literature, which demonstrated that ascorbic acid was mutagenic in the classic Ames test. Careful examination of the methodologies indicated that ascorbic acid alone is not mutagenic. In the earlier studies, metal ions were inadvertently present in the test system. Ascorbic acid, in the presence of transition metals and oxygen, results in the generation of mutagenic free radicals and hydrogen peroxide. Ascorbic acid, in the absence of metal ions, was not mutagenic (128). In addition, in vivo mutagenicity studies with very high intakes of ascorbic acid (5000 mg/kg body weight in guinea pigs) demonstrated that ascorbic acid is not genotoxic (128).

As discussed above, the ability of ascorbic acid to block the formation of mutagenic *n*-nitroso compounds accounts for one aspect of ascorbate's indirect antimutagenic ability (103). The antioxidant capacity of ascorbate may be responsible for decreasing the mutagenic effect of ultraviolet light on mammalian cells in culture (129).

Exposure to mutagenic agents in the workplace can cause adverse changes in chromosome structure and potentially lead to increased cancer risk. Ascorbic acid supplementation of individuals exposed to halogenated ethers resulted in a decrease in the frequency of chromosome defects (130). A similar reduction in chromosome aberrations was found when coal tar workers were supplemented with the vitamin (131). These intervention trials document the effective antimutagenic activity of ascorbic acid.

B. Lipid Metabolism and Cardiovascular Effects

Cardiovascular diseases have been associated with a number of dietary factors including increased fat consumption, high circulating cholesterol levels, as well as decreased circulating levels of high density lipoproteins (HDLs).

Ascorbic acid has been shown to affect cholesterol metabolism; conversion of cholesterol to bile salts is decreased by ascorbic acid deficiency in guinea pigs (132).

Ascorbic acid deficiency also resulted in the formation of atherosclerotic lesions in guinea pigs (133). A major component of atherosclerotic plaques is cholesterol. Supplementation of these guinea pigs with ascorbic acid resulted in the elimination of the atherosclerotic lesion (134).

Epidemiological data indicate that vitamin C status is inversely associated with cholesterol levels and directly related to HDL levels in several studies (135–138). Both a decrease in circulating cholesterol and an increase in HDL levels are thought to be cardioprotective. Of interest is the recent data showing that patients with coronary artery disease and strokes had lower serum and leukocyte vitamin C levels than controls (139–141).

In a large, multinational study, plasma vitamin C levels were shown to be inversely related to mortality due to ischemic heart disease (142).

The mechanisms thought to be involved in the ability of ascorbic acid to lower cardiovascular risks include its role in cholesterol metabolism, effect on lipoproteins, maintenance of the vascular wall integrity due to its requirement for collagen synthesis and its ability to protect against free-radical damage to lipids and other molecules due to its antioxidant function.

C. Effects on Oral Health and Wound Healing

One of the primary effects of scurvy is bleeding gums and loss of dentition. In a carefully controlled study, when young males were given 5 mg/day vitamin C for 4 weeks, the percentage of bleeding gum sites increased significantly. When the subjects were given 605 mg/day, the gums showed very few bleeding sites. In fact, there were fewer sites of bleeding than when the subject were given 65 mg/day (121,143). The mechanism by which vitamin C could protect gums from bleeding may involve its role in collagen formation and the maintenance of basement membranes. This is also the rationale for the importance of vitamin C in wound healing.

Vitamin C deficiency has long been associated with impaired wound healing in animal models and humans (144–146). In addition, clinical studies have shown that supplemental levels of the vitamin (8–50 times the RDA level of 60 mg/day) given before and/or after surgery, significantly increased wound healing (147–149).

Surgery has been associated with a rapid decrease in plasma as well as in the buffy layer (the layer containing the white blood cells) vitamin C levels to approximately half that seen prior to surgery (150). The postoperative decrease is seen even when patients are given supplemental vitamin C (147,148). A decrease in vitamin C status has also been found following myocardial infarction (151) and during acute infections (152). Although the decrease in leukocyte vitamin C level may be due to an increase in the number of white blood cells in the buffy layer, no definitive explanation has been given for the rapid depletion of plasma vitamin C (150). The decrease may be due to an increased utilization of the vitamin under stressful conditions. There may also be a redistribution of the vitamin to the wound site or other tissues.

D. Immune-Related Functions

Ascorbic acid has been shown to have numerous biochemical functions, which impact upon the capacity of the immune system to function optimally (153).

1. Nonspecific Immune Responses

The ability of ascorbic acid to accelerate hydroxlation reactions associated with the formation of collagen is important for the maintenance of the natural barrier provided by the skin and the linings of all the body openings. In laboratory studies, ascorbic acid was shown to be involved in the secretory processes required by immune cells to release immunomodulatory substances (154). In animal models, ascorbic acid supplementation enhanced interferon production (155) and complement component, C1q synthesis (156). Both of these secreted substances are important in protection from infectious agents.

Neutrophils are the key white blood cells involved in the destruction of bacteria. Several aspects of neutrophil function are enhanced by ascorbic acid. These include chemotaxis and protection of neutrophils and surrounding tissue from extracellular free-radical oxidative damage without compromising intracellular bacteria killing capacity (157–159). Furthermore, ascobic acid may be involved in the regulation of 5-lipoxygenase, the enzyme which catalyzes the synthesis of the chemotactic factor leukotriene B4 (160). The concentration of ascorbic acid in these cells is approximately 150 times its concentration in the plasma (89,90,157,161). Ascorbic acid supplementation has also been found to normalize the reduced chemotactic and bactericidal activities of neutrophils from individuals with inherited phagocytosis disorders (162,163) as well as from newborn infants (164). In several instances, clinical improvements were found.

2. Specific Immune Responses

Ascorbic acid–deficient guinea pigs have depressed cell-mediated immune responses, which include delayed hypersensitivity, cytotoxicity, inflammatory and autoimmune responses, and increased survival of skin grafts. Ascorbic acid supplementation has increased lymphocytic proliferation and delayed hypersensitivity responses in some studies with adults (165).

A major biochemical function of ascorbic acid is its capacity to protect vitamin E. Since vitamin E can enhance both nonspecific and specific immune responses, its protection by ascorbic acid indirectly can affect overall immune function (87).

There is, therefore, a large body of data that suggests that ascorbic acid is important for many aspects of immune function.

E. Risk Groups

Epidemiologial and, in some cases, experimental studies have shown that certain population groups have a lower vitamin C status than the rest of the population. These individuals are therefore at risk for developing symptoms of marginal or frank vitamin C deficiency.

1. Smokers

The U.S. National Health and Examination Survery II (NHANES II) documented the significantly lower vitamin C status of adult male and female cigarette smokers who were not taking vitamin C supplements. The highest prevalence of lower vitamin C plasma levels was in adults below the poverty level. The third group identified as at risk for vitamin C deficiency were those who consume diets inadequate in vitamin C–rich foods and do not take a vitamin supplement. In general, males had a lower vitamin C status than females (113).

In the case of smokers, research has shown that smokers absorb vitamin C to a lesser extent than nonsmokers (Fig. 8) and have a higher metabolic turnover of the vitamin C they absorb (166).

2. Elderly

An extensive review of the literature indicates that elderly individuals, either institutionalized or not, have lower vitamin C levels than other adults (167). Plasma and leukocyte vitamin C levels decrease with increasing age in both sexes (168). In addition, elderly men require a higher intake of vitamin C daily to reach the same circulating vitamin C level found in elderly women (169). However, the elderly, regardless of sex, require higher vitamin C intakes to reach the same serum vitamin C levels found in young adults (170). Dietary habits, loss of dentition, and economic considerations may be important in the lowered vitamin C status of the elderly.

The incidence of cataract formation and subsequent loss of vision increases with advancing age. Epidemiological data indicate that the incidence of cataracts correlated inversely with vitamin C status (171). Preliminary data from a recent study in Canada showed that the risk of developing cataracts was significantly reduced in an elderly population that consumed supplements of vitamin C and vitamin E (172).

3. Diabetics

Diabetic patients have an increased turnover rate and decreased vitamin C status compared to nondiabetic individuals. The reason for this may stem from the strong similarity between the chemical structures of glucose and ascorbic acid. Since both molecules use

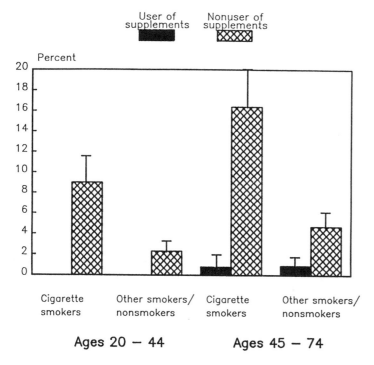

Figure 8 Percentage of American males aged 20–74 years with low serum vitamin C levels (<14 μmol/1 [0.25 mg/dl]) by age group, current cigarette-smoking status, and dietary supplement usage, 1976–1980. (From Ref. 113.)

the same receptor for uptake into leukocytes, it is thought that the high circulating level of glucose in diabetics might decrease the ability of ascorbic acid to enter these cells. Recent studies have shown that glucose infusion in normal adults resulted in a dramatic decrease in the intracellular level of ascorbic acid in peripheral blood leukocytes and a concomitant decrease in functional parameters (173).

4. Others

Other important risk groups with low vitamin C status include alcoholics, hospitalized patients, pregnant and lactating women (174), rheumatoid arthritis and cancer patients, women taking oral contraceptives (175), and individuals exposed to petrochemicals in the workplace (176). As mentioned earlier, patients undergoing surgical procedures have a dramatic decrease in plasma ascorbic acid, which may be detrimental since vitamin C deficiency is associated with impaired wound healing (145). More importantly, vitamin C supplementation has been shown to enhance wound healing (177).

IX. SCURVY

Although well known for several centuries, controlled, experimental vitamin C deficiency in man was first described only in 1940 when H. Crandon placed himself on a diet consisting of cheese, bread, crackers, eggs, beer, black coffee and pure chocolate candy fortified with vitamins A, B1, B2, D, yeast, nictonic acid, and wheat-germ oil for 6 months (178).

The plasma vitamin C level fell rapidly, reaching zero after 41 days on the diet, whereas ascorbic acid in white blood cells was depleted only by day 121. The first sign of scurvy appeared at day 132, when perifollicular hyperkeratotic papules began to develop associated with a marked dryness of the skin. Perifollicular hemorrhages or petechiae could be detected over the lower legs following 161 days. X-ray films of the teeth taken at day 180 revealed interruptions of the lamina dura. At day 182, a 6-cm transverse incision was made in the left midback and compared with a similar experimental injury made on day 85. Ten days later there was no healing of the wound beneath the skin; a drain had to be inserted and the wound was brought together with only silk sutures. A biopsy showed a lack of intercellular substance and capillary formation. At the same time, the subject performed a fatigue test, which consisted of two grades of work, walking and running, on a motor-driven treadmill. The experiment was repeated after 10 days during which the volunteer received daily 1000 mg vitamin C iv remaining on the same deficient diet. During the period of moderate work, the heart rate was 40 beats higher than during the control test and after a higher grade of work the subject was exhausted after 16 seconds compared with 66 second after the vitamin C supplementation. During the recovery period the heart rate fell more rapidly following the administration of vitamin C. All signs of scurvy disappeared within 6 days of vitamin C supplementation, although some hyperkeratotic papules were still present for 14 days. The white cell count remained normal between 3200 and 5000 during the dietary period but rose to 9000 after the beginning of the vitamin C therapy.

Cases of scurvy still occur occasionally (despite improved standards of living) due to inadequate diets and food faddism (179,180). Infantile scurvy or Barlow's disease had been confused with rickets during the second half of the nineteenth century since it presents a different picture from that in adults (181). In a mild form it is scarcely recognizable, typical signs being painful swollen legs (182), and more severe cases may even lead to a sudden death (183).

X. NUTRITIONAL ASSESSMENT

Assessment of vitamin C status is most critical when the physician is confronted with a patient exhibiting signs of deficiency disease. Although scurvy is considered a rare disease in the industrialized world, there have been recent documented cases of adults with edema associated with lower leg pain and profound muscle fatigue, hair follicle abnormalities, vasculitis, systemic bleeding disorders, hyperkeratoses, and loss of teeth which have been corrected by administration of vitamin C (179). The major problem associated with adult scurvy is the misdiagnosis because of the presumed rarity of this nutrient deficiency disease. Plasma ascorbic acid levels below 0.2 mg/dl and leukocyte concentrations below 2 $\mu g/10^8$ cells are indicative of vitamin C deficiency (184). As discussed above, alcoholics and elderly, especially elderly men living alone with marginal economic resources, are at risk of developing overt signs of vitamin C deficiency (179).

Whole blood, serum, and plasma are generally used as biochemical indicators of vitamin C status (185). Blood vitamin C levels reflect the recent intake of vitamin C, in contrast to peripheral blood leukocyte levels, which reflect tissue reserves. Normal plasma levels are 0.8–1.4 mg/dl. Leukocyte vitamin C levels are more difficult to measure than plasma levels. Normal leukocyte vitamin C levels are 20–40 $\mu g/10^8$ cells (186). Red blood cells have significantly lower concentrations of ascorbic acid compared to leukocytes (Table 7). Some investigators have measured urinary vitamin C, however, this is generally regarded as a poor indicator of adequacy because the vitamin does not appear in the urine unless the body pool of ascorbic acid exceeds 1500 mg (9).

Correlation of either plasma or leukocyte levels with vitamin C intake has shown wide variations (187). The range of vitamin C plasma levels in healthy normal individuals was 0.31–2.1 mg/dl and ranged from 0.12 to 1.35 in an elderly population (168). Elderly individuals given 1 g/day vitamin C for 60 days had an average plasma vitamin C level of 1.37 mg/dl, however the range was between 0.45 and 2.66 mg/dl (168).

The vitamin C status of the individuals participating in the NHANES II survey was determined by measuring the plasma level and taking a diet history. The vitamin C status was dramatically affected by cigarette smoking, economic level, and supplement/dietary intake (113) (Fig. 8).

XI. REQUIREMENT

Ascorbic acid is a required, essential nutrient for humans, nonhuman primates, guinea pigs, salmon, trout, catfish, and a small number of other animals. An essential nutrient is one that cannot be synthesized de novo and therefore must be provided in the diet. The level of intake required is, in part, dependent upon the body's handling of the nutrient.

Recently, certain strains of animals normally able to synthesize ascorbic acid have been found with genetic defects that result in a dietary requirement for ascorbic acid. In the rat model (osteogenic disorder or OD rat), the strain has been inbred and a limited number of animals are available for experimentation. Approximately 300 mg/kg of ascorbic acid in the diet is required to prevent deficiency symptoms, whereas more than 300 mg/kg diet is needed to achieve maximum activity of the hepatic drug-metabolizing enzymes (188). An inherited ascorbic acid deficiency in pigs resulted in a decreased cellular immune response, which was normalized when ascorbic acid was given in the diet (189). These new animal models, as well as the guinea pig, are important in elucidating the functional requirements of ascorbic acid.

A. Absorption

In humans, ascorbic acid is absorbed by passive and active transport mechanisms predominantly in the distal portion of the small intestine and to a lesser extent in the mouth, stomach, and proximal intestine (190). Little ascorbic acid is excreted in the feces, even when gram amounts are ingested (191).

B. Metabolism

The size of the body pool and the rate of turnover of vitamin C are used to estimate its metabolic utilization and are therefore important criteria for assessment of vitamin C status. The results of studies using radioactively labeled ascorbic acid indicate that the body pool size of healthy adult males examined was greater than 1400 mg (75,184,192–195). The turnover rate calculated in these studies ranged from 45 to 60 mg/day. At these values, Kallner (75) found a plasma concentration of 0.7–0.8 mg/dl. A significant adverse change in psychological functions was found when the body pool size reached 600 mg (196). Clinical signs of scurvy are associated with a pool size <300 mg (184).

In a study using rhesus monkeys, administration of oral contraceptive agents increased the turnover rate of ascorbic acid. The authors suggest that these drugs may have the same effect in women, consequently increasing their requirement for vitamin C (197).

C. Tissue Concentrations

The adrenal glands and pituitary glands have the highest concentration of ascorbic acid/weight of tissue than any other tissue in the body of animals that synthesize ascorbic acid (rats) a well as in humans (81) (Table 8). Tissue concentrations may be related to the function of the vitamin in the specific tissue.

D. Excretion

The major route of excretion is the urine, and the renal threshold corresponds to a plasma concentration of approximately 0.8 mg/dl. As the plamsa concentration increases, the threshold is exceeded, and ascorbic acid appears in the urine (Table 9). Recent experiments have shown that approximately 2.5% of the vitamin C intake was excreted when greater than 98% of the ascorbate was absorbed (intakes < 60 mg), even though the body pool sizes ranged from 900 to 17,000 mg. The total turnover rate was calculated to be approximately 60 mg/day (75). Based upon these kinetic studies as well as other important considerations, the RDA for vitamin C was established in 1980 as 60 mg/day for adults of both sexes (9) (Table 10).

E. Recommended Intake Levels

The required level of intake to prevent scurvy is approximately 10 mg/day. However, it is well recognized that this level of intake is inadequate for the maintenance of an

Table 8 Tissue Concentrations of Ascorbic Acid

Tissue	Rat (mg/100 g)	Human (mg/100 g)
Adrenal glands	280–400	30–40
Pituitary gland	100–130	40–50
Liver	25–40	10–16
Spleen	40–50	10–15
Lungs	20–40	7
Kidneys	15–20	5–15
Testes	25–30	3
Thyroid	22	2
Thymus	40	
Brain	35–50	13–15
Pancreas		10–16
Eye lens	8–10	25–31
Skeletal muscle	5	3– 4
Heart muscle	5–10	5–15
Bone marrow	12	
Plasma	1.6	0.4–1.0
Saliva		0.07–0.09

Source: Ref. 81.

Table 9 Urinary Excretion of Oral Ascorbic Acid Based Upon Tracer Experiments

Ascorbic acid dosages (mg/day)	Total	Excretion in urine (%)	
		Ascorbic acid	Metabolites
1 × 30	30	6.6	93.4
2 × 30	60	20.3	79.7
2 × 45	90	34.1	65.9
4 × 45	180	61.7	38.3
4 × 250	1000	87.4	17.8
4 × 500	2000	87.9	12.1
2 × 1000	2000	87.0	13.0

Source: Ref. 75.

optimal body pool or optimal health. Since there is not complete agreement on the criteria for assessment of optimal health, the required level of vitamin C has not been conclusively established. In a recent controlled dietary intake study using healthy young men, plasma ascorbic acid levels of less than 0.4 mg/dl were shown to accurately reflect low dietary intake. The calculated intake to reach the maximal body pool size was 138 mg/day (143,198).

Garry (169,170) has estimated that elderly males require 125 mg/day and elderly females need 75 mg/day to maintain plasma ascorbic acid levels at approximately 1.0 mg/dl, which may be the level needed to saturate the body pool of this population group. More than half the elderly men with low plasma vitamin C levels of < 0.3 mg/dl had daily intakes of 40–50 mg (169).

A positive correlation between vitamin C intake and bone density was found in an epidemiological study in postmenopausal women (199). In another study, there was a positive correlation between vitamin C and bone mineral content in postmenopausal women

Table 10 1980 U.S. Recommended Daily Dietary Allowances for Vitamin C

Age group	Amount (mg)
Males	
Adults: 19+ years	60
Females	
Adults: 19+ years	60
Pregnancy, second half	80
Lactation period	100
Children	
Neonates, premature infants	100
Under 1 year	35
1–3 years	45
4–6 years	45
7–10 years	45
11–14 years	50
15–18 years	60

Source: Ref. 9.

whose average intake of vitamin C was 174 mg/day (200). The age- and sex-related losses of bone are the major contributing factors in the development of osteoporosis.

In a preliminary report of an epidemiological study of 113 adults age 40–70 years, the lowest prevalence of cataracts was associated with individuals with the highest vitamin C intakes (171).

Recommended levels of intake for adults of various countries range from 30 to 100 mg/day. Recently, higher intakes have been recommended for smokers in France, Canada, and New Zealand (Table 11). In the elderly population group, there may be evidence for increasing recommended intake levels (170,201).

The ascorbic acid status for newborns and premature infants has been carefully examined. The plasma level of vitamin C declines rapidly to less than one-third the original level after premature birth in infants fed pasteurized pooled human milk. The authors indicate that this is a significant decrease in vitamin C status in the preterm infant (202). Preterm infants have higher requirements than full-term infants for many nutrients, including vitamin C (203).

In a larger population study, low vitamin C status was observed in 27% of infants at 6 months of age and in 30% of infants at one year of age (204). However, in an intervention study, full-term infants given breast milk from mothers supplemented with 90 mg/day vitamin C received approximately twice the RDA level recommended for infants from birth to 6 months of age. The concentration of vitamin C in the breast milk was not increased further by maternal supplementation up to 1000 mg/day (205). The investigators suggest that there may be an optimal threshold level of vitamin C in human milk, which is reached when 90 mg of vitamin C are added to the diet of nursing women. These findings suggest that the recommended intake levels for preterm and full-term infants may need to be reevaluated.

XII. INDUSTRIAL USES

The chemical characteristics of ascorbic acid make it an important agent in the preservation of processed food products. The antioxidant, reducing properties, nitrosamine blocking, and metal sequestering capacities of ascorbic acid have resulted in its use in the production of cured meats, brewed products, stabilization of vegetable oils, animal fats, and margarine as well as a number of other food products (206).

Ascorbic acid can retard the browning of fresh and canned fruits and vegetables. It has been suggested that ascorbic acid be used as a partial replacement for sulfites (206,207).

The ability of ascorbic acid to block the formation of nitrosamines has been used successfully in the preparation of bacon and other cured meat products. The addition of ascorbic acid significantly lowers the level of nitrosamines formed during frying (208). Ascorbic acid is widely used in the baking industry, where its addition results in enhanced quality of the dough and improved appearance of the baked goods (109).

In commercial fisheries, ascorbic acid is added to the fish food. Enhancement in immune responses and decreases in the rate of infection have been shown in fish given supplemental ascorbic acid (209). In addition, fish dipped in ascorbic acid have retarded rancidity and discoloration (109). As mentioned previously, dipping of fresh chicken parts in ascorbic acid solutions decreased microbial growth and increased shelf life (95).

Ascorbic acid has been used as an acid catalyst in the polymer industry, in the production of developer solutions in the photographic industry, in cosmetic formulations, as

Table 11 Recommended Dietary Allowances for Vitamin C for
Various Countries

Country	Allowance (mg/day)	Country	Allowance (mg/day)
Australia	30	Italy	60
Bolivia	60	Japan	50
Brazil	75	Malaysia	30
Bulgaria	95	Mexico	50
Canada	60[b]	New Zealand	60[b]
Colombia	40	Norway	60
Czechoslovakia	60	Philippines	75
Denmark	60	South Africa	60
England	30	South Korea	55
FAO/WHO	30	Spain	60
Finland	60	Sweden	60
France	80[b]	Switzerland	75
DDR	45	Taiwan	60
FRD	75	Thailand	30
Holland	50	Uruguay	30
Hungary	30	U.S.A.	60
India	50	U.S.S.R.	78
Israel	70	Venezuela	60

[a]Recommendations are for moderately active, adult males.
[b]Higher intake recommended for smokers: Canada 80–85; France 120; New
Zealand 75.

a preservative for stored blood, in the production of printing inks, and a wide range of
other applications (109).

XIII. SAFETY

Since some people consume large amounts of vitamin C, there is some concern as to whether
the intake of these supplements has undesirable side effects. Ascorbic acid is considered
as one of the safest constituents of nutrition by the Joint Expert Committee on Food Ad-
ditives of the WHO/FAO. The acceptable daily intake (ADI), defined as the amount of
a food additive which may be ingested without any risk of harm, is 1050 mg for a 70-kg
man (210). Nevertheless, many reports have been published claiming adverse effects of
high intakes of ascorbic acid. Most of these allegations are, however, based on anecdotal
and uncontrolled studies as has been critically reviewed by several authors (211–214).

The most frequently cited adverse effect of high intakes of ascorbic acid concerns
the formation of renal calcium oxalate stones since oxalate is a urinary metabolic end product of vitamin C (215,216). Most of the 30–40 mg oxalate excreted per day is derived
from endogenous metabolic processes, 35–50% for the degradation of ascorbic acid.
Therefore, urine is normally supersaturated with respect to calcium oxalate since its solubility in water is only about 9 mg per liter at 37°C. Glucuronides, peptides, colloids,
phosphates, and other urinary constituents are thought to contribute to the prevention of
stone formation. Individuals who have a tendency to form kidney stones often have normal

oxalate levels and hence no primary disorder of oxalate metabolism. Since the metabolic turnover of ascorbic acid is limited, changes in urinary oxalate excretion evoked by high intakes of ascorbic acid (up to 9 g/day) are in the range of the variability seen in this particular population. Patients with renal insufficiency should restirct their intake of the vitamin to 100–200 mg a day since multiple metabolic and eliminatory processes may be impaired and thus the handling of ascorbate may not be predictable. Recurrent kidney stone formers and patients on chronic hemodialysis should also avoid high doses of ascorbic acid.

Methodological pitfalls account for many discrepancies in findings of varying oxalate levels after vitamin C intake. Inappropriate handling and storage of the samples favor an in vitro conversion of ascorbic acid to oxalic acid. It can therefore be concluded that vitamin C cannot be considered a risk factor for oxalate stones in healthy persons.

A few cases were reported of a conditioning effect of high-dose ascorbic acid intakes upon cessation of the supplementation. However, these reports do not appear to be objectively determined. Controlled studies in guinea pigs and man have failed to reproduce a rebound effect (217).

Ascorbic acid may interfere with nonspecific color reactions of laboratory tests such as the analysis of glucose, uric acid, creatinine, and inorganic phosphate (218). The detection of occult blood may be blocked by ascorbic acid, which appears in the feces when amounts higher than 1 g per day are ingested (219). These unfavorable effects can easily be avoided by using suitable laboratory methods and by appropriate instructions to patients prior to the laboratory assay procedures.

A critical evaluation of the literature dealing with possible side effects of large oral intakes of ascorbic acid allows the conclusion that ingestion of up to 10 g vitamin C per day does not constitute a serious health risk for man.

ACKNOWLEDGMENT

We thank Dr. Urs Hengartner for his comments and suggestions, especially for reviewing all the formulas and Sec. III, "Chemistry."

REFERENCES

1. P. A. Vassal, D'où vient le mot 'scorbut'? *Rev. Path. Gen. Physiol. Clin. 680*:1279–1283 (1956).
2. C. G. King, *World Rev. Nutr. Diet 18*:47–59 (1973).
3. J. E. Halver, R R. Smith, B. M. Tolbert, and E. M. Baker, *Ann. N.Y. Acad.Sci. 258*:81–102 (1975).
4. K. J. Carpenter, *The History of Scurvy and Vitamin C.* Cambridge University Press, Cambridge, 1986.
5. A. F. Hess. *Scurvy, Past and Present.* Philadelphia, J. B. Lippincott Co., 1920.
6. U. Wintermeyer, H. Lahann, and R. Vogel, *Vitamin C.* Deutscher Apotheker Verlag, Stuttgart, 1981.
7. J. Lind, *A Treatise on the Scurvy.* London, 1753 (republished by Edinburgh University Press, Edinburgh, 1953).
8. R. Priestley, *Nutr. Today 4*:18 (1969).
9. *Recommended Dietary Allowences*, 9th Ed. National Academy of Sciences, Washington, D.C., 1980, p. 72.
10. A. Holst and T. Frölich, *J. Hyg.* (Cambridge) *7*:634–671 (1907).
11. T. Smith, Ann. Rep. Bureau of Animal Industry. Washington, D.C.: US Department of

Agriculture, 1895–1896, pp. 166–179.

12. C. Bolle,. *Z. f. die Gesamte physikalische Therapie* (Leipzig) 6:354–356 (1902–1903).
13. K. Hart, *Virchows Archiv.* 208S:367–396 (1912).
14. S. S. Zilva, *Lancet 1*:478–478 (1921).
15. J. C. Drummond, *Biochem. J. 13*:77–80 (1919).
16. J. C. Drummond, *Bochem. J. 14*:660–660 (1920).
17. A. Szent-Györgyi, *Biochem. J. 22*:1387–1409 (1928).
18. J. L. Svirbely and A. Szent-Györgyi, *Biochem. J. 26*:865–870 (1932).
19. C. G. King and W. A. Waugh, *Science 75*:357–358 (1932).
20. W. N. Haworth, and E. L. Hirst, *J. Soc. Chem. Ind. 52*:645–646 (1933).
21. T. Reichstein, A. Grüssner, and R. Oppenhauer, *Helv. Chim. Acta 16*:1019–1033 (1933).
22. IUPAC-IUB Commission on Biochemical Nomenclature. *Biochim. Biophys. Acta 107*:1–4 (1965).
23. The Merck Index, 10th Ed. M. Windholz, S. Budavari, R. F. Blumetti, and E. S. Otterbein (Eds.). Merck & Co., Inc., Rahway, N.J. 1983, p. 120.
24. B. M. Tolbert and J. B. Ward, Dehydroascorbic acid. In *Ascorbic Acid: Chemistry, Metabolism, and Uses*, P. A. Seib and P. M. Tolbert (Eds.). American Chemical Society, Washington, D.C. 1982, pp. 101–123.
25. J. Hvoslef, *Acta Cristallogr. 28*:916–923 (1972).
26. J. Hvoslef, *Acta Cristallogr.* Section B 24:23, 1431 (1968).
27. J. Hvoslef, *Acta Cristallogr.* Sect. B. 25:2214 (1969).
28. J. V. Paukstelis, D. D. Mueller, P. A. Seib, and D. W. Lillard, Jr., NMR spectroscopy of ascorbic acid and its derivatives. In *Ascorbic Acid: Chemistry, Metabolism, and Uses*, P. A. Seib and P. M. Tolbert (Eds.). American Chemical Society, Washington, D.C., 1982, pp. 28.10 125–151.
29. T. Radford, J. G. Sweeny, G. A. Iacobucci, and D. J. Goldsmith, *J. Org. Chem. 44*:658–659 (1979).
30. I. A. Meshal and M. M. A. Hassan, *Anal. Profiles Drug Substances 11*:45–78 (1982).
31. T. Z. Liu, N. Chin, M. D. Kiser, and W. N. Bigler, *Clin. Chem. 28*:2225–2228 (1982).
32. J. S. Lawendel, *Nature 180*:434–435 (1957).
33. Y. Ogata and Y. Kosugi, *Tetrahedron 26*:4711–4716 (1970).
34. K. Mikova and J. Davidek, *Chem. Listy 68*: 715 (1974).
35. K. Niemelä, *J. Chromatogr. 399*:235–243 (1987).
36. D. W. Bradley, G. Emery, and J. E. Maynard, *Clin. Chim. Acta 4*:47–52 (1973).
37. J. R. Cooke and R. E. D. Moxon, The detection and measurement of vitamin C. In *Vitamin C (Ascorbic Acid)*, J. N. Counsell and D. H. Hornig (Eds.). Applied Science, London, 1981, pp. 167–198.
38. T. C. Crawford, Synthesis of L-ascorbic acid. In *Ascorbic Acid: Chemistry, Metabolism, and Uses*, P. A. Seib and P. M. Tolbert (Eds.). American Chemical Society, Washington, D.C., 1982, pp. 1–36.
39. T. Reichstein and A. Grüssner, *Helv. Chim. Acta 17*:311–328 (1934).
40. M. Kulhanek. *Adv. Appl. Microbiol. 12*:11–33 (1970).
41. S. Anderson, C. B. Marks, R. Lazarus, J. Miller, K. Stafford, J. Seymour, D. Light, W. Rastetter, and D. Estell, *Science 230*:144–149 (1985).
42. L. A. Pachla and D. L. Reynolds, *J. Assoc. Off. Anal. Chem. 68*:1–12 (1985).
43. H.O. Beutler and G. Beinstingl, *Dtsch. Lebensm. Rdsch. 76*:69–75 (1980).
44. M. Okamura, *Clin. Chim Acta 103*:259–268 (1980).
45. J. H. Roe and C. A. Kuether, *J. Biol. Chem. 147*:399–407 (1943).
46. O. Pelletier and R. Brassard, *J. Food Sci. 42*:1471–1477 (1977).
47. A. Zloch, J. Cerven, and E. Ginter, *Anal. Biochem. 43*;99–106 (1971).
48. J. Ballantine, and A. D. Woolfson, *J. Pharm. Pharmacol. 32*:353–356 (1980).
49. T. Tono and S. Fujita, *Agric. Biol. Chem. 45*:2947–2949 (1981).

50. K. Matsumoto, K. Yamada, and Y. Osajima, *Anal. Chem. 53*:1974–1979 (1981).

51. M. H. Bui-Nguyen, *J. Chromatogr. 196*:163–165 (1980).

52. M. T. Parviainen, K. Nyyssönen, I. M. Penttilä, K. Seppänen, R. Rauramaa, J. T. S. Salonen, and C. G. Gref, *J. Liq. Chromatogr. 9*:2185–2197 (1986).

53. R. Sasaki, T. Kurokawa, and S. Tero-Kubota, *J. Gerontol. 38*:26–30 (1983).

54. J. W. Erdman, Jr. and B. P. Klein, Harvesting, processing and cooking influences on vitamin C in foods. In *Ascorbic Acid: Chemistry, Metabolism, and Uses*, P. A. Seib and P. M. Tolbert (Eds.). American Chemical Society., Washington, D.C., 1982, pp. 499–532.

55. J. C. Brand, V. Cherikoff, A. Lee, and A. S. Truswell, *Lancet 2*:873–873 (1982).

56. O. O. Keshinro, *Nutr. Reports Internat. 31*:381–387 (1985).

57. K. Milton and R. Jenness, *Experientia 43*:339–342 (1987).

58. F. A. Loewus, and M. W. Loewus, CRC Critical Reviews. *Plant Sciences 5*:101–119 (1987).

59. M. Grün, B. Renstrom, and F. A. Loewus, *Plant Physiol. 70*:1233–1235 (1982).

60. V. R. Franceschi, *Plant Cell Environ 10*:397–406 (1987).

61. K. Saito and Z. Kasai, *Plant Physiol. 76*:170–174 (1984).

62. U. Malipiero, H. P. Ruffner, and D. M. Rast, *J. Plant Physiol. 129*:33–40 (1987).

63. B. Halliwell, Ascorbic acid and the illuminated chloroplast. In *Ascorbic Acid: Chemistry, Metabolism, and Uses*, P. A. Seib and P. M. Tolbert (Eds.). American Chemical Society, Washington, D.C., 1982. pp. 263–274.

64. N. J. Chinoy, Ed., *The Role of Ascorbic Acid in Growth, Differentiation and Metabolism of Plants*. Martinus Nijhoff, The Hague, 1984.

65. P. M. H. Kroneck, F. A. Armstrong, H. Merkle, and A. Marchesini, Ascorbate oxidase: Molecular properties and catalytic activity. In *Ascorbic Acid: Chemistry, Metabolism, and Uses*, P. A. Seib and P. M. Tolbert (Eds.). American Chemical Society, Washington, D.C., 1982, pp. 223–248.

66. I. B. Chatterjee, *Science 82*:1271–1272 (1973).

67. E. C. Birney, R. Jenness and I. D. Hume, *Evolution 24*:230–239 (1980).

68. I.B. Chatterjee, A. K. Majumder, B. K. Nandi, and N. Subramanian, Synthesis and some major functions of vitamin C in animals. In *Second Conference on Vitamin C*, C. G. King and J. J. Burns (Eds.). N.Y. Acad. Sci., New York, 1975, vol. 258, pp. 24–47,

69. P. H. Sato, L. A. Roth, and D. M. Walton, *Biochem. Med. Metabol. Biol. 35*:59–64 (1986),

70. J. J. Burns, Introduction: Overview of ascorbic acid metabolism. In *Second Conference on Vitamin C*, C. G. King and J. J. Burns (Eds.). N.Y. Acad. Sci., New York, 1975, pp. 5–6.

71. J. J. Burns, C. Evans and N. Trousof, *J. Biol. Chem. 227*:785–794 (1957).

72. F. Horio and A. Yoshida, *J. Nutr. 112*:416–425 (1982).

73. U. Moser, Uptake of ascorbic acid by leukocytes. *Third Conference on Vitamin C*, J. J. Burns, J. M. Rivers and L. J. Machlin (Eds.). N.Y. Acad. Sci., New York, 1987, vol. 498, pp. 200–215.

74. M. Khatami, L. E. Stramm, and J. H. Rockey, *Exp. Eye Res. 43*:607–615 (1986).

75. A. Kallner, D. Hartmann, and D. Hornig, *Am. J. Clin. Nutr. 32*:530–539 (1979).

76. D. Hornig, and D. Hartmann, Kinetic behaviour of ascorbic acid in guinea pigs. In *Ascorbic Acid: Chemistry, Metabolism and Uses*, P. A. Seib and P. M. Tolbert (Eds.). American Chemical Society, Washington, D.C., 1982, pp. 293–316.

77. A. Kallner, D. Hornig and R. Pellikka, *Am. J. Clin. Nutr. 41*:609–613 (1985).

78. E. M. Baker, D. C. Hammer, S. C. March, B. M. Tolbert, and J. E. Canham, *Science 173*:826–827 (1971).

79. L. V. Benitez and J. E. Halver, *Proc. Natl. Acad. Sci. USA 79*:5445–5449 (1982).

80. B. W. Tucker and J. E. Halver, *Fish Physiol. Biochem. 2*:151–160 (1986).

81. M. Levine and K. Mortia, Ascorbic acid in endocrine systems. In *Vitamins and Hormones*, vol. 42, G. D. Aurbach and D. B. McCormick (Eds.). Academic Press, Inc., New York, 1985, pp. 1–64.

82. M. Levine, *New Engl. J. Med. 314*:892–902 (1986).

83. A. Bendich, L. J. Machlin, O. Scandurra, G. W. Burton, and D. D. M. Wayner, *Adv. in Free Radical Biology & Medicine 2*:419–444 (1986).

84. C. J. Bates, The function and metabolism of vitamin C in man. In *Vitamin C, (Ascorbic Acid)*, J. N. Counsell and D. H. Hornig (Eds.). Applied Science Publishers, London, 1981, pp. 1–22.

85. V. G. Zannoni, J. I. Brodfuehrer, R. C. Smart, and R. L. Susick, Ascorbic acid, alcohol, and environmental chemicals. In *Third Conference on Vitamin C*, J. J. Burns, J. M. Rivers, and L. J. Machlin (Eds.). N.Y. Acad. Sci., New York, 1987, vol. 498, pp. 364–388.

86. R. N. Williams and C. A. Paterson, *Exp. Eye Res. 43*:7–13 (1986).

87. A. Bendich, P. D'Apolito, E. Gabriel, and L. J. Machlin, *J. Nutr. 114*:1588–1593 (1984).

88. P. Barkhan and A. N. Howard, *Biochem. J. 70*:163–168 (1958).

89. R. M. Evans, L. Currie, and A. Campbell, *Br. J. Nutr. 47*:473–482 (1982).

90. U. Moser and F. Weber, *Internat. J. Vit. Nutr. Res. 54*:47–53 (1983).

91. R. Anderson and P. T. Lukey, A biological role for ascorbate in the selective neutralization of extracellular phagocyte-derived oxidants. *Ann. N.Y. Acad. Sci. 498*:229–248 (1987).

92. Bissell, M. J., C. Hatie, D. A. Farson, R. I. Schwarz, and W. J. Soo, *Proc. Natl. Acad. Sci. 77*:2711–2715 (1980).

93. T. E. Miller. *J. Bacteriol. 98*:949–955 (1969)

94. A. Murata, R. Oyadomari, T. Ohashi and K. Kitagawa, *J. Nutr. Sci. Vitaminol. 21*:261–269 (1975).

95. A. S. Arafa and T. C. Chen, *Poultry Sci. 56*:1345–1349 (1977).

96. S. S. Mirvish. Blocking the formation of N-nitroso compounds with ascorbic acid in vitro and in vivo. In *Second Conference on Vitamin C*, C. G. King and J. J. Burns (Eds.). N.Y. Acad. Sci., New York, 1975, vol. 259, pp. 175–180.

97. E. Bright-See, *Seminars in Oncology 10*:294–298 (1983).

98. S. S. Mirvish, *Cancer 58*:1842–1850 (1986).

99. S. A. Kyrtopulos, *Am. J. Clin. Nutr. 45*:1344–1350 (1987).

100. M. L. Burr, I. M. Samloff, C. J. Bates and R. M. Holliday, *Br. J. Cancer 56*:163–167 (1987).

101. P. I. Reed, K. Summers, C. L. R. Smith, C. L. Walters, B. A. Bartholomew, M. J. Hill, S. Vennitt, D. Hornig, and J. P. Bonjour, *Gut 24*:A492–493 (1983).

102. B. E. Glatthaar, D. H. Hornig, and U. Moser, The role of ascorbic acid in carcinogenesis. In *Essential Nutrients in Carcinogenesis*, L. A. Poirier, P. M. Newberne and M. W. Pariza (Eds.). Plenum Press, New York, 1987, pp. 357–377.

103. E. P. Norkus, and W. A. Kuenzig, *Carcinogenesis 6*:1593–1598 (1985).

104. H. Ohshima, J. C. Bereziat and H. Bartsch, *Carcinogenesis 3*:115–120 (1982).

105. J. H. Weisburger, H. Marquardt, H. F. Mower, N. Hirota, H. Mori, and G. Williams, *Preventive Med. 9*:352–361 (1980).

106. Shin-Hsin, Lu, H. Oshima, H. Fu, Y. Tian, F. Li, M. Blettner, J. Wahrendorf, and H. Bartsch, *Cancer Res. 46*:1485–1491 (1986).

107. H. Ohshima and H. Bartsch, The influence of vitamin C on the in vivo formation of nitrosamines. In *Vitamin C (Ascorbic Acid)*, J. N. Counsell and D. H. Hornig (Eds.). Applied Science, London, 1981, pp. 215–224.

108. H. J. O'Connor, N. Habibzedah, C. J. Schorah, A. T. R. Axon, R. E. Riley, and R. C. Garner, *Carcinogenesis 6*:1675–1676 (1985).

109. J. C. Bauernfeind, Ascorbic acid technology in agricultural, pharmaceutical, food, and industrial applications. In *Ascorbic Acid: Chemistry, Metabolism, and Uses*, P. A. Seib and B. M. Tolbert (Eds.). American Chemical Society, Washington, D. C., 1982, pp. 395–497.

110. D. J. Smithard and M. J. S. Langman, *Br. J. Clin. Pharmac. 5*:181–185 (1978).

111. R. C. Smart and V. G. Zannoni, *Biochem. Pharmacol 35*:3180–3182 (1986).

112. T. K. Basu, The influence of drugs with particular reference to aspirin on the bioavailability of vitamin C. In *Vitamin C, (Ascorbic Acid)*, J. N. Counsell and D. H. Hornig (Eds.). Applied Science Publishers, London, 1981, pp. 273–281.

113. C. Woteki, C. Johnson, and R. Murphy, A Nutritional status of the U. S. Population: Iron, Vitamin C, and Zinc. In *What Is American Eating?*, Natl. Acad. Press, Washington, D. C., 1986, pp. 21–39.

114. L. Hallberg, Effect of vitamin C on the bioavailability of iron from food. In *Vitamin C* (Ascorbic Acid), J. N. Counsell and D. H. Hornig (Eds.). Applied Science Publishers, London, 1981, pp. 49–61.

115. L. Hallberg, M. Brune, and L. Rossander-Hulthen, Is there a physiological role of vitamin C in iron absorption? In *Third Conference on Vitamin C*, J. J. Burns, J. M. Rivers, and L. J. Machlin (Eds.). N.Y. Acad. Sci. New York, 1987, vol 498, pp. 324–332.

116. E. R. Monsen and J. F. Page, *J. Agric. Food Chem. 26*:223–226 (1978).

117. N. W. Solomons and F. E. Viteri, Biological interaction of ascorbic acid and mineral nutrients. In *Ascorbic Acid: Chemistry, Metabolism, and Uses*, P. A. Seib and B. M. Tolbert (Eds.). American Chemical Society, Washington, D.C., 1982, pp. 551–569.

118. C. M. Plug, D. Decker and A. Bult, *Pharm. Weekblad 16*:245–248 (1984).

119. J. J. M. Marx, and J. Stiekema, *Eur. J. Clin. Pharmacol. 23*:335–338 (1982).

120. A. Bendich and M. Cohen, *Toxicology Letters*, in press.

121. R. A. Jacob, S. T. Omaye, J. H. Skala, P. J. Leggott, D. L. Rothman, and P. A. Murray, Experimental vitamin C depletion and supplementation in young men. In *Third Conference on Vitamin C*, J. J. Burns, J. M. Rivers, and L. J. Machlin (Eds.). N.Y. Acad Sci., New York, 1987, pp. 333–346.

122. E. B. Finley and F. L. Cerklewski, *Am. J. Clin. Nutr. 37*:553–556 (1983).

123. P. Altmann, R. F. L. Maruna, H. Maruna, W. Michalica, and G. Wagner, *Wiener Medizinische Wochenschrift 131*:311–314 (1981).

124. P. R. Flanagan, M. J. Chamberlain, and L. S. Valberg, *Am. J. Clin. Nutr. 36*:823–829 (1982).

125. C. H. Hill, Interactions of vitamin C with lead and mercury. In *Micronutrient Interactions: Vitamins, Minerals and Hazardous Elements*, O. A. Levander and L. Cheng (Eds.), N. Y. Acad Sci., New York, 1980, vol. 355, pp. 262–266.

126. M. M. Jones and M.A. Basinger, *J. Toxicol. Environ. Health 12*:749–756 (1983).

127. M. R. S. Fox, R. M. Jacobs, A. O. L. Jones, B. E. Fry, Jr., and C. L. Stone, Effects of vitamin C and iron on cadmium metabolism. In *Micronutrient Interactions: Vitamins, Minerals and Hazardous Elements* O. A. Levander and L. Cheng (Eds.). N.Y. Acad. Sci., New York, 1980, vol. 355, pp. 249–261.

128. E. P. Norkus, W. Kuenzig, and A. H. Conney, *Mutation Res. 117*:183–191 (1983).

129. T. G. Rossman, C. B. Klein, and M. Naslund, *Carcinogenesis 7*:727–732 (1986).

130. R. J. Sram, I. Samkova, and H. Hola, *Hyg. Epid. Microbiol. Immunol. 27*:305–318 (1983).

131. R. J. Sram, L. Dobias, A. Pastorkova, P. Rossner, and L. Janca, *Mutat. Res. 120*:181–186 (1983).

132. E. Ginter, P. Bobek, and M. Jurcovicova, Role of L-ascorbic acid in lipid metabolism. In *Ascorbic Acid: Chemistry, Metabolism and Uses* P. A. Seib and B. M. Tolbert (Eds.). American Chemical Society, Washington, D. C., 1982, pp. 381–395.

133. G. C. Willis, *Can. Med. Assoc. J. 69*:17–22 (1953).

134. G. C. Willis, *Can. Med. Assoc. J. 77*:106–109 (1957).

135. C. Krumdieek and C. E. Butterworth, *Am. J. Clin. Nutr. 27*:866–876 (1974).

136. B. Sokoloff, M. Hori, C. Saelhof, McConnell, and T. Imai, *J. Nutr. 91*:107–118 (1967).

137. J. P. Church, J. T. Judd, C. W. Young, J. L. Kelsay, and W. W. Kim, *Am. J. Clin. Nutr. 40*:1338–1344 (1984).

138. P. F. Jacques, S. C. Hartz, R. B. McGandy, R. A. Jacob, and R. M. Russell *J. Am. Coll. Nutr. 6*:169–174 (1987).

139. J. Ramirez and N. C. Flowers, *Am. J. Clin. Nutr. 33*:2079–2087 (1980).

140. E. Cheraskin and W. M. Ringsdorf, *J. Electrocardial. 12*:441 (1979).

141. R. Hume, B. D. Vallance and M. M. Muir, *J. Clin. Pathol. 35*:195–199 (1982).

142. K. F. Gey, H. B. Stahelin, P. Puska, and A. Evans, Relationship of plasma level of

vitamin C to mortality from ischemic heart disease. In *Third Conference on Vitamin C*, J. J. Burns, J. M. Rivers, and L. J. Machlin (Eds.). N.Y. Acad Sci., New York, vol. 498, pp. 110–120.

143. P. J. Leggott, P. B. Robertson, D. L. Rothman, P. A. Murray, and R. A. Jacob, *J. Periodont. 57*:480–485 (1986).

144. P. L. Schwartz, *J. Am. Diet. Assoc. 56*:497–503 (1970).

145. S. M. Levenson, G. Manner, and E. Seifter, Aspects of the adverse effects of dysnutrition on wound healing. In *Progress in Human Nutrition*, Vol. 1, (S. Margen, Ed.). Avi Publishing Co., Westport, Conn., 1971, pp. 132–156.

146. W. M. Ringsdorf and E. Cheraskin, *Oral Surg. 53*:231–236 (1982).

147. S. P. Shukla, *Experientia 25*:704–704 (1969).

148. T. T. Irvin, D. K. Chattopadhyay, and A. Smythe, *Surg. Gynec. Obstet. 147*:49–55 (1978).

149. A. H. Hunt, The role of vitamin C in wound healing *Br. J. Surg. 28*:436–461 (1941).

150. C. J. Schorah, N. Habibzadeh, M. Hancock and R. F. G. J. King, *Ann. Clin. Biochem. 23*:566–570 (1986).

151. R. Hume, E. Weyers, T. Rowan, *Br. Heart J. 34*:238–243 (1972).

152. R. Hume and E. Weyers, *Scott. Med. J. 18*:3–7 (1973).

153. A. Bendich. *Food Tech. 41*:112–114 (1987).

154. D. J. Morre, F. L. Crane, I. L. Sun, and P. Navas, The role of ascorbate in biomembrane energetics. In *Third Conference on Vitamin C*. J. J. Burns, J. M. Rivers, and L. J. Machlin (Eds.). N.Y. Acad. Sci., New York, 1987, vol. 498, pp. 153–171.

155. B. V. Siegel, *Infect. Immunol 10*:409–410 (1974).

156. C. S. Johnston, G. D. Cartee, and B. E. Haskell, *J. Nutr. 115*:1089–1093 (1985).

157. R. Anderson, Ascorbic acid and immune functions: Mechanism of immunostimulation. In *Vitamin C, (Ascorbic Acid)*, J. N. Counsell and D. H. Hornig (Eds.). Applied Science, London, 1981, pp. 249–272.

158. R. S. Panush and J. C. Delafuente, *World Rev. Nutr. Diet. 45*:97–132 (1985).

159. B. Halliwell, M. Wasil, and M. Grootveld, Elsevier *213*:15–18 (1987).

160. K. H. Schmidt, D. Steinhilber, U. Moser, and H.-J. Roth, *Int. Archs. Allergy Appl. Immun. 85*:441–445 (1988).

161. A. Castelli, G. E. Martorana, E. Meucci, and G. Bonetti, *Acta Vitaminol. Enzymol. 4*:189–196 (1982).

162. R. S. Weening, E. P. Schoorel, D. Roos, M. L. Van Schaik, A.A Voetman, A. A. Bot, A. M. Batenburg-Plenter, C. Willems, W. P. Zeijlemaker, and A. Astaldi, *Blood 57*:856–865 (1981).

163. J. I. Gallin, *Rev. Infect. Dis. 3*:1196–1220 (1981).

164. K. Vohra, A. J. Kahn, W. Rosenfeld, V. Telang, and H. E. Evans, *Pediatr. Res. 17*:340 (1983).

165. R. Anderson, The immunostimulatory, anti-inflammatory and anti-allergic properties of ascorbate. In *Advances in Nutritional Research*, Vol. 6, H. H. Draper (Ed.). Plenum Press, New York, 1984, pp. 19–45.

166. A. B. Kallner, D. Hartmann, and D. Hornig, *Am. J. Clin. Nutr. 34*:1347–1355 (1981).

167. L. Cheng, M. Cohen, and H. N. Bhagavan, Vitamin C and the elderly. In *CRC Handbook of Nutrition in the Aged*, R. R. Watson (Ed.). CRC Press, Inc., Boca Raton, Fla., 1985, pp. 157–185.

168. C. J. Schorah, W. P. Tormey, G. H. Brooks, A. M. Robertshaw, G. A. Young, R. Talukder and J. F. Kelly, *Am. J. Clin. Nutr. 34*:871–876 (1981).

169. P. J. Garry, D. J. Vanderjagt, and W. C. Hunt, Ascorbic acid intakes and plasma levels in healthy elderly. In *Third Conference on Vitamin C*, J. J. Burns, J. M. Riers, and L. J. Machlin (Eds.). N.Y. Acad. Sci., New York, 1987, vo. 498, pp. 90–99.

170. P. J. Garry, J. S. Goodwin, W. C. Hunt, and B. A. Gilbert, *Am. J. Clin. Nutr. 36*:332–339 (1982).

171. P. F. Jacques, J. Phillips, L. T. Chylack, R. B. McGandy, and S. H. Hartz, *J. Am. Coll. Nutr. 6*:435–435 (1987).
172. J. Robertson. The University of Western Ontario, Canada, 1987.
173. R. E. Pecoraro and M. S. Chen, Ascorbic acid metabolism in diabetes mellitus. In *Third Conference on Vitamin C*, J. J. Burns, J. M. Rivers, and L. J. Machlin (Eds.). N.Y. Acad. Sci., New York, 1987, vol. 498, pp. 248–258.
174. C. J. Schorah, Vitamin C status in population groups. In *Vitamin C (Ascorbic Acid)*, J. N. Counsell and D. H. Horning (Eds.). Applied Science Publishers, London, 1981, pp. 23–47.
175. M. I. Irwin and B. K. Hutchins, *J. Nutr. 106*:823–79 (1976).
176. E. B. Dawson, W. A. Harris, W. E. Rankin, L. A. Charpentier, and W. J. McGanity, Effect of ascorbic acid on male fertility. In *Third Conference on Vitamin C*, J. J. Burns, J. M. Rivers, and L. J. Machlin (Eds.). N.Y. Acad. Sci., New York, 1987, pp. 312–323.
177. R. G. Burr and K. T. Rajan, *Br. J. Nutr. 28*:275–281 (1972).
178. J. H. Crandon, C. C. Lund, and D. B. Dill, *New Engl. J. Med. 223*:353–369 (1940).
179. J. B. Reuler, V. C. Broudy, and T. G. Gooney, *JAMA 253*:805–807 (1985).
180. M. Hughes, N. Clark, L. Forbes, and D. G. Colin-Jones, *Br. Med. J. 293*:366–366 (1986).
181. P. R. Evans, *Br. Med. J. 287*:1862–1863 (1983).
182. W. J. Boeve, and A. Martijn, *Skeletal Radiol. 16*:67–69 (1987).
183. W. J. Allender, *J. Anal. Toxicol. 6*:202–204 (1982).
184. R. E. Hodges, E. M. Baker, J. Hood, H. E. Sauberlich, and S. C. March, *Am. J. Clin. Nutr. 22*:535–548 (1969).
185. G. M. Jaffe, Vitamin C in *Handbook of Vitamins*, 1st ed., L. J. Machlin (Ed.). Marcel Dekker, New York, 1984, pp. 199–244.
186. C. J. Schorah, Inappropriate vitamin C reserves: Their frequency and significance in an urban population. In *The Importance of Vitamins to Health* T. G. Taylor (Ed.). MTP Press, Lancaster, England, 1979, pp. 61–72.
187. T. K. Basu and C. J. Schorah, In *Vitamin C in Health and Disease*. Avi Publishing Co., Westport, Conn. 1982, pp. 61–92.
188. F. Horio, K. Ozaki, A. Yoshida, S. Makino, and Y. Hayashi, *J. Nutr. 115*:1630–1640 (1985).
189. B. Kristensen, P. D. Thomsen, B. Palludan, and I. Wegger, *Acta Vet. Scand. 27*:486–496 (1986).
190. E. P. Norkus and W. Kuenzig, in press.
191. D. Hornig, J. P. Vuilleumier, and D. Hartmann, *Intern. J. Vitamin Nutr. Res. 50*:309–314 (1980).
192. E. M. Baker, J. C. Saari, and B. M. Tolbert, *Am. J. Clin. Nutr. 19*:371–378 (1966).
193. E. M. Baker, R. E. Hodges, J. Hood, H. E. Sauberlich, and S. C. March, *Am. J. Clin. Nutr. 22*:549–558 (1969).
194. E. M. Baker, R. E. Hodges, J. Hood, H. E. Sauberlich, S. C. March, and J. E. Canham, *Am. J. Clin. Nutr. 24*:444–454 (1971).
195. R. E. Hodges, J. Hood, J. Canham, H. E. Sauberlich, and E. M. Baker, *Am. J. Clin. Nutr. 24*:432–443 (1971).
196. R. A. Kinsman, and J. Hood, *Am. J. Clin. Nutr. 24*:455–464 (1971).
197. J. Weininger and J. C. King. *Am. J. Clin. Nutr. 35*:1408–1416 (1982).
198. R. A. Jacob, J. H. Skala, S. T. Omaye ,and J. R. Turnlund, *J. Nutr. 117*:2109–2115 (1987).
199. M. F. R. Sowers, R. B. Wallace, and J. H. Lemke, *Am. J. Clin. Nutr. 41*:1045–1053 (1985).
200. J. L. Freudenheim, N. E. Johnson, and E. L. Smith, *Am. J. Clin. Nutr. 44*:863–876 (1986).
201. H. M. V. Newton, C. J. Schorah, N. Habibzadeh, D. B. Morgan, and R. P. Hullin, *Am. J. Clin. Nutr. 42*:656–659 (1985).
202. K. Heinonen, I. Mononen, T. Mononen, M. Parviainen, I. Penttila, and K. Launiala, *Am. J. Clin. Nutr. 43*:923–924 (1986).
203. S. A. Udipi, A. Kirksey, K. West, and G. Giacoia, *Am. J. Clin. Nutr. 42*:522–530 (1985).

204. J. S. Vobecky, J. Vobecky, D. Shapcott, and R. Blanchard, *Am. J. Clin. Nutr. 29*:766–771 (1976).
205. L. O. Byerley and A. Kirksey, *Am. J. Clin. Nutr. 41*:665–671 (1985).
206. B. Borenstein, *Food Tech. 41*:98–99 (1987).
207. M. Liao and P. A. Seib, *Food Tech. 41*:104–107 (1987).
208. J. I. Gray, S. K. Reddy, J. F. Price, A. Mandagere, and W. F. Wilkens, *Food Tech. 36*:39–45 (1982).
209. V. S. Durve and R. T. Lovell, *Can. J. Fish Aquat. Sci. 39*:948–951 (1982).
210. Wld. Hlth. Org. Techn. Rep. Ser. 1972, No. 505, Wld. Hlth. Org. Techn. Rep. Ser. 1974, No. 539.
211. W. F. Körner and F. Weber, *Int. J. Vit. Nutr. Res. 42*:528–544 (1972).
212. D. H. Hornig and U. Moser, The safety of high vitamin C intakes in man. In *Vitamin C (Ascorbic Acid)*, J. N. Counsell and D. H. Hornig (Eds.)., Applied Science, London, 1981, pp. 225–248.
213. A. Hanck, *Int. J. Vit. Nutr. Res. Suppl. 23*:221–238 (1982).
214. J. M. Rivers, Safety of high-level vitamin C ingestion. In *Third Conference on Vitamin C* J. J. Burns, J. M. Rivers, and L. J. Machlin (Eds.). N.Y. Acad. Sci., New York, 1987, pp. 445–454.
215. U. Moser and D. Hornig, *Trends Pharmacol. Sci. 3*:480–483 (1982).
216. H. Gerster, *Nutrition 10*:614–617 (1986).
217. H. Gerster and U. Moser, Nutr. Res., 8:1327–1332 (1988).
218. G. Siest and W. Appel, *J. Clin. Chem. Clin. Biochem. 16*:103–110 (1978).
219. D. P. Ganick and J. R. Close, *Lancet 2*:820–821 (1977).
220. M. Olliver, Ascorbic Acid: Estimation. In *The Vitamins*, vol. I., W. H. Sebrell and R. S. Haris (Eds.). Academic Press, New York, 1967, pp. 338–359.
221. J. S. Lawendel, *Nature 178*:873–874 (1956).
222. J. Tillmans, P. Hirsch, and J. Jackish, *Z. Untersuch. Lebensm. 63*:241–267 (1932).
223. B. Hubmann, D. Monnier, and M. Roth, *Clin. Chim. Acta 25*:161–166 (1969).
224. A. E. Burgess and J. M. Ottaway, *Analyst 97*:357–362 (1972).
225. V. R. White and J. M. Fitzgerald, *Anal. Chem. 44* 1267–1269 (1972).
226. K. K. Verma and A. K. Gulati, *Analt. Chem. 52*:2336–2338 (1980).
227. J. V. Lloyd, P. S. Davis, and H. Lander, *J. Clin. Path. 22*:453–457 (1969).
228. L. L. Stookey, *Anal. Chem. 42*:779–781 (1970).
229. N. Burger and V. Kara-Gasparec, *Talanta 20*:782–785 (1973).
230. V. Zannoni, M. Lynch, S. Goldstein, and P. Sato, *Biochem. Med. 11*:41–48 (1974).
231. M. M. Aly, *Anal. Chim. Acta 106*:379–383 (1979).
232. H. Shieh and T. R. Sweet, *Anal. Biochem. 96*:1–5 (1979).
233. M. Schmall, C. W. Pfifer, and E. G. Wollish, *Anal. Chem. 25*:1486–1490 (1953).
234. M. J. Deutsch and C. E. Weeks, *J. Assoc. Off. Agric. Chem. 48*:1248–1256 (1965).
235. S. P. Perone and W. J. Keeflow, *Anal. Chem. 28*:1760–1763 (1966).
236. B. Roe and J. H. Bruemmor, *Proc. Florida St. Hort. Soc. 87*:210–213 (1975).
237. Mapson, L. W. and S. M. Partridge, *Nature 164*:479–480 (1949).
238. C. C. Sweeley, R. Bentley, M. Makita, and W. W. Wells, *J. Am. Chem. Soc. 85*:2497–2507 (1963).
239. J. C. Saari, E. M. Baker, and H. E. Sauberlich, *Anal. Biochem. 18*:173–177 (1967).
240. M. Vecchi and K. Kaiser, *J. Chromatogr. 26*:22–29 (1967).
241. K. Schmidt, H. Oberritter, G. Bruchelt, V. Hagmaier, and D. Horning, *Internat. J. Vit. Nutr. Res. 53*:77–86 (1983).
242. J. Geigert, D. S. Hirano, and S. L. Neidleman, *J. Chromatogr. 206*:396–399 (1981).
243. S. Garcia-Castineiras, V. D. Bonnet, R. Figueroa, and M. Miranda, *J. Liq. Chromatogr. 4*:1619–1640 (1981).
244. Lee, W., P. Hamernyik, M. Hutchinson, V. A. Raisys, and R. F. Labbe, *Clin. Chem.*

28:2165–2169 (1982).

245. M. Olliver, Ascorbic Acid: Occurrence in food. In *The Vitamins*, vol. I, W. H. Sebrell and R. S. Harris (Eds.). Academic Press, New York, 1967, pp. 359–367.

246. A. A. Paul and D. A. T. Southgate, *McCance and Widdowson's The Composition of Foods*, 4th ed. Medical Research Council's Special Report No. 297, London, HMS, 1978.

247. S. Nobile and J. M. Woodhill. *Vitamin C: The Mysterious Redox System, A Trigger of Life*. MTP Press, Boston, 1981, pp. 38–55.

248. F. M. Finn and P. A. Johns, *Endocrinology 106*:811–817 (1980).

249. E. J. Diliberto, Jr., G. D. Heckman, and A. J. Daniels, *J. Biol. Chem. 258*:12886–12894 (1983).

250. M. Khatami, W. Li, and J. H. Rockey, *Invest. Ophthalmol. Vis. Sci. 27*:1665–1671 (1986).

251. J. R. Wright, V. Castranova, H. D. Colby, and P. R. Miles, *J. Appl. Physiol. 51*:1477–1483 (1981).

252. E. I. Cullen, V. May, and B. A. Eipper, *Mol. Cel. Endocrinology 48*:239–250 (1986).

253. P. M. Royce, U. Moser, and B. Steinmann, *Matrix 9*:147–149 (1989).

254. P. A. Seib, *Int. J. Vit. Nutr.Res. Suppl. 27*:259–306 (1985).

6
Thiamin

Clark Johnson Gubler
Brigham Young University
Provo, Utah

I. HISTORY

The history of the discovery of thiamin is intriguing and unique in that the present vitamin concept was first conceived and developed from early studies of the "antiberiberi factor," and the class name, vitamin, was derived from early work on its chemical nature. For detail on this fascinating history, see Refs. 1–5.

The disease beriberi (or *Kakke*), prevalent in many parts of the world—particularly Asia—where milled or polished rice is a staple in the diet, has been recognized for centuries and has extracted a great toll in human suffering and death. The first real breakthrough came in 1885, when Dr. K. Takaki, then surgeon general of the Japanese Navy suggested that the carbon/nitrogen ratio of the diet should be decreased from around 32 to 16 by increasing the protein intake. Implementation of this suggestion resulted in the virtual elimination of beriberi in ships' crews in the Japanese navy. However, Takaki's views were not widely accepted or generally implemented, because they ran counter to the generally accepted views of the medical profession on the causes of the disease. Because of the then relatively recent wide acceptance of Pasteur's work on the microbial cause of disease, it was felt that a disease must have a positive etiology, that is, be caused by a microorganism or a toxin. When the infectious theory of its etiology had to be discarded relatively quickly for lack of demonstration of a causative organism, the toxin theory gained widespread acceptance, i.e., the idea that certain kinds of rice associated with berberi contained a toxin that caused the disease. It had been shown that rice bran, and also whole (nonmilled) rice, could alleviate the symptoms of the disease. The explanation was that these substances contained an antagonist to the toxin. However, no toxin could be isolated.

Christian Eijkman, a Dutch medical officer stationed in Java, first discovered that a polyneuritis resembling beriberi could be produced in chickens fed on polished rice. He and his successor, Gerrit Grijns, further demonstrated (1900) that this polyneuritis could be prevented or cured by feeding "kitchen scraps" and, later, by rice bran or polishings. This was really the first adventure in the experimental characterization of a nutritional deficiency and led the way, by providing an animal model, to the isolation of the lacking nutritional factor. These workers were able to show that this "polyneuritis preventive factor" was destroyed in meat or bran by heating at 120–130 °C. Grijns went further and extracted the factor from rice bran, showing that it was water soluble. He obtained some active concentrates but no pure factor. In 1911, a decade after these first attempts of Grijns, Casimir Funk, a young chemist at the Lister Institute in London, obtained a crystalline sustance from rice bran extracts. He was convinced that he had finally isolated the active antiberiberi principle, and it appeared to possess an amine function. He thus coined the name *vitamine*, or an amine essential for life (4). Although these crystals were soon shown to have little antineuritic activity, the name vitamine struck a responsive chord and probably did more to focus attention on the concept of "deficiency diseases" than anything else. In fact, this term was later adopted after dropping the final e, as *vitamins*, a term used to designate the whole class of trace nutritional factors.

In 1910, Captain Edward B. Veddder, with the U.S. Army in Manila in the Philippines, became convinced that the then very prevalent beriberi was indeed caused by a nutritional deficiency and began in earnest to pursue the isolation of the active factor. He enlisted the help of Robert R. Williams of the Bureau of Science in Manila. Dr. Williams became so intensely interested in the problem that he continued in his efforts for a quarter of a century, to the exent of working nights and weekends on his own time and often paying for the research expenses out of his own pocket. In 1926, two Dutch chemists, B. C. P. Jansen and W. Donath (6), again in Java, succeeded in isolating and crystallizing 200 mg of the substances from rice bran extracts. They were aided in this by making use of the demonstrated affinity of Fuller's earth for this substance (7) and by developing a better animal model of the disease, in the form of the rice birds, *Munia maja*, which beame polyneuritic very rapidly. This assay was thus quicker and more reliable than that using pigeons and chickens.

In the meantime, Williams, now in the United States, was continuing his isolation efforts. He and those working with him could not repeat Jansen and Donath's isolation. With modification to minimize losses during the process, they finally succeeded in 1933 in obtaining about 450 mg of crystalline material from 100 kg of rice bran (1,2).

Unfortunately, Jansen and Donath had missed the sulfur atom in the published formula of their original crystalline product: $(C_{18}H_{18}ON_4)Cl_2$. This threw everyone off the track for some time, until Windaus and co-workers (1,2) discovered the presence of an atom of sulfur in 1932, thus making the empirical formula $(C_{12}H_{18}ON_4S)Cl_2$ for the hydrochloride. This seemed to give Windaus and his group the advantage for deriving the structure. However, Williams and his group discovered that the molecule could be split quantitatively by sulfite into a 6-amiopyrimidine sulfonic acid (I) and a base (II) containing a sulfur and a free hydroxyl group:

$$C_{12}H_{16}N_4OS \xrightarrow{\text{H}_2\text{SO}_3} \underset{\text{I}}{C_6H_9N_3SO_3} + \underset{\text{II}}{C_6H_9NOS}$$

Structure II was soon shown to be a thiazole, and Williams published his first formula for the material, which was then called vitamin B_1, as

On the reduction of the pyrimidine moiety with Na in liquid NH_3, Williams and Cline got a dimethylaminopyrimidine that they then identified as 2,5-dimethyl-6-aminopyrimidine. Thus, the presence of an ethyl group was ruled out, and by January of 1936, Williams and his group had a good idea of the final stucture of B_1, including the methylene bridge between the two ring systems. His group then synthesized the 2-methyl-5-ethoxymethyl-6-oxypyrimidine and converted it to the corresponding 5-methylsulfonic acid. This proved to be identical with the deaminated sulfonic acid product of the sulfite cleavage of B_1. Hence, Williams and his group was able to publish the final correct formula for B_1-

on May 23, 1936, at which time they already had some of the first biologically active synthetic material available and proposed the name thiamine.

It was then only a short time (July 1936) until Williams' group accomplished the complete synthesis by building up each ring independently (the pyrimidine having a $-CH_2Br$ group in the 5 position) and then linking the two together. The synthetic product was shown to be identical with the natural thiamine by ultraviolet (UV) spectrum, thiochrome test, and biological tests on microorganisms and animals. Todd and Bergel in England followed in February 1937 with a different synthetic approach and Andersag and Westphal in Germany in October by still another approach (1,2).

The chemical industry did not show much interest in this substance during these early years. However, in 1934, a change in attitude became evident, sparked possibly by Reichstein's synthesis of ascorbic acid on a technical scale and other developments. Merck & Co. in the United States and Hoffmann-LaRoche in Switzerland began to show interest in and encouragement of the work on its characterization and synthesis. Shortly after the synthesis had been established, technical production was started in the spring of 1937 by these two firms and developed into a successful operation by the end of 1937. This was quite an accomplishment, since at the time even the starting materials had to be synthesized, and to commercially synthesize an organic compound with 15–17 different steps was unheard of in the pharmaceutical industry. The demand and production rose rapidly, which resulted in a rather precipitous drop in price per kilogram. This is shown in Table 1 for the years 1937–1967. Publication of production figures was discontinued after 1960. Production has undoubtedly continued to rise, worldwide, but inflation has caught up with the price, which was listed at $35–40 per kilogram in 1978.

The first breakthrough on the physiological functions of thiamin came when Thompson and Johnson (8) in 1935 demonstrated a high blood pyruvate level in B_1 deficiency. Peters and co-workers (9–11) then showed, between 1936 and 1938, that thiamin was essential for carbohydrate, and specially for pyruvate metabolism. Lohmann and Schuster (12) then discovered that the active coenzyme form of the vitamin was the pyrophosphate ester:

$$
\begin{array}{c}
\text{CH}_3 \\
\text{N} = \text{C} - \text{NH}_2 - \text{HCl} \qquad | \\
| \qquad | \qquad\qquad \text{C} = \text{C} - \text{CH}_2\text{CH}_2\text{OP}_2\text{O}_6\text{H}_3 \\
\text{CH}_3 - \text{C} \quad\ \text{C} - \text{CH}_2 - \overset{+}{\text{N}} \qquad | \\
\| \qquad \| \qquad\qquad\ \ \text{CH} - \text{S} \\
\text{N} - \text{CH} \qquad \text{Cl}^- \ \text{CH} - \text{S}
\end{array}
$$

This was shown to be the coenzyme for yeast pyruvic decarboxylase (then called carboxylase, hence the name cocarboxylase for the coenzyme). This discovery was then followed by the finding that thiamin diphosphate was the coenzyme also for pyruvate and α-ketoglutarate dehydrogenase complexes in animals and for transketolase in plants and animals.

II. CHEMISTRY

A. Isolation

Prior to 1926, Grijns, Funk, and Williams and co-workers had tried diligently to isolate the antiberiberi factor but had succeeded only in concentrating it. As indicated above, Jansen and Donath first succeeded in obtaining the material in purified crystalline form in 1926. Some of this material was sent to a chemical laboratory in Scotland for further

Table 1 Production and Price of Thiamin

Year	Kilograms	Price ($/kg)	Approximate value ($)
1937	100	—	—
1939	1600	1000	1,600,000
1940	3700	600	2,220,000
1951–1955	100,000–120,000	145	15,000,000
1956	120,000	70	8,400,000
1960	150,000	36	5,400,000
1967	200,000 (est.)	15	3,000,000

characterization, but for some inexplicable reason it was set on a shelf and forgotten. It took another 8 years (1932) before Windaus et al. were able to obtain the crystalline vitamin from yeast concentrates supplied them by I.G. Farbenindustrie in Germany. It was not until a year later that Williams and co-workers were finally successful in obtaining crystalline vitamin from rice polishings (4.2–4.9 g from 1000 kg polishings) (1,2).

As soon as the procedure for the chemical synthesis of thiamin was developed, its isolation from natural sources (rice bran, yeast extracts, or rice and wheat germ) could not compete with production by chemical synthesis, and hence is only of historical interest as far as commercial production is concerned.

The original isolation of thiamin depended on the discovery that it is adsorbed on such materials as Fuller's earth (7), a preparation of hydrated aluminum silicate. This principle is used for the preliminary separation of thiamin from interfering substances in complex extracts of plant and animal tissues prior to spectrophotometric or fluorometric assay by well-established methods (13–15). The preparation most widely used currently is produced by the Permutit Co. and sold in an activated form as Permutit-T or Thiochrome Decalso. Thiamin in the cationic form is absorbed on this material; anionic and nonionic substances pass through the column. The thiamin is then eluted with hot acidic KCl.

Separation and detection of thiamin and its phosphate esters and some analogs by various column chromatographic procedures has been reported using a weak cation exchanger (Amberlite IRC50) with gradient elution (16); a strong cation exchanger (Dowex 1 × 8) using two columns in tandem (17) or one column (18); Dowex 2 × 8 with elution using 0.01 M formic acid followed by 0.5 M sodium formate (19); Dowex 1-x-4, acetate form, with successive elution with H_2O, 0.1 M acetate buffer, pH 4.5, and 1.0 M acetate buffer, pH 4.5 (20); and DEAE Sephadex A-25, H^+ form followed by elution successively with 0.1, 0.2, and 0.3 M formic acid (21,22).

Siliprandi and Siliprandi (16) also achieved excellent separations using chromatography on Whatman #1 paper with N-propanol: 1.0 M acetate buffer, pH 5.0:H_2O (70:20:10) or Munktell #00 paper with N-propanol: 0.5 M acetate buffer pH 4.50 (60:40). Kiessling (23) also described a procedure that separates thiamin and its esters well and separates thiamin phosphates from nucleotide phosphates using Whatman #1 paper and isobutyric acid: 1 N NH_4OH:0.1 M EDTA (100:60:1.6) as solvent. R_f values were 0.87, 0.77, 0.68 and 0.55 for thiamin, thiamin monophosphate, thiamin diphosphate, and thiamin triphosphate, respectively. Camiener and Brown (24) separated thiamin and its esters and also thiazole and thiazole phosphate on Whatman #1 paper and N-propanol: 1 M acetate buffer, pH 5.0:H_2O (70:10:20); Carlson and Brown (25) described the separation of thiamin and hydroxyethylthiamin. More recently a separation by ascending chromatography on Whatman 3 MM paper using either isobutyric acid: (conc.) NH_4OH:0.1 M NaH_2PO_4:H_2O (198:3:40:58 v/v) or N-propanol:H_2O:1 M acetate buffer, pH 5.0 (7:2:1 v/v) as solvents has been described (26) with R_f values of 0.84, 0.70, and 0.54 with the first solvent and 0.60, 0.27, and 0.06 with the second for thiamin HCl, thiamin monophosphate, and thiamin diphosphate, respectively.

Thin-layer chromatography has also been used successfully to separate thiamin and its esters and products (27–32) on plates of Kiesel gel G (silica gel G′) with a variety of solvents. These have the advantages of using smaller amounts of material and being much more rapid.

Electrophoresis can also be used effectively for separation of thiamin and its phosphate esters. Siliprandi and Siliprandi (16) used Munktell 20 paper ad 0.05 M acetate buffer, pH 5.44. Thiamin and the monophosphate then migrated toward the negative pole and the di- and triphosphates toward the positive with excellent separations. Rossi-Fanelli et al. (33) and Patrini and Rindi (34) used electrophoresis on a column packed with powdered cellulose with ammonium formate buffer, 0.05 M, pH 5.1, as the solvent.

Hemming and Gubler (35–37) and more recently Ishii et al. (38), Sanemori et al. (39), Kimura et al. (40) Barnes (41), and Bettendorff et al. (42) have described the separation of thiamin and its phosphate esters and some thiamin analogs by high-performance liquid chromatography. Echols et al. (43) have described a gas chromatographic determination of thiamin.

B. Structure and Nomenclature

Empirical formula (hydrochloride): $C_{12}H_{17}N_4OSCl \cdot HCl$
Chemical name: 3-(4′amino-2′-methyl-pyrimidin-5′-ylmethyl)-
5-(2-hydroxyethyl)-4-methylthiazolium chloride hydrochloride
Structure:

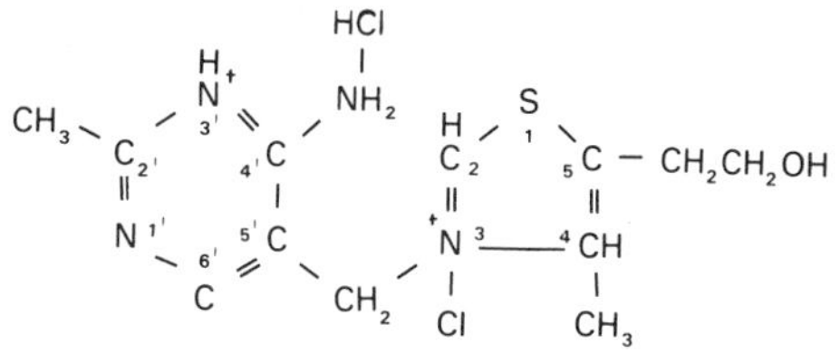

Nomenclature
Accepted terms: thiamin (or thiamine) (United States) (thiamin now the suggested spelling); aneurin (United Kingdom)
Obsolete terms: vitamin B_1; oryzamin, torulin, polyneuramin, vitamin F, antineuric vitamin, antiberiberi vitamin

C. Commercial Forms

The two most common commercial preparations of thiamin in the United States and Europe are the hydrochloride and the nitrate. The discovery, in 1951, by Fujiwara, Watanabe, Matsukawa and co-workers (3,66) that treatment of thiamin with an extract of garlic (or other *Allium* species) converted it into a product that did not give the thiochrome reaction but was very active biologically opens the door to another type of thiamin preparation. This was called allithiamin and was later shown to be a mixed thiamin allyl disulfide (TAD). A larger variety of thiamin alkyl disulfides have since been synthesized and studied. Of these the most important commerical forms, which are used in Japan, Europe, and other parts of the world, but are not yet approved in the United States, are TAD, thiamin prophyldisulfide (TPD), thiamin tetrahydrofurfuryl disulfide (TTFD), and O-benzoyl thiamin disulfide (see Table 2). These forms are less water soluble and more lipid soluble and appear to be more rapidly absorbed and better retained in the body than thiamin hydrochloride. They are readily converted in vivo to thiamin (66,67).

D. Structures of Important Analogs, Antagonists, and Commercial Forms

Thiamin analogs and antagonists can be classified in a number of ways (see Refs. 44–46 for more detailed review.) For the purpose of this review they will be classified as follows (This is a modification of Roger's categories 2,44–46):

1. Substitutions on the pyrimidine or thiazole rings
2. Modifications of the pyrimidine or thiazole rings

Table 2   Structures of Thiamin Alkyl Disulfides[a]

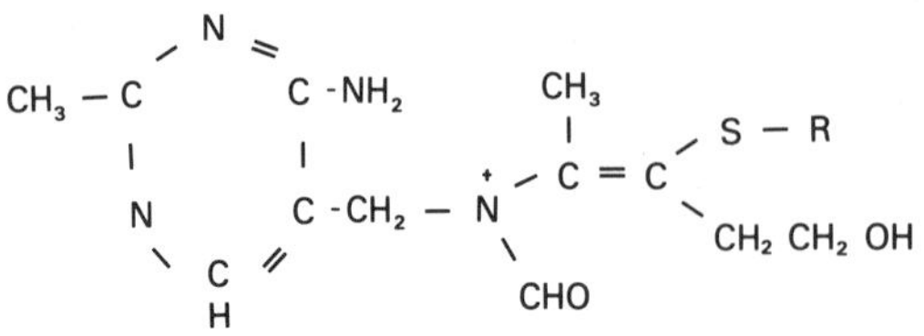

CH₃ — C ... N ... C -NH₂ ... C -CH₂ — N ... C = C ... S — R ... CH₂ CH₂ OH ... CHO ... CH₃ ... C H

Name	R
Allithiamin	-CH₂=CH-CH₂
Thiamin propyldisulfide	-CH₂-CH₂-CH₃
Thiamin tetrahydrofurfuryldisulfide	-CH₂-CH₂(CH₂)₂-CH₂
O-Benzoylthiamin disulfide	—

[a]Another analog frequently mentioned is *O-benzoylthiamin disulfide:

CH₃ — C ... N ... C -NH₂ ... C -CH₂ — N ... C = C — S⁻ ... CH₃ ... CH₂ CH₂ O-C-OC₆H₅ ... C H ...]₂

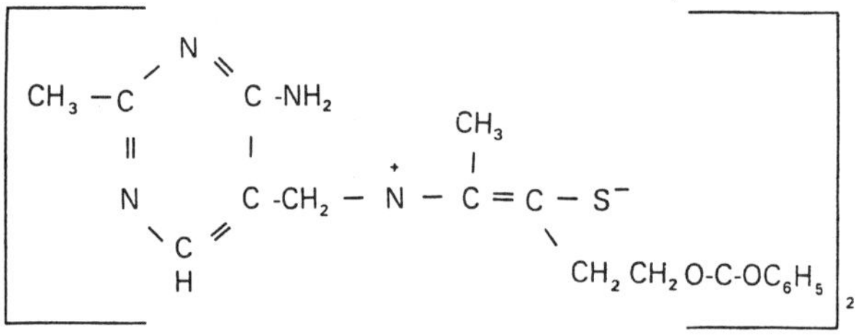

3. Anticoccidial inhibitors
4. Thiaminases and antithiamin substances

Groups 1 and 2 include the "classic thiamin antagonists of Roger's classification. They are more complex and resemble thiamin more closely than those in group 3, which do not have the hydroxyethyl side chain.

1. Group 1

The best known representatives of group 1 are listed in Table 3, where the substitutions of the various ring positions are compared with thiamin.

It is now well known that the principal catalaytic function of thiamin is in carbonyl activation followed by splitting of the affected carbon-to-carbon bond. Extensive studies of thiamin-catalyzed reactions in both nonenzymatic and enzymatic systems by Breslow and Krampitz (see Ref. 2) have shown that the catalytic function involves the 2 carbon of the thiazole with its ability to form a carbanion as a result of its peculiar environment in the thiazole ring. Hence, any substitution (i.e., a methyl) at C-2 (III, Table 3) completely eliminates both its catalytic and biological activity. In general, the mechanism involves the binding of the thiazole C-2 with a 2-carbonyl group (2-ketoacid or 2-ketosugar) accompanied by the ejection of CO_2 or an aldehyde. The remaining adduct, at the oxidation stage of an aldehyde, can then react further in one of several ways: (1) by protonation to give an active aldehyde addition product (decarboxylases); (2) by direct oxidation with suitable electron acceptors to give a high-energy 2-acyl addition product, or by reaction with oxidized lipoate to form an acyldihydrolipoate product (oxidases or dehydrogenases); or (3) by addition to an aldehyde carbonyl, thus producing a new ketol (e.g., transketolase, phosphoketolase, a carboligases). Although free thiamin, and even some thiazolium compounds, can catalyze many of these reactions at a slow rate under appropriate conditions,

Table 3 Structures of Thiamin Analogs Compared to Thiamin

Number	Name	R_1	R_2	R_3	R_4	R_5	R_6
I	Thiamin	H	CH_3	NH_2	CH_3	H	H
II	Oxythiamin	H	CH_3	OH	CH_3	H	H
III	2-Methylthiamin	H	CH_3	NH_2	CH_3	CH_3	H
IV	2′-Ethylthiamin	H	C_2H_5	NH_2	CH_3	H	H
V	2′-Propylthiamin	H	C_3H_7	NH_2	CH_3	H	H
VI	2′-Butylthiamin	H	C_4H_9	NH_2	CH_3	H	H
VII	6′-Methylthiamin	H	H	NH_2	CH_3	H	CH_3
VIII	2′-Trifluoromethylthiamin	H	CF_3	NH_2	CH_3	H	H
IX	2′-Methylthiothiamin	H	CH_3S	NH_2	CH_3	H	H
X	2′-Methoxythiamin	H	CH_3O	NH_2	CH_3	H	H

[a]*Source*: From Ref. 2.

the active coenzyme has a pyrophosphate bound on the hydroxyethyl group at the C-5 of the thiazole (19). This group, along with Mg^{2+}, participates in the binding of the coenzyme with apoenzyme. Hence, for any analog to be an effective antagonist of thiamin-dependent enzymes, it must contain this hydroxyethyl group and be phosphorylated by thiamin pyrophosphokinase. Thus, this group is included in all the analogs of Table 3. A methyl at the 2′ position on the pyrimidine ring (I) is important but not absolutely essential, since the 2′-ethyl analog (IV) ranges in activity from slightly inferior to greater than the 2′-methyl in various systems, the 2′-propyl (V) is devoid of either coenzyme or antagonist activity, but the 2′-butyl (VI) analog is a highly protent antagonist. Other modifications at the 2′-carbon, i.e., 2′-methylthio (IX), 2′-methoxy (X), and 2′-trifluoromethyl (VII) have been shown to exhibit antagonism in some systems (45,46). The pyrimidine 4′-NH_2 group plays an essential role in the release of the aldehyde adduct from the thiazole C-2 after splitting of the —C—C— bond. Hence, oxythiamin (II) diphosphate can bind with thiamin-dependent apoenzymes but cannot complete the reaction, so it is a potent antagonist. If the methyl is shifted from the 2′ to the 6′ position on the pyrimidine (VII), the compound is essentially inactive.

2. Group 2

The best-known representatives of group 2 are shown in Table 4. Of the structures of Table 4, double changes in the thiamin structure (XII and XIV) lead to complete inactivity either as coenzyme or antagonists, as does substitution of O for S in the thiazole ring (XIII), an imidazolium for a thiazolium structure (XV), or a pyridine ring for the pyrimidine (XVI). Of the group in Table 4, only pyrithiamin, in which a —CH=CH— has been substituted for S (or a pyridinium ring for the thiazolium) (XI), has potent activity as a thiamin antagonist.

Of the classic antagonists, only oxythiamin (II) (OTh) and pyrithiamin (neopyrithiamin) (XI) (PTh) have been studied extensively (44–49). 2′-Butylthiamin (VI) has been shown to produce neurologial symptoms similar to those caused by pyrithiamin. The effects of

Table 4 Structures of Thiamin Analogs with Alterations of the Pyrimidine and Thiazole Ring

Number	Name	R_1	R_2	R_3	R_4	X	Y
XI	Pyrithiamin	H	CH_3	NH_2	CH_3	-CH=CH-	N
XII	1'-n-Butylpyrithiamin	H	n-C_4H_9	NH_2	CH_3	-CH=CH-	N
XIII	Oxazolethiamin	H	CH_3	NH_2	CH_3	O	N
XIV	Oxypyrithiamin	H	CH_3	OH	CH_3	-CH=CH-	N
XV	N-Acylimidazolium analog	H	CH_3	NH_2	CH_3	N-acyl	N
XVI	Darnow analog	H	CH_3	NH_3	CH_3	S	C

the antagonists OTh and PTh in animals are summarized in Table 5 and compared with those associated with thiamin deprivation. Oxythiamin produces most of the usual symptoms and biochemical changes associated with thiamin deficiency, but never the neurological symptoms, whereas pyrithiamin produces chiefly the neurological syndrome. The anorexia and inanition after oxythiamin treatment appear much earlier and are more severe than with either thiamin deprivation or pyrithiamin treatment. The lack of neurologial involvement with oxythiamin is undoubtedly related to its inability to cross the blood-brain barrier (50). On the other hand, thiamin deficiency and pyrithiamin treatment appear to break down this barrier (51,52).

An interesting variation of this type is the nonquaternary phenylthiazino-thiamin:

This compound has been reported to produce neuromuscular symptoms in rats (53).

3. Group 3: Anticoccidial Inhibitors

A larger number of chick anticoccidial compounds of varying potency have been produced (44–46). These have the pyrimidine ring similar to thiamin, and this is combined through the methylene bridge to a quaternary nitrogen of a pyridine ring. They thus resemble pyrithiamin, but do not have the hydroexyethyl group, and hence cannot be pyrophosphorylated. Thus, they are not substrates for thiamine pyrophosphokinase and so are not good inhibitors of the thiamin diphosphate–dependent enzymes. The variations in this group are made by various substitutions on the pyrimidine and pyridine rings. These have been shown to inhibit thiamin transport across the chick intestinal wall and also across bacterial cell walls. In small doses, they affect chiefly bacterial thiamin transport and hence exert anticoccidial action. At the larger dosage levels, they can also produce thiamin deficiency and growth retardation in the chicks. A typical example, and the product most extensively used commerically, is amprolium: 1-(4-amino-2-n-propyl-5-pyrimidinylmethyl)-

Table 5 Comparison of Effects of Thiamin Deprivation and of OTh and PTh Treatment

Symptom or effect	Thiamin deprivation	OTH Treatment	PTH Treatment
Anorexia (loss of appetite)	+	+++	± (?) last stages
Weight loss (inanition)	+	++	+ not until terminal
Bradycardia	+	++	+ last stages
Heart enlargement	+	++	+ last stages
Adrenal hypertrophy	+	++	+ last stages
Elevation of blood corticosterone	++	++ to - with later exhaustion	+ last stages
Elevation of blood pyruvate	+	+++	± except in convulsions
Penetration of antagonist into brain	NA	− to slight	+++
Increased urinary thiamin excretion	decrease	+	+++
Depletion of tissue thiamin	++	±	+++
Inhibition of TPK	NA	+ very weak	+++
Phosphorylation to -PP	NA	+++	± (?)
Inhibition of ThDP-dependent enzymes by inhibitor diphosphate			
Decrease in tissue enzyme activity			
PyDH			
Liver	+++	++	++
Heart	+++	+++	++
Brain	+	0	+++
αKgDH			
Liver	++	0	0
Heart	+++	++	+
Brain	0	0	++
Neurological effect (ataxia, convulsions)	±	0	+++

[a]Abbreviations: Oth = oxythiamin; PTh = pyrithiamin; TPK = thiamin pyrophosphokinase; PyDH = pyruvate dehydrogenase; αKgDH = α-ketoglutarate dehydrogenase; TdDP = thiamin diphosphate. NA = not applicable.
Source: From Refs. 48, 49.

2-picolinium bromide hydrobromide:

The proposed modes of action of PTh, OTh, and amprolium are summarized in Figure 1.

4. Group 4: Thiaminases and Antithiamin Substances

Since the original discovery that Chastek paralysis in foxes fed raw carp was due to the destruction of dietary thiamin by an enzyme named thiaminase, a great deal of work

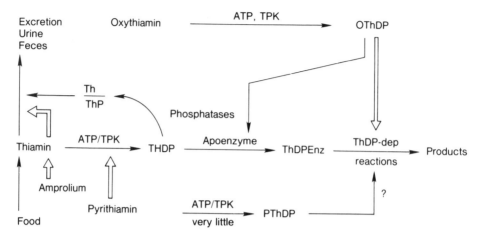

Figure 1 Summary of present information on the modes of action of OTh, PTh, and amprolium in antagonism of ThDP-dependent systems. Abbeviations: Th, thiamin; ThP, thiamin monophosphate; ThDP, thiamin diphosphate; PThDP, pyrithiamin diphosphate; OThDP, oxythiamin diphosphate; TPK, thiamin pyrophosphokinase. (Modified from Ref. 47).

been done in this area. Thiamin-destroying or inactivating factors have been discovered in fish, shelfish, ferns, tea, betel nuts, and a variety of vegetables. (For more details see Refs. 3, 45, 54–65). Two thiaminases have been described (see Ref. 54). Thiaminase I is found in fresh fish and shellfish, ferns, and some bacteria and catalyzes a base exchange between the thiazole and another base:

A variety of bases have been shown to activate this reaction and exchanges. Thaiminase II is a hydrolytic enzyme that hydrolyzes the methylene-thiazole-*N* bond:

$$CH_3-C \overset{N}{\underset{N}{\diagdown}} \overset{}{C}-NH_2 \quad HC \overset{S}{\underset{N}{\diagdown}} C-CH_2CH_2OH$$

$$\underset{\overset{|}{C}H}{N} \quad C-CH_2-\overset{+}{N}----C \qquad + HOH \longrightarrow$$

$$CH_3 \quad$$

$$CH^3-C \overset{N}{\underset{N}{\diagdown}} C-NH^2 \quad + \quad HC \overset{S}{\underset{}{\diagdown}} C-CH_2CH_2OH \quad + H^+$$

$$\underset{\overset{|}{C}H}{N} \quad C-CH_2OH \quad N----C$$

$$CH_3$$

This type is found chiefly in certain species of bacteria. Table 6 summarizes the substrate specificities of thiaminases I and II. The decomposition of thiamin and its analogs by thiaminase II is identical to that shown for sulfite.

Some relatively simple compounds that simulate parts of the thiamin molecule, i.e., 2- and 4-methylthiazolium salts, in which the quaternizing group is either 2-aminobenzyl or 2-aminoethyl, are typical examples (45,59) of compounds that inhibit the type I thiaminases.

In addition to the thermolabile thiaminases, thermostable factors that inactivate thiamin have been demonstrated in fern, tea, betel nut, and a larger number of other plants and vegetables and some animal tissues as well. In animal tissues they are generally thought to be hemin products that bind thiamin. The product will not form thiochrome but is biologically available. In plants 3,4-dihydroxycinnamic acid (caffeic acid) has been shown to be one of the thermostable antithiamin factors (54–65).

Tannic acid is most likely the substance in tea that inactivates thiamin by forming a tannin–thiamin adduct. Somogyi's group (57,58) has shown that a large variety of polyphenols, particularly diphenols in addition to caffeic acid, are powerful inhibitors of thiamin. The most active have the second hydroxyl in the *ortho* position. Most dihydroxy derivatives of tyrosine are active except those with an aldehyde or nitro group in the *para* position. Some flavinoids, such as quercetin and rutin, were also reported to be active. It would thus appear that the group of thermostable antithiamins (thiamin inactivators) may include a rather large variety of naturally occurring substances. The exact mechanism of the reaction involved in this type of thiamin inactivation has not been elucidated, and it may well involve several reactions. In some cases, a significant amount of thiamin disulfide has been produced. Also, 2-methyl-4-amino-5-amino-methylpyrimidine has been isolated from reaction mixtures, indicating a destruction of the thiazole portion. Since the presence of O_2 increases the amount of thiamin inactivated, it appears that oxidative mechanisms are involved. Generally, these types of antithiamin reactions result in a product (or products) that are both thiochrome negative and microbiologically inactive.

E. Synthesis

1. Chemical

The original synthesis of thiamin was accomplished almost simultaneously in 1936–1937 by Williams and co-workers, Todd and Bergel and Andersag and Westphal by slightly different procedures, which are used today with only slight modifications (1,2). Either

Table 6 Substrate Specificities for Thiaminase I and II

	Substrates			Decomposition by thiaminase I		Decomposition by thiaminase II
	R_1	R_2	R_3	Shellfish	B. Thiaminolyticus	B. Aneurinolyticus
Thiamin	NH_2	CH_3	CH_2CH_2OH	+++	+++	+++
Oxythiamin	OH	CH_3	CH_2CH_2OH	±	±	++
4'-Methylaminothiamin	$NH \cdot CH_3$	CH_3	CH_2CH_2OH	−	−	+
2'-Hydroxymethylthiamin	NH_2	CH_2OH	CH_2CH_2OH	+++	+++	+++
2'-Ethylthiamin	NH_2	CH_2OH_3	CH_2CH_2OH	++	+++	++
	NH_2	CH_3	CH_2CH_2OAc	++	++	
	CH_2	CH_3	$COOCH_2CH_3$	++	++	
	CH_2	CH_3	CH_2CH_2Cl	+++	+++	+++
Thiamin pyrophosphate	NH_2	CH_3	$CH_2CH_2O\text{-}P\text{-}O\text{-}P$	+++	+++	−
S-thiamin				−	−	+++
S-S-thiamin				−	−	+++
Pyrimidinyl pyrimidine	NH_2	CH_3		+++	++	++

the pyrimidine and thiazole rings can be prepared separately and condensed via the bromide or the pyrimidine ring can be synthesized and the thiazole ring formed in situ on it (2,45,46,68,69). This latter procedure is probably the one of choice. It is as follows:

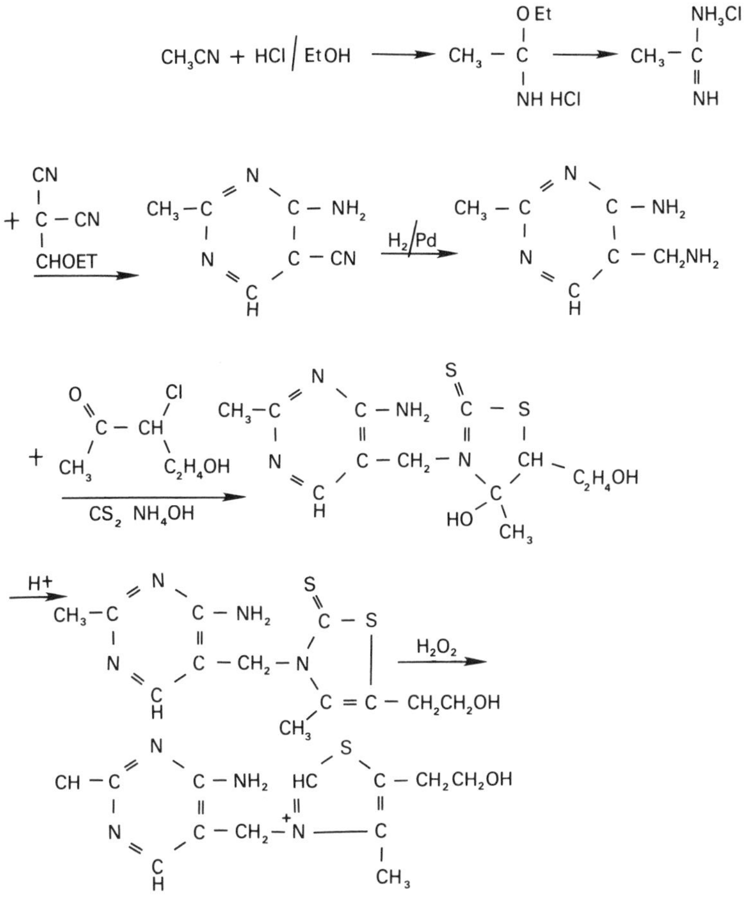

$$CH_3CN + HCl \big/ EtOH \longrightarrow CH_3 - \underset{\underset{NH\,HCl}{|}}{\overset{\overset{OEt}{|}}{C}} \longrightarrow CH_3 - \underset{\underset{NH}{\|}}{\overset{\overset{NH_3Cl}{|}}{C}}$$

2. Biosynthesis

Thiamin cannot be synthesized to any significant extent by animals, although it is synthesized by their symbiotic gut microflora. Many microbial species are autotrophic with respect to thiamin, others can synthesize it if the pyrimidine and thiazole are available, and still others have a dependence on the complete molecule. Higher plants can synthesize the vitamin de novo. In these organisms the pyrimidine precursor of thiamin is synthesized by a different pathway than the pyrimidine precursor of the pyrimidine nucleotides. With the pyrimidine and thiazole available or synthesized, they are generally condensed according to the scheme shown in Figure 2 (3,4,8,69–71).

F. Chemical Properties

Thiamin hydrochloride crystallizes into colorless monoclinic needles, usually as the hemihydrate. It has a very characteristic odor and a slightly bitter taste. It is very soluble

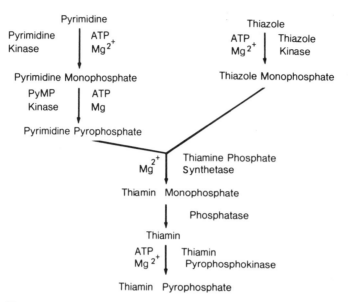

Figure 2 Biosynthetic pathway for thiamin pyrophosphate.

in water, only partly soluble in alcohol and acetone, and insoluble in ether, benzene, hexane, chloroform, and other fat solvents. The chloride hydrochloride crystallizes readily from alcohol-H_2O or acetone–H_2O as the hemihydrate. On exposure to air of average humidity, the compound absorbs H_2O corresponding to about 1 mol/mol. This can be removed by heating at 100 °C or in a vacuum over H_2SO_4 or P_2O_5. In the dry form it is stable at 100 °C. A 5% aqueous solution of the hydrochloride has a pH of about 3.5. The equivalent solution of the mononitrate has a pH of 6.5–7.1. Aqueous solutions are quite stable below pH 5.5 to heat (even autoclaving) and to oxidation. Above pH 5.0 thiamin is destroyed relatively rapidly by autoclaving and at pH 7.0 or above by boiling or even at room temperature. At pH 8.0 or above thiamin turns yellow and is destoryed by a complex series of irreversible reactions (72). In strongly alkaline solution in the presence of oxidizing agents [$Fe(CN)_6^{2-}$, $HgCl_2$, cyanogen bromide, and others] thiamine is converted to thiochrome, which has a characteristic blue fluorescence. This is the basis for the most common assay procedures (see Sec. III). Thiamin gives a number of other color reactions, i.e., a pink color with diazotized sulfanilic acid and formaldehyde, a red-purple color with diazotized p-aminoacetophenone, and an orange-red precipitate with potassium bismuth iodide. Picrolonic acid, gold chloride, mercuric chloride, and iodine also give colored precipitates with thiamin. It is precipitated by tannins, various alkaloid reagents, picric acid, quinine, strychnine, and iron and ammonium citrates. Thiamin is readily ruptured at the methylene bridge into pyrimidine and thiazole by sulfite treatment at pH 6.0 or above. Below pH 5.0 the rate of destruction is greatly reduced. Thiamin in aqueous solutions at pH 5.0 exhibits two absorption maxima at 235 and 267 nm, respectively. The absorption values are somewhat pH-dependent, so below pH 3.0 only one peak at 247 nm is observed. Thiamin forms esters at the hydroxyethyl side chain with various acids, the most important being the mono,-, di-, and triphosphoric esters (73). Above pH 5, and particularly at mild alkaline pH, the thiazole ring can be opened to form thiolthiamin.

This can then react with suitable alkyl compounds to form S-alkyl-thiamines or with alkysulfides to form mixed thiamin-alkyl disulfides (see Ref. 3 for further details):

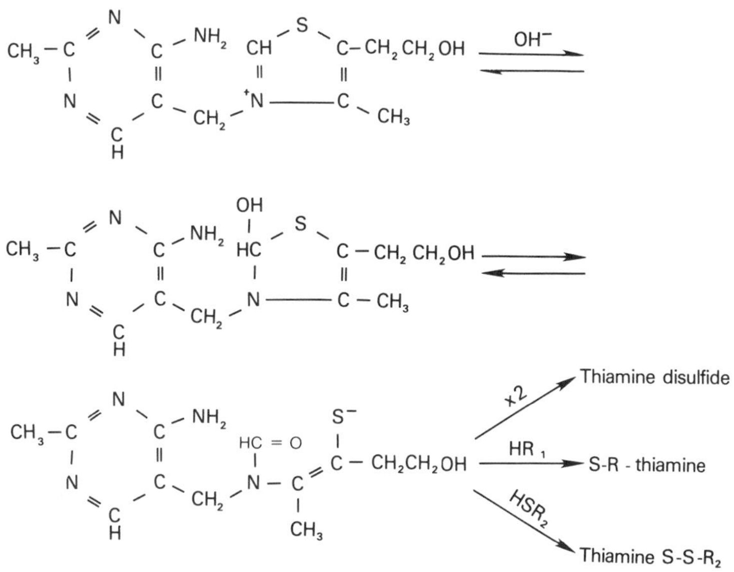

Thiamine disulfide

S-R - thiamine

Thiamine S-S-R$_2$

III. ANALYTICAL PROCEDURES

It has been known since 1935 that alkaline oxidation of thiamin by ferricyanide gives a product with an intense blue fluorescence, which has been named thiochrome:

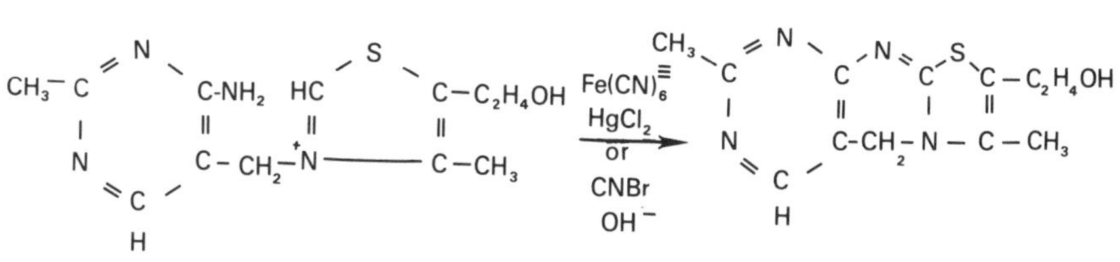

Many modifications based on this method have been described, and it is at present by far the most widely used method for determining thiamin in foods, feeds, pharmaceutical preparations, and other substances. It is the basis for the official standard method of the Association of Official Agricultural Chemists (74) and the Association of Vitamin Chemists (75). Other more detailed descriptions of methods of assay can be found in Refs. 13–15.

A. Extraction Procedures

In animal tissues, thiamin occurs principally as the phosphate esters, with about 80% as the diphosphate, only traces as the monophosphate and free thiamin, and about 10% as the triphosphate. In plants, a larger proportion is present as free thiamin. In both cases a significant part of the thiamin is protein bound. Hence, extraction procedures must be designed to free thiamin and its products from protein. A suitable sample of solid or liquid materials is finely ground or homogenized in a volume about 10–15 times its weight of 0.1 N HCl and heated on a steam or boiling water bath for 30–60 min. More acid should be added if the pH rises above 2.0 during extraction. For total thiamin the extract is then neutralized to pH 4.5 (usually with sodium acetate) and treated with an enzyme preparation containing phosphatase (ie., Takediastase, Park-Davis; Diastase, Merck & Co.; Polidase, Schwartz Laboratories; Mutase, Wallerstein Labs; or Clarase, Takamine Labs) and incubated 4–5 hr at 40–50 °C to hydrolyze the phosphate esters. Though the phosphate esters also form thiochrome, the thiochrome phosphates are not soluble in isobutanol, and hence are not extracted and measured. If only free thiamin is to be measured, the enzymatic step is eliminated. Enzymatic treatment of plant materials also aids by hydrolysis of excess starch. Centrifugation or filtration can be used to separate the extract from insoluble materials. Special extraction procedures are described in Ref. 13.

B. Further Purification

With most complex biological materials, further treatment is necessary to remove interfering materials. Thus, a suitable volume of the extract is put on a prepared and washed column of ion exchanger (aluminum silicate preparation designated variously as Permutit T., Thiamin Decalso, Decalso F, or Zepolit S/E). The column is then washed several times with hot distilled water to wash out impurities, followed by elution of the thiamin with 25 ml (in two to three aliquots) of a hot solution of 25% KCl in 1.0 N HCl. Generally the eluate is then made up to a suitable volume (usually 50 ml).

C. Thiochrome Formation and Fluorescence Measurement

A suitable aliquot of the above eluate is transferred to each of two test tubes. To one is added 3 ml alkaline ferricyanide solution [3 ml 1% $K_3Fe(CN)_6$] diluted to 100 ml with 15% NaOH, prepared fresh daily with efficient shaking. To the other is added 3.0 ml 15% NaOH (blank). Both are then vigorously extracted with 15 ml fluorescence-free isobutanol. Both are centrifuged and the isobutanol layer carefully taken off. If necessary the isobutanol solution can be shaken with dry Na_2SO_4 to remove H_2O and clarify. The clear isobutanol extract is then read in a photofluorometer or a spectrophotofluorometer at an incident light wavelength (excitation) of 365 nm and emission wavelength of 436 nm. This is sometimes standardized with a known quinine standard, but a suitable thiamin standard should also be carried through the various steps for comparison. An improved, simplified modification of this procedure has recently been described by Edwin (76) and Edwin and Jackman (77). Some authors feel that $HgCl_2$ or cyanogen bromide is preferable to ferricyanide as oxidant for conversion to thiochrome. With some modifications, H_2O_2 is added before fluorescence measurement to remove excess $Fe(CN)_6$. Methods have been reported for the simultaneous assay of thiamin, hydroxyethylthiamin, and pyrithiamin in the same sample (78–80) by the proper choice of oxidizing conditions and wavelengths for excitation and emission. Thiochrome and pyrichrome fluorescence is significantly intensified in the presence of alcohol; hence, the extraction into isobutanol serves two purposes: (1) further separation of the thiochrome from interfering substances, and (2) increasing the sensitivity of the assay.

D. Other Methods

Thiamin can also be determined spectrophotometrically by measuring its UV absorbance at 266 nm, but this is only feasible in the absence of significant amounts of other materials absorbing at 265 nm, i.e., nucleic acids. For molar extinction coefficients for thiamin and some analogs, see Ref. 81.

A spectrophotometric colorimetric method has also been described by Prebluda and McCollum (82) and improved by Melnick and Field (83). This is based on the color production of a diazotized aromatic amine (*p*-amino-acetophenone) with thiamin. This method is much less sensitive and less specific than the fluorometric thiochrome method and hence has not found widespread use.

IV. BIOASSAY PROCEDURES

A. Using Animals

As indicated above, all the earlier assays for thiamin during its initial isolation and purification were performed using chickens and later pigeons and rice birds. The early work of Peters and co-workers on the relation of thiamin (B_1) to pyruvate metabolism utilized chiefly pigeon assays. Later, assays were described using rats and measuring either growth rate or relief of bradycardia as measures of the available thiamin. These methods suffer from a high variability and require relatively large amounts of material and long periods of time for the results, hence are mostly of historical interest. It may be useful or necessary at times to use animal assays to establish the biological activity or availability of a new preparation. (For further details see Refs. 13,83, and 84).

B. Microbiological Assays

A large variety of microorganisms have been shown to require thiamin for growth and reproduction. Some for which thiamin assays have been described are *Phycomyces blakeslecanus*, *Kloeckera brevis*, *Ochromonas danica*, *Lactobacillus viridescens*, and *Lactobacillus fermenti*. Some are not entirely specific since they will respond to the thiazole and pyrimidine precursors as well as to thiamin. Assays based on *L. viridescens* and *L. fermenti* are at present the methods of widest choice and use, partly because these two organisms respond only to intact thiamin. Microbiological assays are simple, inexpensive, and very sensitive (detection of 5–50 ng of thiamin is possible). Their chief drawback is that it takes longer periods to obtain the results. The values obtained usually compare favorably with those obtained by the thiochrome procedure. (For more details see Refs. 13, 67, and 84).

V. CONTENT IN FOODS

A. Distribution

In most animal products, 95–98% of the thiamin occurs in phosphorylated form (thiamin mono-, di, and triphosphates) with about 80–85% as the diphosphate, which is the active coenzyme form. In plant products most of the vitamin occurs in the nonphosphorylated form. Thiamin has widesprad distribution in foods, but the content is relatively low in most foods. It is essentially absent in oils and fats and some highly refined foods, such as refined sugars, and the content of green vegetables, fruits and sea foods is relatively quite low. For the thiamin content of a large variety of natural and processed foods reference can be made to tables published by H.J. Heinz Co. (85) and the U.S. Department of

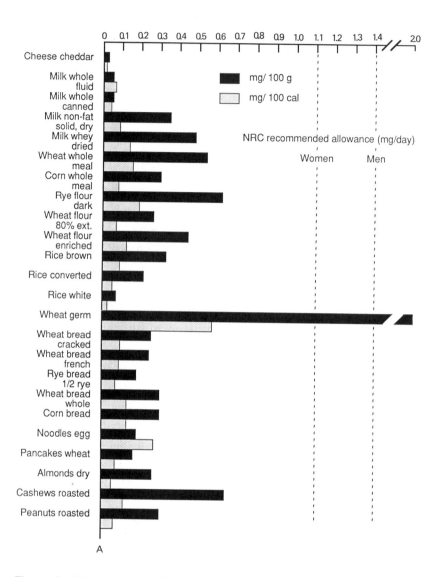

Figure 3 Thiamin content of selected foods.

of Agriculture (86). The thiamin contents of selected foods has been compiled from these sources in Figure 3 as mg thiamin per 100 g edible portion and mg thiamin per 100 cal. As can be seen, the highest source of thiamin is dried brewer's yeast. Other good sources are dried baker's yeast, pork (particularly liver), cereal germs, whole grains and products derived from them, nuts, and dried legumes.

In cereal grains the thiamin is very unevenly distributed, being quite low in the endosperm (the starchy interior) and quite high in the germ. The highest area is the scutellum, the thin layer between the germ and the endosperm. As was indicated in the section on the history of beriberi and the discovery of the vitamin, this nutritional deficiency arises from the milling or polishing of brown rice to produce the more esthetically pleasing white

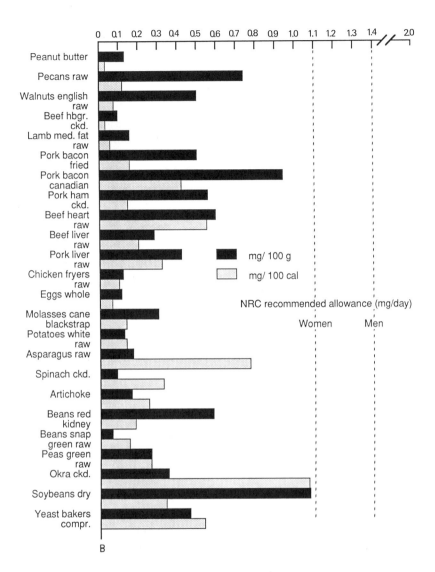

rice, in which the germ has been removed with the bran. The same thing happens in the high milling of wheat to produce white flour, which has a relatively low content of thiamin. By regulating the degree of milling, or most generally by fortifying the white rice or white flour with thiamin (and other B vitamins), the nutritional quality can be raised to the original or acceptable levels without sacrificing the esthetic quality. However, with the present emphasis on the importance of fiber in the diet, it would seem preferable to use whole-grain products, which would eliminate the need for artificial fortification and intake of separate fiber preparations. One reason for removal of the germ is, of course, related to the keeping quality of the processed products (e.g., flour). The unsaturated oils in the germ become rancid easily and also are more attractive to weevils and other vermin. Most white rice and white flour used in developed countries is now enriched or fortified. (For further details, see Refs. 45,85–91.)

In a recent study, the thiamin content of a variety of prepared food dishes, both raw and cooked, as served in the military dining halls, has been published (91). In general, these values agree well with those presented in Figure 3.

B. Stability and Availability

Factors that affect the availability of thiamin in the final product after handling and processing the foods are (1) pH, (2) temperature, (3) solubility, (4) oxidation, (5) radiation, (6) presence of stable thiamin-destroying substances, and (7) thiaminases. The volume of literature dealing with these effects on the availability of thiamin in foods is so voluminous that the studies cannot be treated individually. Detailed reviews have been made by Farrer (90), Dwivedi and Arnold (92), Burger and Walters (93), and Engler and Bowers (94).

1. pH

It has long been known that thiamin is very stable at acid pH (3), still quite stable at pH 5–6, but becomes quite unstable at pH 7 and is rapidly destroyed, largely irreversibly, above pH 8 (see Ref. 95). The rate of destruction at any temperature is accelerated at higher pH. Thus, the addition of sodium bicarbonate to peas or green beans to better retain the green color or to dried beans to soften the skins can lead to large losses of thiamin during cooking. Similarly, in vegetables and meats that have a pH above 7, greater destruction occurs at higher temperatures than occurs in acidic vegetables and fruits. A large number of products have been identified after alkaline treatment of thiamin, among which are thiochrome (in the presence of oxidizing agents), thiamin sulfide, thiamin disulfide (or mixed disulfides in the presence of other RSH compounds), products resulting from the rupture of the methylene bridge between the pyrimidine and thiazole rings, and many other identified and nonidentified products.

2. Thermal Degradation of Thiamin

It has been shown that the thermal degradation of thiamin follows the Arrhenius equation:

$$K = I - \frac{E}{RT}$$

where K = the rate constant, I = a constant, E = energy of activation, R = gas constant, and T = absolute temperature. This also applies to thermal destruction during processing of foods. This is, of course, accelerated at higher pH, as indicated above, especially in the presence of oxidizing conditions. Thiamin bound to protein, as in tissues, is more stable to thermal destruction than is free thiamin. Farrer (90) gives extensive figures on losses of thiamin on cooking and canning of meats, with losses of from 25 to 85%, depending on temperature, time, and type of meat product. Cooking by microwave leads to much smaller losses. Baking of breads leads to losses of 5–35%. The presence of starch seems to exert some protective effect. Losses on cooking of vegetables also varied from 0 to 60%, but here again the degree was related to temperature, time of exposure, and pH. Losses are greater with vigorous boiling or with other types of agitation than with simmering at the same temperature. This effect no doubt relates to an accompanying oxidation. In the processing of milk the following losses have been reported: pasteurization, 9–20%; sterilization, 30–50%; spray-drying, 10%; roller-drying, 15%; and condensing (canning), 40%. As with processing of vegetables, higher temperatures for shorter periods of time for pasteurization gave smaller losses of thiamin. Foods can be stored frozen for long periods without significant loss of thiamin, but losses are significant on thawing, chiefly because of loss in the drip fluid. Losses reported on storage of canned fruits and vegetables vary widely from worker to worker and also with type. At room temperature losses ranged from negligible to 20% for a year, with green beans and peaches more susceptible than peas, lima beans, and citrus fruits or tomatoes. Losses rise sharply with rise in storage temperatures.

Thiamin losses in dehydrated products and pharmaceutical preparations are very low if the materials are kept dry. Thiamin mononitrate is preferable to the hydrochloride for thiamin fortification, since it has been found to be more stable under storage and processing conditions.

3. Solubility

High water solubility is an important factor in the losses of the B vitamins in general, and thiamin in particular, from foods. Thus, the Asian practice of cooking rice in an excess of water leads to large losses of thiamin, particularly in highly milled and fortified rice. Extensive washing can also lead to losses. The practice of parboiling rice, especially fortified rice, causes the added thiamin to be distributed throughout the kernal rather than on the surface. This leads to greater thermal stability and smaller losses due to washing or leaching of the thiamin. Relatively small losses occur if rice (and other cereals and vegetables) are cooked in just enough water to be taken up. One of the most significant losses in home cooking of vegetables arises from the use of excess cooking water, which is then discarded. Overcooking of vegetables and other foods is also a factor in thiamin loss. As mentioned above, the chief loss of thiamin in frozen products occurs on thawing with loss of soluble thiamin in the drip juices.

4. Oxidation

As indicated above, processing at higher pH and temperatures in the presence of oxygen or other oxidants can form thiamin sulfides and disulfides that are still biologically active, but when thiochrome and other oxidation products are formed, the vitamin activity is irreversibly lost.

5. Radiation

Thiamin is susceptible to destruction by x-rays, γ-rays, and UV Irradiation. UV irradiation leads to the production of 2-methyl-4-amino-5-aminoethyl pyrimidine. Ultrasonic irradiation has also been shown to lead to some destruction.

6. Presence of Antithiamins or Thiamin-Destroying Substances

It was discovered early in the race for the isolation of thiamin that it was readily destroyed by sulfites, which rupture the methylene bridge, thus splitting the pyrimidine and thiazole rings apart. This is very slow at pH 3.0, much faster at 5.0, and occurs rapidly above pH 6.0. Hence, the treatment of fruits during dehydration with SO_2 effectively destroys most of the thiamin present. The reaction is as follows:

As discussed above under thiamin antagonists, the presence of naturally occurring thiamin-destroying substances (thiaminases and other antithiamines) in raw fish, coffee, tea, ferns, betel nuts, and a large variety of other plants can lead to thiamin destruction in foods during processing or in the gut after ingestion (see Refs. 3,45,54–56). This is evident by the large number of documented instances of frank thiamin deficiency in both animals and humans resulting from ingestion of these antithiamin-containing feeds or foods. This may occur by destruction of thiamin or by conversion to a product that is biologically unavailable or unabsorbed from the gut.

VI. METABOLISM OF THIAMIN

A. Absorption

Extensive work by Rindi and co-workers (96–97) using inverted jejunal sacs has shown that both rat and human jejunal mucosa absorb thiamin at low concentrations by a saturable active carrier-mediated process that can accumulate thiamin against a concentration gradient. The process follows Michaelis-Menten kinetics, with a K_m of 0.16–0.38 μM. This is of the same order of magnitude as the K_m of thiamin pyrophosphokinase for pyrophosphorylation of thiamin, and thus a close association between transport and phosphorylation was assumed (see also Ref. 98). Studies by Schenker and co-workers (see Refs. 99,102–104) and Komai et al. (100) have shown that there are two transport systems in intestinal mucosa, one by passive diffusion when the thiamin concentrations exceed 2 μM. Pyrithiamin (2 μM), dinitrophenol (200 μM), norethylmaleimide (100 μM), and ouabain (100 μM) all inhibited thiamin absorption at <2 μM but had no effect at 20 μM concentrations. Anoxia, Na^+ deficiency, and low temperatures also decreased the intestinal uptake of thiamin at low but not at high concentrations of thiamin. The above authors conclude that the active absorption (transport) of thiamin across the mucosal cell is not associated with or dependent upon phosphorylation. The presence of a specific carrier is implied, and this is supported by the isolation of a thiamin-binding protein from *Escherichia coli* (101,105,106), which is associated with thiamin transport into and out of the cell. It is well known that excessive alcohol ingestion is associated with a deficiency of thiamin, and Schenker and co-workers have shown that ethanol, either orally or intravenously administered, inhibits intestinal thiamin uptake. The 4-NH_2 and the imidazole quaternary nitrogen are necessary for uptake of thiamin of its analogs by the rat small intestine, and the 2-methyl and 5-hydroxyethyl appear to be necessary for binding of the substance to the carrier protein. The active site for coenzyme function, the thiazole C-2, plays no essential role in transport. Active thiamin absorption is greatest in the jejuneum and ileum. It is confined, in the rat, to the proximal 22 cm of the small intestine and is negligible in the distal portion and in the stomach and large intestines. Thus, thiamin produced by gut microflora is mostly produced in the cecum of the rat intestine and is unavailable to the animal except by coprophagy. The role of thiamin pyrophosphokinase (or thiamin kinase), if any, in thiamin absorption and transport in the small intestine is not yet clear. A high percentage of the thiamin in the epithelial cells is phosphorylated, yet the thiamin arriving on the serosal side of the mucosa is largely as free thiamin. Thus, "entry of thiamin into the mucosal cell is linked with a carrier-mediated system which is dependent either on thiamin phosphorylation-dephosphorylation coupling or on some metabolic energetic mechanism, possibly activated by Na" (97). Thiamin exit from the mucosal cell on the serosal side is dependent on Na⁺ and on the normal function of AT-Pase at the serosal pole of the cell.

Thiamin preparations with greater lipid solubility (i.e., thiamin alkyldisulfides) are much more readily absorbed, and thus result in higher blood and tissue levels, than with thiamin hydrochloride (3,66,67). These are most probably absorbed by a process of diffusion.

B. Transport

The principles discussed above relating to thiamin absorption appear to apply to thiamin transport in most other cells as well, i.e., in *E. coli* (101,106), liver (103), and brain slices (105). On the other hand, thiamin seems to be transported into red blood cells by a facilitated diffusion process (104).

C. Tissue Deposition and Storage

There have been numerous reports on the thiamin contents of and distribution in organs and tissues of many species of animals, including humans (for details see Refs. 3,87, and 88). It is beyond the scope of this chapter to do more than summarize order of magnitude and relationships. The values in the same organ or tissue may vary quite widely between species, i.e., in liver it varies from 1.33 mg per 100 g in the mouse, to 0.22 in the human, to 0.03 in codfish. In general the heart has the highest thiamin content (0.28–0.79 mg per 100 g), followed by the kidney (0.24–0.58), liver (0.20–0.76), and brain (0.14–0.44), with lesser amounts in other tissues. The levels are generally lower in the human than for the corresponding tissue of other mammals. Of special interest is the relatively quite high level of thiamin in pork muscle (0.8–1.2 mg per 100 g) as compared with 0.1–0.2 mg per 100 g for muscle of other species and 0.2–0.4 mg per 100 g for port liver. In general, in the spinal cord and brain, the thiamin level is about double that of the peripheral nerves (88). The whole-blood thiamin varies from 5 to 12 μg per 100 ml, 90% of which is in the red cells and leukocytes. Leukocytes have a 10 fold higher concentration than red cells. Rat liver cell fractions contain the following approximate percentages of the total thiamin: nuclei 10%; mitochondria, 35%; microsomes, 5%, and soluble, 50% (for further details, see Ref. 45). Thiamin has a relatively high turnover rate in the body and is not stored in large amounts or for any period of time in any tissue. Hence, a continuous supply is necessary. Relatively short periods of time with inadequate intake can lead to biochemical, followed shortly by clinical, signs of deficiency. It is thus relatively easy to produce a severe deficiency in a short time even in adult experimental animals, as shown in Figure 4 for rats. During thiamin deprivation the brain is the last tissue to lose its thiamin stores. A normal adult rat on a thiamin intake of 40–60 μg per 100 g body weight per day has a total thiamin concentration of about 2 μg/g body weight (3). In the human it is only half this concentration. Though the muscle concentration is low as compared to brain, liver, kidney, and heart, its content makes up 40% of the total body thiamin due to the large bulk. The main storage organ is the liver. Figure 5 shows the relation of thiamin intake in rats to tissue concentrations (3). When the intake is about 60 μg per 100 g body weight and the total body thiamin reaches 2 μg/g, a plateau is reached in most tissues, so that further increases in intake do not result in further increases in tissue concentrations. Figure 6 shows the relation of tissue thiamin concentrations to the appearance of various symptoms in rats (3). Thiamin entering the body by absorption or parenteral

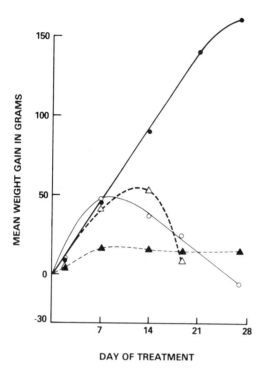

Figure 4 Typical growth curves for rats with thiamin deficiencies produced by thiamin deprivation and treatment with oxythiamin (OTh) and pyrithiamin (PTh): ●———●, Control; ○———○, thiamin-deprived; ▲———▲, OTh; △———△, PTh.

administration is rapidly deposited in the liver, muscle, and other organs and there converted to the diphosphate by thiamin pyrophosphokinase and ATP (see Refs. 107–109):

$$\text{Thiamin} + \text{ATP} \xrightarrow[\text{Mg}^{2+}]{\text{TPK}} \text{thiamin diphosphate} + \text{AMP}$$

The small amount of the monophosphate present probably arises by hydrolysis of the terminal phosphate by thiamin diphosphatase. An enzyme, thiamin pyrophosphate-ATP phosphoryltransferase, has been described that pyrophorylates thiamin diphosphate to thiamin triphosphate. This could account for the approximately 10% of the total thiamine reported as thiamin triphosphate in some tissues (111).

D. Metabolism

As indicated above, thiamin taken by oral or parenteral routes is quickly converted to the diphosphate and to a smaller extent the triphosphate esters in the tissues. All thiamin in excess of tissue needs and binding and storage capacity is rapidly excreted in the urine. Thus, there is a relationship between tissue needs and urinary excretion, and urinary

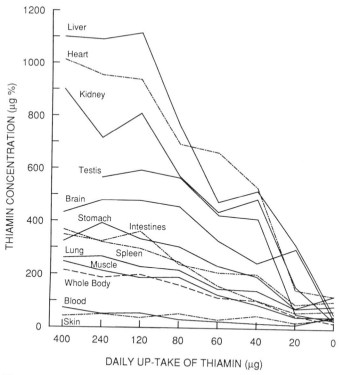

Figure 5 Relation of thiamin intake to tissue concentrations. (Adapted by permission from Ref. 3.)

excretion following a test dose of thiamin has been extensively used as one measure of adequacy of thiamin stores. It has been shown in rats that a parenteral intake of thiamin of 10 μg per 100 g body weight is adequate for growth (3,49) but leads to lower than normal tissue levels. The three phosphate esters are hydrolyzed by their respective phosphatases, resulting in free thiamin, which is then rapidly excreted or metabolized. The factors that regulate this process in apposition to the pyrophosphorylation of the thiamin are not known. It has been repeatedly demonstrated, since the early work of Von Muralt, that stimulation of nerves, as well as treatment with nerve-blocking agents (e.g., tetrodotoxin, ouabain, acetylcholine, etc.), cause the release of thiamin or thiamin monophosphate with a concomitant decrease in the tri- and diphosphates (110,112). Administration of the antagonist pyrithiamin also causes a rapid decrease in the levels of total thiamin and phosphorylated thiamines with increase of thiamin excretion. This most probably is the result of blocking of thiamin phosphorylation so that the rapid turnover leads to the drop in the phosphorylated forms.

E. Excretion

In addition to free thiamin, a small amount of thiamin diphosphate, thiochrome, and thiamin disulfide, about 20 or more metabolites of thiamin have been reported in the urine of rats and humans. Of these, only six have really been identified: 2-methyl-4-amino-5-pyrimidine carboxylic acid, 4-methyl-thiazole-5-acetic acid, 2-methyl-4-amino-5-hydroxymethyl

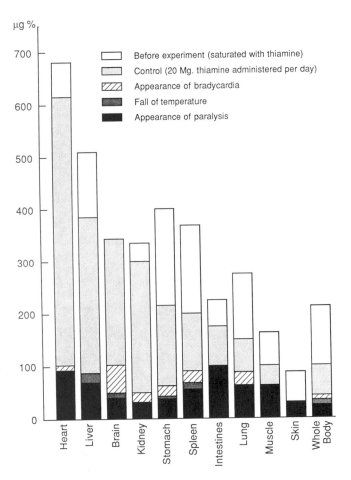

Figure 6 Relationship of tissue concentrations of thiamin to first appearance of various symptoms. (Adapted by permission from Ref. 3)

pyrimidine, 5-(2-hydroxyethyl)-4-methyl-thiazole, [3,(2′-methyl-4-amino-5′pyrimidinyl-methyl)-4-methylthiazole-5-acetic acid], and 2-methyl-4-amino-5-formylaminomethyl-pyrimidine (113). The same labeling pattern of metabolites is found when either ^{14}C pyrimidine– or ^{14}C thiazole–labeled thiamin are administered to rats. This would suggest that most of the metabolites have both rings still coupled together. Of these 20 or more metabolites of thiamin observed in the urine, only six are of quantitative importance. The relative proportion of metabolites to thiamin excreted increases with decreasing thiamin intake (113–115).

VII. BIOCHEMICAL FUNCTIONS

At the present time (see Refs. 45,116–118), the only known biologically active coenzyme form of thiamin is the diphosphate ester (thiamin pyrophosphate, thiamin diphosphate, or cocarboxylase) (12). Thiamin monophosphate is completely inactive, and any coenzyme activity previously attributed to the triphosphate undoubtedly results from partial conversion to the diphosphate by hydrolysis of the terminal phosphate ester bond by thiamin triphosphatase. Thiamin diphosphate has been shown then to act as coenzyme in the following reactions.

A. Straight Decarboxylation of α-Ketoacids to the Corresponding Aldehyde Moiety

This system occurs only in yeast and some other microorganisms and applies chiefly to the decarboxylation of pyruvate. The initial reaction is the binding of the pyruvate by nucleophilic attack at the thiazole C-2 carbon to form "active pyruvate" or 2-(α-hydroxy-α-carboxyethyl)-thiamin diphosphate. Decarboxylation of the activated pyruvate then leads to 2-α-hydroxyethyl thiamin diphosphate ("active aldehyde") (see Ref. 119).

This product is then open to several reactions according to the system involved (see Fig. 7). In fermentation, the acetaldehyde is released and reduced to ethanol. In some microorganisms and with animal tissues in vitro in the presence of acetaldehyde or other aldehydes, the "nascent" acetaldehyde can react with them to form acetoin or acyloins, respectively. In the presence of excess pyruvate, acetolactate can be produced.

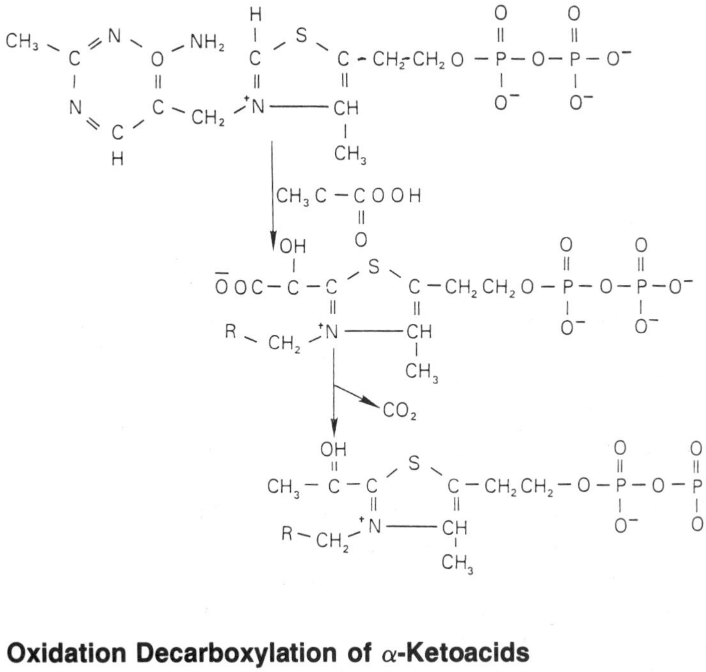

B. Oxidation Decarboxylation of α-Ketoacids

In animal tissues tthe decarboxylation of pyruvate is accompanied by oxidation to give acetylocoenzyme A, which then enters the TCA cycle where the acetate can be further oxidized to CO_2 and H_2O. This oxidative decarboxylation is accomplished bya multienzyme complex bound to the mitochondrial membrane called pyruvate dehydrogenase complex (also pyruvate dehydrogenase or, earlier, pyruvate oxidase). It is composed of three enzymes, i.e., a thiamin diphosphate–dependent pyruvate decarboxylase, a lipoic acid-bound dihydrolipoyl transacetylase, and a dihydrolipoyl dehydrogenase, an FAD-dependent enzyme to reoxidize the reduced lipoic acid (120–123). The proposed mechanism is

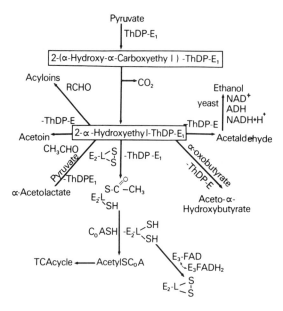

Figure 7 Summary of metabolic pathways for pyruvate.

summarized in Figure 8. Another reaction in the TCA cycle, the oxidative decarboxylation of α-ketoglutarate to succinyl-SCoA, involves an analogous series of reactions catalyzed by α-ketoglutarate dehydrogenase complex to form succinyl SCoA. It is interesting
to note that the entry of pyruvate into the TCA (Krebs) cycle by oxidative decarboxylation via the pyruvate dehydrogenase complex is regulated by the phosphorylation and
dephosphorylation of the complex by a protein kinase and phosphatase to produce an inactive and active form of the enzyme, respectively (121,124). It has been claimed that
the activity of the α-ketoglutarate dehydrogenase complex is not regulated by this
mechanism (121).

More recently it has been shown that the decarboxylation of the three branched-chain
α-ketoacids derived from the deamination of leucine, isoleucine, and valine, namely, α-
ketoisocaproic, α-keto-β-methyl valeric, and α-ketoisovaleric acids, are also oxidatively
decarboxylated by a multienzyme complex analogous to those for pyruvic and α-ketoglutaric
acids, but more specific for these branched-chain α-ketoacids. Although some earlier studies
suggested the existence of three enzymes, each specific for one of the three branched-
chain α-ketoacids, the latest evidence indicates a single enzyme, cospecific for all three
α-ketoacids with only limited activity for pyruvate. This enzyme activity plays an important role in the normal metabolism of these α-ketoacids, as evidenced by the severe
metabolic and physiological disturbances found in individuals with Maple Syrup Urine
Disease (branched-chain ketoaciduria), who have a genetic inability to synthesize this
enzyme. In this disease the enzyme, not the coenzyme (thiamin diphosphate), is lacking
or faulty, although one variant of the disease responds to large doses of thiamin or its
diphosphate (see Refs. 122,125–127).

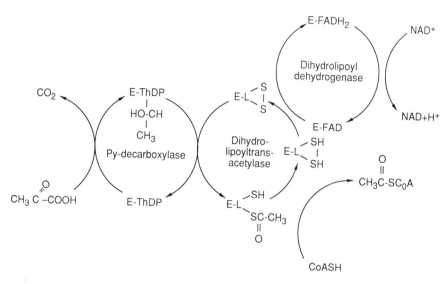

Figure 8 Summary of reactions catalyzed by the pyruvate dehydrogenase complex. (Adapted from Ref. 120.)

C. Transketolase Reactions

In the transketolase reactions, the transketolase ThDP reacts with appropriate ketosugars to break the carbon–carbon bond between C-2 and C-3 to form the ThDP-glycolaldehyde intermediate ("active glycolaldehyde"), which is then transferred to a suitable acceptor aldehyde in the so-called pentose or hexose monophosphate shunt pathway for oxidation of glucose, as shown in Figure 9 (see Refs. 128–130). This metabolic pathway for glucose as an alternate to the glycolysis-Krebs cycle pathway is important, not so much for energy production as for production of pentoses for RNA and DNA synthesis and NADPH for biosynthesis of fatty acids and other products. It can also supply intermediate sugars for glycolysis.

D. Other Functions

Since the early work of Von Muralt (112), it has repeatedly been demonstrated that stimulation of nerves or treatment with certain neuroactive drugs results in a decrease in the level of thiamin diphosphate and particularly thiamin triphosphate in the nerve concomitant with a release of thiamin monophosphate, and particularly free thiamin, into the surrounding medium. It has thus been postulated that thiamin, probably as thiamin triphosphate, plays an essential role in nerve transmission, apart from its enzymatic role in the Krebs cycle and the pentose pathway. It is at present believed that this nerve conduction function involves a role in the gating mechanism for Na^+, and K^+ transport via the Na^+, K^+-dependent ATPase. This is supported by the fact that nerves contain a rather constant and significant level of thiamin triphosphate (10%) and also by the fact that patients with Leigh's disease (subacute necrotizing encephalomyelopathy) have a deficiency of thiamin triphosphate (but normal levels of the diphosphate), and this is accompanied by severe neurological involvement. The presence of an inhibitor of thiamin triphosphate synthesis from thiamin diphosphate is thought to be the contributing factor (see Refs. 131–134). Thiamin has also

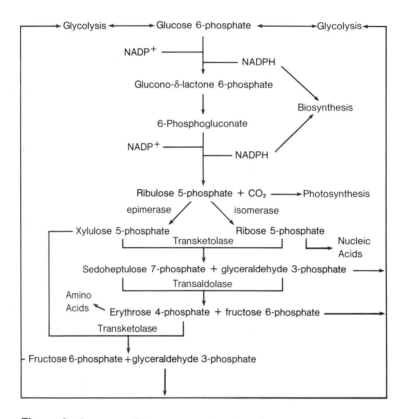

Figure 9 Summary of hexose monophosphate shunt pathway.

been shown to bear a relationship to the levels and function of various neurotransmitters, i.e., serotonergic (135), adrenergic (136), and cholinergic (152,135,137) systems. Whether or to what extent these changes are responsible for the neurological symptoms of thiamin deficiency remains to be established.

VII. DEFICIENCY SIGNS

In both animals and humans the most prominent signs of thiamin deficiency can be divided into a triad of symptoms: (1) loss of appetite (anorexia) and associated weight loss, (2) heart involvement, and (3) neurological symptoms. The degree and manifestations of the individual symptoms may vary from species to species and with individuals and type of diet, but all three types are generally present to some degree (see Tables 4 and 7).

A. Animals

Fowl (e.g., pigeons and chickens) are much more susceptible to the neuromuscular effects of thiamin deficiency than most mammals. This manifests itself as a peculiar head retraction called "opisthotonos." This condition has also been reported in young animals but is not usual. Generally, in the calf, pigs, rats, mice, rabbits, and monkeys, neurological involvement expresses itself as ataxia and incoordination progressing to convulsions and death. Rats on a severely thiamin-deficient synthetic diet will usually die of other things before the brain is sufficiently depleted for neurological symptoms to become manifest. If the diet is less deficient or if small supportive amounts of thiamin are given, neurological symptoms can be made to appear. As shown in Table 4, treatment with the antagonist oxythiamin never results in neurological involvement, but treatment with pyrithiamin or butylthiamin invariably gives rise chiefly to neurological signs. The biochemical lesion or lesions responsible for the neurological symptoms are still not known. One might expect that, since the oxidative decarboxylation of pyruvate and α-ketoglutartate are essential steps in energy production via the Krebs cycle and this cycle plays a prominent role in metabolism in the brain, the neurological dysfunction could be attributed to failure of this cycle. However, it has been shown that the decrease in activity of the pyruvate and α-ketoglutarate dehydrogenase systems does not seem to be great enough to explain the severe neurological involvement (52,138). Although operation of the Krebs energy cycle is reduced in thiamin deficiency, regional concentrations of ATP and creatine phosphate are normal or even slightly elevated (139-142). It has also been suggested that the accumulation of pyruvate might be toxic. However, the evidence available suggests that this is not so (131). Since less pyruvate is converted to acetyl CoA, which is a precursor for acetylcholine, a deficiency of this important neurotransmitter could be the responsible factor. It has been repeatedly shown that either there is no change in available acetylcholine in the brains of rats with neurological symptoms or the reduction is rather small, and the acethylcholine levels seemed to show no correlation with appearance or severity of symptoms (52). More recent work (see Ref. 137) has supported the importance of the cholinergic system in the neurological manifestations of thiamin deficiency.

The accumulation of α-ketoglutarate resulting from failure of its oxidative decarboxylation might also be expected to change the γ-aminobutyric and glutamic acids, two more neuroactive substances, in the brain. Again, changes observed do not correlate with the development of the neurological symptoms in rats (116-118).

Transketolase activity seems to be affected more quickly by deficiency than that of the α-ketoacid decarboxylases. Thus, it has been suggested that the appearance and severity of the neurological symptoms may be related to the decrease in transketolase activity (131,132,134). However, subsequent studies cast doubt on the significance of changes in the transketolase activity for the development of the neurological symptoms (48,132,134,142). In fact, it remains to be shown what actual significance, if any, the pentose pathway has in brain metabolism and function.

The work of Von Muralt (112) and later of Cooper and co-workers (133,144,145) has suggested a nonmetabolic role of thiamin in brain function, more specifically in nerve transmission. When nerves are stimulated, the levels of thiamin tri- and diphosphates decrease and thiamin monophosphate and free thiamin are released into the surrounding medium. This is believed to involve sodium and potassium transport at the membrane (146).

Recent work by Plaitakis et al. (135) has suggested that severe thiamin deficiency effects the serotonergic system and its interplay with other transmitter systems and that such disturbances may contribute to the neurological symptoms of thiamin deficiency.

The cardiac symptoms include hypertrophy (enlargement), bradycardia (slowing of heart rate), and changes in the electrocardiogram, along with fatty degeneration and necrosis of cardiac muscle fibers and heart failure in advanced deficiency (3,45,147-149). Again the biochemical changes responsible for the cardiac symptoms are not known. Neither the high pyruvate and lactate levels nor a lack of available ATP or creatine phosphate appear to be responsible (148). In fact, the bradycardia persists in the isolated perfused deficient heart. Electrocardiogram changes usually attributed to thiamin deficiency have been shown to largely result from the associated inanition (148). However, development of heart changes was shown to correlate well with the reduction of activities of pyruvate and α-ketoglutarate dehydrogenases in the cardiac muscle.

The anorexia (loss of appetite) associated with thiamin deficiency seems to be more severe and more specific than that associated with other deficiencies. This would suggest some specific biochemical lesion in the gut or the central appetite center to be responsible. As shown in Table 4, treatment of rats with the antagonist, oxythiamin, elicits earlier and more severe anorexia than does thiamin deficiency per se while pyrithiamin treatment results in little or no evidence of anorexia except possibly in the terminal stages. Since oxythiamin does not cross the blood-brain barrier but pyrithiamin readily does, this seems to rule out any effect directly on the appetite center and suggests a peripheral effect on the gut. It has been shown that the development of anorexia correlates well with decreases in mucosal transketolase activity but not with changes in pyruvate dehydrogenase activity (150–152). Recent experience with forced feedings has also been shown that the anorexia is associated with an inability to assimilate food (150–152). The anorexia is associated with weight loss, unthrifty appearance, and ultimate death. Figure 4 gives typical weight gain curves in rats subjected to thiamin deprivation and oxythiamin and pyrithiamin administration. A summary of characteristic thiamin deficiency symptoms in animals is presented in Table 7.

B. Humans

The classic pathological syndrome or disease resulting from naturally occurring thiamin deficiency in humans is called beriberi (see Refs. 3,5,113,115,153). This disease, seldom seen in the Western world, is prevalent in the Orient, where polished white rice is the dietary staple. It has been endemic there for 4000 years. Three main types of beriberi have been recognized: (1) "dry" or neuritic beriberi; (2) "wet" or edematous beriberi; and (3) infantile or acute beriberi. The signs and symptoms vary, depending on age, individual, diet, duration and severity of the deficiency, and abruptness of onset. Dry beriberi

Table 7 Summary of Main Effects of Thiamin Deficiency in Animals

Summary	Effect
Intestinal tract	Loss of appetite, mucosal inflammation, ulcers, hemorrhages
General	Weight loss, unthrifty appearance, general weakness, death
Heart	Fatty degeneration and necrosis of fibers, bradycardia, enlargement, electrocardiogram changes, heart failure
Liver	Fatty degeneration and hemorrhages
Central nervous system	Incoordination, ataxia, progressive paralysis leading to death; in birds, typical neck retraction (opisthotonos)
Skin	Skin edema, cyanosis
Muscle	Diffuse degeneration with fiber swelling and vacuolation, muscle weakness

occurs chiefly in older adults and is characterized by marked wasting, particularly of the lower extremities, with less cardiac involvement. In wet beriberi, cardiac involvement is more pronounced, leading to edema that progresses from the lower extremities upward until, if severe, it reaches the heart and causes heart failure. *Infantile beriberi* occurs most frequently in breast-fed infants between 2 and 6 months of age. The nursing mother may or may not show mild signs of deficiency. The condition has a very rapid onset and fulminating course and may result in death, usually from heart failure, in a matter of hours. It is often accompanied by a characteristic cry changing from a loud piercing one to a thin weak or inaudible one (aphonia) shortly preceding death. Vomiting and convulsions may also occur. These infants suffer from anorexia, and milk is regurgitated. Abdominal distention indicates difficulty in assimilating food taken in (3).

In wet, or *cardiac beriberi*, cardiovascular and respiratory symptoms predominate, with edema and other signs of principally right-sided heart failure as prominent signs. It may vary from chronic onset to an acute fulminating type called *shoshin*, or acute pernicious beriberi heart, which is a serious threat to life if immediate treatment is not undertaken. Edema of the extremities and organs is present in varying degrees and masks the wasting away of the tissues. In dry, or *neuritic beriberi*, wasting away of the tissues is a prominent sign along with ascending symmetrical bilateral peripheral neuritis.

General symptoms of beriberi include anorexia, heart enlargement, and tachycardia (as contrasted to bradycardia in animals), lassitude and muscle weakness, paresthesia, hyperesthesia or anesthesia of skin, loss of knee and ankle jerks with subsequent foot and wrist drop, ataxia due to muscle weakness, and dyspnea on exertion.

Beriberi has been largely eliminated in those progressive countries where fortification of rice is practiced but is still prevalent in those countries where unfortified polished rice is widely used. Frank thiamin deficiency is seldom seen in Western countries. However, with better tests available to diagosis, it is becoming evident that subclinical thiamin insufficiency is more widespread than previously realized, especially among the elderly and other groups who consume snacks and highly refined and processed foods or who have digestive or other problems that prevent the assimilation or utilization of thiamin.

The most frequently encountered type of thiamin deficiency in Western countries, and particularly in the United States, is associated with alcohol abuse or alcoholism and is the well-known Wernicke-Korsikoff syndrome or Wernicke's encephalopathy. Manifestations range from mild confusion to coma and include ophthalmoplegia with sixth nerve weakness and lateral or vertical nystigmus, cerebellar ataxis, psychosis, confabulation, and severe impairment of retentive memory and cognitive function. This is generally thought to result from a high intake of "empty" calories in the form of ethanol, coupled with a low intake of nutritionally adequate foods. In both naturally occurring and experimental thiamin deficiency in humans, emotional and psychotic disturbances are often encountered, including intolerance to noise, inability to concentrate, inattention to details, memory defects, irritability, nervousness, anxiety, depression, insomnia, and uncooperativeness.

IX. METHODS OF NUTRITIONAL ASSESSMENT

Frank thiamin deficiency in humans in the form of beriberi or Wernicke-Korsikoff syndrome and experimental deficiency in animals are quite readily recognized and diagnosed. However, even in such cases, the symptoms may mimic other diseases and it is helpful to have laboratory support for the diagnosis. On the other hand, it is becoming increasingly evident that there exist, even in developed countries, many cases of subclinical or borderline thiamin inadequacy that affect the individual's performance and well-being without showing overt signs of deficiency. In order to discover such cases, and to make earlier diagnosis of impending clinical deficiency disease, various biochemical procedures have been developed and used over the years, based on the premise that the biochemical lesion or change precedes the manifest symptoms and thus can detect preclinical thiamin deficiency and assess thiamin nutritional status. To accomplish this one must obtain some measure of the thiamin available in the tissues or measure some disturbance of intermediary metabolism resulting from the unavailability of thiamin in the tissues. In humans, this change must be manifest in material that is readily obtainable, such as blood or urine. (For further details, see Refs. 45,115,147,154–156.)

The following tests have been tried to determine the adequacy of thiamin status in animals and humans.

A. Blood Thiamin

The level of thiamin in whole blood or its components has been extensively investigated as one possible measure of thiamin nutritive status. For this to be a reliable index, one must assume or prove that blood levels are a true reflection of tissue levels. This has been shown to be true in experimental animals but must still be assumed in humans. The blood contains only about 0.8% of the total body thiamin and the concentration is very low (6–12 μg/100 ml). Since most of the blood thiamin occurs in the formed elements, the serum level is still much lower. The concentration in leukocytes is about 10 times that of the red cells. If whole-blood thiamin is measured, the hematocrit must then be taken into consideration in the interpretation of the levels measured. Due to difficulty in the assay of such small quantities of thiamin by the thiochrome procedures in the presence of large amounts of other materials, day-to-day individual variability, the relatively small changes in thiamin-deficient individuals, and some other problems, the use of blood thiamin determinations as a measure of thiamin status or to detect thiamin deficiency has not found wide acceptance. However, Baker et al. (157) have developed a highly sensitive, accurate, and reproducible microbiological method using *Ochromonas danica*, which can be used with whole blood, red cells, leukocytes, or any other body fluid or tissues and which they feel is a better diagnostic tool than other methods, even the blood transketolase method. They have used it successfully for the past 15 years. They claim it is particularly useful in mild or borderline deficiency and especially in the presence of liver disease. Recently developed more sensitive and reliable HPLC methods for assay of thiamin or thiamin diphosphate (41,158) may make the assay of blood or red cell thiamin more favorable.

B. Urinary Thiamin Excretion

Until recently the most commonly used procedure for assessment of thiamin status was the determination of urinary excretion levels by the thiochrome method or by microbiological assay. A number of large nutrition surveys have used this method. It has been adequately established that there is a reasonably close correlation between the degree of thiamin deficiency (availability of thiamin in the tissue) and the decrease in thiamin excretion in the urine. Urinary excretion decreases with decreasing intake until a critical low level is reached, after which further lowering of intake has little effect on the level of excretion. Any decrease in intake below this level then leads to depletion of tissue stores. A direct measure of 24-hr excretion is preferred, but this is not practical with large groups and with field surveys. Hence, many surveys have used 4-hr excretion levels related to the simultaneously excreted creatinine. Some have also preferred to use excretion of a test dose of thiamin. Because of the variability with individuals and between individuals and the fact that urinary excretion or load tests are probably not a reliable index of thiamin status and certainly give no indication of disturbances in metabolism, urinary thiamin levels have not been widely accepted as a reliable index of thiamin status.

Some interest has been shown in the use of excretion of some thiamin metabolites as a test for thiamin status. Some 20 metabolites have been separated from urine, but as yet no acceptable procedure has been developed. More work needs to be done in this area.

Both blood levels and urinary excretion of thiamin are really only a reflection of the immediately preceding intake and other factors and may not be a reliable index of tissue stores, distribution, or actual biochemical functioning, and hence are of limited value for interpretation of actual thiamin status.

C. Blood Pyruvate and Lactate Levels

The early extensive work of Peters and co-workers showed that thiamin was required for pyruvate metabolism and that blood pyruvate and lactate levels increased significantly in thiamin-deficient animals and humans. This would be a good example of a result of biochemical disturbance and hence should be a good measure of thiamin functional status in the tissues. However, a part of the increase in pyruvate is due to increased activity of the adrenals from the stress of inanition, and many other conditions give rise to increased blood pyruvate and lactate levels. Hence, great care must be exercised before the increase can be attributed to thiamin deficiency. This is particularly true with borderline or subclinical insufficiency. The test can be made more favorable for diagnosis if blood pyruvate levels are measured after a test dose of glucose. By determining pyruvate and lactate after combining a test dose of glucose with a regulated mild exercise, Horwitt and Kreisler (159) developed a concept called the carbohydrate metabolism index (CMI), which they claim gives a more reliable indication of a disturbance in glucose metabolism through pyruvate. However, this test has also not found widespread use as an index of thiamin status.

D. Blood Transketolase Activity and the ThDP Effect

The most reliable index of the functional state of thiamin would be the activity of a thiamin-requiring enzyme in a representative body tissue (see Refs. 154–156,160,161). Brin and co-workers (160–162) were able to show that blood (particularly red cell) transketolase activity is a reliable index of the availability of the coenzyme thiamin diphosphate, and hence correlated well with the degree of deficiency in both animals and humans. They measured transketolase activity by either the disappearance of pentose (ribose-5-phosphate plus xylulose-5-phosphate) or the appearance (accumulation) of hexose. These were determined by the appropriate colorimetric carbohydrate assays. The method was made more sensitive and specific by measuring the activity before and after the addition of the coenzyme (thiamin diphosphate). The difference is the percent thiamin diphosphate effect. Generally, even in subclinical thiamin deficiency, the transketolase activity is reduced below normal and is returned to normal levels on the addition of the coenzyme, in vitro, thus indicating that the low level is generally due to loss of the coenzyme. However, in severe deficiency, particularly the chronic type associated with alcoholism, the activity is low and is only partially restored by addition of the coenzyme, thus indicating a deficiency of coenzyme along with lower level of apoenzyme as well. This is one complication of the method that can give erroneous results if not properly interpreted. Some prefer to run the test before and after in vivo administration of thiamin or thiamin diphosphate to get the thiamin diphosphate effect. Brin recommends that a thiamin diphosphate effect, "TPP-effect," of < 15% denotes adequate thiamin status, 15–25% = mild deficiency and >25% = severe deficiency. Dreyfus (163) claims that the colorimetric determination of sedoheptulose production is a better and more consistent measure of transketolase activity. Warnock (164) has described a modification of this method. Extensive studies in both animals and humans have shown good correlations between tissue thiamin levels and also urinary excretion levels with erythrocyte transketolase activity and also a negative correlation with the thiamin diphosphate effect. Erythrocyte transketolase seems to be one of the first systems to become affected by a lack of coenzyme, and hence is a very useful index of early subclinical thiamin deficiency. This indicates that the biochemical lesion precedes the clinical symptoms. As Sauberlich (153,154) has said, "Of the few tests available, erythrocyte transketolase activity measurement appears the most convenient, feasible, specific and sensitive" of the various methods used to assess thiamin adequacy and status. More recently Takeuchi et al. (165) have described an improved transketolase activity assay in erythrocytes based on Brin's and Dreyfus's methods.

More direct spectrophotometric methods have been suggested, based on the change in absorption at 340 mμ due to the decrease or increase in NADH in reactions coupled with glyceraldehyde-3-phosphate oxidation or reduction with the appropriate auxiliary enzymes (166,167). This method has the advantage that it is measuring the reaction directly rather than measuring an end product after a period of time, which itself can be further metabolized. Waring et al. have proposed an automated method for assay of erythrocyte transketolase activity (168).

X. NUTRITIONAL REQUIREMENTS

A. Animals

As with most of the water-soluble vitamins, thiamin cannot be stored to any great extent by the animal body. Because of this lack of storage capability, coupled with a relatively large daily requirement and the daily excretory losses, a constant intake is needed. Hence it is relatively easy to produce a thiamin deficiency even in nongrowing adult animals. When the intake exceeds a certain level the tissues become saturated and any excess is excreted as intact thiamin or its metabolites. It is difficult to decide on an exact criterion for determining the requirement of an animal for a nutrient. Growth curves are often used. However, the influence of the thiamin content of the diet on the growth rate of rats is an asymptotic one, and it is difficult to say what is the maximum or "normal" growth rate, much less the "optimum" rate. Rats receiving 10 μg thiamin per 100 g body weight per day on a synthetic diet grow equally as well as similar age rats on a "complete" rat chow (Purina) diet (138) (see also Fig. 4). However, tissue levels on this intake were only about 20–25% of the levels in the chow-fed rats (80). Even at these low tissue levels no clinical or biochemical signs of deficiency could be detected. Does this reflect the minimum requirement? Shimozono and co-workers (3) and Murdock and Gubler (80,169) have shown that an intake of about 60 μg/100 g/day is necessary to saturate the tissues at a maximum or "ceiling" level. At this intake level, the whole-body thiamin concentration levels off at about 2 μg/g body weight. This has been illustrated in Figure 5. As shown in Figure 6, different symptoms appear at different degrees of tissue deficiency, but these occur at around 15–20% of the ceiling levels. Thus, rats on 10 μg per 100 g/day must be right on the borderline of deficiency.

Many factors influence the requirement for thiamin. Some that have been studied in more detail (see Ref. 45) are as follows:

1. The size of the animal: Cowgill demonstrated that the thiamin requirement of animals is proportional to their size.
2. Composition of diet: Since thiamin is specifically involved in carbohydrate metabolism through both the tricarboxylic acid cycle and the pentose pathway, the level of carbohydrate in the diet relative to other energy-supplying components influences the thiamin requirement. The "thiamin-sparing" effect of fats has long been known. High levels of sorbitol, ascorbic acid, and some other relatively nonabsorbable carbohydrates have been shown to exert a "thiamin-sparing" effect. However, this was shown to result from greater production of thiamin by the gut microflora followed by coprophagy. Excessive alcohol consumption leads to thiamin deficiency as a result of decreased availability due to poor diet and also decreased absorption of the thiamin ingested. Mention has been made of the effects of thiaminases and antithiamin substances present in the diet leading to a decrease in the available thiamin to the extent that cases of outright thiamin deficiency have been reported under these circumstances.
3. Physical state of the animal: Conditions that increase the metabolic rate (e.g., rapid growth, fever, hyperthyroidism, pregnancy, and lactation) increase the thiamin requirement. Likewise, such conditions as diahrrea and malabsorption increase the requirement.
4. The temperature of the environment (climate): It has been reported that both elevation and lowering of the environmental temperature increase the thiamin requirement. The opposite has also been reported. Hence, other facts related to temperature must affect the requirement.
5. Intestinal microflora: Some organisms produce thiamin in significant quantitites above their own requirements. However, since this takes place in the lower bowel where little thiamin absorption occurs, this can oly be of benefit to the animal if it practices coprophagy. Other microorganisms may consume thiamin or produce thiaminases, thus making the ingested thiamin unavailable to the animal.
6. Individual genetic factors: It is becoming increasingly evident that some individuals require greater thiamin intake than others to satisfy their requirements. This has been demonstrated with different strains of rate and pigeons, and individual variations in requirements are well known to nutrition researchers. However, it has been difficult to separate true genetic differences from other factors.
7. Performance of muscular work: If the chief source of energy for the work is carbohydrate, an increase in muscular activity will increase the thiamin requirement. If fat or other noncarbohydrate materials serve as the energy source, the work will have less impact on the thiamin requirement.
8. Age of the animal: It is evident that during periods of growth and greater metabolic activity, the relative requirement for thiamin will be increased. It is interesting that the requirement has also been claimed to be increased in old age in both rats and humans. This is most probably related to less efficient utilization of the vitamin.

Undoubtedly other factors influence the requirement, but they have not been adequate' studied. It is evident from the above list that it is difficult to ascertain and state the e' thiamin requirements of animals, particularly without defining the conditions.

It is also obvious that life is possible at different levels of thiamin intake and storage. Is the optimal intake that which will support all life processes, or that which keeps the tissue concentrations at the "ceiling level"? There is a relatively wide difference between the amount needed for "normal" growth and tissue enzyme activities and that needed to keep the tissue concentrations at the saturation levels. As stated by Jansen (see Ref. 45), "We cannot tell whether this maximal intake of thiamin has any advantage to the animal or not."

B. Humans

It is even more difficult in humans than in animals to ascertain the minimum and optimum requirements for a nutrient. Many studies have been made on human thiamin requirements, by both nutrition surveys and experimental deficiency. On the basis of these, the minimum requirement appears to be between 0.20 and 0.23 mg per 1000 cal. In order to allow a factor of safety the value of 0.50 mg per 1000 cal has thus been recommended as adequate for most persons. However, as with animals, other factors must be considered with individual cases. Tables 8 and 9 present the recommended allowance for humans of various age groups and sex for the United States and the variations in these recommendations in various countries, respectively. These values have been calculated also as micrograms thiamin required per kilogram body weight. The average value of 20–30 μg/kg weight for humans is in contrast to the 500–600 μg/kg weight found for mice and rats, as indicated above. (See Refs. 170–172).

XI. FACTORS THAT INFLUENCE THIAMIN STATUS AND IDENTIFICATION OF GROUPS AT GREATEST RISK OF DEFICIENCY

A. Dietary Practices

Some dietary factors or customs that influence thiamin status and increase the risk of deficiency have been discussed in preceding sections, such as the high intake of carbohydrate, particularly of carbohydrate that has been refined or processed in such a way as to remove much of the thiamin (e.g., polished rice, overmilled wheat flour, or refined sugar), and the customs of chewing betel nuts or fermented tea leaves, excessive intake of tea or coffee, and the eating of some types of raw seafood and raw bracken fern, all of which supply factors that tie up thiamin or destroy it, thus making it unavailable. Groups that subsist largely on snack foods and unbalanced fad diets are also at increased risk.

B. Disease

Disease can affect thiamin status in the following ways:

1. By decreasing the intake: Diseases or conditions that cause loss of appetite, nausea, vomiting, or excessive pain limit the intake of food and thus of the vitamin. Intake is also often limited in diets prescribed for various diseases, which are often followed for prolonged periods, thus affecting the quantity and nutritional quality of the diet.
2. By preventing normal absorption: Examples of individuals at greater risk of deficiency are patients with diarrhea, dysentery, sprue, ulcerative colitis, cancer, achlorhydria, biliary disease, and alcoholism.

Table 8 Recommended Daily Dietary Allowances of Thiamin

Category	Age (yr)	Weight kg	Weight lb	Calories	Thiamin mg/day	Thiamin mg/1000 cal
Infants	0–0.5	6	14	kg × 115	0.3	—
	0.5–1.0	9	20	kg × 105	0.5	—
Children	1–3	13	28	1300	0.7	0.54
	4–6	20	44	1700	0.9	0.53
	7–10	30	66	2400	1.2	0.52
Males	11–14	44	97	2700	1.4	0.52
	15–18	61	134	2800	1.4	0.50
	19–22	67	147	2900	1.5	0.52
	23–50	70	154	2700	1.4	0.52
	51–75	70	154	2400	1.2	0.50
	76+	—	—	2050	1.2	0.58
Females	11–14	44	97	2200	1.1	0.50
	15–18	54	119	2100	1.1	0.52
	19–22	58	128	2100	1.1	0.52
	23–50	58	128	2000	1.0	0.50
	51–75	58	128	1800	1.0	0.56
	76+	—	—	1600	1.0	0.62
	Pregnant	—	—	+300	+0.4	0.61
	Lactating	—	—	+500	+0.5	0.52

Source: From Food and Nutrition Board National Academy of Sciences-National Research Council-*Recommended Daily Dietary Allowances-Revised*, 1974. Designed to provide for individual variations among most individuals in the United States, under environmental stresses, for good nutrition of practically all healthy people.

Table 9 Comparative Recommended Daily Allowances[a] for Thiamin in Various Countries

Country	Male mg/day	Male mg/1000 cal	Female mg/day	Female mg/1000 cal
United States	1.4	0.50	1.0	0.50
FAO/WHO	1.3	0.40	0.9	0.40
Australia	1.2	0.43	0.8	0.38
Canada	0.9	0.31	1.7	0.29
Japan	1.5	0.50	1.2	0.50
The Netherlands	1.2	0.40	1.0	0.42
Norway	1.7	0.50	1.3	0.52
South Africa	1.0	0.33	0.8	0.35
United Kingdom	1.2	0.40	1.0	0.40
USSR	2.0	—	2.0	—
East Germany	1.6	0.59	1.4	0.60
West Germany	1.2	0.67	0.9	0.68
Philippines	1.2	0.50	0.9	0.50

[a]For ages 20–30 years for moderate activity.
Source: From National Academy of Sciences, *Recommended Daily Allowances*, 7th Ed., National Academy of Sciences, Washington, D.C., 1968.

3. By interference with utilization: This is encountered in diseases associated with liver dysfunction (e.g., hepatitis or cirrhosis) and possibly diabetes.
4. By increasing requirements, such as in psychosis associated with hyperactivity, fevers, and infection, hyperthyroidism (thyrotoxicosis), or conditions with diuresis (diabetes insipidus and diabetes mellitus or treatment with diuretic drugs) in which excretion is increased.

C. Parasites

Intestinal parasites could affect the availability of ingested thiamin by causing diarrhea with consequent decrease in absorption or by decreasing availability of thiamin as a result of its utilization by the parasites.

D. Drugs

Drugs that cause nausea and lack of appetite, induce diuresis, or increase intestinal motility decrease the availability of thiamin.

E. Alcohol

In Western societies, the chief group at risk of thiamin deficiency comprises those with excessive intake of alcohol (ethanol), often expressed in Wernicke's encephalopathy, Korsikoff's psychosis, or combined Wernicke-Korsikoff syndrome (5) (see also Ref. 173). Thiamin deficiency in chronic alcoholism appears to have a triple origin: (1) inadequate intake resulting from decreased intake of a balanced diet due to the contribution of the ethanol to the caloric intake, to loss of appetite, for economic reasons, and others; (2) decreased absorption; and (3) decreased utilization. Chronic alcoholics have repeatedly been shown to have decreased transketolase levels and above-normal thiamin diphosphate effect, which return to normal on rehabilitation regimens and particularly after thiamin administration. Some more chronic cases, especially with cirrhosis, may have lowered levels of apotransketolase as well as of coenzyme (thiamin diphosphate) and hence respond more slowly or incompletely with respect to restoration of transketolase activity. Blass and Gibson (174) have shown that at least some patients with Wernicke-Korsikoff syndrome have a genetically determined abnormal transketolase with a higher K_m for thiamin diphosphate that would, in effect, require a higher concentration of the coenzyme to saturate the apoenzyme.

F. Heavy Metals and Thiamin

Since the early work of Peters and co-workers, which shows that the neurological symptoms of poisoning by arsenical war gases closely resembled those of thiamin (aneurin) deficiency, it is common knowledge that poisoning by other heavy metals likewise exhibits many of the same neurological symptoms as thiamin deficiency. These metals, however, do not act directly on the sulfur of the thiamin diphosphate in the pyruvate decarboxylase function of the pyruvate dehydrogenase complex but on the second enzyme, lipoic transacetylase, in the complex. The net result is still the blocking of pyruvate metabolism through the TCA cycle. These effects cannot be effectively reversed by normal monothiols (e.g., cysteine or glutathione) but can by dithiols, such as British Antilewisite (dimercaptopropanol; BAL), by chelating with the metal and freeing the lipoic acid for its coenzymatic function. More recently it has been found that penicillamine (p,p-dimethylcysteine) is less toxic and more effective in removing Cu in Wilson's disease or Pb in lead poisoning (126).

G. Smoking

Little information is available on the possible effects of smoking on thiamin functions and metabolism. However, it has been shown that thiamin and nicotine exhibit a mutual antagonism in the guinea pig atrium (174) and nicotine decreases tissue thiamin in the developing chick embryo (176,177). Strauss and Scheer (178) report a marked reduction in thiamin excretion in heavy smokers.

H. Age

It is generally assumed that elderly persons have an increased requirement for the B vitamins, including thiamin. This may result mostly from generally poor appetite and eating habits or low income of the elderly, thus necessitating vitamin supplementation. However, it has been demonstrated that old rats require more thiamin per gram of food eaten than young rats (179), and Lazarov (189) found a significantly lower transport of thiamin across the intestine in older than in younger rats. Raffsky and colleagues (181,182) reported a lowered excretion of thiamin in elderly humans, thus suggesting lower levels in the tissues. Blass and co-workers (183) have reported decreased levels of pyruvate dehydrogenase activity in the brain of Alzheimer's disease patients.

I. Genetics

It is common knowledge that the thiamin requirements vary for different species, and even for different strains or individuals within a species (45). Genetic mutations can also result in modifications of or inability to synthesize thiamin-dependent enzymes, thus leading to certain signs of deficiency, most notably alterations in pyruvate metabolism with resulting neurological symptoms such as have been observed in maple syrup urine disease (branched-chain α-ketoaciduria) (126) or diseases associated with pyruvate and/or α-ketoglutarate dehydrogenase complex deficiencies (184–186). It was also reported above that Blass and Gibson (174) demonstrated an abnormal transketolase in certain alcoholics. Some variants of these hereditary disorders related to thiamin functions can be treated effectively with high doses of thiamin, but most of them cannot.

J. Stress

Little definitive work has been done on this point. It has been reported that stress, such as higher temperatures (environmental and fevers), cold exposure, infections, and excessive muscular work (fatigue), results in increased requirements for thiamin (5,45). Much of the earlier work in this area is inconclusive or contradictory, which points to the need for better-controlled studies.

K. Other Dietary Factors

Note has already been made of the dependence of the thiamin requirement on the type of diet, i.e., the requirement is higher as the carbohydrate is increased and lower as the fat content is increased. In addition, it is becoming more evident as more studies are done that the metabolism and functions of thiamin are modified by changes in the level of other nutrients, particularly Mg^{2+} and Ca^{2+} and some others of the B vitamins 43,187,188). Mg^{2+} deficiency leads to a decrease in tissue thiamin levels as well as to a disturbance in thiamin functions. Deficiencies of vitamins B_6 and B_{12} result in decreased levels of thiamin in tissues (189), and folate deficiency results in malabsorption of thiamin (190).

XII. PHARMACOLOGY OF THIAMIN

Large doses given intravenously to animals cause vasodilatation, fall in blood pressure, bradycardia, and respiratory arrhythmia and depression. The evidence suggests that the effect on blood pressure is a combination of three effects: on the vascular smooth muscle, on the central vasomotor center, and on the heart (bradycardia). It is not known whether bradycardia results from the direct action of thiamin on the cardiac vagus or on the cardiac center in the CNS. Very large doses of thiamin depress the transmission of impulses at the neuromuscular junction, i.e., they have a curarelike action. It has been claimed that acetylthiamin has an acetylcholinelike effect and that there is an interdependence between the two. Thiamin also has an inhibitory effect on acetylcholinesterase at high concentrations. The physiological importance of this interaction is still a matter of controversy. Thiamin in doses of 15–30 mg/kg has been reported to cause blockage of the sympathetic cervical ganglia in the cat. Some of the effects reported earlier were shown to be chiefly due to the acidity of thiamin hydrochloride solutions and other factors that were not properly controlled. (See Refs. 5 and 45 for further details.)

XIII. EFFECTS AND HAZARDS OF HIGH DOSES OF THIAMIN

Extensive studies on acute toxicity and the evidence against cumulative toxicity indicate a very large margin of safety between effective therapeutic and toxic doses of thiamin. The ratio between the daily requirement for thiamin and its lethal dose has been estimated at between 600 and 70,000, depending on the route of administration. On intravenous injection, the lethal doses were 125, 250, 300, and 350 mg/kg for mice, rats, rabbits, and dogs, respectively (45,191,192). The ratio of lethal doses by the intravenous route to those by subcutaneous and oral routes were found to be 1:6:40. In monkeys up to 600 mg/kg was required to produce toxic symptoms. Death is due to depression of the respiratory center. With artificial respiration the lethal dose can be much higher. Dogs and monkeys seem to be less sensitive than rodents to thiamin intoxication. However, rabbits receiving intravenous doses of 50 mg/kg daily for 4 weeks failed to show any toxic manifestations or pathological tissue changes. Rats have been maintained for three generations on daily intakes of 0.08–1.0 mg thiamin without any untoward effects. This is about 50–100 times the daily requirement.

In humans, no toxic effects, other than possibly some gastric upset, have been reported even with high oral doses. Also, large parenteral doses are generally well tolerated even up to 100–500 mg. Few if any toxic effects have been noted with thousands of injections by subcutaneous, intramuscular, or intravenous routes of doses as high as 100–200 times the recommended daily requirements. Most of the reported instances of toxic reactions have been following repeated parenteral injections and were undoubtedly due to sensitization and anaphylactic shock. For this reason, parenteral administration of thiamin is now used only in special cases.

REFERENCES

1. R. R. Williams, *Toward the Conquest of Beriberi*. Harvard University Press, Cambridge, Mass., 1961.
2. H. M. Wuest (Ed.), Unsolved problems of thiamin. *Annals N.Y. Acad. Sci., 98*:385 (1962).
3. N. Shimozono and E. Katsura (Eds.), *Review of Japanese Literature on Beriberi and Thiamin* (1961).
4. C. Funk, *J. Physiol., 43*:395 (1911).
5. F. Bicknell and F. Prescott, *The Vitamins in Medicine*, 3rd ed. Grune and Stratton, New York, 1953, pp. 183–284.
6. B. C. P. Jansen and W. F. Donath, *Proc. Kon. Ned. Akad. Wetensch.*, Amsterdam *29*:1390 (1926).
7. A. Seidell, *Publ. Health Rep. (U.S.), 31*:364 (1916).
8. R. H. S. Thompson and R. E. Johnson, *Biochem J., 29*:694 (1935).
9. R. A. Peters, *Lancet, 1*:1161 (1936).
10. R. A. Peters, *Biochem. J., 31*:2240 (1936).
11. G. J. McGowan and R. A. Peters, *Biochem. J., 31*:1637 (1937).
12. K. Lohmann and P. Schuster, *Biochem Z, 224*:148 (1937).
13. P. Gyorgy and W. N. Pearson (Eds.), *The Vitamins, Chemistry, Physiology, Pathology and Methods*, Vol. VI and VII, 2nd ed., Academic Press, New York, 1967.
14. R. Strohecker and H. M. Henning, *Vitamin Assay. Tested Methods*, Verlag Chemie, Weinheim, 1965, pp. 65–97.
15. *Methods of Vitamin Assay*. 2nd Ed. Ass'n of Vitamin Chemists, Inc., Interscience Inc., New York, 1951.
16. D. Siliprandi and H. Siliprandi, *Biochim. Biophys. Acta, 14*:52 (1954)
17. L. DeGiuseppe and G. Rindi, *J. Chromat., 1*:545 (1958).
18. G. Rindi and L. Degiuseppe, *Biochem. J., 78*:602 (1961).
19. A. Schellenberger and G. Heubner, *Hoppe-Seylers Zeitschr. Physiol. Chem., 343*:189 (1965).
20. H. Koike, T. Wada, and H. Minakami, *The Journal of Biochem. (Jap.), 62*:492 (1967).
21. H. Nakamura, K. Sanada, and E. Katsura, *Vitamin (Jap.), 37*:1-4 (1968).
22. T. Matsuda and J. R. Cooper, *Anal. Biochem. 117*:203 (1981).
23. K. H. Kiessling, *Acta Chem. Scand., 10*:1356 (1956).
24. G. W. Camiener and G. M. Brown, *J. Biol. Chem., 235*:2404 (1960).
25. G. L. Carlson and G. M. Brown, *J. Biol. Chem., 236*:2099 (1961).
26. L. M. Lewin and R. Wei, *Anal. Biochem. 16*:29 (1966).
27. H. Ganshirt and A. Malzacher, *Naturwiss., 47*:279 (1960).
28. S. David and H. Hirschfeld, *Bull. Sco. Chim. (France), 5*:1011 (1963).
29. D. B. Johnson and T. W. Goodwin, *Biochem. J. 88*:62P (1963).
30. T. Ono and M. Hara, *Bitamin (Jap.), 33*:512 (1966).
31. P. P. Waring, W.C. Gould, and Z. Ziporin, *Anal. Biochem., 24*:185 (1968).
32. C. Levorato and L. Cima, *J. Chromatog., 32*:771 (1968).
33. A. Rossi-Fanelli, H. Siliprandi, D. Siliprandi, and P. Ciccarone, *Biochem. Biophys., 58*:237 (1955).
34. C. Patrini and G. Rindi, *Int. J. Vitam. Nutr. Res., 50*:10 (1980).
35. B. C. Hemming and C. J. Gubler, *Fed. Proc., 37*:1346 (#422) (1978).
36. B. C. Hemming and C. J. Gubler, in *Methods in Enzymology*, Vol. 62-D, McCormick and Wright (Eds.), Academic Press, New York, 1979, p. 63.
37. B. C. Hemming and C. J. Gubler, *J. Liquid Chromatography 3*:1967 (1980).
38. K. Ishii, K. Sarai, H. Sanemori, and T. Kawasaki, *Anal. Biochem., 97*:191 (1979).
39. H. Sanemori, H. Ueki, and T. Kawasaki, *Anal. Biochem., 107*:451 (1980).
40. M. Kimura, T. Fujita, S. Nishida, and Y. Itokawa, *J. Chromat., 188*:417 (1980).
41. M. Barnes, *Clin. Chim. Acta, 153*:43 (1985).

42. L. Bettendorff, C. Grandfils, F. Schoffeniels, J. Bontemps, D. Schmartz, and G. Dandrifosse, in Mol. Basis of Nerve Action, Proc. Intern. Symp. Mem. D. Nachmanson, J. P. Changeux (Ed.), pp. 479–490.

43. R. E. Echols, R. H. Miller, and L. Thompson, *J. Chromat., 347*:89 (1985).

44. E. F. Rogers, *Ann N.Y. Acad. Sci., 98*:412 (1962).

45. W. H. Sebrell and R. S. Harris (Eds.), *The Vitamins—Chemistry, Physiology, Pathology and Methods*, Vol. V., Academic Press, New York, 1973, pp. 98–162.

46. E. F. Rogers, in *Methods of Enzymology*, Vol. XVIII A., D. B. McCormick and L. D. Wright (Eds.), Academic Press, New York, 1970, pp. 245–258.

47. E. P. Steyn-Parvé, in *Thiamine Deficiency, Biochemical Lesions and Their Clinical Significance*. Ciba Study, Gp. #28, G. E. W. Wolstenholme and M. O'Connor (Eds.), London, 1967.

48. C. J. Gubler, in *Thiamin*, C. J. Gubler, M. Fujiwara and A. M. Dreyfus (Eds.) Wiley and Sons, New York, 1986, pp. 121–139.

49. C. J. Gubler, *Intern. Zeitscher, Vitaminforsch, 3*:287 (1968).

50. G. Rindi, L. De Guiseppe, and U. Ventura, *J. Nutr., 81*:147 (1963).

51. L. G. Warnock and V. J. Burkhalter, *J. Nutr., 94*:256 (1968).

52. D. C. Cheney, C. J. Gubler and A. W. Jaussi, *J. Neurochem., 16*:1283 (1969).

53. M. Moreta, T. Kanaga, and T. Mineshita, *J. Vitaminol. (Kyoto), 14*:223 (1968).

54. K. Murata, in *Review of Japanese Literature on Beriberi and Thiamin*, Vitamin B₁ Research Committee of Japan, Tokyo, 1965, p. 220.

55. K. Murata, M. Yamaoka, and A. Ichikawa, *J. Nutr. Sci. Vitaminol., 22*:(Suppl.) 7 (1976).

56. K. Murata, R. Tanaka, and M. Yamaoka, *J. Nutri. Sci. Vitaminol., 20*:351 (1974).

57. J. C. Somogyi, *Bibl. "Nutritio et. Dieta.", 8*:74 (1966).

58. J. C. Somogyi, *J. Vitaminol, 17*:165 (1971).

59. R. R. Sealock and R. L. Goodland, *J. Am. Chem. Soc., 6*:507 (1944).

60. S. Vimokesant, S. Nakornchai, K. Rungruangsak, S. Dhanamitta, and D. M. Hilker, *J. Nutri. Sci. Vitaminol., 22*:(Suppl.) 1 (1976).

61. D. M. Hilker, *J. Nutr. Sci. Vitaminol, 22*:(Suppl.) 3 (1976).

62. K. Rungruangsak, P. Tosukhowong, G. Panijpan, and S. L. Vimokesant, *Am. J. Clin. Nutr., 30*:1680 (1977).

63. S. Vimokesant, S. Kunyara, K. Rungrnangsak, S. Nakamchai, and B. Panijpan, *Ann. N.Y. Acad. Sci., 378*:123 (1982).

64. D. M. Hilker and J. C. Somogyi, *Ann. N.Y. Acad Sci., 378*:137 (1982).

65. K. Murata, *Ann. N.Y. Acad. Sci., 378*:146 (1982).

66. M. Fujiwara, *J. Nutr. Sci. Vitaminol., 22*:(Suppl.) 57 (1976).

67. H. Baker and O. Frank, *J. Nutr. Sci.Vitaminol., 22*:(Suppl) 63 (1976).

68. D. B. McCormick and L. D. Wright (Eds.), *Methods in Enzymology*, Academic Press, New York, 1979, pp. 51–125.

69. M. F. Florkin and E. H. Stotz (Eds.), *Comprehensive Biochemistry*, Vol. 11 Elsevier Pub. Co., New York, 1963, pp. 3–22.

70. G. M. Brown, *Ann. N.Y. Acad. Sci., 98*:479 (1962).

71. M. Florkin and E. H. Stotz, (Eds.), *Comprehensive Biochemistry*, Vol. 21, Elsevier Pub. Co., pp. 1–9. Elsevier Pub. Co., New York, 1971.

72. G. D. Maier and D. E. Metzler, *J. Am. Chem. Soc., 79*:4386 (1957).

73. M. Viscontini, G. Bonetti, and P. Karrer, *Helv. Chim. Acta, 32*:1478 (1949).

74. Association of Official Agricultural Chemists, "Official and Tentative Methods of Analysis," 9th ed., Washington, D.C., 1960, p. 655.

75. "Methods of Vitamin Assay," 3rd ed. Assoc. Vitamin Chemists, Wiley New York, 1966.

76. E. E. Edwin, in *Methods in Enzymology*, Vol. 62. D. B. McCormick and L. D. Wright (Eds.), Academic Press, New York, 1979, pp. 51–54.

77. E. E. Edwin and R. Jackman, *Analyst, 100*:689 (1975).

78. M. Morita, J. Kanaya, and T. Minesita, *J. Vitaminol., 14*:67 (1968).

79. M. Morita, J. Kanaya and T. Minesita, *J. Vitaminol., 15*:116 (1969).

80. D. S. Murdock and C. J. Gubler, *J. Nutr. Sci. Vitaminol., 19*:43 (1973).

81. J. H. Wittorf and C. J. Gubler, *Eur. J. Biochem., 22*:544 (1971).

82. H. J. Prebluda and E. V. McCollum, *J. Biol. Chem., 127*:495 (1939).

83. D. Melnick and H. Field, *J. Biol. Chem., 127*:505 (1939).

84. C. I. Bliss and P. Gyorgy, in *Vitamin Methods*, P. Gyorgy (Ed.), Vol. 2. Academic Press, New York, 1951, pp. 179-201.

85. B. T. Burton, *The Heinz Handbook of Nutrition*. McGraw Hill, New York, 1965.

86. B. K. Watt and A. L. Merril, *Composition of Foods*, U. S. Dept. of Agriculture Handbook No. 8, Washington D. C., U.S. Dept. of Agriculture, 1963.

87. Texas University Studies on the Vitamin Content of Tissues II. Texas University Publication #4237, Texas University, Austin, TX, 1942.

88. C. Long, *Biochemistry Handbook*, Van Nostrand, Princeton, N.J., 1961.

89. A. Von Muralt, *Vitamins and Hormones, 5*:93 (1947).

90. K. T. H. Farrer, in *Advances in Food Research* Vol. 6, E. M. Mark and G. F. Stewart (Eds.). Academic Press, New York, 1955, pp. 257-306.

91. M. H. Dong, E. L. McGown, B. W. Schwenneker, and H. E. Sauberlich, *J. Am. Dietetic. Assn., 76*:156 (1980).

92. G. R. Dwivedi and R. G. Arnold, *J. Agric. Food Chem., 21*:54 (1973).

93. I. H. Burger and C. L. Walters, *Proc. Nutr. Soc., 32*:1 (1973).

94. P. P. Engler and J. A. Bowers, *J. Am. Diet. Assoc., 69*:253 (1976).

95. R. G. Yount and D. E. Metzler, *J. Biol. Chem. 234*: 738 (1959).

96. G. Rindi and U. Ventura, *Physiol. Rev., 52*:821 (1972).

97. V. Basilico, G. Ferrari, G. Rindi, and G. D'Andrea, *Arch. Int. Physiol. Biochem., 87*:981 (1979).

98. K. Schaller and H. Hoeller, *Int. J. Vitam. Nutr. Res., 44*:443 (1974).

99. A. M. Hoyumpa, Jr., H. M. Middleton, III, F. A. Wilson, and S. Schenker, *Gastroenterology, 68*:1218 (1975).

100. T. Komai, K. Kawai, and H. Shindo, *J. Nutr. Sci. Vitaminol., 20*:163,179 (1974).

101. A. Matsura, A. Iwashima, and Y. Nose, *Biochem. Biophys. Res. Commun., 51*:241 (1975).

102. A. M. Hoyumpa, Jr., K. J. Breen, S. Schenker, and F. A. Wilson, *J. Lab. Clin. Med., 86*:803 (1975).

103. A. M. Hoyumpa, Jr., K. J. Breen, S. Schenker, and F. A. Wilson, *Am. J. Clin. Nutr., 31*:938 (1978).

104. A. M.Hoyumpa, Jr., *Am. N.Y. Acad. Sci., 38*:123 (1982).

105. Y. Nose, A. Iwashima, and A. Nishino, in *Thiamine*, C. J. Gubler, M. Fujiwana, and P. Dreyfus (Eds.), John Wiley & Sons, New York, 1976, pp. 157-168.

106. Y. Itokawa, M. Kimura, and K. Nishino, *Ann. N.Y. Acad. Sci., 378*:327 (1982).

107. J. W. Peterson, C. J. Gubler, and S. A. Kuby, *Biochim. Biophys. Acta, 397*:377 (1975).

108. C. J. Gubler, G. Fleming, and S. A. Kuby, *Ann. N.Y. Acad. Sci., 378*:459 (1982).

109. A. I. Voskoboyev and Y. M. Ostrovsky, *Ann. N.Y. Acad. Sci., 378*:161 (1982).

110. K. Nishino, Y. Itokawa, N. Nishino, K. Piros, and J. R. Cooper, *J. Biol. Chem., 248*:11871 (1983).

111. J. H. Pincus, G. B. Solitare, and J. R. Cooper, *Arch. Neurol., 33*:759 (1976).

112. A. Von Muralt, *Ann. N.Y. Acad. Sci., 98*:499 (1962).

113. R. A. Neal and H. F. Sauberlich, in *Modern Nutrition in Health and Disease*, 5th ed., R. S. Goodhart and M. E. Shils (Eds.). Lea and Febiger, Philadelphia, 1973, p. 186.

114. M. Balaghi and W. N. Pearson, *J. Nutr., 91*:9 (1967).

115. W. N. Pearson, *Am. J. Clin. Nutr., 20*:514 (1967).

116. L. O. Krampitz, *Ann. Rev. Biochem., 38*:213 (1969).

117. L. O. Krampitz, *Thiamin Diphosphate and Its Catalytic Functions*, Marcel Dekker, New York, 1970.

118. D. E. Metzler, in *The Enzymes*, 2nd ed., D. Boyer, H. Lardy and K. Myrbaeck (Eds.). Academic Press, New York, 1960, pp. 295–337.

119. J. Ullrich, *Ann. N.Y. Acad. Sci., 378*:287 (1982).

120. L. J. Reed, in *Thiamine Deficiency. Biochemical Lesions and Their Clinical Significance*, G. E. W. Wolstenholme and M. O'Connor (Eds.), Ciba Study Group, #28, London, 1967.

121. L. J. Reed, *Acta. Chem. Res., 7*:40 (1974).

122. M. Koike, M. Hamada, K. Koike, T. Hiraoka, and Y. Nakaula, in *Thiamine*, C. J. Gubler, M. Fujiwara and P. M. Dreyfus, (Eds.). John Wiley and Sons, New York, (1976), pp. 5–18.

123. M. Koike and K. Koike, *Ann. N.Y. Acad. Sci., 378*:225 (1982).

124. L. J. Reed, in *Thiamine*, C. J. Gubler, M. Fujiwara and P. M. Dreyfus (Eds.). John Wiley and Sons, New York, 1976, pp. 19–27.

125. L. J. Elsas, II, D. J. Danner and B. L. Rogers, in *Thiamine*, C. J. Gubler, M. Fujiwara, and P. M. Dreyfus (Eds.). John Wiley and Sons, New York, 1976, pp. 335–349.

126. J. B. Stanbury, J. B. Wyngaarden, and D. S. Fredrickson (Eds.), *The Metabolic Basis of Inherited Diseases*. McGraw-Hill, New York, 1972, pp. 426–429.

127. F. H. Pettit, S. J. Yeaman, and L. J. Reed, *Proc. Natl. Acad. Sci., USA, 75*:4881 (1978).

128. B. L. Horecker, in *Reflections on Biochemistry*, A. Kornberg, L. Cornudella, B. L. Horecker, and J. Ono (Eds.) Pergamon Press, 1976, pp. 65–72.

129. D. E. Metzler, Biochemistry, Ch. 9, 1977, pp. 543–546.

130. L. Stryer *Biochemistry*, 2nd ed., Ch. 15. W. H. Freeman and Co., San Francisco, 1981, pp. 333–342.

131. K. Kanig, *Die Bedeutung der B-Vitamine für das Nervesystem* in Wissenschaftiche Berichte, #4 E. Merck, (Ed.) 1968, p. 118.

132. P. M. Dreyfus and G. Hauser, in Proceedings of the Fifth International Congress of Neuropathology, F. Luethy and A. Bischoff (Eds.), Zurich, 1965, p. 429.

133. J. R. Cooper and J. H. Pincus, *Neurochem. Res., 4*:223 (1979).

134. P. M. Dreyfus, *J. Neuropathol. Exp. Neurol., 24*:119 (1965).

135. A. Plaitakis, E. Chung Hwang, M. H. Van Woert, P. I. A. Szilagyi, and S. Berl, *Ann. N.Y. Acad. Sci., 378*:367 (1982).

136. R. G. Mair, C. D. Anderson, P. J. Langlais and W. J. McEntee, *Brain Res., 360*:273 (1985).

137. G. E. Gibson, L. Barclay, and J. Blass, *Ann. N.Y. Acad. Sci., 378*:382 (1982).

138. C. J. Gubler, *J. Biol Chem., 236*:3112 (1961).

139. J. Holowach, F. Kauffman, M. G. Ikossi, C. Thomas, and D. B. McDougal Jr., *J. Neurochem., 15*:621 (1968).

140. D. W. McCandless and S. Schenker, *J. Clin. Invest., 47*:2268 (1968).

141. A. Ine, S. Shim, and H. Iwata, *J. Neurochem., 17*:1373 (1970).

142. D. W. McCandless, *Ann. N.Y. Acad. Sci., 378*:355 (1982).

143. C. J. Gubler, B. L. Adams, B. Hammond, E. C. Yuan, C. M. Guo, and M. Bennion, *J. Neurochem., 22*:831 (1974).

144. J. R. Cooper, *Biochim. Biophys. Acta, 156*:368 (1968).

145. Y. Itokawa, J. R. Cooper, Y. Yoshitoshi, and N. Shibata, *Biochim. Biophys. Acta, 196*:274 (1970).

146. R. L. Barchi, in *Thiamine*, C. J. Gubler, M. Fujiwara, and P. M. Dreyfus (Eds.). John Wiley and Sons, New York, 1976, pp. 283–305.

147. S. Yamashita, *Jpn. Heart J., 2*:42 (1961).

148. D. J. B. Sutherland, A. W. Jaussi, and C. J. Gubler, *J. Nutr. Sci. Vitaminol., 20*:35 (1974).

149. J. A. Marks, *Guide to the Vitamins*, University Park Press, Baltimore, 1975.

150. C. J. Gubler, P. Bai, and M. Bennion, *J. Nutr., 101*:731 (1971).

151. C. J. Gubler, *J. Nutr. Sci. Vitaminol. (Supp.), 22*:33 (1976).

152. R. A. Bitter, C. J. Gubler, and R. W. Heninger, *J. Nutr., 98*:147 (1969).

153. H. E. Sauberlich, *Am. J. Clin. 20*:528 (1967).
154. H. E. Sauberlich, R. P. Dowdy, and J. H. Skala, *Laboratory Tests for the Assessment of Nutritional Status*, CRC Press, Cleveland, 1974.
155. J.C. Somogyi, *J. Nutr. Sci. Vitaminol. (Suppl), 22*:29 (1976).
156. D. Hoetzel and R. Bitsch, *J. Nutr. Sci. Vitaminol. (Suppl.), 22*:41 (1976).
157. H. Baker, O. Frank, J. J. Fennelly, and C. M. Leevy, *Am. J. Clin. Nutr., 14*:197 (1964).
158. B. Bötticher and D. Bötticher, *Intern. J. Vit. Nutr. Res., 56*:155 (1986).
159. M. K. Horwitt and O. Kreisler, *J. Nutr., 37*:411 (1949).
160. M. Brin, M. Tai, A. S. Ostashever, and H. Kalinsky, *J. Nutr., 71*:273 (1960).
161. M. Brin, *Ann. N.Y. Acad. Sci., 98*:528 (1962).
162. M. Brin, in *Methods in Enzymology*, Vol. 9, W. A. Woods (Ed.). Academic Press, New York, 1966, p. 506.
163. P. M. Dreyfus, *Biochim. Biophys. Acta, 65*:181 (1962).
164. L. G. Warnock, *Clin. Chem. 21*:432 (1975).
165. T. Takeuchi, K. Nishino, and Y. Itokawa, *Clin. Chem., 30*:658 (1984).
166. E. H. J. Smeets, H. Muller, and M.DeWeal, *Clin. Chim. Acta, 33*:379 (1971).
167. K. P. Vo-Kachtu, R. H. Clayburgh, and H. H. Sandstead, *J. Lab. Clin. Med., 81*:983 (1974).
168. P. P. Waring, D. Fisher, J. McDonnell, E. L. McGown, and H.E. Sauberlich, *Clin Chem., 28*:2206 (1982).
169. D. S. Murdock and C. J. Gubler, *J. Nutr. Sci. Vitaminol., 19*:237 (1973).
170. C. Bhuvaneswaren and A. Sreenivasan, *Ann. N.Y. Acad. Sci., 98*:576 (1962).
171. G. E. W. Wolstenholme and M. O'Connor (Eds.), *Biochemical Lesions and Their Clinical Significance*, Ciba Study Gp. #28, J. and A. Churchill, Ltd., London, 1967.
172. National Academy of Science, *Recommended Dietary Allowances*, 8th ed., National Academy of Sciences, Washington, D.C., 1974.
173. C. M. Leevy, *Ann. N.Y. Acad. Sci., 378*:316 (1982).
174. J. P. Blass and G. E. Gibson, *N. Engl. J. Med., 297*:1367 (1977).
175. H. Iwata and A. Inoue, *Nippon Yakurigaku, 64*:46 (1968).
176. S. Kato, *Folia Pharmacol. Jpn., 55*:5 (1959).
177. S. Kato, *Nippon Yakurigaku Zashi, 55*:138 (1959).
178. L. H. Strauss and P. Scheer *Intern. Z. Vitaminforsch., 9*:39 (1939).
179. C. A. Mills, E.Cottingham, and E. Taylor, *Arch. Biochem., 9*:221 (1946).
180. J. Lazarov, *J. Expt. Gerontol., 12*:75 (1977).
181. H. A. Raffsky, B. Newman, and N. Jolliffe, *J. Lab. Clin. Med., 32*:118 (1947).
182. H. A. Raffsky and B. Newman, *Gastroenterology, 1*:737 (1943).
183. Ran-Fu Rex Shen, Young-Tai Kim, J. P. Blass, and M. E. Weksler, *Ann. Neurol., 17*:444 (1985).
184. J. P. Blass and G. E. Gibson, in *Advances in Neurology*, Vol. 21, R.A.P. Kark, R. N. Rosenberg and L.J. Schut (Eds.). Raven Press, New York, 1978, pp. 181–198.
185. J. P. Blass, *Neurology, 29*:280 (1979).
186. M. K. Abboud, D. A. Alexander, and S. S. Najjar, *J. Pediatrics, 107*:537 (1985).
187. M. Kimura and Y. Itokawa, *J. Neurochem. 28*:389 (1977).
188. L. Zieve, *Ann. N.Y. Acad. Sci., 162*:732 (1969).
189. K. Nishino and Y. Itokawa, *J. Nutr., 107*:775 (1977).
190. L. Howard, C. Wagner, and S. Schenker, *J. Nutr., 104*:1024 (1974).
191. H. Molitar and W. L. Sampson, *E. Merck's Jahresbericht, 57*:3 (1963).
192. G. Hecht and H. Weese, *Klin. Wochenschr., 16*:414 (1937).

7
Riboflavin

Jack M. Cooperman and Rafael Lopez*

New York Medical College
Valhalla, New York

---

*Present affiliation: Our Lady of Mercy Medical Center, Bronx, New York

I. HISTORY

Vitamin B was originally considered to have two components, a heat-labile vitamin B_1 and a heat-stable vitamin B_2. In the 1920s, vitamin B_2 was thought to be the factor necessary for preventing pellagra.

In 1927, Paul Györgi in Heidelberg was investigating egg white injury in rats. The curative factor for this condition was called vitamin H. Since both pellagra and vitamin H deficiency were associated with dermatitis, Györgi decided to test the effect of vitamin B_2 on vitamin H deficiency in the rat. He enlisted the services of Wagner-Jauregg in Kuhn's laboratory at the Kaiser Wilhelm Institute for Medical Research in Heidelberg (1). Initially, yeast and liver were used as the starting materials, but these proved difficult to work with. Egg white was then used, and crystalline ovoflavin was subsequently obtained at the end of 1932. This preparation was effective in promoting growth in the rat.

It was shown at about this time, in another laboratory, that a whey concentrate was similar to the ovoflavin preparation. Wagner-Jauregg then used his method to isolate the vitamin from milk with the aid of a cheese factory in Bavaria and succeeded in isolating 1 g of vitamin B_2.

When Warburg and Christian discovered the "yellow enzyme" in 1932, as a flavin-containing enzyme, the biological significance of vitamin B_2 was made apparent. The yellow enzyme was necessary for the oxidation of glucose-6-phosphate. These authors studied the photochemical oxidation of riboflavin to lumiflavin. The structure of the latter compound proved useful to Kuhn and his co-workers for elucidating the structure of riboflavin, which they subsequently synthesized in 1934. Karrer and his co-workers also synthesized riboflavin in 1934.

II. CHEMISTRY

A. Isolation

Riboflavin can be isolated from natural products by a combination of solvent extraction, absorption on columns, and elution by solvents (1).

Such solvents as acetone, methanol, ethanol, and butanol, either at room temperature or at the boiling point, liberate the vitamin from bound forms and extract the free riboflavin. The extract can be put on a column containing Florisil, Fuller's earth in acid solution, Floridin XXF, or Frankonit in neutral solution. An excellent eluent is pyridine diluted with aqueous methanol or ethanol. Other eluents that have been used are 80% acetone, boiling 60% ethanol, ammonia, and triethanolamine.

Although charcoal binds riboflavin tightly, it is difficult to elute the vitamin from this absorbant. Riboflavin in the eluate is crystallized by solvent extraction and precipitation. An aqueous acetone–petroleum ether mixture has been used successfully to crystallize riboflavin.

Reduced riboflavin is very insoluble, and advantage is taken of this in crystallizing the vitamin. For example, in the commercial preparation of riboflavin from bacterial synthesis, sodium dithionite is added to the broth after fermentation ceases and the reduced riboflavin is precipitated. This is harvested and purified, and then oxidized back to riboflavin.

B. Structure and Nomenclature

Chemically riboflavin is 7,8-dimethyl-10-(1'-D-ribityl) isoalloxazine. Its structure with the new numbering system is shown in Figure 1. The International Union of Nutrition Sciences Committee on Nonmenclature and the Commission of Biochemical Nomenclature IUPAC-IUB have designated *riboflavin* as the name for this vitamin.

Among the various names formerly used for this vitamin are vitamin B_2, vitamin G, ovoflavin, lactoflavin, lyochrome, uroflavin, and hepatoflavin. In Great Britain the common spelling is riboflavine.

C. Structure of Important Analogs, Antagonists, and Commercial Forms

None of the analogs of riboflavin have had experimental or commercial importance. The antagonist D-galactoflavin, 7,8-dimethyl-10-(d-1'-dulcityl)isoalloxazine, has been used experimentally in animals and humans to hasten the development of riboflavin deficiency. All the analogs and homologs have been described in a recent review (1).

The two important derivatives of riboflavin are the coenzymes riboflavin 5'-phosphate and flavin adenine dinucleotide.

Riboflavin is sold commercially as crystalline riboflavin. Since it is sparingly soluble in water at room temperature, 10–13 mg per 100 ml, solutions for oral or parenteral administration required the addition of such compounds as tryptophan and nicotinamide to increase its solubility. Now, however, the sodium salt of riboflavin 5'-phosphate (FMN) is commercially available. It has a high solubility and is as active as riboflavin in both animals and humans.

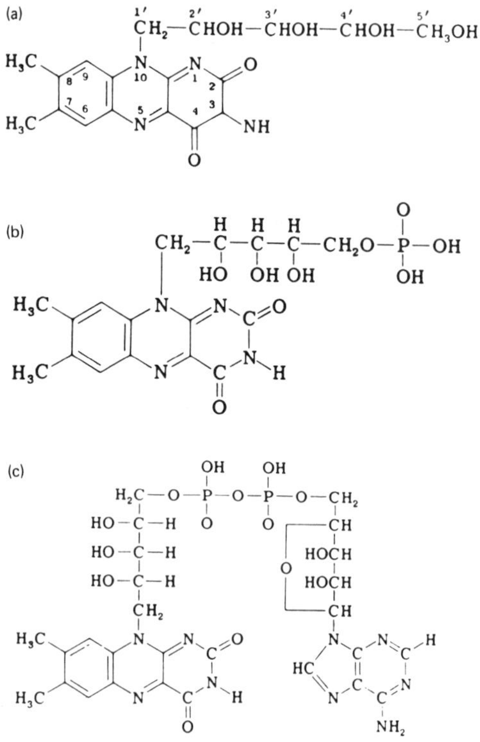

(a)

(b)

(c)

Figure 1   (a) Riboflavin (new numbering system);
(b) riboflavin 5′-phosphate (FMN); (c) flavin adenine
dinucleotide (FAD).

D. Synthesis

Most of the commercially available riboflavin is made by bacterial synthesis, a cheap and
convenient way to produce crystalline riboflavin.

The basic synthetic method for the preparation of riboflavin involves the condensation of 1,2-dimethyl-4-amino-5-(D-1′-ribitylamino)benzene with alloxan. Boric acid
catalyzes the reaction.

A detailed discussion of this and other synthetic methods has been presented (1).

E. Chemical and Physical Properties

Riboflavin has a molecular weight of 376.4 daltons. Its empirical formula is $C_{17}H_2ON_4O_6$,
with an elemental analysis of C 54.25%, H 5.36%, and N 14.89% (Fig. 1). The decomposition point is 278°C, with darkening occurring at 240°C. It is an orange powder, and
water solutions have intense greenish yellow fluoresence with a maximum at 565 nm. Optimal fluorescence is at pH 3–8 and is quenched by the addition of acid or alkali. The
amphoteric compound has dissociation constants at 6.3×10^{-12} (K_a) and 0.5×10^{-5} (K_b).
Riboflavin has little optical activity in neutral or acidic solutions. In basic solutions the
optical rotation is concentration dependent.

The vitamin is relatively heat stable. It is very light sensitive, especially at acidic pH, where it is converted to lumichrome (7,8-dimethylalloxazine). In alkaline solution, light decomposition forms lumiflavin (7,8,10-trimethylisoalloxazine).

Riboflavin can be reduced by sodium dithionite to dihydroriboflavin, a colorless compound, which can be reoxidized by shaking in air.

III. ANALYTICAL PROCEDURES

The riboflavin content of tissues and biological fluids is determined by either a fluorometric or a microbiological assay. Although the microbiological method is more sensitive, it requires 1–3 days for completion, whereas the fluorometric assay can be completed within a working day. Details for both methods have been given elsewhere (2). Both FMN and FAD (Fig. 1), the enzymatic forms of riboflavin in tissue, are bound to protein and must be liberated before analysis. This is accomplished by either enzyme or acid treatment.

In the fluorometric method, finely homogenized tissue or fluids are treated with dilute trichloroacetic acid to separate the flavins from protein. Incubation of materials containing FAD with trichloroacetate results in hydrolysis of FAD to FMN. On a molar basis, riboflavin and FMN have equal fluorescence but FAD has fluorescence only 14% of that value. In some procedures, extracts are treated with dilute $KMnO_4$ to oxidize substances whose fluorescence may interfere with the procedure. In other procedures the extracts are passed through Florisil column and eluted with a pyridine–acetic acid solution. The fluorometer is set with a fluorescein standard and the samples read before and after the addition of a sodium hydrosulfite solution. The latter quenches the fluorescence of riboflavin, and this makes it possible to distinguish riboflavin from any substance in the sample that also fluoresces.

Free riboflavin is very soluble in benzyl alcohol, but FMN and FAD are not. Therefore, extracting with this solvent permits the measurement of free riboflavin. Alternatively riboflavin, FMN and FAD may be separated by high-performance liquid chromatography (HPLC) and each fraction measured by fluorescence spectrometry (3,4).

The microbiological assay for riboflavin was the first practical microbiological assay for a vitamin. Samples are prepared by autoclaving a finely divided specimen in 0.1N HCl to liberate the flavins. Riboflavin, FMN, and FAD are equally active in the microorganism on a molar basis. Alternatively, the sample may be treated with an enzyme, such as Clarase, to release the flavins. The solution is filtered through paper to eliminate traces of fatty acids, which interfere with bacterial growth. A solution of pure riboflavin is run so that a standard curve may be drawn plotting concentration against acid produced or light transmittance.

The medium for the assay supports the growth of the assay microorganism *Lactobacillus casei* upon the addition of riboflavin. The turbidity due to the growth of the bacteria can be read in a colorimeter after 16–24 hr incubation at 37 °C. If turbid or colored solutions are to be assayed, the incubation period is extended to 72 hr, and the lactic acid produced by the bacteria from glucose is titrated with dilute alkali. The concentration of riboflavin in the samples is determined from the standard curve.

IV. BIOASSAY PROCEDURES

The first widely used rat bioassay for riboflavin was devised by Bourquin and Sherman (4) in 1931. The diet contained natural materials and was also lacking in other vitamins. These were added as they became available.

The original diet was eventually replaced by a purified semisynthetic diet containing all the nutrients known to be required by the rat with the exception of riboflavin. Weanling rats are fed the deficient diet for 2–3 weeks, when growth ceases. The rats are then divided into groups balanced for weight and sex. The material to be tested is then added to the diet at different levels. The test period is usually 4 weeks. From the average growth of the control groups a standard dose-response curve is drawn. The value for the test material is determined from interpolation of the growth curve.

Bioassays using chicks have also been devised. The bioassay works fairly well for high-potency material. However, with low-potency material, too much must be added to the diet. This may dilute out known nutrients and may also change the fat and carbohydrate content, both of which affect the riboflavin requirements.

The microbiological assay, once introduced, became the method of choice, since it was less costly and less time-consuming and provided results comparable with those obtained with animal bioassays.

V. CONTENT IN FOODS

A. Distribution

The best natural source of riboflavin is yeast, but it is not normally part of a dietary regimen. Milk and meat are the best contributors to dietary riboflavin in the United States. Although fruits and vegetables are moderately good sources of this vitamin, they are not consumed in sufficient quantities to meet the daily requirements. Rapidly growing, green, leafy vegetables are a particularly good source. Table 1 lists food sources of riboflavin on a milligrams per 100 g and on a milligrams per serving basis (5). It has been estimated that milk and milk products contribute almost one-half the riboflavin in the American diet, with meat, eggs, and legumes contributing abot 25%. Fruits and vegetables and cereal grains contribute about 10% each (6).

B. Stability and Availability

Riboflavin is remarkably stable during heat processing. However, considerable loss may occur if foods are exposed to light. Thus, sun drying of foods will destroy most of the riboflavin. Exposure of milk in glass bottles will result in loss of riboflavin. Cooking eggs or meat in pots open to light also causes destruction.

Such processes as pasteurization, evaporation, or condensation have little effect on the riboflavin content of milk.

Riboflavin in meat is relatively stable during cooking, canning, and dehydration. However, since it is water soluble, some will be found in juices and drippings of meat as well as in the water in which the meat is cooked. Riboflavin is stable in these products during storage if kept out of high-temperature environments.

Blanching of fruits and vegetables results in little loss of riboflavin content. Boiling in water results in leaching of the vitamin into the water, which should be used for sauces.

Cereal grains, though poor sources of riboflavin, are important for those living in areas of the world where cereals constitute the major dietary component. Milling of rice and wheat results in considerable loss of riboflavin, since most of the vitamin is in the germ and bran, which are removed during this process. About one-half the riboflavin content is lost when rice is milled. White flour contains about 35% the riboflavin of whole wheat. However, vitamin-enriched white flour, which is widely used by bakers, contains more

Table 1 Riboflavin Content of Foods

Food	Riboflavin (mg/100 g)	Riboflavin (mg per average serving)
Milk and diary products		
Milk	0.17	0.41 (1 cup)
Yogurt	0.16	0.39 (1 cup)
Skim milk	0.18	0.44 (1 cup)
Cheddar cheese	0.46	0.13 (1 ounce)
Cottage cheese (creamed)	0.25	0.61 (1 cup)
Cottage cheese (uncreamed)	0.28	0.56 (1 cup)
American cheese	0.43	0.12 (1 ounce)
Ice cream	0.21	0.28 (1 cup)
Meats		
Liver	3.5	2.37 (2 ounces)
Beef (cooked)	0.24	0.18 (3 ounces)
Hamburger (broiled)	0.24	0.20 (3 ounces)
Chicken (cooked, flesh only)	0.19	0.16 (3 ounces)
Lamb (cooked)	0.22	0.25 (4 ounces)
Pork (cooked)	0.27	0.18 (2.3 ounces)
Ham (cured and roasted)	0.19	0.16 (3 ounces)
Veal (roast)	0.31	0.26 (3 ounces)
Eggs (large)	0.30	0.15 (1 egg)
Fish and Seafood		
Bluefish	0.09	0.08 (3 ounces)
Salmon (canned)	0.19	0.16 (3 ounces)
Shad (baked)	0.26	0.22 (3 ounces)
Sardines (canned)	0.20	0.27 (3 ounces)
Tuna (canned)	0.12	0.10 (3 ounces)
Swordfish (broiled)	0.05	0.04 (3 ounces)
Clams (raw)	0.18	0.15 (3 ounces)
Oysters (raw)	0.18	0.43 (1 cup)
Vegetables		
Asparagus (cooked)	0.18	0.11 (4 spears)
Beets (cooked)	0.04	0.04 (2 beets)
Beet greens (cooked)	0.15	0.22 (1 cup)
Broccoli (cooked)	0.20	0.36 (1 stalk)
Cabbage (raw)	0.06	0.04 (1 cup)
Cabbage (cooked)	0.06	0.03 (1 cup)
Carrots (raw)	0.06	0.03 (1 carrot)
Cauliflower (cooked)	0.08	0.10 (1 cup)
Collards (cooked)	0.19	0.37 (1 cup)
Corn (cooked)	0.06	0.08 (1 ear)
Lima beans (cooked	0.10	0.17 (1 cup)
Potatoes (baked)	0.04	0.04 (1 potato, medium)
Spinach	0.14	0.25 (1 cup)
Tomato	0.04	0.07 (1 tomato, medium)
Turnip greens (cooked)	0.23	0.33 (1 cup)
Fruit		
Apple	0.01	0.02 (1 apple)
Avocado	0.15	0.43 (1 avocado)

Continued

Table 1 *Continued*

Food	Riboflavin (mg/100 g)	Riboflavin (mg per average serving)
Fruit (continued)		
Banana	0.04	0.07 (1 banana, medium)
Cantaloupe	0.02	0.06 (½ cantaloupe)
Orange	0.03	0.05 (1 orange)
Peaches	0.04	0.05 (1 peach, medium)
Prunes (cooked)	0.07	0.18 (1 cup)
Strawberry (raw)	0.07	0.10 (1 cup)
Watermelon (raw)	0.01	0.13 (1 wedge)
Cereal grains		
White bread, enriched	0.20	0.05 (1 slice)
Whole wheat bread	0.11	0.03 (1 slice)
Rye bread	0.08	0.02 (1 slice)
Oatmeal (cooked)	0.02	0.05 (1 cup)
Rice (unenriched, cooked)	0.01	0.02 (1 cup)
Rice (enriched, cooked)	0.01	0.02 (1 cup)
Dried beans and nuts		
Beans, navy (cooked)	0.07	0.13 (1 cup)
Beans, red kidney (cooked)	0.04	0.11 (1 cup)
Cow peas (cooked)	0.04	0.11 (1 cup)
Split peas (cooked)	0.09	0.22 (1 cup)
Peanuts (roasted)	0.09	0.22 (1 cup)
Walnuts	0.11	0.14 (1 cup)
Snack foods		
Brownies	0.10	.02 (1 brownie)
Candy, milk chocolate	0.36	0.10 (1 ounce)
Pretzel	Trace	Trace
Pizza	0.16	0.12 (1 slice)
Popcorn	0.17	0.01 (1 cup)
Beverages		
Beer	0.03	0.11 (a 12 ounce can)
Colas	0	0 (a 12 ounce can)
Soda	0	0
Wine	0.02	0.02 (1 glass)
Yeast (dry)	5.4	0.38 (1 package)

Sources: B. K. Watt and A. L. Merrill, *Composition of Foods*, Agriculture Handbook No. 8, Agricultural Research Service, USDA, Washington, D.C., 1963, and C. F. Adams, *Nutritive Value of American Foods in Common Units*, Agricultural Handbook No.456, Agricultural Research Service, USDA, Washington, D.C., 1975.

riboflavin than whole wheat flour. Rice is not enriched with riboflavin since the yellow color of the vitamin would present problems. However, converted or parboiled rice, in which the whole brown rice is steamed, thereby driving the vitamins in the germ and aleurone layers into the endosperm prior to milling, retains most of the vitamin content of the whole rice.

Animal sources of riboflavin are better absorbed and hence more available then vegetable sources.

VI. METABOLISM

Riboflavin exists in mammalian tissues primarily as FMN and FAD and as free riboflavin in the eye and urine. Thus, the metabolism discussed in this section concerns all three forms and their interconversion.

A. Absorption

Riboflavin occurs in food as FAD, FMN, and free riboflavin. All three can fulfill the requirement for this vitamin.

Experimental studies of free riboflavin + FMN absorption have been done in rats and humans mostly utilizing supraphysiological doses. Under these conditions, FMN is hydrolyzed in the upper gastrointestinal tract to free riboflavin, which then enters the mucosal cells of the small intestine. In the mucosal cells riboflavin is phosphorylated to FMN by the following mechanisms:

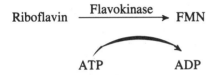

FMN then enters the portal system, where it is bound to plasma albumin, and transported to the liver, where it is converted to FAD. Presumably, dietary riboflavin is absorbed in the same way, except that a large portion of it is in the form of FAD, which must be hydrolyzed to free riboflavin before absorption (7).

Absorption does not occur by simple diffusion but involves an active, saturable transport system. When riboflavin or FMN is given orally with food, absorption is increased, since the vitamin is at the absorption sites for a longer period of time. Bile salts also increase the absorption of riboflavin, but the mechanism is unknown. In children with biliary atresia absorption of this vitamin is decreased (8,9).

B. Transport

In humans, about one-half the free riboflavin and 80% of the FMN in plasma are bound to proteins, primarily to albumin. The degree of binding varies with the species, with less bound in dog and rat plasma. Although the significance of this protein binding is not fully understood, it may have a role in transporting riboflavin from plasma into the central nervous system (46). Certain drugs, such as ouabain, theophylline, and penicillin, may displace riboflavin from binding protein and thus inhibit transport to the central nervous system. It has been shown that when boric acid, which occupies the same albumin-binding site, is fed to humans or rats, riboflavinuria and riboflavin deficiency occur. Some of the effects of boric acid toxicity can be overcome by feeding riboflavin.

The binding of FMN and riboflavin to albumin involves hydrogen bonding, which is not as strong as the bond of flavin to flavoproteins in tissues. The latter binding is so strong that, in experimental riboflavin deficiency, a significant portion remains in the liver even though the animals succumb to the deficiency.

A genetic disease of chicken, renal riboflavinuria, is characterized by lack of plasma protein binders and results in excess urinary loss of riboflavin. Affected hens lay eggs with a low riboflavin content, and the embryos usually succumb within 2 weeks of incubation.

Bovine and chicken plasma contain a number of proteins that may bind riboflavin. During pregnancy in cows, another binding protein appears in the plasma (67).

A riboflavin-binding immunoglobulin has been isolated from a patient with multiple myeloma (68). Immunoglobulins in normal humans were also found to bind riboflavin and may be the major cause of variations in riboflavin binding in human plasma (10). A riboflavin-binding protein has been crystallized from hen egg white (11).

C. Tissue Deposition and Storage

Riboflavin and FMN are converted to FAD in the tissues where binding to specific flavoproteins occurs. In vitro studies with rat hepatocytes indicate that uptake of riboflavin is by facilitated diffusion followed by rapid phosphorylation by flavokinase (12). The liver, the major site of storage, contains about one-third the total body flavins. The liver, kidney, and heart have the richest concentration of this vitamin, and 70–90% is in the form of FAD (Table 2). Free riboflavin constitutes less than 5% of the stored flavins (13).

A significant amount of free riboflavin exists in retinal tissue, but its function there is not known. Photo-dynamic damage to rat lenses occurs when they are cultured in a medium with riboflavin, light, and oxygen (14).

In the human brain, the riboflavin content is higher in the basal ganglia and temporal cortex than in the frontal cortex (15).

D. Metabolism

In tissues, FAD can be hydrolyzed to FMN and free riboflavin by phosphatases and nucleotidases. Flavins bound to protein are resistent to hydrolysis, and this probably accounts for the fact that significant stores of flavin remain in the livers of animals that die of riboflavin deficiency. When the proteins are saturated with flavins, the unbound FAD is subjct to degradation:

$$\text{FAD} \xrightarrow{\text{FAD pyrophosphatase}} \text{FMN} \xrightarrow{\text{FMN phophatase}} \text{riboflavin}$$

E. Excretion

Riboflavin is excreted primarily in the urine, with bile and sweat the minor routes of excretion. Studies of turnover rate of riboflavin in normal rat tissue have shown that the half-life is about 16 days. In the deficient rat the turnover rat is much slower. Riboflavin is excreted primarily unchanged, since no decomposition product has been found in either tissues or urine. When radioactive riboflavin was fed in physiological doses to rats, close to quantitative recoveries of radioactivity, as riboflavin was obtained with only traces as

Table 2 Flavin Composition of Rat Tissues, Weight (μg/g)

Tissue	FAD	FMN	Riboflavin
Liver	59.0	8.4	0.8
Kidney	46.2	13.5	1.6
Heart	35.5	2.0	0.1
Spleen	9.9	0.2	1.1
Brain	6.0	0.9	0.2

radioactive CO_2. Degradation products of riboflavin may occur in feces due to bacterial degradation. The kidney excretes both riboflavin and FMN, but FMN is dephosphorylated in the bladder (16).

The urinary excretion of riboflavin is about 200 μg per 24 hr in normal adults. In riboflavin deficiency this excretion decreases to 40–70 μg per 24 hr. The Interdepartmental Committee on Nutrition for National Defense (ICNND) lists excretions of less than 24 μg of riboflavin per gram of creatinine as an indicator of riboflavin deficiency in adults.

Nearly all of a large oral dose of riboflavin is excreted in the urine of normal adults. The peak of excretion occurs within 2 hr. This is graphically illustrated in individuals who take a dose of riboflavin, either in a vitamin pill or in enriched foods. After about 2 hr the color of urine will change from straw color to an orange-yellow hue. This is also observed in the diapers of infants given vitamin drops containing riboflavin.

The renal clearance of riboflavin is 270–310 ml/min, is dose related, and exceeds the glomerular filtration rate. This is evidence of active tubular secretion.

In humans, less than 1% of orally administered riboflavin is excreted in the bile, and there is some question about whether an enterohepatic circulation of the vitamin exists. In the rat, a considerable portion of administered riboflavin is excreted in the bile and the excretion is dose dependent.

Excretion in sweat is negligible. Adults in whom sweat was induced thermally, only 12 μg riboflavin was secreted in 400 ml in an hour. This is not sufficient to induce riboflavin deficiency in the tropics.

In the rat, less than 5% of an oral dose appeared in the feces. This is probably not an important route of excretion.

VII. BIOCHEMICAL FUNCTION

Riboflavin in its coenzyme forms of FMN and FAD acts as an intermediary in the transfer of electrons in biological oxidation-reduction reactions. Those that function aerobically are called oxidases, and those that function anaerobically are called dehydrogenases (17).

The oxidases are soluble enzymes found in the cell cytoplasm and transfer hydrogen directly to molecular oxygen to form hydrogen peroxide. The best known oxidase is the old yellow enzyme of Warburg. This is an FMN-containing flavoprotein that takes part in the oxidation of glucose to gluconic acid. NADP is the initial hydrogen acceptor, and it passes the hydrogen to the flavoprotein, which then reacts with oxygen to form hydrogen peroxide.

Another glucose oxidase isolated from *Penicillium notatum* is an FAD-containing flavoprotein. This reacts with glucose to form gluconic acid and hydrogen peroxide. NADP does not take part in this reaction. This stable enzyme is used in the determination of glucose because of its great specificity for this sugar.

Two other enzymes, which are flavoproteins that react directly with substrate, are D-amino acid oxidase and L-amino acid oxidase. These enzymes oxidize α-amino acids to keto acids. The D-amino acid oxidase specific for D-amino acids contains FAD as the prosthetic group. The L-amino acid oxidase specific for L-amino acids is an FMN flavoprotein.

Xanthine oxidase differs from the other flavin oxidases since it contains the metals molybdenum and iron. This enzyme, which is found in milk and liver, utilizes a variety of purines as substrates. It converts hypoxanthine to xanthine and the latter to uric acid. It also reacts with aldehydes to form acids, a notable example being the conversion of retinal (vitamin A aldehyde) to retinoic acid.

The flavoproteins that react anaerobically are important parts of the chain that links substrate oxidation with phosphorylation and the synthesis of ATP. This pathway usually involves NAD, and the cytochromes, and the hydrogen resulting from substate oxidations is converted to H_2O.

Cytochrome reductase, an FAD-containing flavoprotein, oxidizes NADH and the hydrogen is passed through the cytochrome system to combine with oxygen to form water. NADH is formed during the oxidation of intermediaries in carbohydrate metabolism.

Succinic dehydrogenase, an FAD flavoprotein, can react with succinic acid, an intermediary in the Krebs cycle. The hydrogen is then passed on to the cytochrome system. When a hydrogen goes directly from a substrate to a flavoprotein and then through the cytochromes, two ATP molecules are formed. This contrasts with three ATP molecules formed when a hydrogen goes from substrate to NAD and then FAD and cytochrome system.

An FAD flavoprotein is an important link in fatty acid oxidation. This includes the acyl-coenzyme A dehydrogenases, which are necessary for the stepwise degradation of fatty acids in the Knoop mechanism, in which two carbon units are removed at one time. The hydrogen the FAD acquires in this pathway also passes through the cytochrome system to unite with oxygen to form water. ATP is generated in this pathway.

A FMN flavoprotein is required for the synthesis of fatty acids from acetate. Thus, flavoproteins are necessary for both the degradation and synthesis of fatty acids.

Other flavin enzymes include mitochondrial α-glycerophosphate dehydrogenase, an FAD flavoprotein, and lactic acid dehydrogenase, an FMN flavoprotein. These are part of the shuttle mechanism in which reducing equivalents are passed from the cytoplasm to the mitochondria. This mechanism is necessary to carry hydrogen across the mitochondrial membrane, which is impermeable to NAD and NADH.

Erythrocyte glutathione reductase, an FAD-containing enzyme, has been shown to reflect the riboflavin nutritional status of both rats [18] and humans [19,20] and has been used as a biochemical indicator of riboflavin deficiency.

The foregoing discussion is not a complete catalog of flavin enzymes, but it does point out the biochemical role of flavoproteins as hydrogen acceptors and thus their key role in the biological oxidations and reductions. Flavoproteins are essential for the metabolism of carbohydrates, fats, and lipids. In addition, these enzymes are essential for the conversion of pyridoxine and folic acid into their coenzyme forms.

Multiple acyl-CoA dehydrogenation deficiencies have been described in several patients, and the defect has been located in the electron transfer flavoprotein and/or electron transfer flavoprotein dehydrogenase [21].

VIII. DEFICIENCY SIGNS

Signs of riboflavin deficiency have appeared in individuals who have subsisted on a nutritionally poor diet for extended periods of time. The signs observed under these conditions may not necessarily be specific for riboflavin deficiency, since the regimen may be lacking in several nutrients.

Experimental studies have been done in animals and in volunteers in which diets lacking only in riboflavin were fed or in which riboflavin antagonists were fed. Under these conditions the signs observed are more likely to be specific for riboflavin deficiency.

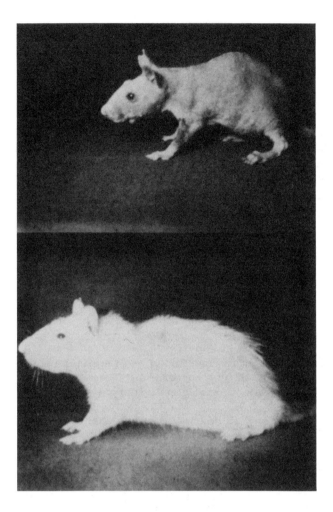

Figure 2 Riboflavin deficiency in the rat. Note growth failure, dermatitis, and keratitis of the cornea. Bottom picture shows rat after 2 months of riboflavin therapy.

A. Animals

In all animal studies, riboflavin deficiency results in lack of growth, failure to thrive, and eventual death. During the course of the deficiency, specific signs in various organs and systems have appeared as follows.

1. Rat

The riboflavin-deficient rat has an unkempt appearance, with uneven and ragged fur and areas of alopecia with an incrustation of red material on the skin (Fig. 2). The skin is characterized by a seborrheic inflammation. Tissue studies revealed a moderate hyperkeratosis of the epidermis with atrophic sebaceous glands.

Mouth changes include red and swollen lips and abnormal changes in the papillae of the tongue. Severe eye changes include blepharitis, conjunctivitis, corneal opacity, and vascularization. There is some question as to whether riboflavin deficiency cause cataracts in the rat.

The severity of the deficiency may be aggravated by feeding a high-fat diet. Under these conditions, paralysis of the legs is induced, characterized by degeneration of the myelin sheaths of the sciatic nerves, axis cylinder swelling, and fragmentation. In the spinal cord, myelin degradation and gliosis have been observed.

In the reproductive system, severe deficiency results in anestrus. Dams given less than adequate levels of riboflavin give birth to litters with multiple anomalies of the skeletal system. These include shortening of the mandible, cleft palate, fusion of the ribs, and abnormalities of the fingers, toes, tibia, fibula, radius, and ulna. In addition to skeletal changes, hydrocephalus, eye lesions, malformation of the heart, and hydronephrosis occurs (22).

Mice made riboflavin deficient show lesions similar to those of the riboflavin-deficient rat.

2. Birds (Poultry)

A good portion of the riboflavin produced commercially is used in poultry diets (23). The riboflavin-deficient chick develops a paralysis with degenerative changes in the myelin sheaths of the nerve roots, pyramidal tract, and cranial nerves. Curled toe paralysis is the prominent feature of chronic deficiency.

The riboflavin-deficient hen lays fewer eggs, and the eggs have reduced hatchability. In the deficient turkey, severe dermatitis is seen. The duck develops no deficiency signs but dies within a week after being given a riboflavin-deficient diet.

3. Canines

Experimental riboflavin deficiency in the dog results in growth failure, weakness, ataxia, and inability to stand (23). The animals collapse, become comatose, and die. During the deficiency state a dermatitis develops on the chest, abdomen, inner thigh, axilla, and scrotum. A hypoplastic anemia with fatty infiltration of the bone marrow also occurs. Cardiological effects include bradycardia and sinus arrythmia with respiratory failure. Corneal opacity has also been observed.

Foxes on a riboflavin-deficient regimen have signs similar to those seen in the deficient dog. In addition, the fur color is bleached. This has important implications for commercially bred foxes.

4. Pigs

Pigs fed a riboflavin-deficient diet grow poorly and develop a scaly dermatitis with loss of hair and bristles (23). Other signs are corneal opacity, lenticular cataracts, hemorrhagic adrenals, fatty degeneration of the proximal convoluted tubules of the kidney, inflammation of the mucous membrane of the gastrointestinal tract, and nerve degeneration. If not treated with riboflavin, the pigs collapse and die.

5. Ruminants

Ruminants do not require a dietary source of riboflavin, since bacteria in their rumens synthesize the vitamin (23). However, the newborn calf whose rumen flora is not yet established requires dietary riboflavin. This is usually supplied by the mother's milk or artificial milks. Failure to provide riboflavin results in redness of the buccal mucosa, lesions in the corner of the mouth, loss of hair, diarrhea, excessive salivation and tearing, and loss of appetite.

6. Rhesus Monkeys and Baboons

Experimental riboflavin deficiency has been studied in rhesus monkeys fed a purified diet lacking in riboflavin, and it was found that riboflavin deficiency develops relatively slowly (24,25). Weight loss appears after 6–8 weeks on the diet. Dermatological changes in the skin, mouth, face, legs, and hands appear after 2–6 months, reached a peak after 8 months. If not supplemented with vitamin, the monkeys suddenly collapse and die. A normocytic hypochromic anemia is observed following a freckled type of dermatitis.

Post-mortem studies revealed the presence of a fatty liver with about one-third the normal amount of riboflavin present. Interestingly, the animals do not develop anorexia and the signs cannot be attributed to inanition.

Experimental riboflavin deficiency in the baboon results in skin lesions after 8–12 weeks. The early signs resemble scurvy, with edematous and bleeding gums. The muzzle, chin, and face develop a seborrheic dermatitis. A red cell aplasia appears after 8–30 months, resulting in anemia. The adrenal cortex becomes cirrhotic, and response to ACTH is suppressed. Although blepharitis occurs, vascularization of the cornea is not observed.

B. Humans

Riboflavin deficiency signs have been observed in humans consuming nutritionally poor diets and under experimental conditions. In the latter, volunteers were fed a purified diet complete in all respects except for riboflavin or given in addition to such a diet the riboflavin antagonist, galactoflavin, to hasten the onset of the vitamin deficiency (26).

Several of the deficiency signs originally attributed to riboflavin deficiency, observed in subjects from areas where poor diets are consumed, have been shown not to be specific for a deficiency of this vitamin. The signs attributed to riboflavin deficiency in such subjects are seborrheic dermatitis around the nose and mouth, dermatitis and pruritus of the scrotum and vulva, cheilosis, stomatitis, and geographic tongue (Fig. 3). Eye changes include reduced tearing, photophobia, circumcorneal infections, limbic proliferation, corneal opacity, and ulceration and presenile cataracts.

Under experimental conditions without antagonist supplements, deficiency signs appear after 94–130 days (27). These include lesions of the lips and mouth and seborrheic dermatitis similar to that described above. The signs disappeared within a month after supplementation of the diet with 5 mg of riboflavin per day.

In studies in which the experimental diet was supplemented with galactoflavin, the volunteers were patients with colon cancer whose nutritional status was good. In these subjects, cheilosis and angular stomatitis appeared after 1.5–7 weeks on the regimen. Oral mucosal changes consisting of hyperemia and edema of the posteria pharynx, fauces, uvula, and buccal mucosa appeared after 2–5 weeks. Glossitis with flattening followed by disappearance of the filiform papillae occured after 2–6 weeks. The fungiform papillae became enlarged, and the tongue color changed to magenta or beefy red. The tongue of these subjects is sore, and loss of taste sensation develops. Seborrheic dermatitis of the face, trunk, extremities, and scrotum becomes apparent after 2–7 weeks.

Anemia with a reticulocytopenia was seen after 3–9 weeks on the diet. The resulting normocytic, normochromic anemia with hemoglobin levels of 3–9.7 g per 100 ml made transfusions necessary. Leukopenia and thrombocytopenia were also present. Changes in bone marrow morphology involving an increased percentage of pronormoblasts with nuclear

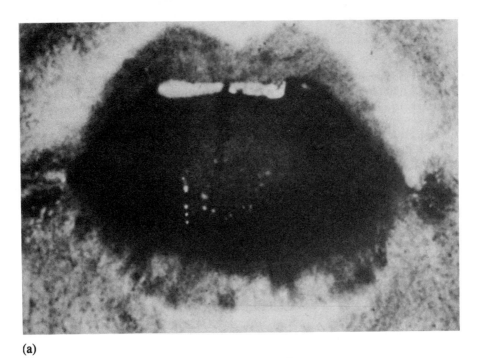

(a)

Figure 3 Signs of riboflavin deficiency in a male maintained for 1 year on a diet containing 0.55 mg riboflavin per 1000 cal. (a) Note the angular stomatitis and cheilosis. (b) The subject had a scaly pruritic dermatitis in the anterior aspect of the scrotum. [From O.W. Hills, E. Liebert, D. L. Steinberg, and M. K. Horwitt, Clinical aspects of dietary depletion of riboflavin, *Arch. Intern. Med.*, 87:682–693 (1951). Copyright 1951 American Medical Association.]

vacuoles occurred after the second week of the diet. No megaloblastosis was found, indicating that folic acid and vitamin B_{12} metabolism were not disturbed. The myeloid and megakaryocytic series were normal.

Peripheral neuropathy of the hands and feet occurred after 90 days on this regimen, characterized by hyperesthesia, coldness, and pain. There was also decreased perception to touch, pain, temperature, vibration, and position. Recovery was slow after riboflavin administration.

Those who were able to maintain an adequate food intake were able to maintain their weight. Liver and renal function and serum proteins were unaffected by the diet.

Overt clinical signs of riboflavin deficiency are rarely seen among inhabitants of the developed countries. However, the so-called subclinical stage of the deficiency characterized by a change in biochemical indices is common. The Ten State Nutritional Survey recently completed in the United States revealed considerable biochemical evidence of riboflavin deficiency. The introduction of the erythrocyte glutathione reductase test has helped uncover riboflavin deficiency in a variety of conditions in which the overt changes described above were not evident. Such subject's intake of riboflavin may be sufficient to prevent clinical signs but not sufficient to keep the flavoproteins saturated for optimal metabolism rates. In children this may result in less than normal growth.

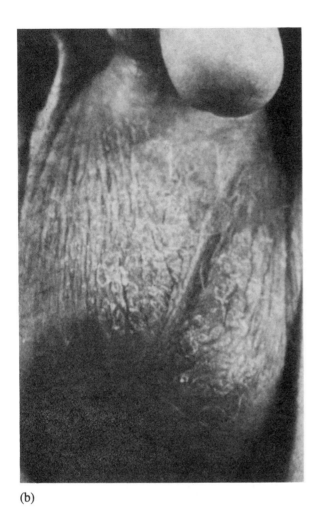

(b)

Riboflavin deficiency with biochemical changes but not necessarily with clinical signs has been observed in women taking oral contraceptive agents, diabetics, children and adolescents from low socioeconomic backgrounds, children with chronic heart disease, the aged, and infants undergoing prolonged phototherapy for hyperbilirubinemia.

C. Effect of Riboflavin Deficiency on Metabolism

Riboflavin deficiency in the experimental animal results in enlarged liver weight in relation to body weight, with increased fat deposition. Liver cell mitochondria increase in size with increase in the number and length of the cristae. The effect of this on the function of the mitochondria is still not elucidated.

Glucose, fatty acid, and amino acid metabolism are affected by riboflavin deficiency. For example, the unsaturated fatty acids, linoleic, linolenic, and arachidonic, are reduced in the liver and plasma probably because of reduction in dehydrogenation activity.

The metabolism of tryptophan is also affected, with an increase in urinary excretion of anthranilic and xanthurenic acids. This results from the fact that riboflavin coenzymes are necessary for the conversion of pyridoxine to pyridoxal, which is the coenzyme form required in several steps in the conversion of tryptophan to niacin.

Certain liver flavoproteins, such as glycolate oxidase, D-amino acid oxidase, xanthine oxidase, and succinic acid dehydrogenase, are decreased in the riboflavin-deficient rat.

In both the rat and human, erythrocyte glutathione reductase activity decreases during deficiency.

IX. METHODS OF NUTRITIONAL ASSESSMENT

Several methods have been used to assess nutritional status of riboflavin. These include clinical signs, blood and urine levels of the vitamin, and measurement of enzymatic coenzyme activity at the cellular level (28). Clinical signs are difficult to assess and appear only after prolonged ingestion of a diet low in the vitamin.

Biochemical methods are more quantitative and often can detect the deficiency state before clinical signs appear. Originally, urinary excretion and blood levels were used as indices of the deficiency state. Urinary excretion of riboflavin has been studied extensively in normal adults and in volunteers fed diets low in this vitamin.

The normal adult excretes 120 μg or more per 24 hr; excretions of less than 40 μg per 24 hr were characteristic of deficiency (29). Results were often expressed in terms of micrograms riboflavin per gram creatinine, and this made it possible to collect less than 24 urine samples. Riboflavin was determined by either microbiological assay or by fluorometric techniques. As can be seen from Table 3, the urinary excretion per gram creatinine varies with age, since children excrete more riboflavin per unit creatinine.

Table 3 Biochemical Indices of Riboflavin Deficiency

Subjects	Deficient (high risk)	Low (medium risk)	Acceptable (low risk)
Creatine (μg/g)			
1 to 3 years	< 150	150–499	> 500
4 to 6 years	< 100	100–299	> 300
7 to 9 years	< 85	85–269	> 270
10 to 15 years	< 70	70–199	> 200
Adults	< 27	27–79	> 80
Pregnant, 2nd trimester	< 39	39–119	> 120
Pregnant, 3rd trimester	< 30	30–89	> 90
Creatinine (μg per 24 hr), adults μ/24 hr	< 40	40–119	> 120
Creatinine (μg per 6 hr), adults	< 10	10–29	> 30
Load test (μg in 4 hr), return in adult of 5 mg riboflavin dose	< 1000	1000–1399	> 1400
Erythrocyte riboflavin (μg per 100 ml cells),	< 10.0	10.0–14.9	>15.0
EGR activity coefficients, all ages	> 1.3	1.21–1.3	< 1.2

The urinary excretion of riboflavin has limited use as an indicator of deficiency, since it tends to reflect current intake rather than flavin stores. Furthermore, in experimental studies, adults given 0.8–0.9 mg riboflavin per day, levels less than the daily requirements to provide the optimal body stores, excreted normal levels of riboflavin in the urine. In addition, urinary excretions are affected by age, physicial activity, body temperature, sleep, stress, and nitrogen balance. The method had been used extensively in population surveys when better methods were not available.

Plasma levels of riboflavin tend to be variable and reflect current intake (20). At best, plasma levels of riboflavin and other vitamins can be used to determine whether an individual's dietary regimen places him or her at risk to develop a vitamin deficiency.

Erythrocyte levels have been used more often than plasma levels, since this is presumably a storage site of the vitamin and should not depend upon current intake. Levels less than 10 μg riboflavin per 100 ml packed erythrocytes were considered to indicate deficiency. Erythrocyte riboflavin was determined by fluorometric assay. In long-term studies with volunteers fed diets low in riboflavin, the change in erythrocyte-riboflavin levels appeared much later than changes in other indices. In addition, the difference between levels for normals and for deficients were small and no greater than twofold. In infants and children, neither plasma nor erythrocyte levels were satisfactory indices of deficiency.

A newer biochemical method has recently been introduced and is based upon the change in activity of erythrocyte glutathione reductase (EGR), an FAD-containing enzyme. Experimental studies in rats and volunteers have shown that EGR activity is a more sensitive and specific indicator of riboflavin deficiency. Tests are based upon the following reaction,

$$\text{NADPH} + \text{H}^+ + \text{GSSG} \xrightarrow{\text{EGR}\cdot\text{FAD}} \text{NADP}^+ + 2\text{GSH}$$

where GSSG = oxidized glutathione. During dietary deprivation of riboflavin, EGR loses its saturation with FAD, and less NADPH is used in the foregoing reaction. NADPH has a high absorbancy at 340 nm, and the disappearance of absorbancy is measured using a spectrophotometer. The enzyme can be resaturated by the addition of exogenous FAD. After a hemolysate is prepared from venous blood erythrocytes, the test is set up in two cuvettes. In the first cuvette, the hemolysate, the source of EGR•FAD, is added to a solution containing buffer, GSSG, and NADPH. To the second cuvette, in addition to the foregoing ingredients, FAD is added. The cuvettes are intitially placed in a spectrophotometer to obtain optical density (OD) units and then incubated 10 min at 37 °C, after which time another reading is taken. If an individual's EGR is saturated with FAD, the difference in initial and final absorbancy in OD units should be the same in both cuvettes. If the EGR is not saturated, the addition of FAD to the second cuvette results in utilization of more NADPH in this stoichiometric reaction. The results are expressed in activity coefficient (AC) units:

$$\text{AC} = \frac{\Delta_{\text{OD}} \text{ with added FAD in 10 min}}{\Delta_{\text{OD}} \text{ without added FAD in 10 min}}$$

The AC is a measurement of the saturation of EGR with FAD, and normal values ranged from 0.9 to 1.2 (19). Values of 1.21–1.3 represent a medium risk and values over 1.3 a high risk (Table 3).

The method described above has been shown to be a valid index of riboflavin deficiency in infants (30), children (30), adolescents (3), pregnant and lactating women (32), and the aged (33). It is unaffected by degree of anemia or stress. The method has recently been evaluated for dose-response relationships and for rate and specificity of response (68,69).

X. NUTRITIONAL REQUIREMENTS

A. Animals

Riboflavin is required by both invertebrates and vertebrates. Experimental studies to determine requirements have been limited to vertebrates. There is considerable variation in requirements even among members of the same species due to difference in body size and age. However, if the requirements are stated in terms of milligrams riboflavin per kilogram diet, a more uniform pattern emerges. From Table 4 it is apparent that, except for the hamster, which requires 6 mg, the riboflavin requirement for the various species is between 1 and 4 mg/kg diet. Increased dietary fat or protein increases the requirements for riboflavin in rats and chickens. In a poikilotherm, the rainbow trout, the requirement for maximum growth was 3.6 mg/kg diet although it required 6 mg/kg diet for liver and kidney flavin saturation. These values were not dependent on temperature of water or genetic differences and were similar to those of homeothermic species (34).

B. Humans

The requirements of humans for riboflavin have been determined from experimental studies with adults and infants. The minimum requirement was defined as that level which would prevent clinical signs of deficiency and would allow for a normal urinary excretion. In adults, consumption of 0.55 mg/day resulted in clinical signs of riboflavin deficiency and reduced urinary excretion. Levels of 0.8–0.9 mg/day prevented the appearance of clinical signs, but the urinary excretion was still below normal. It was therefore assumed that this level was insufficient to provide saturation of tissue deposits.

Table 4 Riboflavin Requirements of Animals

Animal	Riboflavin (mg/kg diet)
Mouse	1–3
Hamster	6
Rat	2.5
Guinea pig	3
Cat	3–4
Dog	2.2
Chick	3–4
Duck	3
Swine	2–4
Calf	1
Monkey (rhesus)	1

Source: Reports of the Committee on Animal Nutrition, *Nutritional Requirements of Domestic Animals*, National Academy of Sciences, National Research Council, Washington, D.C., 1980.

Since individual differences were found in the requirements based on weight and food intake, the requirement was given in terms of milligrams riboflavin per 1000 Cal food intake. Under these conditions, a level of 0.5 mg per 1000 Cal was estimated to be the minimum requirement for adults to maintain a normal urinary excretion. On similar basis, the infant's minimum daily requirement was estimated as 0.6 mg per 1000 Cal.

Recommended Dietary Allowances (RDA) are made by the Food and Nutrition Board of the National Research Council, the National Academy of Sciences. These allowances are defined as the levels of nutrients considered to be adequate to meet the known nutritional needs of practically all healthy people. For an individual, the allowances may be higher than the minimum requirements. The main uses of RDA are for planning and procuring food supplies to meet the total needs of a population. The recommended daily allowance for riboflavin is 0.6 mg per 1000 Cal for all ages, and the allowances for men and women at each age group is shown in Table 5. For the adult male, the allowance varies from 1.4 to 1.8 mg/day, depending upon age. For the female, the range is 1.2–1.3, depending upon age.

Urinary excretion studies have shown that pregnant women excrete less riboflavin than nonpregnant women of the same age group and require more energy than nonpregnant women. The allowance has been increased 0.3 mg to meet the additional requirements of pregnancy.

The estimated amount of riboflavin secreted in milk is 0.34 mg. Since the utilization of additional riboflavin for milk was determined to be 70%, the allowance for lactating women was raised to 1.8 mg/day for the first 6 months and 1.7 mg/day for the second 6 months.

Table 5 Recommended Dietary Allowances for Riboflavin

Category	Age (yr)	Riboflavin (mg per 1000 cal)	Riboflavin (mg/day)
Infants	0–0.5	0.6	0.4
	0.5-1	0.6	0.5
Children	1–3	0.6	0.8
	4–6	0.6	1.1
	7–10	0.6	1.2
Males	11–14	0.6	1.5
	15–18	0.6	1.8
	19–24	0.6	1.7
	25–50	0.6	1.7
	51+	0.6	1.4
Females	11–14	0.6	1.3
	15–18	0.6	1.3
	19–24	0.6	1.3
	25–50	0.6	1.3
	51+	0.6	1.2
Pregnant		0.7	+1.6
Lactating	(1st 6 mo)	0.7	+1.8
	(2nd 6 mo)	0.7	1.7

Source: Food and Nutrition Board, *Recommended Dietary Allowances*, 9th Revised Ed., National Research Council, National Academy of Sciences, Washington, D.C., 1980.

XI. FACTORS THAT INFLUENCE VITAMIN STATUS AND IDENTIFICATION OF GROUPS AT GREATER RISK OF DEFICIENCY

A. Drugs

Antibiotics, such as tetracycline, penicillin, and streptomycin, reduce the requirements of several animal species for riboflavin. They may inhibit microorganisms in the gut that compete for riboflavin and other nutrients. The effect of antibiotics on the human requirement for riboflavin is not known.

Anticholinergic drugs delay gastric emptying and decrease intestinal transit rate. For these reasons, administration of anticholinergic drugs increases the absorption of riboflavin by allowing the vitamin to remain at intestinal absorption sites for longer periods of time (16).

Ingestion of boric acids may induce riboflavin deficiency, since it displaces riboflavin from plasma-binding sites and results in increased urinary excretion of the vitamin (35). It has been shown that patients with boric acid overdose have signs of riboflavin deficiency (36).

Probenecid inhibits gastrointestinal absorption and renal tubular secretion of riboflavin. The latter results in decreased urinary excretion of riboflavin.

It has been shown that women taking oral contraceptive agents may develop riboflavin deficiency (37). This is especially true of those on marginal diets who have been on these agents for a year or more. In view of the teratogenic effects of riboflavin deficiency, women who have been on oral contraceptive agents should wait at least 6 months after stopping intake of the drugs before they become pregnant.

Chlorpromazine is a structural analog of riboflavin. Studies with rats have shown it to be an antagonist of riboflavin, preventing the incorporation of the vitamin into FAD. It also blocks the enhancement of the conversion of riboflavin to FAD by thyroxine (38).

It has been postulated that antimalarial drugs work through interference of riboflavin metabolism (39).

Vegetables and cereal grains are not good sources of riboflavin. Vegans are at high risk for developing riboflavin deficiency. The milk of lactating vegans has been shown to be significantly lower in riboflavin content than the milk of omnivores (71).

A riboflavin coenzyme is essential for the conversion of methemoglobin to hemoglobin. In riboflavin deficiency, methemoglobin has been shown to accumulate in erythrocytes (72,73).

Riboflavin has been used as a drug marker to check adherence to a therapeutic drug regimen. The drug is prescribed in combination with riboflavin, and an examination of the urine collected 2–4 hr after ingestion of the drug for the orange color owing to urinary riboflavin excretion will reveal whether the drug was actually taken (40).

B. Disease

1. Thyroid Disease

Thyroid disease has a profound effect upon riboflavin metabolism and physiology. Thyroxine stimulates intestinal motility. As a consequence, riboflavin absorption is decreased in hyperthyroidism and increased in hypothyroidism.

Rivlin (41) has elucidated the role of thyroid hormone on riboflavin metabolism. He has shown that thyroxine regulates flavokinase, the enzyme that converts riboflavin to

FMN. In the hypothyroid rat, flavokinase activity is reduced, resulting in a diminished conversion to FMN. Hepatic levels of FMN and FAD are reduced to the levels found in riboflavin-deficient rats. Hyperthyroidism in the rat results in increased flavokinase activity, but FMN and FAD do not rise above normal levels. The mechanism for thyroid hormone regulation is in the synthesis of flavokinase rather than its degradation (42).

Riboflavin in turn may affect deiodination of thyroid hormone:

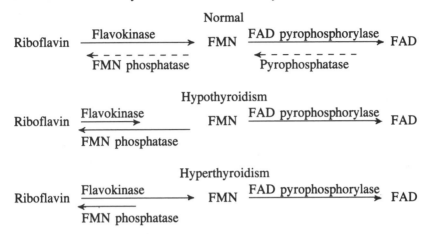

In the human hypothyroid adult, levels of erythrocyte glutathione reductase activity were found to be similar to those observed during riboflavin deficiency (43). However, in the hypothyroid neonate such activity was in the range for normals. This indicates that the regulation of FAD synthesis in the fetus is not thyroxine dependent since thyroxine does not cross the placenta and human thyroid does not begin functioning until the third month of gestation. Another regulatory mechanism involving riboflavin carrier protein may account for fetal FAD synthesis (44).

2. Diabetes

The prevalence of riboflavin among diabetics is significantly higher than among nondiabetics of the some socioeconomic level (45). Among the factors that may contribute to this deficiency is the increased urinary excretion of riboflavin observed in diabetes. In addition, many diabetics who are overweight are given a calorie-restricted diet to control the disease, and this may lead to decreased riboflavin intake. The role of insulin in the regulation of riboflavin metabolism has not been studied.

3. Congenital Heart Disease

A high prevalence of riboflavin deficiency has been noted in children with congenital heart disease in congestive failure (46). This may be due to the fact that these children have a diminished food intake, as well as malabsorption. This condition is not only associated with riboflavin deficiency, but deficiency of other vitamins as well.

4. Biliary Atresia in Children

In the absence of bile salts, gastrointestinal transit time is decreased. Under these conditions riboflavin is not at intestinal absorption sites long enough to be completely absorbed. In infants with biliary atresia (in whom bile is absent), there is evidence that riboflavin malabsorption occurs (16).

5. Hyperbilirubinemia

Phototherapy is often prescribed for infants with mild hyperbilirubinemia. Light degrades bilirubin to soluble substances that can then be excreted. The degradation of bilirubin is caused by singlet oxygen generated by light-activated riboflavin. During this process riboflavin also undergoes degradative changes.

Riboflavin in the plasma of neonates with hyperbilirubinemia was shown to be significantly reduced during phototherapy (47,74). Breast-fed newborns were more prone to riboflavin deficiency after phototherapy, primarily because human milk contains one-third the riboflavin content of cow's milk (75). In vitro studies demonstrated that the addition of theophylline to the medium accelerated the light destruction of bilirubin by riboflavin (66).

Riboflavin deficiency was prevented when neonates received 0.3 mg riboflavin daily during phototherapy (76). Supplementation with riboflavin results in more rapid destruction of serum bilirubin. However, such treatment should be approached cautiously, since in vitro studies have revealed that the photodynamic action of riboflavin may induce alterations in the intracellular DNA that may have mutagenic or carcinogenic potential.

6. Akee Nut Toxicity

Children in Jamaica who eat unripe akee nuts become hypoglycemic, develop stomach pain with vomiting and convulsions, go into coma, and die within 12–20 hr. It has been shown that akee nut contains a toxin, hypoglycin, that is a potent riboflavin antagonist (25). The symptoms of akee nut poisoning can be prevented or ameliorated by the parenteral administration of riboflavin.

In animal studies, hypoglycin has been shown to inhibit gluconeogenesis and fatty acid oxidation. Riboflavin can prevent the hypoglycemia and mitochondrial swelling associated with this toxicity when given before or during administration of hypoglycin. The mechanism for this antagonism is not known.

C. Parasites

There is no specific disease linking parasites to riboflavin deficiency. However, any parasite that causes diarrhea and affects absorption of nutrients may cause riboflavin deficiency.

Riboflavin is an essential nutrient for the *Coccidia* parasite of the chick. The riboflavin antagonist, 5-deazariboflavin, is a potent coccidiostat and has been used to treat coccidiosis in chickens.

D. Alcohol

Studies have shown that there is a high prevalence of riboflavin deficiency among those with chronic alcoholism. There is presently no evidence that alcohol interferes with riboflavin metabolism. In one investigation, reduced erythrocyte glutathione reductase activity could be corrected with riboflavin administration even in those who shortly thereafter succumbed to liver failure (48). The deficiency may be related to poor dietary habits of alcoholics, who are known to have multiple nutritional deficiencies.

E. Heavy Metals

Divalent metals, including Cu^{2+}, Zn^{2+}, Co^{2+}, Fe^{2+}, Mn^{2+}, and Cd^{2+}, form chelates with riboflavin and more avidly with FMN. These chelates are less well absorbed than the unchelated vitamins from the gastrointestinal tract. Ingestion of pharmacological doses of these metals may induce riboflavin deficiency (16).

F. Age

Riboflavin deficiency frequency occurs among the aged. This is probably due to the fact that this population eats less of the foods rich in riboflavin, such as milk, eggs, meat, and green, leafy vegetables, than the younger population. In addition, the aged are likely to have chronic diseases, such as diabetes and heart disease, which may contribute to this deficiency (33). There is no evidence that aging affects riboflavin metabolism. Administration of riboflavin reverses the deficiency.

Surveys of the dietary intake of the aged are of little help in determining their nutritional status. Only biochemical tests can determine the prevalence of riboflavin deficiency.

G. Genetics

Some genetic defects of blood cell riboflavin enzymes have been reported. For example, the neutrophils of patients with chronic granulomatous disease lack an FAD-containing enzyme necessary to form superoxide (49). It was suggested that pharmacological doses of riboflavin may be helpful in this condition.

A genetic disease characterized by the lack of erythrocyte glutathione reductase, an FAD-containing enzyme, is unresponsive to riboflavin therapy.

Erythrocyte pyruvate kinase deficiency, a genetic disease, is associated with low levels of erythrocyte glutathione reductase. Riboflavin therapy is ineffective in alleviating the signs of this deficiency.

H. Stress

Acute starvation, hard work, and heat stress result in increased urinary riboflavin excretion. Chronic stress may lead to riboflavin deficiency, especially if the dietary intake of the vitamin is marginal (25). Exercise increases the riboflavin requirements of young women (50).

Patients undergoing hemodialysis lose water-soluble vitamins, which include riboflavin, and should receive vitamin supplements.

When children receive parenteral nutrition that lacks riboflavin, biochemical evidence of riboflavin deficiency appears within 2 weeks (51).

Studies with experimental animals have shown that wound healing is retarded in the presence of riboflavin deficiency.

There are several interrelationships between riboflavin and tumor growth (25). It has been shown by several investigators that mice and rats fed a riboflavin-deficient diet, either with or without the addition of a riboflavin antagonist, showed a regression of a variety of tumors. However, when azo dyes are used to induce cancer, riboflavin deficiency may enhance liver tumor growth. This is because riboflavin coenzymes are necessary to catabolize the cancer-producing chemicals, thus delaying the elimination of the toxic agents. In the baboon, riboflavin deficiency results in metaplasia of the squamous mucosa of the esophagus. The changes seen are similar to those in primary esophageal cancer in humans and may be considered as precancerous.

Feeding a riboflavin-deficient diet plus a riboflavin antagonist to humans with advanced cancer was unsuccessful in that there was no evidence of cancer regression. However, this regimen did not produce any clear-cut signs of riboflavin deficiency (26).

I. Other Nutrients

Riboflavin coenzymes are necessary to convert several vitamins to their active coenzyme. For example, the FMN-containing enzyme, pyridoxamine phosphate oxidase, is necessary for the conversion of pyridoxine phosphate to pyridoxamine phosphate (52), a coenzyme necessary for the conversion of tryptophan to niacin. During vitamin B_6 deficiency this pathway is disrupted, and xanthurenic acid is excreted in the urine.

Riboflavin coenzymes are also necessary for the conversion of folic acid to its reduced coenzyme form. The serum folate levels in the riboflavin-deficiency baboon are reduced. Riboflavin-deficient rats excrete a larger portion of parenterally administered radioactive folic acid than do normal rats.

The relationship between riboflavin and vitamin B_{12} is not based on reduced activity of riboflavin-containing enzymes but on structural similarity. Both riboflavin and vitamin B_{12} contain the benzimidazole moiety. Riboflavin can partially replace the requirements of the rat and chick for vitamin B_{12} (53).

J. Photosensitization

Riboflavin is a potent photosensitizer which generates singlet oxygen and superoxide anion radicals when exposed to ultraviolet of 290–320 nm and 320–400 nm. This results in photodegradation of ascorbic acid in milk (54), carotenoids, vitamin B_6 and folic acid in human plasma (55–57), and single strand breaks in intracellular DNA in human cell cultures (58). The same mechanism accounts for the photodegradation of bilirubin and development of riboflavin deficiency in the jaundiced newborn (47).

Riboflavin also has photochemical action on quercetin (59), phenylalanine (60), sulfa drugs (61), and tryptophan (62).

XII. EFFICACY OF PHARMACOLOGICAL DOSES

There are no known pharmacological effects of either riboflavin or FMN in humans. FAD has produced hypotensive effects in rabbits, but this effect may be the result of the known hypotensive effects of the AMP portion of the molecule (16).

Riboflavin is rapidly excreted in the urine, to which it imparts a yellow fluorescent color (67). For this reason it is often prescribed with drugs so it can act as a marker to determine whether a patient took the medication.

XIII. HAZARDS OF HIGH DOSES

Riboflavin has a low toxicity, and no case of riboflavin toxicity in humans has been reported (63,76). This is probably because the transport system necessary for the absorption of riboflavin across the gastrointestinal mucosa becomes saturated, limiting the amount of the vitamin that can be absorbed.

Oral doses of 10 g/kg body weight in the rat and 2 g/kg body weight in the dog produced no toxic effects.

The LD_{50} is about 560 mg/kg body weight in rats given the riboflavin intraperitoneally. Death, which occurs in 2–5 days, results from concretion of riboflavin crystals in the kidney, leading to anuria and azotemia. When the blood level of riboflavin exceeds 20 μg/ml, riboflavin will precipitate in the rat's kidneys. Urinary levels of 150 μg/ml may be a sign of imminent toxicity.

When 125 or 500 mg of the sodium salt of riboflavin was injected intraperitoneally in rats, cytological changes were noted in the heart, pancreas, and pituitary gland, in addition to the concentration of riboflavin crystals in the kidney.

When mice were given 340 mg riboflavin per kilogram body weight, there was no apparent toxicity.

REFERENCES

1. T. Wagner-Jauregg, in *The Vitamins*, Vol. 5, 2nd ed., W. H. Sebrell and R. S. Harris (Eds.), Academic Press, New York, 1972, Ch. II, p. 3.
2. H. Baker and O. Frank, in *Riboflavin*, R. S. Rivlin (Ed.), Plenum Press, New York, 1975, p. 49.
3. P. Nielsen, P. Rauschenbach, and A. Bacher, *Methods Enzymol.*, *122*:209 (1986).
4. A. Bourquin and H. C. Sherman, *J. Am. Chem. Soc.*, *53*:3501 (1931).
5. B. K. Watt and A. L. Merrill, *Composition of Foods*, USDA Handbook, #8, USDA, Washington, D.C., 1950.
6. S. M. Hunt, in *Riboflavin*, R. S. Rivlin (Ed.), Plenum Press, New York, 1975, p. 199.
7. J. A. Campbell and A. B. Morrison, *Am. J. Clin. Nutr.*, *12*:162 (1963).
8. G. Levy and W. J. Jusko, *J. Pharm. Sci.*, *55*:285 (1966).
9. W. J. Jusko and G. Levy, *J. Pharm. Sci.*, *56*:58 (1967).
10. W. S. Innis, D. B. McCormick, and A. H. Merrill, Jr., *Biochem. Med.*, *34*:151 (1985).
11. D. Zanette, H. L. Monaco, G. Zanotti, and P. Spadon, *J. Mol. Biol.*, *180*:185 (1984).
12. T. Y. Aw, D. P. Jones, and D. B. Mc Cormick, *J. Nutr.*, *113*:1249 (1983).
13. P. Cerletti and P. Ipata, *Biochem. J.*, *75*:119 (1960).
14. H. M. Jernigan, *Exp. Eye Res.*, *41*:121 (1985).
15. H. Baker, D. Frank, T. Chen, S. Feingold, B. De Angelis, and E. Baker, *J. Neurosci. Res.*, *11*:419 (1984).
16. W. J. Jusko and G. Levy, in *Riboflavin*, R. S. Rivlin (Ed.), Plenum Press, New York, 1975, p. 99.
17. M. K. Horwitt and L. A. Witting, in *The Vitamins*, Vol. 5, 2nd ed., W. H. Sebrell and R. S. Harris (Eds.), Academic Press, New York, 1972, Ch. IX, p. 53.
18. J. A. Tillotson and H. E. Sauberlich, *J. Nutr.*, *101*:1459 (1971).
19. D. Glatzle, W. F. Körner, S. Christeller, and O. Wiss, *Int. J. Vitamin. Res.*, *40*:166 (1970).
20. J. A. Tillotson and E. M. Baker, *Am. J. Clin. Nutr.*, *25*:425 (1972).
21. N. Gregersen, *J. Inherited Metab. Dis.*, *8*: Suppl 1, 65 (1985).
22. J. Warkany, in *Riboflavin*, R. S. Rivlin (Ed.), Plenum Press, New York, 1975, p. 279.
23. M. K. Horwitt, in *The Vitamins*, Vol. 5 2nd ed., W. H. Sebrell and R. S. Harris (Eds.), Academic Press, New York, 1972, Ch. X, p. 73.
24. J. M. Cooperman, H. A. Waisman, K. B. McCall, and C. A. Elvehjem, *J. Nutr.*, *30*:45 (1945).
25. H. Fey and V. Mbaya, *Prog. Food Nutr. Sci.*, *2*:357 (1977).
26. M. Lane, C. P. Alfrey, C. E. Mengel, M. A. Doherty, and J. Doherty, *J. Clin. Invest*, *43*:357 (1964).
27. M. K. Horwitt, C. C. Harvey, W. S. Rothwell, J. L. Cutler, and D. Haffron, *J. Nutr.* (Suppl.) *60*: (1956).
28. H. E. Sauberlich, J. H. Skala, and R. P. Dowdy, *Laboratory Tests for the Assessment of Nutritional Status*, CRC Press, Cleveland, Ohio (1974).
29. M. K. Horwitt, C. C. Harvey, O. W. Hills, and E. Liebert, *J. Nutr.*, *41*:247 (1950).
30. R. Lopez, H. S. Cole, M. F. Montoya, and J. M. Cooperman, *J. Pediatr.*, *87*:420 (1975).
31. R. Lopez, J. V. Schwartz, and J. M . Cooperman, *Am. J. Clin. Nutr.*, *33*:1283 (1980).
32. J. M. Cooperman, H. S. Cole, M. Gordon, and R. Lopez, *Proc. Soc. Exp. Biol. Med.*, *143*:326 (1973).
33. R. Lopez, L. V. Fisher, and J. M. Cooperman, *Fed. Proc.*, *38*:451 (1979).

34. B. Woodward, *J. Nutr.*, *115*:78 (1985).

35. D. A. Roe, D. B. McCormick, and R. T. Lin, *J. Pharm. Sci.*, *61*:1081 (1972).

36. J. Pinto, Y. P. Huang, R. McConnell, and R. S. Rivlin, *J. Lab. Clin. Med.*, *92*:126 (1978).

37. L. J. Newman, R. Lopez, H. S. Cole, and J. M. Cooperman, *Am. J. Clin. Nutr.*, *31*:247 (1978).

38. J. Pinto, M. Wolinsky, and R. S. Rivlin, *Biochem. Pharmacol.*, *28*:597 (1979).

39. P. Dutta, J. Pinto, and R. S. Rivlin, *Lancet 1*:679 (1986).

40. L. M. Young, C. M. Haakenson, K. K. Lee, and J. P. van Eckhout, *Controlled Clin. Trials*, *5*:497 (1984).

41. R. S. Rivlin, *N. Engl. J. Med.*, *283*:463 (1970).

42. S. Lee and D. B. McCormick, *Arch. Biochem. Biophys.* *237*:197 (1985).

43. J. A. Cimino, S. Jhangiani, E. Schwartz, and J. M. Cooperman, *Proc. Sci. Exp. Biol. Med.*, *184*:151 (1987).

44. J. A. Cimino, R. A. Noto, and C. L. Fusco, and J. M. Cooperman, *Am. J. Clin. Nutr.*, *47*:481 (1988).

45. H. S. Cole, R. Lopez, and J. M. Cooperman, *Acta Diabet. Latina*, *13*:25 (1976).

46. M. Steier, R. Lopez, and J. M. Cooperman, *Am. Heart J.*, *92*:139 (1976).

47. D. S. Gromisch, R. Lopez, H. S. Cole, and J. M. Cooperman, *J. Pediatr.*, *90*:118 (1977).

48. W. S. Rosenthal, N. F. Adham, R. Lopez, and J. M. Cooperman, *Am. J. Clin. Nutr.*, *26*:858 (1973).

49. G. M. Babior and R. S. Kipnes, *Blood, 50*:517 (1977).

50. A. Z. Belko, E. Obarzanek, H. J. Kalkwarf, M. S. Rotter, S. Bogusz, D. Miller, J. D. Haas, and D. A. Roe, *Am. J. Clin. Nutr.*, *37*:509, (1983).

51. H. L. Greene, in *Total Parenteral Nutrition: Premises and Promises*, H. Ghadimi (Ed.), John Wiley and Sons, New York, 1975, p. 351.

52. H. Wada and E. E. Snell, *J. Biol. Chem.*, *236*:2089 (1961).

53. J. M. Cooperman, B. Tabenkin, and R. Drucker, *J. Nutr.*, *46*:367 (1952).

54. C. Allen and O. W. Parks, *J. Dairy Sci.*, *62*:1377 (1979).

55. D. A. Roe, *Fed. Proc.*, *46*:1886 (1987).

56. R. F. Branda and J. W. Eaton, *Science, 201*:625 (1978).

57. N. Rudolph, A. J. Parekh, J. Hittelman, J. Burdige, and S. L. Wong, *Am. J. Dis. Child,* *139*:812 (1985).

58. J. F. Ennever and W. T. Speck, *Pediatr. Res.*, *17*:234 (1983).

59. U. Takahama, *Photochem. Photobiol.*, *42*:89 (1985).

60. S. Ishimitsu, S. Fujimoto, and A. Ohara, *Chem. Pharm. Bull.*, *33*:1552 (1985).

61. O. W. Parks, *J. Assoc. Off. Anal. Chem.*, *68*:1232 (1985).

72. J. Bhatia and D. K. Rassin, *J. Parenter. Enteral Nutr.*, *9*:491 (1985).

63. D. B. McCormick, *Nutr. Rev.*, *30*:75 (1972).

64. M. K. Horwitt, in *The Vitamins*, Vol. 5, 2nd ed., W. H. Sebrell and R. S. Harris (Eds.), Academic Press, New York, 1972, Ch. XI, p. 85.

65. R. Spector, *J. Neuro Chem.*, *35*:209 (1980).

66. R. Spector, *J. Clin. Invest.*, *66*:821 (1980).

67. A. F. Merrill, *J. Biol. Chem.*, *254*:9362 (1979).

68. M. Y. Chang, F. K. Friedman, S. Beychok, J. Shyong, and E. F. Osserman, *Biochemistry*, *20*:2916 (1981).

69. A. M. Prentice and C. J. Bates, *Br. J. Nutr.*, *43*:37 (1981).

70. A. M. Prentice and C. J. Bates, *Br. J. Nutr.*, *45*:53 (1981).

71. J. Hughes and T. A. B. Sanders, *Proc. Nutr. Soc.*, *38*:95A (1979).

72. H. J. Power and D. I. Thurman, *Br. J. Nutr.*, *46*:257 (1981).

73. M. Hirano, T. Matsuk, K. Tamishima, M. Takeshita, S. Shimizu, Y. Nagamura, and Y. Yoneyama, *Br. J. Hematol.*, *47*:353 (1981).

74. G. Cocchi, S. Gualandi, M. Barbaati, F. Corsini, and G. P. Salvioli, *Minerva Pediatr.*, *32*:1069 (1980).

75. L. Hovi, R. Hekali, and M. A. Siimes, *Acta Pediatr. Scand.*, *68*:567 (1979).

76. P. Meisel, I. Amon, H. Hüller and K. Jährig, *Biol. Neonate*, *38*:30 (1980).

77. K. L. Tan, M. T. Chow, and S. M. M. Karim, *J. Pediatr.*, *93*:494 (1978).

8
Nicotinic Acid

Jan van Eys

University of Texas
M. D. Anderson Cancer Center
Houston, Texas

I. HISTORY

Nicotinic acid was synthesized by the oxidation of nicotine and related compounds long before it was considered to be a vitamin. The original description of nicotinic acid came from Huber in 1867 (1). In 1873 Weidel described the elemental analysis and crystalline structure of the salts and other derivatives of nicotinic acid in some detail (2). It was only some 50 years later that nicotinic acid was isolated for the first time from natural sources (3).

The disease pellagra was first described by Thiery. He called the disease "mal de la rosa" (4). It became recognized as associated with populations that ingested large amounts of corn (maize). The studies of Goldberger (5) demonstrated that pellagra was a dietary deficiency disease. The nutrients that were helpful were referred to as the pellagra preventative factor (PP) and later identified as niacin.

This identification was not possible until an animal model was found that allowed more detailed experimentation. Goldberger and Wheeler (6) reported on black tongue of dogs as an experimental model for the human disease pellagra. Elvehjem and co-workers (7) then showed the effectiveness of nicotinic acid and nicotinic acid amide to cure canine black tongue.

It is of interest that nicotinamide was already found to be an integral part of the coenzymes for metabolism, coenzymes 1 (8) and 2 (9,10). They were later named diphosphopyridine and triphosphopyridine nucleotide (DPN and TPN), and now are called nicotinamide adenine dinucleotide and nicotinamide adenine dinucleotide phosphate (NAD and NADP).

Parallel with the discovery of nicotinic acid as a curative agent, a form of vitamin PP, the observations were made that the nature and the quality of protein influenced the development of pellagra. There is a strong association epidemiologically between corn and pellagra. In fact, dietary protein quality and quantity are more important than is the nicotonic acid content of the diet.

An experiment of nature exists that shows clearly the interrelationship of tryptophan to nicotinic acid and pellagra. Hartnup's disease (11), named after the first family described, is an affliction that shows all the signs of pellagra. The defect is the lack of absorption or the increased renal excretion of tryptophan. The disease is associated with poor nutrition, and nicotinamide deficiency is a major etiological component (12).

This relationship between tryptophan and niacin is similar to other amino acid nutrient pairs. Thus, methionine and choline, and lysine and carnitine have similar relationships.

However, it is still not as simple as a precursor-product relationship. The association of corn and pellagra is very clear, but it is not totally explainable on the basis of tryptophan and niacin content. For instance, corn is higher in nicotinic acid than is rice. Wilson (13) postulated that corn is deficient in protein of good biological value. Carl Funk coined the word *vitamine* in order to explain the effect of corn in generating pellagra (14). However, Funk later revised this postulate by saying "it may either be a vitamin deficiency, a protein deficiency, or both" (15).

Attempts were made to demonstrate that niacin is in a bound form in cereals to explain the unique role of corn. However, the concept of amino acid imbalance in the diet as a precipitating factor of relative tryptophan deficiency is now widely held (16).

In addition, the fat content of the diet seems to affect the niacin requirement in mice and rats (17,18).

The history of niacin and pellagra is rich. An interesting compilation of historical papers has recently been published (19). Nicotonic acid and nicotinamide are nutrients, but only essential under certain circumstances that are generically understood, but not totally explained.

The story became even more complex when it was discovered that nicotinic acid is also an active pharmacologic agent with toxic potential. A large body of literature has appeared on the use of nicotonic acid, an agent that affects the vascular tone and affects hyperlipidemia. Nicotinamide, on the other hand, has entirely different properties through a influence on NAD synthesis.

This chapter will discuss the chemistry and biology of nicotinic acid and nicotinamide. The word vitamin can be applied to these substances, especially since they represent the active principle of Funk's postulate of a vitamin. However, because of their different properties and metabolic pathways it is necessary to be certain that terms are clearly defined. The term niacin is: "the generic description for pyridine 3-carboxylic acid and derivatives exhibiting qualitatively the biological (nutritional) activity of nicotinic acid. Thus, phrases such as "niacin activity" and "niacin deficiency" represent preferred usage. The compound pyridine 3-carboxylic acid..., also known as niacin or vitamin PP, should be designated nicotinic acid" (20,21).

II. CHEMISTRY

A. Natural Occurrence

Nicotinic acid and nicotinamide occur widely in nature. Much of the nicotinic acid derivatives are in the form of pyridine nucleotides. A variety of substances exist intermediate in the biosynthesis of the pyridine nucleotides from nicotinic acid and tryptophan. In addition, a large number of metabolic substances occur in nature as products of the degradative pathways of nicotinic acid and nicotinamide. The substances found in urine of animals depends greatly on whether nicotinic acid is administered in physiological quantities or whether pharmacological quantities have been administered.

B. Structure and Nomenclature

Figure 1 shows the basic structures of nicotinic acid and nicotinamide.

1. Nicotinic Acid

Nicotinic acid is pyridine 3-carboxylic acid. As mentioned before, a wide variety of names have been attributed to the substance, including a large number of commercial names for its vitamin or pharmacological activity. If the term niacin is used for other than a generic vitamin activity, it is applied to nicotinic acid. Table 1 shows the synonyms used in Chemline, the computerized data base.

2. Nicotinamide

Nicotinamide is pyridine 3-carboxamide. This substance is also marketed under a large number of generic names. If the term analogous to niacin is applied as a chemical substance, niacinamide is used.

3. Coenzyme Forms of Nicotinic Acid and Nicotinamide

Nicotinamide Adenine Dinucleotides (NAD and NADP).   Figure 2 shows the structure of nicotinamide adenine dinucleotide and nicotinamide adenine dinucleotide phosphate. Historically these have been known as coenzyme 1 and coenzyme 2, DPN and TPN. They occur in nature in the oxidized and reduced form. Reduction takes place at the 4 position of the pyridine ring. It is a two-electron reduction with a hydride ion attaching to the 4 position, balanced by the loss of the positive charge at the quaternary pyridine ring in the oxidized form.

Biosynthetic Intermediates.   In the biosynthesis of tryptophan to NAD or the incorporation of exogenous nicotinic acid and nicotinamide into NAD and NADP, a number of analogs occur. These include the nicotinic acid analog of NAD wherein nicotinic acid substitutes for the nicotinamide moiety. In addition, both nicotinic acid and nicotinamide mononucleotides are found in nature. These have the structures indicated in Figure 2.

4. Excretory Products

A number of conjugates occur in the urine of animals. Figure 3 shows the structures of nicotinuric acid, nictinoyl glucuronide, and dinicotinoyl ornithine. All these are products of excessive administration of nicotinic acid and constitute detoxification products. On hydrolysis of the urine, nicotinic acid is recover.

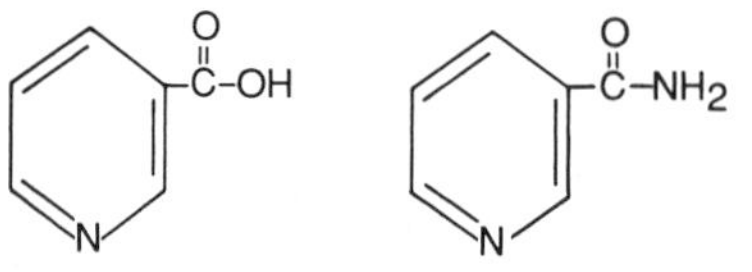

Nicotinic Acid   Nicotinamide

Figure 1   Nicontinic acid and nicotinamide structures.

Table 1 Synonyms and Trade Names for Nicotinic Acid

Acide Nicotinique (French)	Nicamin	Nicotine acid
Acidum Nicotinicum	Nicangin	Nicotinic acid
AI13-18994 (USDA)	Nico	Nicotinipca
Akotin	Nico-Span	Nicotinipca
Apelagrin	Nico-400	Nicotinsaüre
Bionic	Nicobid	NICYL
Caswell No. 598	Nicocap	Nyclin
Daskil	Nicocidin	Pellagra Preventive Factor
Davitamon PP	Nicocrisina	Pellagrin
Direktan	Nicodelmine	Pelonin
Efacin	Nicolar	Pyridine-beta-carboxylic acid
EPA Pesticide Chemical Code	Niconacid	Pyridine-Carboxylique-3 (French)
056701 (NLM)	Niconat	SK-Niacin
HSDB 3134 (NLM)	Niconazid	Tinic
LINIC	Nicosan 3	Vitaplex N
Niac	Nicosyl	Wampocap
Nicacid	Nicotamin	3-Carboxylpyridine
Niacin	Nicotene	3-Pyridinecarboxylic acid
Niacin (USAN)		

Abbreviations as listed in Chemline.

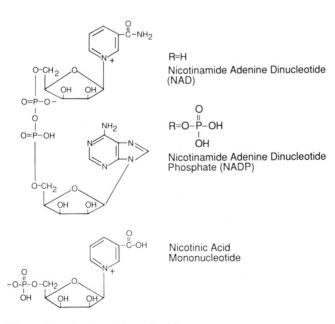

R=H
Nicotinamide Adenine Dinucleotide
(NAD)

$$R=O-\overset{\overset{\textstyle O}{\|}}{\underset{\underset{\textstyle OH}{}}{P}}-OH$$

Nicotinamide Adenine Dinucleotide
Phosphate (NADP)

Nicotinic Acid
Mononucleotide

Figure 2 Nicotinamide nucleotides.

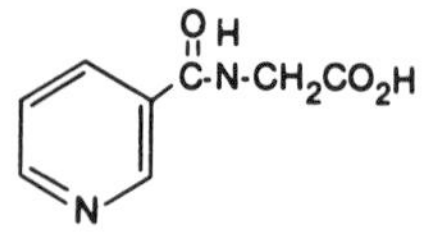

Nicotinuric acid

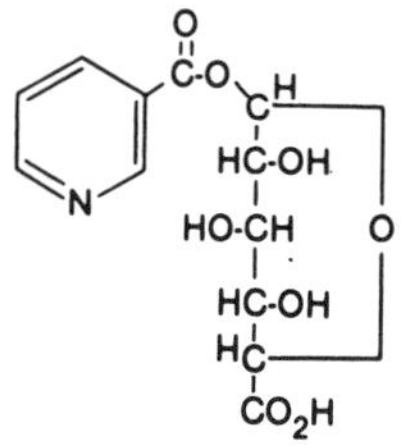

Nicotinoyl glucuronide

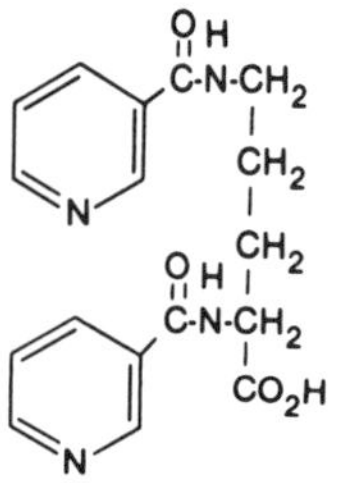

Di-Nicotinolyl Ornithine

Figure 3 Nicotinic acid detoxification products.

Figure 4 shows in addition a number of derivatives that are the result of metabolism. These substances are chemically detectable, but do not support niacin activity on biological tests. The substances that can be found include nicotinamide N'-oxide, 6-hydroxynicotinamide, and N'-methylnicotinamide, the 4 and 6 pyridones of N'-methylnicotinamide (N'-methyl-3-carboxamide- 4-pyridone and N'-methyl-2-pyridone-5-carboxamide), and 6-hydroxynicotinic acid.

C. Structural Analogs

Because of the simple structures of nicotinic acid and nicotinamide, numerous substituted pyridines and substituted heterocyclic compounds have been tested for their biological effect on nicotinic acid and nicotinamide nutriture or metabolism. Furthermore, the nicotinamide moiety of nicotinamide adenine dinucleotides has been substituted with a variety of related pyridine, imidazole, thiazole, or thiodiazole compounds to generate the corresponding base-adenine-dinucleotide analog of NAD. This has resulted in a voluminous literature on niacin analogs. The majority of these analogs mimic or inhibit the biologic effects of NAD in vitro.

A number of substances are important in whole animals as antivitamins.

Figure 5 shows the structure of the antivitamins that have been studied in some detail.

Acetylpyridine has primarily antiniacin toxicity. It can be converted to nicotonic acid, but is readily incorporated into NAD analogs. The result is a serious neurotoxicity. The action can be prevented by the administration of nicotonic acid or nicotinamide before or simultaneously with the drug (22) or by addition of extra tryptophan in the diet (23).

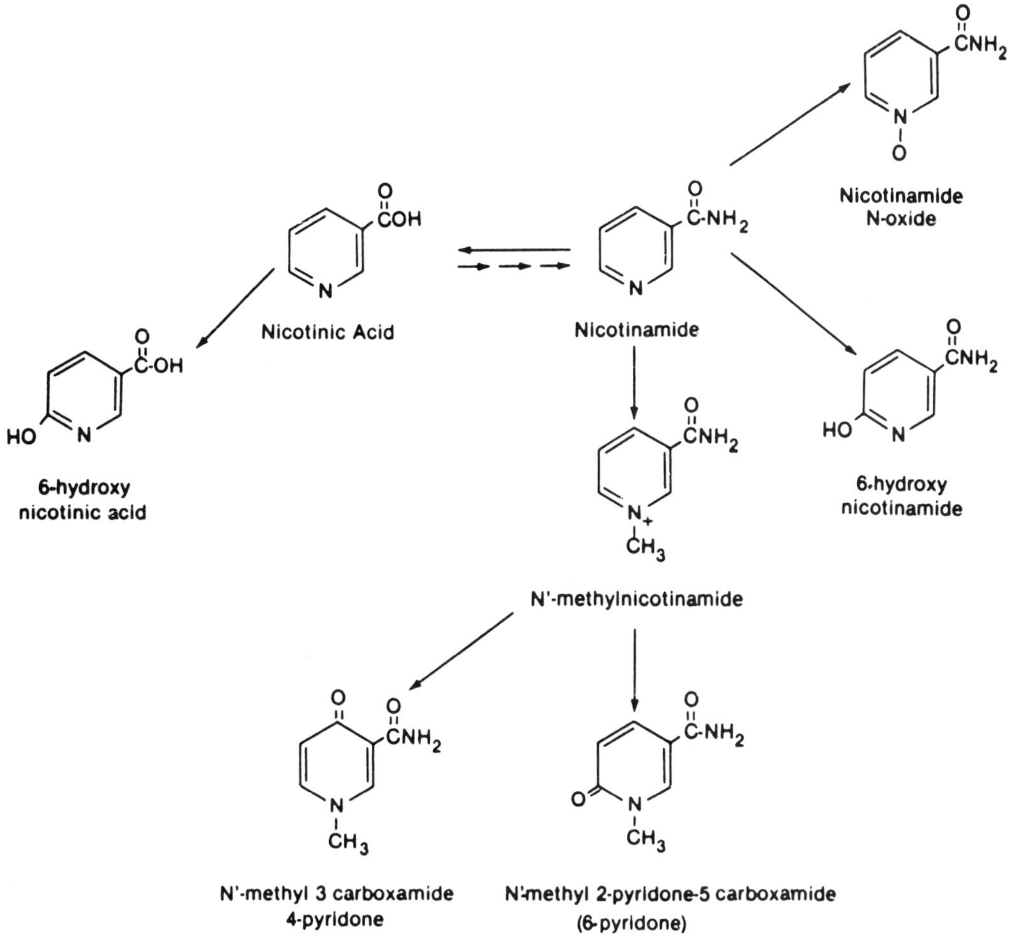

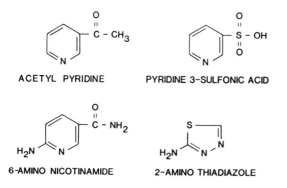

Figure 4 The metabolism of nicotinic acid and nicotinamide in mammals.

Figure 5 The structure of active niacin antagonists.

6-Aminonicotinamide also has a toxicity that can be prevented with nicotinic acid, nicotinamide, or tryptophan (24,25).

The compound has been proposed as an antineoplastic agent and is active in a variety of experimental tumor models. However, the drug is too toxic for human use (26,27).

2-Amino-1,3,4-thiadiazole is the parent compound of a serious of derivatives that have marked antitumor activity in animals. The antitumor activity can be reversed by nicotinamide and nicotinic acid (28–32). This drug has been tested in humans and seems to show modest promise.

D.   Synthesis

Nicotinic acid can be synthesized by construction of the pyridine ring or oxidation of substituted pyridines (33,34).

Nicotinamide is made by the aminolysis of esters of nicotinic acid.

Nicotinic acid is an odorless, nonhygroscopic white crystalline substance (molecular weight, 123.11) that is stable in air. It is resistant to autoclaving. It is soluble in water, glycerol, propylene glycol, dilute acids, alkaline solutions, and ethanol. It is almost insoluble in ethers. Nicotinic acid is stable in the presence of the usual oxidizing agents. However, in alkaline medium it will undergo decarboxylation at high temperature. The melting point is 235–237 °C. It can be sublimated in a vacuum.

Nicotinamide is likewise an odorless, white crystalline compound. The melting point is 129–131 °C. The molecular weight is 122.12. It is soluble in water, acetone, amyl alcohol, butanol, chloroform, ethanol, ethylene glycerol, and glycerol. It is stable in the dry state below 50 °C. When treated with alkali or acid, it is converted into nicotinic acid. Nicotinamide, as well as esters of nicotinic acid, reacts readily with acids or alkyl halides to form quaternary salts.

III.   ANALYTICAL PROCEDURES

A.   Introduction

Nicotinic acid and nicotinamide do not occur free in nature in large quantities. Much of the niacin activity in tissues is bound in the adenine dinucleotides. In addition, a number of degradation and detoxification products occur, as already mentioned. When analytical methods are discussed, therefore, it is extraordinarily important that one be clear whether nicotinic acid itself is to be measured, whether one wants niacin activity, or whether one wants the sum total of all nicotinic acid and nicotinamide derivatives that occur in biological materials. Finally, if one wants to assess the nutritional adequacy of a given foodstuff for niacin activity, one needs to take into account tryptophan content as well.

B.   Chemical Methods

The determination of nicotinic acid and nicotinamide itself by chemical means can be done by the Koenig reaction, which involves the degradation of the pyridine ring, utilizing cyanogen bromide. The open-ring olefinic dialdehyde can then react with an aromatic amine to form a colored product. This reaction can also be used for quinolinic acid, a substance of significance in the transformation of tryptophan to nicotinic acid.

The most widely used methods employ as the chromophore-generating base *p*-methylaminophenol sulfate (Metol) (35) or sulfanilic acid (36). Barbituric acid has also been used as chromogen, but that method is more widely used in pharmaceutical analysis (37). It has been said that the chromogen obtained with p-aminobenzoic acid does not extract organic solvents when bound niacin in cereals is being measured. Therefore, the distinction between free and bound niacin could be made with this assay method (38). In all reactions the color yield for nicotinamide is significantly lower than for nicotinic acid, and acid hydrolysis is therefore often used. This method of hydrolysis is not as reproducible as is optimally desired. Therefore enzymatic deamidation to nicotonic acid is recommended. A method based on that principle has been proposed by Fuller (39) using chromatographically separated nicotinamide, deamidation by the nicotinamide deaminase from *Saccharomyces cerevisiae*, in determination of nicotinic acid. The sensitivity of these methods is in the range of 1–10 μg per sample.

The sensitivity of the nicotinamide assay can be greatly increased by converting nicotinamide to N′-methylnicotinamide and utilizing the fluorescent properties of the adducts at the 4 position. Utilizing acetophenone as the carbonyl compound that forms the adduct, a phenol-substituted naphthyridine derivative can be formed. Nicotinamide is first converted to N′-methyl nicotinamide with methyl iodide (40). The method is sensitive to picomole amounts.

C. Pharmaceutial Preparation Analysis

The same methodology that is used for free nicotinic acid and nicotinamide can be used in pharmaceutical preparations. In the past methodologies based on this approach have been used and even automated (41,42).

Liquid chromatographic assays of multivitamin/mineral preparations have been found to be highly reliable (43). High-performance liquid chromotography has shown excellent agreement with manual methods and automated analysis. A substantial number of such assays are beginning to appear in the literatue (43,44).

IV. ANALYTICAL PROCEDURES FOR METABOLITES

A. Pyridine Nucleotides

1. Chemical Methodology

 A common method for the determination of all quaternary pyridine derivatives is the adduct formation with cyanide. The cyanide reaction is the basis of the determination of the complete variety of nicotinamide containing nucleotides and coenzymes (45,46). This methodology does not readily measure nicotinic acid nucleotides because the reaction between cyanide and nicotinic acid nucleotides is very slow to develop (47,48).

The same reaction that was described for the determination of niacin after methylation can be used for the determination of all quaternary pyridine nucleotides. Both N′-methylnicotinamide (49) and pyridine nucleotides (50) can be determined by the adducts of acetone to the quaternary pyridine derivative and the subsequent fluorometric determination of the naphthyridine derivatives. More reliable conversions are seen with methylethyl ketone and most determinations in natural material are based on the utilization of that reagent (51–53).

These methods do not differentiate among nicotinamide adenine dinucleotides or dinucleotide phosphates, nicotinamide mononucleotides, nicotinamide riboside or

N'-methylnicotinamide. To determine those substances individually it is necessary to separate the various pyridine nucleotides by chromatographic methods.

The oxidized and reduced form of nicotinamide coenzymes can be determined separately because NAD and NADP are alkali labile while NADH and NADPH are acid labile. The methodology for separate extractions have been described for NAD by Pinder et al. (54) and NADP by Birch (55).

2. Enzymatic Methods

It is possible to quantitate the coenzymes by their enzymatic properties. Because of their spectral properties and fluorescence of reduced nicotinamide adenine dinucleotides, the extracted material can be directly tested by the addition of a suitable substrate and enyzme. However, there are methodologies to magnify the consequence of the presence of pyridine nucleotides through cycling assays. These have been discovered and made practical by Lowry and co-workers (56). The principle is based on the sharing of the coenzyme by a pair of dehydrogenases by which the enzyme alternately oxidizes the substrate of one enzyme and reduces that of the other. After a period of cycling, if the latter enzyme reaction is irreversible, the product of the second enzyme can be measured, usually in the reverse direction with extra added pyridine nucleotides utilizing the fluorescent properties of the reduced nucleotide. Because of the magnification process and the inherent sensitivity of the fluorometric methodology, exquisitely sensitive assays can be devised. Direct reduction without cycling has a sensitivity of about 3×10^{-6} M. The chemical methods utilizing fluorescene of the alkali or methylethyl ketone derivatives have a sensitivity of about 10^{-7} M, as does the direct determination of reduced pyridine nucleotides with fluorescence. The cycling methods have a sensitivity from 10^{-10} to 10^{-15} M. Much of the methodology has been reviewed and detailed by Pinder et al. (54).

B. Degradation Products

The most important substance that needs to be determined is the presence of N'-methylnicotinamide in the urine. A rapid determination using methylethyl ketone has been described by Pelletier and Campbell (57).

One of the metabolites of nicotinic acid and nicotinamide is 1-methyl-2-oxypyridine-5-carboximide (6-pyridone). The determination is possible, but cumbersome (58).

The niacinamide metabolites can be separated by high-pressure liquid chromatography (59). This methodology can be used for both preparative and analytical purposes.

V. BIOLOGICAL ASSAYS FOR NIACIN ACTIVITY

A. Microbiological Assays

The microbiological techniques for the assays of vitamins and coenzymes have enjoyed great popularity. They have the advantage that multiple forms of a vitamin may be assayed simultaneously, so that vitamin activity can be assessed. For vitamins that have complex transformations and are inherently unstable, this is a great advantage. Even though vigorous hydrolysis of tissue samples will convert will niacin-containing substances to nicotinic acid, the distinction between free and bound niacin in grain and other differential growth-promoting activities could allow the utility of microbiological assays for differentiation niacin activity assessment. The assay has remained popular because of the ready applicability to natural materials. Pearson, in a general review of microbiological assays, utilized the assay for niacin as the paradigm (60).

Microbiological assays for tryptophan have been described, but they are not in general use anymore since the current chromatographic methodology is quite accurate while the extraction methods are about the same.

B. Bioassay Procedures

When fed niacin-deficient purified rations, chicks grow slowly and develop typical deficiency symptoms of inflammation of the crop, mouth, and upper part of the esophagus. The administration of nicotinic acid clears the deficiency symptoms in a few days, and it reestablishes growth. This has been used as a bioassay procedure (61).

However, it must be remembered that the relationship of tryptophan to niacin is valid for birds as well. Furthermore, at least in ducklings, β-picoline, pyridine-3-carbinol, and pyridine-3-aldehyde are active as niacin (62).

Black tongue in dogs was the classical model for pellagra in humans. The same caveats pertain. β-Picoline is partially effective in healing black tongue in dogs (63). Furthermore, in the dog tryptophan serves as a source for niacin as well.

Finally, the balance of other amino acids has a great deal of influence on the precipitation of niacin deficiency in experimental animals. This has been touched upon in the introduction and will be discussed at some greater detail later.

For all these reasons there is no place for whole animal assays in the accurate determination of nicotinic acid and its derivatives.

C. Evaluation of Nutritional Adequacy of Niacin Intake

Whether a patient has adequate niacin nutrition can be evaluated before overt symptoms and signs of niacin deficiency occur by measuring the levels of excreted niacin metabolites or the levels of pyridine nucleotides and accessible tissues. There is considerable variation in niacin metabolite excretion in animals of various species. In humans, excreted niacin metabolites in a healthy well-nourished adult include 4–6 mg of N'-methylnicotinamide. The next most common metabolite is the 6-pyridone. The ratio of pyridone to N'-methylnicotinamide has been used as an assessment of nutritional adequacy. However, it is more common to utilize the single determination of N'-methylnicotinamide because other metabolites are difficult to assess in the field.

VI. NIACIN CONTENT IN FOOD

A. Food Composition

The distribution of niacin in food is as wide as are the ubiquitous cofactors in which it is found. However, most food tables indicate the niacin equivalents. Niacin represents the sum of milligrams of niacin (nicotinic acid plus nicotinamide) plus 1/60 mg of tryptophan. For most dietetic purposes, this calculation is adequate, but for more detailed studies it is inaccurate. The presence of bound niacin and the amino acid imbalances may lower the actual availability of niacin.

It is also important to realize that certain species cannot use tryptophan as a source of niacin. The best known example is the cat (64). The mink (65) is also not able to do so. The rat has similar niacin equivalents for tryptophan as do humans. Therefore, data from rats can be extrapolated to human nutrition.

B. Elemental and Parenteral Preparations

The contents of various elemental diets and proprietary formulas are beginning to be a major concern in the nutriture of the very sick. There are a large number of formulations, and their indications for use vary according to the nutritional status of the patient. All formulas seem to contain adequate protein (tryptophan) and niacin. To date no pellagralike symptoms have been recorded with their use in adequate quantities.

Intravenous hyperalimentation is now frequently used to satisfy the nutritional requirements of sick patients. Here the tryptophan content of the various amino acid sources varies widely. Ranges in tryptophan–leucine ratio have been reported from 1–12.7 through 1–3.5. However, pellegralike symptoms have rarely been described in patients on total parenteral nutrition to date.

VII. METABOLISM

A. Introduction

The metabolism of nicotonic acid is extraordinarily complex. Tryptophan is converted to nicotinic acid and nicotinamide. Secondly, nicotinic acid and nicotinamide, when supplied exogenously, have different pathways to their incorporation into the pyridine nucleotide coenzymes. There is a specific biosynthetic pathway to the formation of pyridine nucleotides and their degradation. Nicotinic acid is widely transformed after ingestion. Furthermore, the excretory compounds are different when nicotinic acid is administered in pharmacologic doses than it is after physiologic doses.

Finally, the biosynthesis of nicotinic acid in plants and microorganisms is different from that in higher organisms.

In the context of this chapter the emphasis will be on the metabolism of the nicotinic acid derivatives in animals.

B. Biosynthesis of Nicotinic Acid from Tryptophan

The average daily intake of tryptophan in the American diet is 800–1000 mg (66,67). The minimum daily requirements for tryptophan is estimated to be 245 mg for adults (68). Part of the excess of tryptophan is converted to nicotinic acid derivatives. Figure 6 shows the pathway of the conversion of tryptophan to niacin. The yield of niacin is only 1 mg/60 mg of tryptophan metabolized, or a molar yield of only 2.75%. The major pathway for tryptophan after its metabolism to 3-hydroxykynurenine is degradation to carbon dioxide and water. Only because one step in this degradation pathway is rate limiting is niacin produced in any significant quantity. Cats have 50 times higher activity of this pathway than do humans and rats. Therefore, they cannot utilize tryptophan to satisfy their niacin requirements.

The first step in the metabolism is the conversion of tryptophan to N'-formylkynurenine. The conversion of tryptophan to N'-formylkynurenine is catalyzed by an enzyme called tryptophan pyrrolase (L-tryptophan 2,3,-dioxygenase). This enzyme is hormonally induced by glucocorticoids and tryptophan itself (69). It is the rate-limiting enzyme in the sequence when not induced.

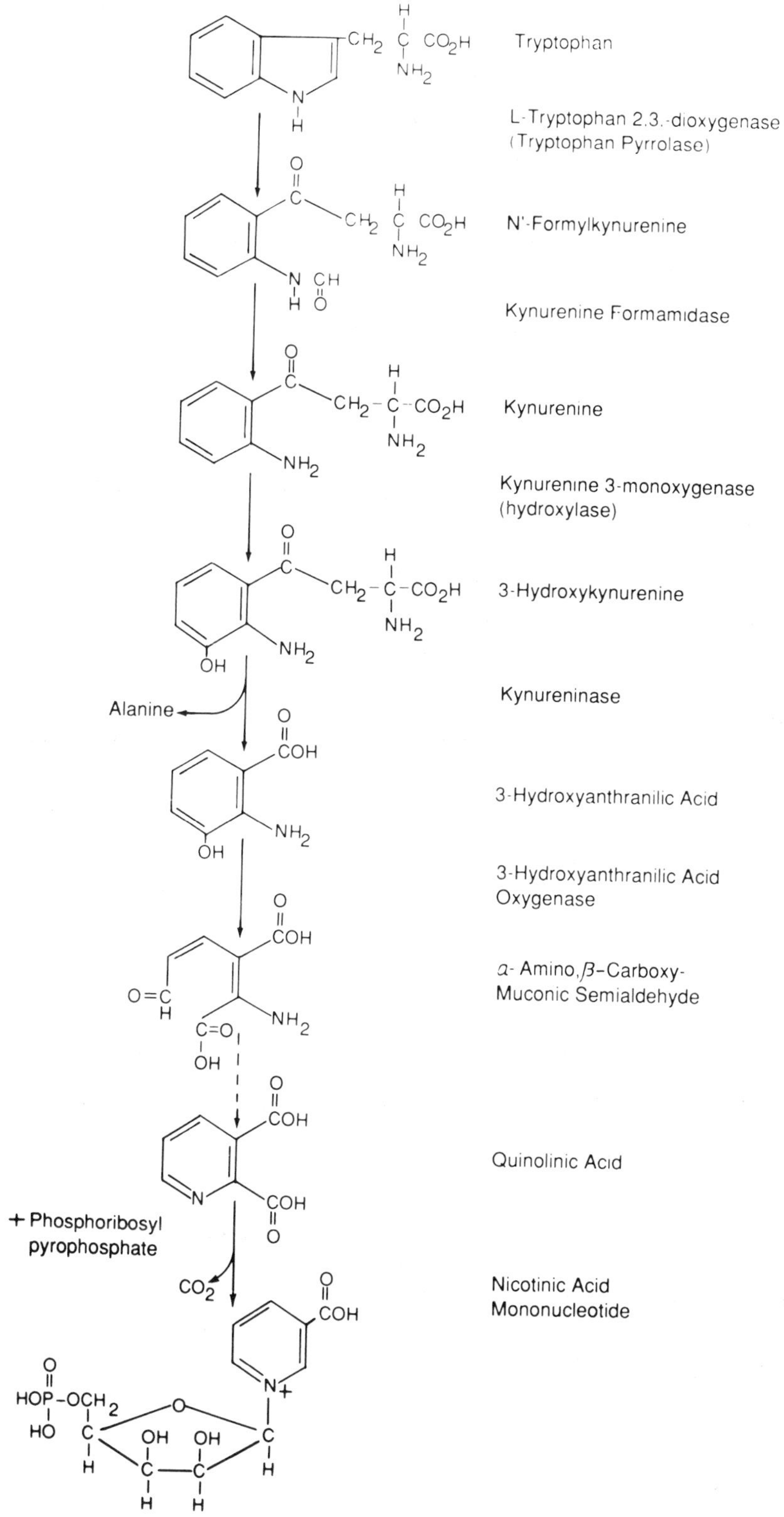

Figure 6 The pathway of the conversion of tryptophan to 3-nicotinic acid.

Figure 7 shows a number of competing pathways for the formation of nicotinic acid.

3-Hydroxyanthranilic acid is the most immediate precursor for nicotinic acid. In the conversion of 3-hydroxyanthranilic acid to nicotinic acid, quinolinic acid was thought for many years to be an intermediate. However, it is now clear that conversion from 3-hydroxyanthranilic acid yields nicotinic acid mononucleotide. The enzyme quinolinate phosphoribosyltransferase converts quinolinic acid to nicotinic acid mononucleotide by simultaneous decarboxylation (70).

The pathway from tryptophan to niacin is sensitive to a variety of nutritional, hormonal, and pathological alterations, as well as the iatrogenic effects of drug therapy.

The most important of these is vitamin B_6. The pathway from tryptophan to niacin has many steps dependent on vitamin B_6. In addition, copper, iron, and magnesium all have roles in the transformation (Fig. 8).

The pathway is sensitive to oral contraceptives, though there is no real reason for concern over the adequacy of niacin nutrition in women taking oral contraceptives. Isonicotinic acid hydrazide can act as a functional B_6 antagonist and therefore can disturb the pathway. Cases of pellagra have been reported on isoniazid therapy, which responded to combined vitamin B_6 and niacin treatment (71). In India, isonicotinic acid hydrazide (INH) has been called a potential "final straw" in the development of pellagra (72).

Riboflavin is involved in the pathway through its conversion to flavin adenine dinucleotide.

Copper deficiency can inhibit the conversion of tryptophan to niacin. Penicillamine has been demonstrated to inhibit the tryptophan niacin pathway in humans (73,74), and this may be due to the copper chelating effect, though vitamin B_6 binding could also be responsible.

C. Preformed Nicotinic Acid

1. Bioavailability

Nicotinic acid is widely distributed in nature. However, it occurs in a variety of forms that may be less available than free nicotinic acid. The primary impetus for this claim comes from the absence of pellagra in Central America, where corn is routinely steeped in lime water before consumption as compared to areas where pellagra was endemic with an equal corn consumption. This has been experimentally tested in animals, and most studies seem to support that claim (75–77), though those studies cannot be unequivocally repeated by everyone (78). Immature corn may have more readily available niacin activity than does older corn (79).

Claims for "alkali-labile" niacin precursors in corn have been made (80,81), but that same precursor occurs in wheat (81,82). Clais of isolation of the specific substance have been made, and the term niacytin has been used for this substance. Other peptide bound niacins have been called niacynogens (83). All these claims for bound niacin still require a great deal of further investigation. Newer varieties of corn have allowed growth in children for whom corn is the only staple (84,85).

2. Uptake

When nicotinic acid is administered in a readily available form in a single dose of "drug" magnitude (i.e., about 1 g) the resulting peak plasma levels are of the order of 25 μg/ml of nicotinic acid itself (86) and about 115 μg/ml of "nicotinic acid" by bioassay (87). The specific nicotinic acid peak is achieved in about a half hour and falls with a half-life

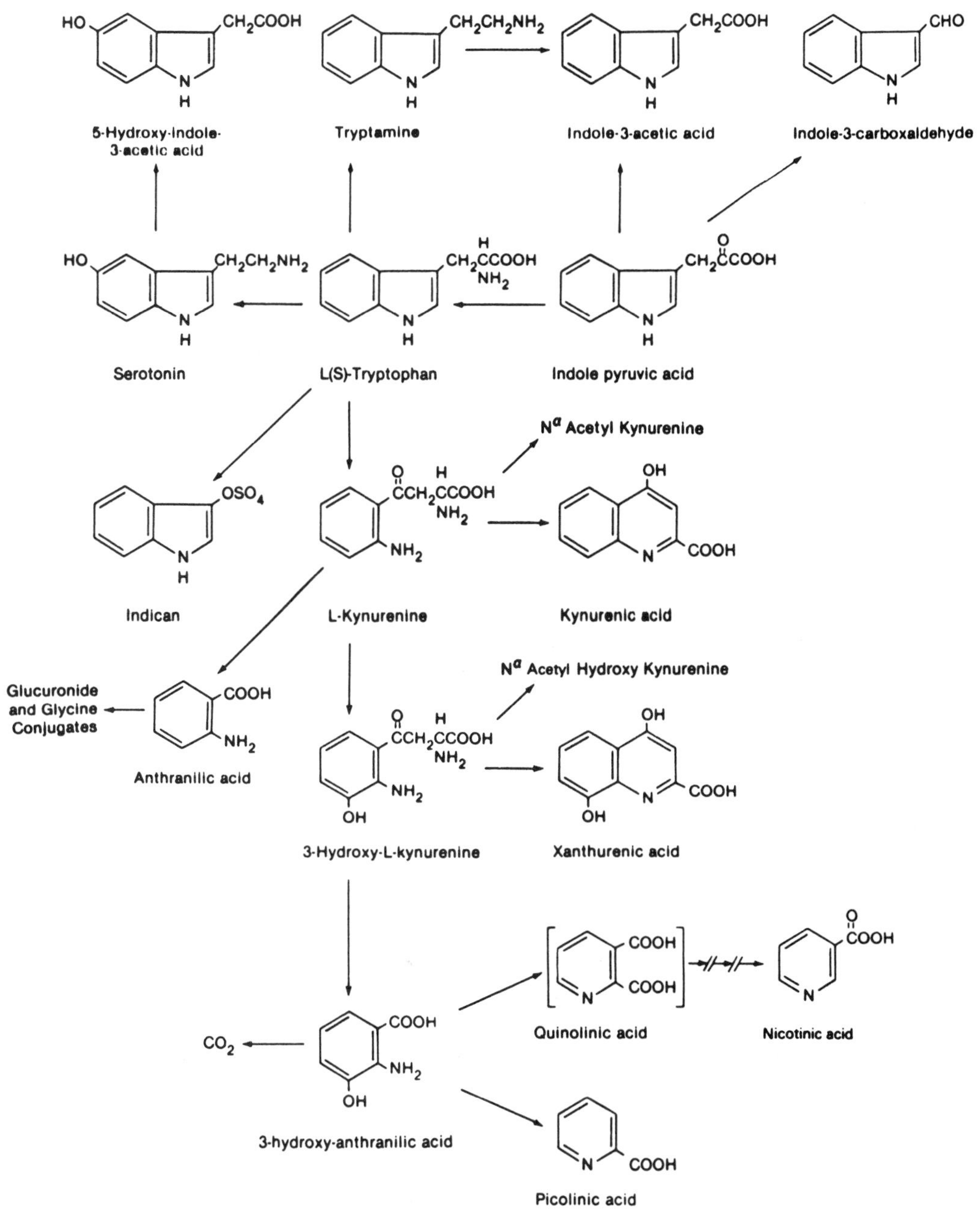

Figure 7 Competing pathways of tryptophan metabolism in animals and man.

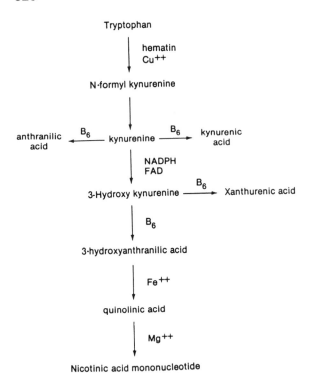

Figure 8 The interaction between vitamin B_6 and metals and the conversion of tryptophan to niacin.

of about 45 min, while microbiological assay levels are higher after 4 hr than after 2 hr, and fall off with a half-life of about 4 hr. The time of peak levels after oral dosage varies with species, being about ½ hr in rats and 1½ hr in dogs. In man the range is from ½ to 2 hr after dosage. Nicotinic acid preparations are rapidly and completely absorbed (88). With relatively large pharmacological doses, a larger fraction of the absorbed material escapes first-pass metabolism, and the plasma and urine levels of unchanged drug are consistent with this rapid and complete absorption (89). Nicotinic acid is absorbed mostly in a nonionic form (90).

About 15–30% of free nicotinic acid in plasma is protein bound (91).

3. Nicotinic Acid Metabolism After Pharmacologic Doses

Careful distinction must be made between the physiological disposition of nicotinic acid in the state of suboptimal to normal nutrition, and the disposition of nicotinic acid when given in pharmacologic doses. It must be remembered that biosynthesized nicotinic acid does not result in free nicotinic acid, but rather is utilized directly to form nicotinic acid nucleotides. When excess nicotinic acid is administered, it is handled in part like benzoic acid and is converted into a series of "detoxification" products. (Figure 3 indicated some of these substances.) Nicotinuric acid was isolated as early as 1913 from the urine of dogs fed nicotinic acid (92). The substance is present in traces only in normal human urine (93).

Other substances found are the gluconuride in rats (94) and chicken (95). In birds the various ornithine conjugates are also formed (95,96). However, most excess nicotinic acid and nicotinamide given acutely is excreted unchanged in rats (97,98) (Fig. 9).

Physiological amounts of nicotonic acid are metabolized in a variety of ways (Fig. 4). The most important ones are N'-methylnicotinamide (99) and N'-methyl-6-pyridone-2-carboxamide (100).

N'-Methyl-3-carboxamide-4-pyridone is also seen in normal mice metabolism (101–103). Hydroxylated metabolites of nicotinic acid or nicotinamide are also seen (104).

These substances are seen as minor metabolites following the injection or ingestion of carbon-labeled nicotinic acid and nicotinamide.

In man the sum of N'-methylnicotinamide and the 6-pyridone gives a satisfactory measure of niacin status (105). On a controlled diet providing 11.3 mg of niacin and 885 mg of tryptophan, the average amount excreted by normal women balanced the intake and measured as N'-methylnicotinamide and the 6-pyridone (106).

4. Nicotinamide-Containing Coenzymes

When nicotinic acid is formed from tryptophan the product is nicotinic acid mononucleotide rather than free nicotinic acid. Preformed nicotinic acid is incorporated into nicotinic acid adenine dinucleotide by first being converted to nicotinic acid mononucleotides which in turn reacts with ATP to form nicotinic acid adenine dinucleotide plus pyrophosphate. The nicotinic acid adenine dinucleotide is then converted to nicotinamide adenine dinucleotide with ATP and glutamine (107).

Figure 10 summarizes the pathways involved. The nicotinamide riboside phosphorylases and hydrolases are nonspecific enzymes and act also on adenosine (108). There is a structural similarity between adenosine and nicotinamide riboside that makes this a reasonable dual function of the enzymes (109).

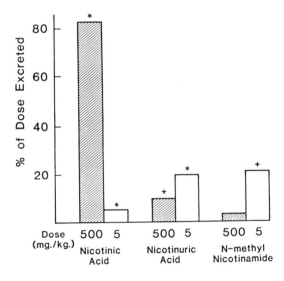

Figure 9 Urinary excretion following [^{14}C] nicotinic acid i.p. in rats. (*) = Major excretion in first 2 hr; (+) = Gradual excretion over 8+ hr.

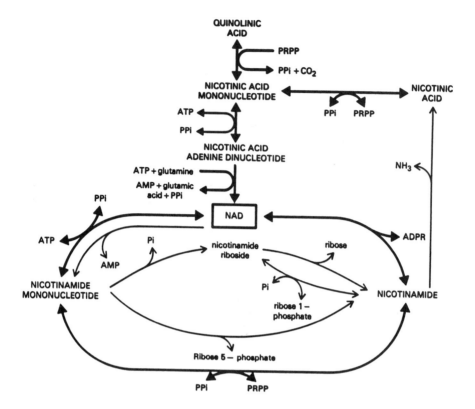

Figure 10 NAD metabolism.

   The NAD cycle as depicted has two degradative routes: via pyrophosphatase to form AMP and nicotinamide mononucleotide, and via hydrolysis to yield nicotinamide adenosine diphosphate ribose. Both enzymes have greater importance than merely degradative activity to balance synthesis and breakdown. The pyrophosphatases yield nicotinamide mononucleotides. A nicotinamide mononucleotide glycohydrolase is part of the transport system which yields free intracellular nicotinamide (110).

   The NAD glycohydrolases, which convert NAD to nicotinamide and adenosine diphosphate ribose, are a group of enzymes that have assumed major importance in molecular biology. These enzymes form poly-ADPR and in so doing influence metabolism of DNA widely.

   The administration of nicotinamide results in increase of up to 10-fold in liver NAD content (111).

5. Homeostasis

All tissues can incorporate nicotinamide into NAD and actually prefer nicotinamide to nicotinic acid. Nicotinamide is the primarily circulating form of the vitamin (112,113). In the liver nicotinic acid is incorporated into NAD, which is then again broken down into nicotinamide. The primary regulatory substance of the homeostasis in whole animals is nicotinamide itself. The levels in blood are buffered by the liver by being converted into a storage form of NAD. The total NAD level in liver is greater than the functional NAD (114). Excess nicotinamide, formed by the hydrolysis of excess NAD, can be converted to numerous inert excretion products.

In peripheral tissues nicotinamide is incorporated and metabolized to NAD. There is a feedback inhibition through NAD levels. A major utilization and regeneration of nicotinamide is through the formation of adenosine diphosphate ribose derivatives, which are necessary for growth and differentiation regulation. Nicotinamide inhibits that process. In fact, nicotinamide is toxic in tissue cultures at concentrations that increase NAD above normal (115).

VIII. DIETARY REQUIREMENTS

A. Tryptophan Requirements

The concept that some amino acids are indispensable while others are not is a relatively old notion. However, only after purified diets were possible could the modern concept of essential amino acids be generated. While the essential/nonessential dichotomy is not absolute, tryptophan falls in the category of absolute dietary essential. The lability of tryptophan to acid hydrolysis made it possible to demonstrate this even before purified diets were available. On the other hand, tryptophan does withstand alkaline hydrolysis. However, the amino acid is racemized in that process. This is an important consideration, because the human seems to use the D-isomer of tryptophan poorly (116).

The quantitative need for tryptophan has been assessed utilizing nitrogen balance techniques on diets with adequate nicotinic acid intake. An accurate measure of minimal daily requirement is not possible. It is usually recommended that the safe intake for an adult male is 500 mg/day (117). However, the total amount that is required is dependent upon the nitrogen intake. It is usually considered that 3–5 mg/tryptophan/kg body weight is appropriate because at about 5 mg/kg the body appears saturated (118). For women, the requirement was 160 mg/day, compared to the requirement for men to stay in balance at about 200 mg/day. However, when the total nitrogen supplied was diminished, the requirement dropped as low as 50 mg/day (119).

Children have different requirements during growth (120–127). Table 2 shows the quantitative tryptophan requirements in man. Recommended dietary allowances are generally set at 30% above those commonly reported as requirements.

B. Requirements of Tryptophan Plus Niacin

The actual requirement of free niacin depends on the quantity of tryptophan in the diet and the efficiency of the conversion. Tryptophan is able to reverse the symptoms of pellagra in humans, but such observations are not sufficiently quantitative to allow estimates of conversion. One can measure in normal men the conversion to niacin metabolites from a test dose of tryptophan and compare that to metabolite levels following a test dose of niacinamide. Usually N'-nicotinamide and N'-methyl-2-pyridone-5-carboxyamide, the 6-pyridone, are used. When the assumption is made that D-tryptophan is not converted to niacin metabolites, the data averaged to a conversion of 55.8 mg tryptophan to 1 mg of nicotinamide, with a range of 33.7–86.3 mg tryptophan (128–130). Similar data are obtained when subjects have been kept on diets deficient in both tryptophan and niacin (131,132). Currently a ratio of 60:1 is usually cited.

Table 2 Quantitative Tryptophan Requirement of Man

Subject	Criteria	Estimated requirement	Ref.
Infants	N-retention, growth	12-40 mg/kg	120
	N-retention, growth	13–16 mg/kg	121
Schoolchildren	N-retention	60–120 mg/day	122
Adult males	N-retention	6–9 mg/kg	123
	Urinary retention	3–6 mg/kg	123
	N-retention	150–250 mg/day	124
	N-retention	225 mg/day	125
	Plasma levels	3 mg/kg	118
	N-retention	2–2.6 mg/kg	118
Adult females	N-equilibrium	82–157 mg/day	119
	N-retention	50 mg/day	126
Elderly (male and female)	Plasma levels	2 mg/kg	127

When there is calorie restriction the excretion of N′-methylnicotinamide increases two- to fivefold, so that the 60:1 ratio may not hold under such conditions (133). Also, when patients are deficient, it takes a while to saturate the body. The conversion ratio does not get established immediately. Nevertheless, in spite of those caveats, the conversion ratio of 60:1 is generally accepted.

Knowing the conversion rate and knowing the tryptophan requirement so that subjects could be kept in nitrogen balance, it became possible to establish the niacin requirement for men. The niacin requirement could be defined as that amount of niacin needed if no conversion from tryptophan were to occur. If tryptophan is ingested, then for each 60 mg of tryptophan one can assume that 1 mg of niacin is obtained. That basic assumption implies that the conversion rate is independent of tryptophan intake, an assumption that is true as long as amino acid imbalances do not change the niacin conversion rate and the patient is in nitrogen balance.

Niacin deficiency was induced by Goldsmith in a number of persons utilizing a corn-based diet. The diets that induced pellagra furnished 3.4–5.4 mg niacin and 151–207 mg tryptophan per day. Therefore, the niacin equivalent of the deficient diets ranged from 5.9 to 8.8 mg/day. The subjects who did not develop pellagra had intakes of 7.4–10.6 mg/day (134–137).

Utilizing diets not containing corn gave somewhat different figures. Interpretations were complicated by the fact that the amount of calories were different between the two sets of experiments. The amount of tryptophan needed to stay in nitrogen balance differs according to the caloric intake. However, in the second set of experiments without corn no subject developed pellagra with a niacin equivalent of 9.2–12.3 mg/day (131). If all data are combined, a minimum requirement of about 4.5 mg/1000 calories of 0.15 mg/kg body weight appears to be a valid estimate.

In infants, niacin equivalent of 6 mg tryptophan/1000 calories in a casein niacin free formula was considered adequate while 4 mg tryptophan/1000 calories was inadequate, as judged by excretion levels of N′-methylnicotinamide (138). When human milk is used as a gauge, 8 mg niacin equivalents per 1000 calories must be adequate, two thirds of which come from tryptophan (139).

The recommended allowances for niacin are summarized in Table 3. The estimates for pregnancy and lactation are based on assumptions that the increased excretion of trypto-phan metabolites in pregnancy might indicate an increased deficiency in conversion of tryptophan to niacin (140). In other words, more tryptophan is needed per se but the higher niacin equivalent is present. However, an opposing idea is that more methylation of nico-tinamide to N'-methylnicotinamide occurs, and that therefore more niaicin is needed (139,141). During lactation there is a loss of about 1.6 mg of performed niacin per 850 ml (140). The actual increases recommended are based more on the increased caloric de-mand than a known increased requirement. In pregnancy the recommended increased energy intake is 300 calories daily or 2 niacin equivalents. In lactation the recommended increase in caloric intake is 500 kcal, thus suggesting an increase in 3.3 mg niacin equivalents. This coupled with the 2.6 mg daily loss in milk suggests an increase of 5 mg niacin equivalents.

Animal data vary widely. The rat is the primary animals for which experimental data are obtained in order to understand mammalian nutrition in general and human nutrition in particular. It is fortuitous that the rat has similar niacin equivalence for L-tryptophan and that therefore data can be translated to humans. For poultry the range for requirements is very wide: 27 mg/kg of diet for growing chickens, 55 mg/kg for ducklings, and 70 mg/kg for turkeys and pheasants (142). As already mentioned in the introduction, certain species cannot utilize tryptophan as a niacin precursor. This is due to the ratio of the rate of 3-hydroxyanthranilic acid conversion to α-amino-β-carboxymuconic-ϵ-semialdehyde

Table 3 Recommended Daily Dietary Allowances[a]

	Age (yr)	Weight (kg)	Height (cm)	Niacin (mg NE)[b]
Infants	0.0–0.5	6	60	5
	0.5–1.0	9	71	6
Children	1–3	13	90	9
	4–6	20	112	12
	7–10	28	132	13
Males	11–14	45	157	17
	15–18	66	176	20
	19–24	70	177	19
	25–50	70	178	19
	51+	70	178	15
Females	11–14	46	157	15
	15–18	55	163	15
	19–22	55	163	15
	23–50	55	163	15
	51+	55	163	13
Pregnancy	—	—	—	17
Lactating	—	—	—	20

[a]The allowances are intended to provide for individual variations among most normal per-sons as they live in the United States under usual environmental stresses. Diets should be based on a variety of common foods in order to provide other nutrients for which human re-quirements have been less well defined.
[b]NE (niacin equivalent) is equal to 1 mg niacin or 60 mg of dietary tryptophan.
(Adapted from Ref. 68)

vs. the formation of quinolinic acid. If the ratio is too high not enough intermediate accumulates to allow the spontaneous conversion to quinolinic acid (143). The end product of the major pathway of 3-hydroxyanthranilic acid includes picolinic acid. The activity of the picolinic acid carboxylase seems to correlate with the dietary need of nicotinic acid (144).

C. Amino Acid Imbalance and Niacin Nutriture

Amino acid imbalance is a term commonly used to designate the relative deficiency of one essential amino acid when one or more amino acids are in excess (145). While amino acid imbalances can be created in a variety of ways, thereby generating relative deficiencies for a number of amino acids, the most frequently cited and investigated problem is the effect of such imbalance on the tryptophan requirement and, thus, the niacin requirement. Initially it was thought that amino acid supplemented 9% casein diets increased the niacin requirements. The specific amino acids most markedly affecting the niacin tryptophan requirements are threonine, cystine/methionine, and leucine. Isoleucine will counteract leucine's effect. If leucine is raised, high valine is also required to counteract the effect.

What is seen in purified diets is not always reproducible, utilizing cereals. Amino acid unavailability from plant proteins is a significant complicating factor.

Corn has an excess of leucine. The toxicity of leucine in a tryptophan marginal diet has been postulated as an etiological factor in pellagra (146). Those claims are not uniformly accepted. While there is significant evidence for the effect of leucine and isoleucine in the experimental setting, the extrapolation to the etiology of pellagra is still tenuous. Balance studies in humans show that there is no consistent effect of L-leucine or vitamin B_6 supplements on the excretion of any of the metabolites of tryptophan measured (146).

D. Deficiency Syndromes

1. Pellagra

Pellagra is a noncontagious, nonhereditary clinical syndrome that can occur at any age in either sex and any race. Prodromal symptoms are insomnia, loss of appetite, weight and strength loss, soreness of the tongue and mouth, indigestion, diarrhea, abdominal pain, burning sensations in various parts of the body, vertigo, headache, numbness, nervousness, distractability, flights of ideas, apprehension, mental confusion, and forgetfulness. Patients have no diagnostic sign of pellagra when they are first seen by the physician in that state.

Classical pellagra shows typical dermal lesions. They are most frequent found over sites of irritation, such as the dorsum of the hands, wrists, elbows, face, neck, under the breasts, knees, feet, and in the perineal region. The lesions are symmetrical and are sharply demarcated from healthy skin. In the early stages the areas closely resemble sunburn and are often accompanied by burning and itching. As the disease progresses the area becomes swollen, tense, and more red. Vesicles and bullae may form and rupture. Even after repletion of the diet, some of the lesions may not disappear. The alimentary tract shows characteristic glossitis and stomatitis. Nausea and vomiting may appear early in the course of the disease.

The central nervous system shows all the signs seen in the prodrome. Numbness, later paralysis of the extremities, particularly of the legs, is a common finding. The more advanced cases of pellagra are characterized by tremor and a spastic or ataxic or ataxic gait which is frequently associated with peripheral neuritis. If the patient is not treated, severe thought disorders can ensue (147).

The occurrence of frank pellagra in human populations is rare in western society. However, Hartnup's disease is a genetic deficiency in the absorption of tryptophan. Such patients have a typical pellagra and the symptoms come intermittently but grow milder with increasing age. There is a marked skin rash usually made worse by sunlight. Neurological symptoms are prominent with unsteadiness, clumsiness, nystagmus, tremor, and diploplia as in cerebellar ataxia. Psychiatric disturbances are seen up to frank delirium. The disease is associated with poor nutrition; nicotinamide deficiency is a major etiological component (12).

Pellagralike syndrome symptoms are seen in malnourished alcoholics.

2. Animal Diseases

A variety of animals have been given the symptoms and signs of combined tryptophan and niacin deficiency. Because of the varying diets that have been used, it is hard to compare these with pure niacin deficiency. The cat, when fed niacin-free rations, develop deficiency signs that include body weight loss, diarrhea, and death. There are no skin or oral lesions. The administration of niacin readily reverses such symptoms (148). That is an important model because of the previously mentioned inability from the part of the cat to convert tryptophan to niacin.

3. The Symptoms of Nicotinic Acid Antagonists

It is of interest that many of the niacin antagonsists give neurological symptoms. For instance, when acetylpyridine is administered to animals, the symptoms are mostly neurological and there are histological abnormalities demonstrable in the hippocampus (149–151).

IX. PHARMACOLOGY

A. Introduction

Nicotinic acid is unusual among the vitamins in that doses in excess of nutritional requirements result in a number of readily recognizable pharmacological responses. Some of those have therapeutic significance. These responses can be broadly classified as vascular and metabolic. The phenomena can be provoked in acute settings and in chronic therapeutic application. Finally, some of these pharmacological effects can result in toxic responses. Few if any of the considerable pharmacological actions of nicotinic acid are shared with nicotinamide. As nutrients the two are quite interchangeable, but in therapeutic settings, the two are very dissimilar. Furthermore, the toxicity of the two substances when administered in excessive quantities are very dissimilar. However, some of the pharmacological effects of nicotinic acid can be blocked by pretreatment of a large dose of nicotinamide.

B. The Effect of Nicotinic Acid on Hyperlipidemia

The initial interest in the action of nicotinic acid on atherosclerosis was related to its effect on the total serum cholesterol levels. Adequately large doses of nicotinic acid can reduce serum cholesterol levels. Even single doses can produce detectable effects (152) though more impressive results are seen after weeks with treatment with divided daily doses of the order of 2–4 g. Continuing treatment remains effective for years. In addition, the effects of nicotinic acid on serum lipids include a lowering of free fatty acids and total lipid levels. In normal subjects, one gram of nicotinic acid three times a day for a month lowered serum cholesterol level by 15% and triglyceride levels by 27%. The major drop was in lipids transported as LDL and VLDL, while HDL cholesterol actually increased by 23% (153).

C. Effects on Vascular Tone

It has long been known that there is a flush reaction to nicotinic acid. This reaction can be seen in humans seconds after as little as 1 mg intravenously and within minutes of somewhat larger dose orally (155). The flush response of nicotinic acid is seen primarily with a rising nicotinic acid blood level and may not persist during a maintained plateau level (155,156). Nicotinic acid has been used in a variety of conditions presumed to be due to impaired circulation.

D. Nicotinic Acid–Induced Fibrinolysis

Nicotinic acid gives a marked fibrinolytic activation when administered intravenously (157,158). The duration of the fibrinolytic response is very short, in spite of its potency. It rarely lasts as long as one hour. A tolerance develops after the initial response to a single dose, so that a second dose is ineffective until days to weeks after the initial effective dose (159,160). For this reason, fibrinolysis is only observed in human subjects in blood drawn 5–20 min after intravenous or intraarterial dose of 10–100 mg of nicotinic acid. Intramuscular doses are more weakly and less consistently effective. Oral doses are ineffective, even in large quantities (6g/day) for a month. Nicotinic acid does not work when added in vitro to blood or plasma. Nicotinamide does not induce lytic activity, but its prior administration blocks the usual response to a subsequent parenteral dose of nicotinic acid. The phenomenon is not seen in a variety of other species, such as the rabbit, dog, rat, or guinea pig.

Patients with hepatic disease differ from normal in their fibrinolytic response to nicotinic acid (161). In such patients repetitive doses are effective and oral doses produce an effect. The phenomenon of nicotinic acid–induced fibrinolysis remains a medical curiosity rather than a therapeutic weapon of known utility.

E. Nicotinic Acid–Related Drugs

Certain derivatives of nicotinic acid and nicotinic acid analogs share some of the pharmacological effects of nicotinic acid. The most important one is β-pyridylcarbinol, which is potentially oxidizable to nicotonic acid. Its clinical use is primarily as a vasodilator (162,163) but it also seems to have some effects on hyperlipidemia (164).

F. Nicotinic Acid in Mental Diseases

The resemblance of the mental disturbances seen in pellagra to schizophrenia have for years suggested that nicotinic acid or nicotinamide might be helpful in the treatment of schizophrenia. However, a review of all the relevant individual controlled studies show that there is no evidence that nicotinic acid is an antipsychotic agent. This statement has now entered textbooks (165), but as late as 1985 review articles still were thought to be necessary to suppress that notion (166).

However, one must remain aware that niacin deficiency does in fact cause psychosis. A recent case of niacin deficiency induced by maintenance hemodialysis underscores this well-documented but nearly forgotten fact (167).

X. TOXICITY

A. Introduction

Both nicotinic acid and nicotinamide can be toxic when administered in excessive quantities. However, the toxicity is entirely different, as might be expected from the pharmacological effects that are exhibited by nicotinic acid and not shared by nicotinamide. Furthermore, the entrance into metabolism of nicotinic acid and nicotinamide are very different. Therefore, they have to be discussed separately.

B. Nicotinamide Toxicity

It has already been mentioned that nicotinamide is toxic to cells at concentrations that increase NAD above normal. When it is fed at levels of 5.3–6.8 μmoles/kg and at levels greater than 10 μmols/kg, rats actually lose weight (168). The LD50 of nicotinamide for young rats is 13.8 μmoles/kg (169). Nicotinamide can enhance the effect of streptozotocin in producing pancreatic islet cell tumors (170–172). The antitumor effect of anticancer agents can also be potentiated by nicotinamide (173).

Chronic administration of nicotinamide at 3g/day for 3–36 months had various side effects such as heartburn, nausea, headaches, hives, fatigue, sore throat, dry hair, tautness of face, and inability to focus the eyes (174).

C. Nicotinic Acid

Nicotinic acid has been given to adults in high doses as part of hyperlipidemia studies. A high percent of patients discontinue the drug due to intolerance. At 1 g tid 24% discontinued the drug. Another 10% dropped after having taken the drug more than a year (175). In a large study only 28% of patients remained on the full initial target dose of 4 g/day (176).

Acute flushing is very common and has been mentioned. Less common are dryness, pruritis, and keratosis nigricans. Hypertension and transient headaches may occur. Sometimes a decreased glucose tolerance is seen. Some degree of increased uric acid level is often noted.

Nicotinic acid frequently causes gastrointestinal symptoms attributable to local irritation. Administering the drug with antacids or administering nicotonic acid as aluminum salts alleviates these effects (177).

There have been concerns about hepatic toxicity. In a large study 10% of patients developed liver function abnormalities (176). However, all jaundiced patients recovered on withdrawal of the drug. In another large study no unusual incidence of jaundice or elevation of liver enzymes was seen (178,179). Nevertheless, this remains a concern. A recently reported case of nicotinic acid–induced fulminant hepatic failure in a 46-year-old man taking 3 g of nicotinic acid daily for hypercholesterolemia should serve as a warning (180).

D. Toxicity of Tryptophan

While the toxicity of tryptophan per se is beyond the scope of this article, it must be noted that a high dietary intake of tryptophan in rats (5.9 g/kg diet) led to a considerable increase in liver pyridine nucleotides and also in urinary excretion of niacin metabolites.

The utilization of nicotinamide and nicotinic acid from nucleotide synthesis is limited, but there seems to be little or no limitation of pyridine nucleotide synthesis from tryptophan through the transformation of quinolic acid to nicotonic acid mononucleotide (181).

REFERENCES

1. C. Huber, *Ann. der Chemic und Pharmacie, 65*:271 (1867).
2. H. Weidel, *Ann. der Chemic und Pharmacie, 165*:328 (1873).
3. Y. Suzuki, T. Simanura, and S. Odale, *Biochem. Zeitschr. 43*:89 (1912).
4. F. Thiery, *Jour. de Med., Chir., et. Pharm.* (Paris, 1755), p. 337.
5. J. Goldberger, C. H. Waring, and D. G. Willits, *Public Health Report, 30*:3117 (1915).
6. J. Goldberger, and G. A. Wheeler, *Public Health Report, 43*:172 (1928).
7. C. A. Elvehjem, R. J. Madden, F. M. Strong, and D. W. Woolley, *J. Am. Chem. Soc., 59*:1767 (1937).
8. H. von Euler, H. Ahlers, and F. Schlenk, *Z. Physiol. Chem., 124*:113 (1936).
9. O. Warburg and W. Christian, *Biochem. Zeitschr., 274*:112 (1934).
10. O. Warburg and W. Christian, *Biochem. Zeitschr., 275*:464 (1935).
11. D. N. Baron, C. E. Dent, M. Harris, E. W. Hart, and J. B. Lepson, *Lancet, 1*:421 (1956).
12. K. Halvorsen and S. Halvorsen, *Pediatrics, 31*:29 (1963).
13. W. H. Wilson, *J. Hyg., 20*:1 (1921).
14. C. Funk, *Münch. Med. Wochenschr., 60*:2614 (1913).
15. C. Funk, in *The Vitamins*, Williams and Wilkins, Baltimore, 1922.
16. C. Gopalan, and K. S. J. Rao, *Vitamins and Hormones, 33*:505 (1975).
17. W. N. Pearson, J. S. Valenzuela, and J. van Eys, *J. Nutr., 66*:277 (1958).
18. N. V. Shasti, and M C. Nath, *J. Vitaminol., 18*:200 (1972).
19. K. J. Carpenter, *Pellagra*, Hutchinson Ross Publishing Co, Stroudsburg, PA, 1981.
20. AIN Committee on Nomenclature, *J. Nutr., 105*:134 (1975).
21. E. H. Todhunter, in *A Guide to Nutrition Terminology for Indexing and Retrieval*, U.S. Government Printing Office, Washington, D. C., 1970, p. 270.
22. D. W. Woolley, *J. Biol. Chem., 157*:455 (1945).
23. D. W. Woolley, *J. Biol. Chem., 162*:179 (1946).
24. W. J. Johnson, and J. D. McColl, *Science, 122*:834 (1955).
25. W. J. Johnson and J. D. McColl, *Fed. Proc., 15*:284 (1956).
26. C. P. Peilis, S. Kofman, M. Sky-Peck, and S. G. Taylor, III, *Cancer, 14*:644 (1961).
27. F. P. Herta, S. G. Weissman, H. G. Thompson, Jr., G. Hyman, and D. S. Martin, *Cancer Res., 21*:31 (1961).
28. T. J. Oleson, *Fed. Proc. 15*:372 (1956).
29. D. M. Shapiro, M. E. Shotts, R. A. Fugman, and I. M. Friedland, *Cancer Res., 17*:29 (1957).
30. M. M. Ciotti, N. O. Kaplan, A. Goldin, and J. M. Vendetti, *Proc. Am. Ass. Cancer Res., 2*:287 (1957).
31. M. M. Ciotti, S. R. Humphreys, J. M. Vendetti, N. O. Kaplan, and A. Goldin, *Cancer Res., 20*:1195 (1960).
32. T. Matsumoto, K. Ootsu, and Y. Okada, *Cancer Chem. Rep. 58: (Part I)*: 331 (1974).
33. J. M. Hundley, in *The Vitamins*, Vol. II, W. H. Sebrell Jr. and R. S. Harris (Eds.), Academic Press, New York, 1954, p. 452.
34. C. D. Rio-Estrada, and H. W. Dougherty, *Kirk-Orthmer Encycl. Chem. Technol., 2nd ed.*, Interscience, New York, 1970, p. 509.
35. F. E. Friedemann and E. J. Frazier, *Arch. Biochem. 26*:361 (1950).
36. Association of Official Agricultural Chemists, in *Official Methods of Analysis, 8th ed.*, W. Horwitz (Ed.), Washington, D.C., 1955, p. 826.
37. O. Pelletier, and J. A. Campbell, *J. Pharm. Sci., 50*:926 (1961).
38. M. L. Das and N. C. Ghosh, *Ind. J. Med. Res., 45*:631 (1957).

39. L. Fuller, in *Methods in Enzymology*, Vol. 66, D. B. McCormick and L. D. Wright (Eds.), Academic Press, New York, 1980, p. 3.
40. B. R. Clark, in *Methods in Enzymology*, Vol. 66, D.B. McCormick and L. D. Wright (Eds.), Academic Press, New York, 1980, p. 5.
41. R. E. Albright and E. F. Degner, *Automat. Anal. Chem. Technicon Symp.*, *3rd, 1*:461 (1967).
42. R. H. Y. S. Bryant, F. J. Burger, R. L. Henry, and F. B. Trenk, *J. Pharm. Sci.*, *6*:1717 (1971).
43. M. Amin and J. Reush, *Analyst 112*:989 (1987).
44. F. L. Lamb, J. J. Holcombe, S. A. Fusari, *J. Ass. Off. Anal. Chem.*, *67*:1007–1011 (1984).
45. M. M. Ciotti and N. O. Kaplan, in *Methods in Enzymology 3*, S. P. Colowick and N. O. Kaplan (Eds.), Academic Press, New York, 1957, p. 890.
46. S. P. Colowick, N. O. Kaplan, and M. M. Ciotti, *J. Biol. Chem.*, *191*:447 (1951).
47. M. Lamborg, F. E. Stolzenbach, and N. O. Kaplan, *J. Biol. Chem.*, *231*:685 (1958).
48. M. Lamborg, as quoted in N. O. Kaplan, *Rec. Chem. Progr.*, *16*:186 (1955).
49. J. W. Huff and W. A. Perlzweig, *J. Biol. Chem.*, *167*:157 (1947).
50. N. Levitas, J. Robinson, F. Rosen, J. W. Huff, and W. A. Perlzweig, *J. Biol. Chem.*, *167*:169 (1947).
51. H. B. Burch, C. A. Storvick, R. L. Bicknell, H. C. Kung, L. G. Alejo, W. A. Everhart, O. H. Lowry, C. G. King, and O. A. Bessey, *J. Biol. Chem.*, *212*:897 (1955).
52. K. H. Carpenter and E. Kodicek, *Biochem. J.*, *46*:421 (1950).
53. G. A. Goldsmith and O. N. Miller, in *The Vitamins*, 2nd ed., *Volume VII*, P. György and W. N. Pearson (Eds.), Academic Press, New York, 1967, p. 137.
54. S. Pinder, J. B. Clark, and A. L. Greenbaum, in *Methods in Enzymology*, Vol. 66, D. B. McCormick, and L. D. Wright, (Eds.), Academic Press, New York, 1980, p. 23.
55. H. B. Burch, in *Methods in Enzymology*, Vol. 66, D. B. McCormick and L. D. Wright (Eds.), Academic Press, New York, 1980, p. 11.
56. O. H. Lowry, J. V. Passoneau, D. W. Schultz, and M. Y. Rock, *J. Biol. Chem.*, *236*:2746 (1961).
57. O. Pelletier and J. A. Campbell, *Anal. Biochem.*, *3*:60 (1962).
58. F. Rosen, W. A. Perlzweig, and J. G. Leder, *J. Biol. Chem.*, *179*:157 (1949).
59. C. Bernofsky, in *Methods in Enzymology*, Vol. 66, D. B. McCormick and L. D. Wright (Eds.), Academic Press, New York, 1980, p. 23.
60. W. N. Pearson, in *The Vitamins*, Vol. VII, P. Györgi and W. N. Pearson, (Eds.), Academic Press, New York, 1964, p. 1.
61. M. R. S. Fox and G. M. Briggs, *J. Nutr.*, *72*:243 (1960).
62. R. van Reen and F. E. Stolzenbach, *J. Biol. Chem.*, *226*:373 (1957).
63. D. W. Woolley, F. M. Strong, R. J. Madden, and C. A. Elvehjem, *J. Biol. Chem.*, *124*:715 (1938).
64. A. C. DaSilva, R. Fried, and R. C. DeAngelis, *J. Nutr.*, *46*:399 (1952).
65. National Research Council, *Nutrient Requirements of Domestic Animals, No. 7 Nutrient Requirements of Mink and Foxes*. National Academy of Science, Washington, D.C., 1968.
66. M. S. Reynolds, *J. Am. Diet, Ass.*, *33*:1015 (1957).
67. M. L. Orr, and B. K. Watt, *USDA Home Econ. Res. Rept.*, U.S. Government Printing Office, Washington, D. C., 1957.
68. Food and Nutrition Board, Committee on Dietary Allowances, *Recommended Dietary Allowances*, 10th revised ed., National Academy of Sciences, Washington, D. C., 1989.
69. W. E. Knox and M. M. Piras, *J. Biol. Chem.*, *242*:2959 (1967).
70. Y. Nishizuka and O. Hayaishi, *J. Biol. Chem.*, *230*:3369 (1963).
71. P. A. DiLorenzo, *Acta Dermatol. Venereol.*, *47*:318 (1967).
72. P. S. Shankar, *J. Ind. Med. Soc. 54*:73 (1955).
73. I. A. Jaffe, *Ann. N. Y. Acad Sci.*, *166*:57 (1969).
74. L. E. Hollister, F. F. Moore, F. Forrest, and J. L. Bennett, *Am. J. Clin. Nutr.*, *19*:307 (1966).
75. J. Laguna and K. J. Carpenter, *J. Nutr. 45*:21 (1951).

76. W. N. Pearson, S. J. Stempfel, J. Salvador-Valenzuela, M. H. Utley, and W. J. Darby, *J. Nutr., 62*:445 (1957).
77. A. E. Harper, B. D. Punelear, and C. A. Elvehjem, *J. Nutr., 66*:163 (1958).
78. R. O. Cravioto, G. H. Massieu, O. Y. Cravioto, and F. de M. Figueroda, *J. Nutr., 48*:453 (1952).
79. K. J. Carpenter, M. Schelstraete, V. C. Vilicich, and J. S. Wall, *J. Nutr., 118*:165 (1988).
80. D. K. Chaudhuri and E. Kodicek, *Biochem. J., 47*:xxxiv (1950).
81. D. K. Chaudhuri and E. Kodicek, *Nature, 165*:1022 (1050a).
82. W. A. Krehl, and F. M. Strong, *J. Biol. Chem., 156*: (1944).
83. W. J. Darby, K. W. McNutt, and E. N. Todhunter, *Nutr. Rev., 33*:289 (1975).
84. G. G. Graham, D. V. Glover, G. Lopez de Romãna E. Morales, and W. C. MacLean, Jr., *J. Nutr., 110*:1061 (1980).
85. G. G. Graham, R. P. Placko, and W. C. MacLean, Jr., *J. Nutr., 110*:1070 (1980).
86. L. A. Carlson, in *Metabolic Effecs of Nicotinic Acid and Its Derivatives*, K. F. Gey and L. A. Carlson (Eds.), Hans Huber, Bern, 1971, p. 163.
87. J. L. S. Holloman, C. G. Davis, and L. C. Leeper, *J. Am. Geriatr. Sco., 10*:903 (1962).
88. B. Petrack, P. Greengrad, and H. Kalinsky, *J. Biol. Chem., 241*:2367 (1966).
89. L. A. Carlson, and A. Hanngren, *Atherosclerosis 28*:81 (1977).
90. J. Elbert, H. Daniel, G. Rehnrer, *Int. J. Vitam. Nutr. Res., 56*:85 (1986).
91. W. T. Robinson, L. Cosyns, and M. Kraml, *Clin. Biochem., 11*:46 (1978).
92. D. Zeckerman, *Z. Biol, 59*:17 (1913).
93. B. C. Johnson, T. S. Hamilton, and H. H. Mitchell, *J. Biol. Chem. 159*:231 (1945).
94. J. van Eys, O. Touster, and W. J. Darby, *J. Biol. Chem., 217*:287 (1955).
95. M. L. Wu Chang, and B. Conner-Johnson, *J. Biol. Chem., 226*:799 (1956).
96. W. T. Dann and L. W. Huff, *J. Biol. Chem., 168*:121 (1947).
97. B. Petrack, P. Greengaard, and H. Kalinsky, *J. Biol. Chem., 241*:2367 (1966).
98. P. Greengaard, B. Petrack, and H. Kalinsky, *J. Biol. Chem., 242*:152 (1967).
99. J. W. Huff and W. A. Perlzweig, *J. Biol. Chem., 120*:515 (1970).
100. W. E. Knox and W. I. Grossman, *J. Biol. Chem., 168*:363 (1947).
101. M. L. WuChang and B. Connor-Johnson, *J. Biol. Chem., 234*:1817 (1959).
102. M. L. WuChang and B. Connor-Johnson, *J. Biol. Chem., 236*:2096 (1961).
103. M. L. WuChang and B. Connor-Jonnson, *J. Nutr., 76*:512 (1962).
104. Y. C. Lee, R. K. Sholson, and N.Raica, *J. Biol. Chem., 244*:3277 (1969).
105. J. G. Prinsloo, J. P. DuPlessis, H. Kinger, D. J. DeLange, and L. S. de Villier, *Am. J. Clin. Nutr., 21*:98 (1968).
106. E. I. Frazier, M. E. Prather, and E. Hoene, *J. Nutr., 56*:501 (1955).
107. J. Preiss and P. Handler, *J. Biol. Chem., 233*:488 (1958).
108. J. W. Rowen and A. Kornberg, *J. Biol Chem., 193*:497 (1951).
109. J. van Eys, *J. Bacteriol. 80*:386 (1960).
110. A. J. Andreoli, T. W. Okita, R. Bloom, and T. A. Grover, *Biochem. Biophys. Res Comm., 12*:92 (1963).
111. N. O. Kaplan, A. Goldin, S. R. Humphreys, M. M. Ciotti, and F. E. Stolzenbach, *J. Biol. Chem., 219*:287 (1956).
112. S. Chaykin, M. Dagani, L. Johnson, and M. Samli, *J. Biol. Chem., 240*:932 (1965).
113. S. Chaykin, M. Dagani, L. Johnson, M. Samli, and J. Bataile, *J. Biochim. Biophys. Act., 100*:351 (1965).
114. C. Bernofsky, *Mol. Cel. Biochem., 33*:135 (1980).
115. D. A. Gardner, G. H. Sato, and N. O. Kaplan, *Develop. Biol., 28*:84 (1972).
116. R. R. Langner, and C. P. Berg, *J. Biol. Chem., 214*:699 (1955).
117. W. C. Rose, W. J. Haines, and D. T. Warner, *J. Biol. Chem., 206*:421 (1954).
118. V. R. Young, M. A. Hussein, E. Murray, and N. S. Scrimshaw, *J. Nutr., 101*:45 (1971).
119. R. M. Leverton, N. Johnson, L. Pazur, and J. Ellison, *J. Nutr., 58*:219 (1956).

120. A. A. Albanese, J. E. Frankston, and V. Irby, *J. Biol. Chem.*, *100*:31 (1945).

121. S. E. Synderman, A. Boyer, S. V. Phansalkar, and L. E. Holt, Jr., *Am. J. Dis. Child*, *102*:163 (1961).

122. I. Nakagawa, T. Takahashi, T. Suzuki, and K. Kobayashi, *J. Nutr.*, *80*:305 (1963).

123. L. E. Holt, Jr., A. A. Albanese, J. E. Frankston, and V. Irby, *Bull. Johns Hopkins Hosp.*, *75*:353 (1944).

124. M. Womack and W. C. Rose, *J. Biol. Chem.*, *171*:37 (1947).

125. H. R. Baldin and C. P. Berg, *J. Nutr.*, *39*:203 (1949).

126. H. Fisher, M. K., Brush, and P. Griminger, *Am. J. Clin. Nutr.*, *22*:1190 (1969).

127. K. Tonsirin, V. R. Young, M. Miller, and N. S. Scrimshaw, *J. Nutr.* *103*:1220 (1973).

128. G. A. Goldsmith, O. A. Miller, and W. G. Unglaub, *Fed. Proc.* *15*:553 (1956).

129. G. A. Goldsmith, *Am. J. Clin. Nutr.*, *6*:479 (1958).

130. G. A. Goldsmith, O. N. Miller, and W. G. Unglaub, *J. Nutr.*, *73*:172 (1961).

131. M. K. Horwitt, C. C. Harvey, W. S. Rothwell, J. L. Cutler, and D. Haffron, *J. Nutr.*, *60* (Suppl. 1):*43* (1956).

132. V. M. Vivian, *J. Nutr.*, *82*:395 (1964).

133. C. F. Consolazio, H. L. Johnson, H. J. Krzywick, and N. F. Witt. *Am. J. Clin. Nutr.*, *25*:572 (1972).

134. G. A. Goldsmith, H. P. Sarett, U. D. Register and T. Gibbens, *J. Clin. Invest*, *31*:533 (1952).

135. G. A. Goldsmith, H. L. Rosenthal, J. Gibbens, and W. G. Unglaub, *J., Nutr.*, *56*:371 (1955).

136. G. A. Goldsmith, J. Gibbens, Unglaub, W. G., and O. N. Miller, *Am. J. Clin. Nutr.*, *4*:151 (1956).

137. G. A. Goldsmith, *Am. J. Diet, Assn*, *32*:312 (1956).

138. L. E., Holt, Jr. *Arch. Dis. Child*, *31*:427 (1956).

139. K. U. G. Toverd, G. Stearns, and I. G. Macy, in *National Research Council Bull.*, *123*: Nat. Acad. Sci., Washington, D.C.

140. A. M. Wertz, M. B. Derby, P. K. Ruttenberg, and G. P. French, *J. Nutr.*, *68*:583 (1959).

141. W. J. Darby, W. J. McGannity, M. P. Martin, E. Bridgforth, P., M. Densen, M. M. Kaser, P. J. Ogle, J A. Newbill, A. Stockwell, M. E. Ferguson, O. Touster, G. S. McClellan, C. Williams, and R. O. Cannon, *J. Nutr.* *51*:565 (1953).

142. National Research Council, *Nutrient Requirements of Domestic Animals, No. 1. Nutrient Requirements of Poultry,* 6th rev. ed. National Academy of Science Washington, D.C., 1971.

143. L. M. Henderson and P. B. Swan, in *Methods in Enzymology*, Vol. XVIII, D. B. McCormick and L. D. Wright (Eds.)., Academic Press, New York, 1962, p. 1974.

144. R. N. DiLorenzo, Ph.D. thesis, Cornell University, Ithaca, New York, 1972.

145. W. D. Salmon, *Am. J. Clin. Nutr.*, *6*:487 (1958).

146. G. Gopalan and K. S. J. Rao, *Vitamins and Hormones*, *33*:505 (1970).

147. T. P. Spies, in *Clinical Nutrition*, N. Joliffe, F. F. Tizdall, and P. R. Cannon (Eds.), Hoeber, New York, 1950, p. 531.

148. A. C. DaSilva, R. Fried, and R. C. DeAngelis, *J. Nutr.*, *46*:399 (1952).

149. R. E. Coggeshall and P. D. MacLean, *Proc. Soc. Expt. Biol. Med.*, *98*:687 (1958).

150. S. P. Higgs, *Am. J. Path.*, *31*:189 (1955).

151. R. E. Coggeshall and P. D. MacLean, *Proc. Soc. Expt. Biol. Med.*, *52*:106 (1943).

152. R. Altschul, A. Hoffer, and J. D. Stephen, *Arch. Biochem. Biophys.*, *54*:588 (1955).

153. J. Shepperd, C. J. Packard, J. R. Patsch, A. M. Gotto, Jr., and O. D. Taunton, *J. Clin. Invest.* *63*:858 (1979).

154. R. Altschul, Niacin, in *Vascular Disorders and Hyperlipidemia*, C. C. Thomas, Springfield, Ill., 1964.

155. N. Svedmyr, L. Harton, and L. Lundholm, *Clin. Pharmacol. Ther.*, *10*:559 (1969).

156. R. G. G. Andersson, G. Aberg, R. Brattsand, E. Ericsson, and L. Lundholm, *Acta Pharmacol. Toxicol.*, *41*:1 (1977).

157. M. Weiner, K. deKrinis, W. Redisch, and J. M. Steele, *Proc. Soc. Exp. Biol. Med., 98*:755 (1958).
158. P. Meneghini and F. Piccinini, *Arch. E. Maragliano Patol. Clin, 14*:69 (1958).
159. M. Weiner, W. Redisch, and K. deKrinis, *Proc. 7th Cong. Eur. Soc. Haematol. Lond. Part II*:890 (1960).
160. D. R. Rosing, D. R. Redwood, P. Brakman, T. Astrup, and S. E. Epstein, *Thrombosis Res., 13*:419 (1978).
161. M. Weiner, *Am. J. Med. Sci., 246*:79 (1963).
162. W. Redisch and O. Brandman, *Angiology, 1*:312 (1950).
163. *AMA Drug Evaluations*, 3d ed., Publishing Sciences Group, Littleton, Mass., 1977.
164. L. Landholm, L. Jacobson, R. Brattsand, and O. Magnusson, *Atherosclerosis, 29*:217 (1978).
165. H. I. Kaplan, A. M. Freedman, and B. J. Sadock, *Comprehensive Textbook of Psychiatry*, 3rd Ed., Williams & Wilkins, Baltimore, 1980.
166. W. M. Petrie and T. A. Ban, *Drugs, 30*:58 (1975).
167. Y. Waterlot, J. P. Sabot, M. Marchal, J. L. Vanherweghem, *Nephrol Dial. Transplant, 1*:204 (1986).
168. P. Handler and W. J. Dann, *J. Biol. Chem., 146*:357 (1943).
169. F. G. Brozda and R. A. Coulson, *Proc. Soc. Exp. Biol. Med., 62*:19 (1946).
170. A. A. Rossini, N. A. Like, W. L. Chick, M. C. Appel, and G. F. Cahill, *Proc. Natl. Acad. Sci. USA, 74*:2485 (1977).
171. T. Kazumi, G. Yoshino, S. Fujii, and S. Baba, *Cancer Res., 38*:2144 (1978).
172. T. Kazumi, G. Yoshino, Y. Yoshida, K. Doi, M. Yoshida, S. Kaneko, and S. Baba, *Endocrinol., 103*:1541 (1978).
173. G. Calcutt, S. W. Ting, and A. W. Preece, *Brit. J. Cancer, 24*:380 (1970).
174. T. R. Robie, *J. Schiz., 1*:133 (1967).
175. R. C. Charman, L. B. Matthews, and C. Braeuler, *Angiology, 23*:29 (1972).
176. H. K. Schock, in *Drugs Affecting Lipid Metabolism*, W. L. Holmes, L. H. Carlson, and R. Paoletti, (Eds.), Plenum Press, New York, 1969, p. 405.
177. J. L. S. Holloman, C. G. Davis, and L. C. Leeper, *J. Am. Geriatr. Soc., 10*:903 (1962).
178. Coronary Drug Project Research Group, *JAMA, 231*:360 (1975).
179. R. H. Jones, *Adv. Exp. Med. Biol., 82*:656 (1977).
180. G. L. Clementz, A. W. Holmes, *J. Clin. Gastroenterol., 9*:582 (1987).
181. G. M. McGreanor, D. A. Bender, *Brit. J. Nutr., 56*:577 (1986).

9
Vitamin B$_6$

James E. Leklem
Oregon State University
Corvallis, Oregon

I. INTRODUCTION AND HISTORY

Vitamin B_6 is unique among the water-soluble vitamins with respect to the numerous functions it serves and its metabolism and chemistry. Within the past few years the attention this vitamin has received has increased dramatically (1–7). A recent lay publication (8) has also focused on vitamin B_6.

This chapter will provide an overview of vitamin B_6 as related to human nutrition. Both qualitative and quantitative information will be provided in an attempt to indicate the importance of this vitamin within the context of health and diseases of humans. As a nutritionist my perspective no doubt is biased by these nutritional elements of this vitamin. The exhaustive literature on the intriguing chemistry of the vitamin will not be dealt with in any detail, except as related to the function of vitamin B_6 as a coenzyme. To the extent that literature is available, reference will be made to research in humans, and animal or other experimental work included as necessary.

As we approach the end of the second generation of research in vitamin B_6, there may be a tendency to lose the sense of excitement of discovery that Gyorgy and colleagues experienced when they began to unravel the mystery of vitamin B complex. Some of the major highlights of the early years of vitamin B_6 research are presented in Table 1. Paul Gyorgy was first to use the term vitamim B_6 (9). This term was used to distinguish this factor from other hypothetical growth factors B_3, B_4, B_5 (and Y). Some four years later (1938) in what is a fine example of cooperation and friendship, Gyorgy (10) and Lepkovsky (11) reported the isolation of pure crystalline vitamin B_6. Three other groups also reported the isolation of vitamin B_6 that same year (12–14). Shortly after this, Harris and Folkers (15) as well as Kuhn et al. (16) determined that vitamin B_6 was a pyridine derivative and structurally identified it as 3-hydroxy-4,5-dihydroxymethyl-2-methylpyridine. The term pyridoxine was first introduced by Gyorgy (17) in 1939. An important aspect of this early research was the use of animal models in identification of vitamin B_6 (as pyridoxine in various extracts from rice bran and yeast). This early research into vitamin B_6 then provided the groundwork for research into the requirement for vitamin B_6 for humans and the functions of this vitamin.

Identification of the other major forms of the vitamin B_6 group, pyridoxamine and pyridoxal, occurred primarily through the use of microorganisms (18,19). In the process of developing an assay for pyridoxine, Snell and co-workers observed that natural materials were more active in supporting the growth of certain microorganisms than predicted by

Table 1 Historical Highlights of Vitamin B_6 Research

1932	A compound with the formula of $C_3H_{11}O_3N$ was isolated from rice polishings.
1934	Gyorgy shows there was a difference between the rat pellagra preventive factor and vitamin B_2. He called this vitamin B_6.
1938	Lepkovsy reports isolation of pure crystalline vitamin B_6. Keresztesky and Stevens, Gyorgy, Kuhn and Wendt, and Ichibad and Michi also report isolation of vitamin B_6.
1939	Chemical structure determined and vitamin B_6 synthesized by Kuhn and associates and by Harris and Folkers.
1942	Snell and co-workers recognize existence of other forms of pyridoxine.
1953	Snyderman and associates observe convulsions in an infant and anemia in an older child fed a vitamin B_6–deficient diet.

their pyridoxine content as assayed with yeast (19). Subsequently, this group observed enhanced growth-promoting activity in the urine of vitamin B$_6$–deficient animals fed pyridoxine (19). Treatment of pyridoxine with ammonia also produced a substance with growth activity (20). These findings subsequently led to the synthesis of pyridoxal and pyridoxamine (21,22). With the availability of these three forms of vitamin B$_6$ further research into this intriguing vitamin was then possible.

II. CHEMISTRY

Since Gyorgy first coined the term vitamin B$_6$ (9), there has been confusion in the terminology of the multiple forms of the vitamin. Vitamin B$_6$ is the recommended term for the generic descriptor for all 3-hydroxy-2-methylpyridine derivatives (23). Figure 1 depicts the various forms of vitamin B$_6$, including the phosphorylated forms. Pyridoxine (once referred to as pyridoxal) is the alcohol form and should not be used as a generic name for vitamin B$_6$. The trivial names and abbreviations commonly used for the three principal forms of vitamin B$_6$, their phosphoric esters, and analogues are as follows: pyridoxine, PN; pyridoxal, PL; pyridoxamine, PM; pyridoxine 5'-phosphate, PNP; pyridoxal 5'-phosphate, PLP; pyridoxamine 5'-phosphate, PMP; 4-pyridoxic acid, 4-PA. As will be discussed later, other forms of vitamin B$_6$ exist, particularly bound forms.

The various physical and chemical properties of the phosphorylated and non-phosphorylated forms of vitamin B$_6$ are given in Table 2. Detailed data on flourescence (27) and ultraviolet (26) absorption characteristics of B$_6$ vitamers are available. Of importance to researchers and also to food producers and consumers is the relative stability of the forms of vitamin B$_6$. Generally, as a group B$_6$ vitamers are considerable labile, but the degree to which each is degraded varies. In solution the forms are light sensitive (24,28), but this sensitivity is influenced by pH. Pyridoxine, pyridoxal and pyridoxamine are relatively heat-stable in an acid medium, but they are heat-labile in an alkaline medium. The hydrochloride and base forms are readily soluble in water, but they are minimally soluble in organic solvents.

The coenzyme form of vitamin B$_6$, PLP, is found covalently bound to enzymes via a Schiff base with an ε-amino group of lysine in the enzyme. While nonenzymatic reactions with PLP or PL and metal ions can occur (29), in enzymatic reactions the amino group of the substrate for the given enzyme forms a Schiff base via a transimination reaction. Figure 2 depicts the formation of a Schiff base with PLP and an amino acid. Because of the strong electron-attracting character of the pyridine ring, electrons are withdrawn

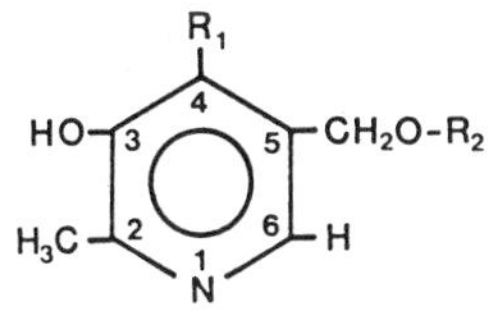

PN ; R$_1$= CH$_2$OH   PNP ; R$_2$=PO$_3^=$
PM ; R$_1$= CH$_2$NH$_2$ PMP ; R$_2$=PO$_3^=$
PL ; R$_1$= CHO   PLP ; R$_2$=PO$_3^=$

Figure 1 Structure of B$_6$ vitamers.

Table 2 Physical Properties of B$_6$ Vitamers

	Molecular weight	Stability to white light[a] pH 4.5		pk		Fluorescence Maxima[b]		Ultraviolet absorption spectra[e]			
								0.1N HCl		pH 7.0	
		8 hr	15 hr	pk1	pk2	Activation (λ)	Emission (λ)	λ$_{max}$	ε$_{max}$	λ$_{max}$	ε$_{max}$
Pyridoxine	16911	97%	90%	5.0	8.9	325	400	291	8900	254	3760
										324	7100
Pyridoxamine	168.1	81%	57%	3.4	8.1	325	405	293	8500	253	4600
										325	7700
Pyridoxal	167.2	97%	68%	4.2	8.7	320	385	288	9100	317	8800
Pyridoxine 5'-phosphate	249.2	—	—	—	—	322	394	290	8700	253	3700
										325	7400
Pyridoxal 5'-phosphate	248.2	—	—	2.5	3.5	330	400	293	900	253	4700
										325	8300
Pyridoxal 5'-phosphate	247.2	—	—	2.5	4.1	330	375	293	7200	388	5500
								334	1300		
4-Pyridoxic acid	183.2	—	—	—	—	325[c]	425[c]	—	—	—	—
						355[d]	445[d]				

[a]Percent stability compared to solution in dark (24). 8 hr, 15 hr = length of time exposed to light.
[b]From Storvick et al. (25); pH 7.0.
[c]pH 3.4, 0.01 N acetic acid.
[d]pH 10.5, 0.1 N NH$_4$OH, lactone of 4-PA.
[e]Data is for PN·HCL, PL·HCL, PM·2HCL, PLP monohydrate, PMP dihydrate (26).

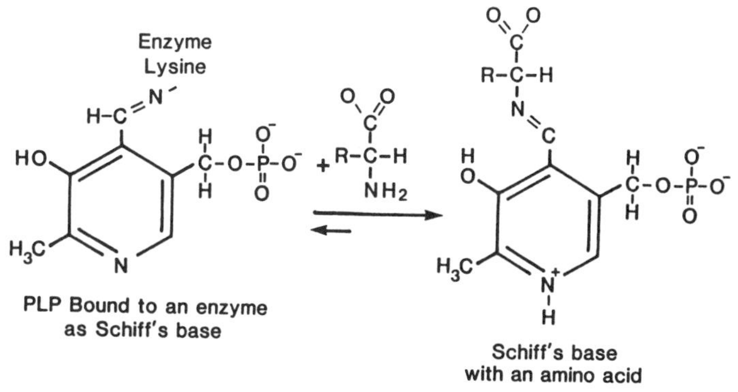

Figure 2 Schiff base formation between pyridoxal-5'-phosphate and an amino acid.

from one of the three substituents (R group, hydrogen, or carboxyl group) attached to the α-carbon of the substrate attached to PLP. This results in the formation of a quinonoid structure. There are several structural features of PLP that make it well suited to form a Schiff base and thus act as a catalyst in a variety of enzyme reactions. These features have been detailed by Leussing (30) and include the 2-methyl group, which brings the pKa of the proton of the ring pyridine closer to the biological range; the phenoxide oxygen (position 3), which aids in expulsion of a nucleophile at the 4 position; the 5'-phosphate group, which functions as an anchor for the coenzyme, prevents hemiacetal formation and the drain of electrons from the ring; and the protonated pyridine nitrogen that is *para* to the aldehyde group aids in delocalizing the negative charge and helps regulate the pKa of the 3-hydroxyl group. A recent publication has extensively reviewed the chemistry of pyridoxal 5'-phosphate (4).

PLP has been reported to be a coenzyme for over 100 enzymatic reactions (31). Of these, nearly half involve transamination-type reactions. Transamination reactions are but one type of reaction which occur as a result of Schiff base formation. The three types of enzyme reactions catalyzed by PLP are listed in Table 3 and are classified according to reactions occurring at the α-, β-, or γ-carbon.

III. OCCURRENCE IN FOODS

To appreciate the function vitamin B$_6$ plays in human nutrition, one must first have knowledge of the various forms and quantities found in foods. A microbiological method for determining the vitamin B$_6$ content of foodstuffs was developed by Atkin in 1943 (32). While this method has been refined (25,33), it still stands as the primary method for determining the total vitamin B$_6$ content of foods and has been the basis for most of the data available on the vitamin B$_6$ content of foods.

There are various forms of vitamin B$_6$ in foods. In general, these forms are some derivative of the three forms: pyridoxal, pyridoxine, and pyridoxamine. Pyridoxine and pyridoxamine (or their respective phosphorylated forms) are the predominant forms in plant foods. Although there are exceptions, pyridoxal, as the phosphorylated form, is the predominant form in animal foods. Table 4 contains data for the vitamin B$_6$ content of a

Table 3 Enzyme Reactions Catalyzed by Pyridoxal 5'-Phosphate

Type of reaction	Typical reaction or enzyme
Reactions involving α-carbon	
Transamination	Alanine $\rightarrow$ pyruvate + PMP
Racemization	D-Amino acid $\rightleftarrows$ L-amino acid
Decarboxylation	5-OH Tryptophan $\rightarrow$ 5-OH tryptamine + CO_2
Oxidative deamination	Histamine $\rightarrow$ imidazole-4-acetaldehyde + NH_4^+
Loss of the side chain	THF + Serine $\rightarrow$ glycine + N5, 10-methylene THF
Reactions involving β-carbon	
Replacement (exchange)	Cysteine synthetase
Elimination	Serine and threonine dehydratase
Reaction involving the γ-carbon	
Replacement (exchange)	Cystathionine $\rightarrow$ cysteine + homoserine
Elimination	Homocysteine desulfhydrase
Cleavage	Kynurenine $\rightarrow$ anthranilic acid

representative sample of food commonly consumed in the United States. Data on the amount of each of the three forms is also listed (34). While the phosphorylated forms are usually the predominant forms in most foods, the microbiological methods used to determine the level of each form measure the sum of the phosphorylated and free (nonconjugated) forms.

In addition to the phosphorylated forms, other conjugated forms have been detected in certain foods. A glycosylated form of pyridoxine has been identified in rice bran (35) and subsequently quantitated in several foods (36). The glycosylated form isolated from rice bran has been identified as 5'-O-(β-D-glucopyranosyl) pyridoxine (37) (Fig. 3). Suzuki et al. have shown that the 5'-glucoside can be formed in germinating seeds of wheat, barley, and rice cultured on a pyridoxine solution (29). In addition a small amount of 4'- glucoside was also detected in wheat and rice germinated seeds, but not in soybean seeds. Also of interest is an as yet unidentified conjugate of vitamin B_6 reported by Tadera and co-workers (38). This conjugate released free vitamin B_6 (measured as pyridoxine) only when the food was treated with alkali and then β-glucosidase. Tadera et al. have also identified another derivative of the 5'-glucoside of pyridoxine in seedlings of podded peas (39). This derivative was identified as 5'-O(6-O-malonyl-β-D-glucopyranosyl) pyridoxine. The role these conjugates play in plants is unknown. Table 5 lists the total vitamin B_6 content of pyridoxine 5'-glucoside content of various foods. There is no generalization that can be made at this time as to a given class of foods having high or low amounts of pyridoxine 5'-glucoside. The effect of the 5'-glucoside of vitamin B_6 nutrition will be addressed in the section on bioavailability and absorption.

Food processing and storage may influence the vitamin B_6 content of food (40–49) and result in production of compounds normally not present. Losses of 10–50% have been reported for a wide variety of foods. Heat sterilization of commercial milk was found to result in conversion of pyridoxal to pyridoxamine (41). Storage of heat-treated milk decreases the vitamin B_6 content presumably due to formation of bis-4-pyridoxyl-disulfide. The effect of various processes on vitamin B_6 content of milk and milk products has been reviewed (49). Losses range from 0 to 70%. Vanderslice et al. have reported an HPLC method for assessing the various forms of vitamin B_6 in milk (50) which should aid in understanding effects of processing on vitamin B_6 content of milk and milk products.

Table 4 Vitamin B$_6$ Content of Selected Foods and Percentages of the Three Forms

Food	Vitamin B$_6$[a] (mg/100 g)	Pyridoxine[b] (%)	Pyridoxal (%)	Pyridoxamine (%)
Vegetables				
Beans lima, frozen	0.150	45	30	25
Cabbage, raw	0.160	61	31	8
Carrots, raw	0.150	75	19	6
Peas, green, raw	0.160	47	47	6
Potatoes, raw	0.250	68	18	14
Tomatoes, raw	0.100	38	29	33
Spinach, raw	0.280	36	49	15
Broccoli, raw	0.195	29	65	6
Cauliflower, raw	0.210	16	79	5
Corn, sweet	0.161	6	68	26
Fruits				
Apples, red delicious	0.030	61	31	8
Apricots, raw	0.070	58	20	22
Apricots, dried	0.169	81	11	8
Avocados, raw	0.420	56	29	15
Bananas, raw	0.510	61	10	29
Oranges, raw	0.060	59	26	15
Peaches, canned	0.019	61	30	9
Raisins, seedless	0.240	83	11	6
Grapefruit, raw	0.034	—	—	—
Legumes				
Beans, white, raw	0.560	62	20	18
Beans, lima, canned	0.090	75	15	10
Lentils	0.600	69	13	18
Peanut butter	0.330	74	9	17
Peas, green, raw	0.160	69	17	14
Soybeans, dry, raw	0.810	44	44	12
Nuts				
Almonds, without skins, shelled	0.100	52	28	20
Pecans	0.183	71	12	17
Filberts	0.545	29	68	3
Walnuts	0.730	31	65	4
Cereals/Grains				
Barley, pearled	0.224	52	42	6
Rice, brown	0.550	78	12	10
Rice, white, regular	0.170	64	19	17
Rye flour, light	0.090	64	22	14
Wheat, cereal, flakes	0.292	79	11	10
Wheat flour, whole	0.340	71	16	13
Wheat flour, all purpose white	0.060	55	24	21
Oatmeal, dry	0.140	12	49	39
Cornmeal, white and yellow	0.250	11	51	38
	—	—	—	—
Bread, white	0.040	—	—	—
Bread, whole wheat	0.180	—	—	—

(continued)

Table 4 *(continued)*

Food	Vitamin B$_6$[a] (mg/100 g)	Pyridoxine[b] (%)	Pyridoxal (%)	Pyridoxamine (%)
Meat/Poultry/Fish				
Beef, raw	0.330	16	53	31
Chicken breast	0.683	7	74	19
Pork, ham, canned	0.320	8	8	84
Flounder fillet	0.170	7	71	22
Salmon, canned	0.300	2	9	89
Sardine, Pacific				
canned, oil	0.280	13	58	29
Tuna, canned	0.425	19	69	12
Halibut	0.430	—	—	—
Milk/Eggs/Cheese				
Milk, cow, homogenized	0.040	3	76	21
Milk, human	0.010	0	50	50
Cheddar	0.080	4	8	88
Egg, whole	0.110	0	85	15

[a]Values from Ref. 34, Table 1.
[b]Values from Ref. 34, Table 2.

DeRitter (51) has reviewed the stability of several vitamins in processed foods, including vitamin B$_6$, and found that the vitamin B$_6$ added to flour and baked into bread is stable. This has been confirmed by Perera et al. (52).

Gregory and Kirk have found that during thermal processing (53) and low-moisture conditions of storage of foods (46), there is reductive binding of pyridoxal and pyridoxal 5′-phosphate to the ε-amino groups of protein or peptide lysyl residues. These compounds are resistant to hydrolysis and also posses low vitamin B$_6$ activity. Interestingly, Gregory (54) has shown that ε-pyridoxyllysine bound to dietary protein has anti-vitamin B$_6$ activity (50% molar vitamin B$_6$ activity for rats).

Another reaction that could compromise the amount of biologically available vitamin B$_6$ is the conversion of pyridoxine to 6-hydroxypyridoxine in the presence of ascorbic acid (52). Food high in vitamin C as spinach, sweet peppers, potatoes, tomatoes, and strawberries when incubated with pyridoxine resulted in the formation of this 6-hydroxy compound. The extent to which this reaction occurs in foods under various processing conditions remains to be determined.

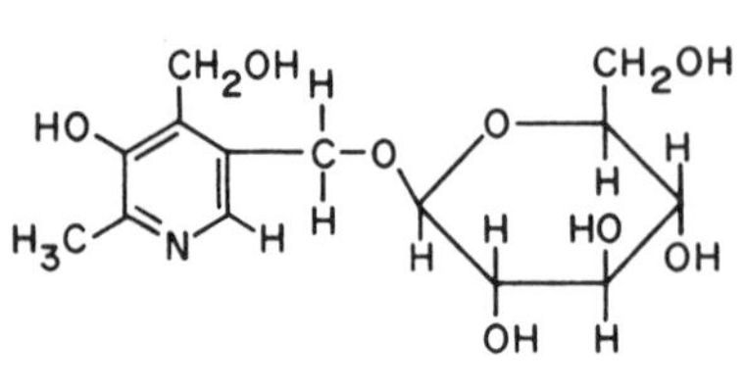

Figure 3 Structure of 5′-O-(β-D-glucopyranosyl) pyridoxine.

Table 5   Vitamin B$_6$ and Glycosylated Vitamin B$_6$ Content of Selected Foods

Food	Vitamin B$_6$ (mg/100 g)	Glycosylated vitamin B$_6$ (mg/100 g)
Vegetables		
Carrots, canned	0.064	0.055
Carrots, raw	0.170	0.087
Cauliflower, frozen	0.084	0.069
Broccoli, frozen	0.119	0.078
Spinach, frozen	0.208	0.104
Cabbage, raw	0.140	0.065
Sprouts, alfalfa	0.250	0.105
Potatoes, cooked	0.394	0.165
Potatoes, dried	0.884	0.286
Beets, canned	0.018	0.005
Yams, canned	0.067	0.007
Beans/Legumes		
Soybeans, cooked	0.627	0.357
Beans, navy, cooked	0.381	0.159
Beans, lima, frozen	0.106	0.039
Peas, frozen	0.122	0.018
Peanut butter	0.302	0.054
Beans, garbanzo	0.653	0.111
Lentils	0.289	0.134
Animal products		
Beef, ground, cooked	0.263	n.d.
Tuna, canned	0.316	n.d.
Chicken breast, raw	0.700	n.d.
Milk, skim	0.005	n.d.
Nuts/Seeds		
Walnuts	0.535	0.038
Filberts	0.587	0.026
Cashews, raw	0.351	0.046
Sunflower seeds	0.997	0.355
Almonds	0.086	-0-
Fruits		
Orange juice, frozen concentrate	0.165	0.078
Orange juice, fresh	0.043	0.016
Tomato juice, canned	0.097	0.045
Blueberries, frozen	0.046	0.019
Banana	0.313	0.010
Banana, dried chips	0.271	0.024
Pineapple, canned	0.079	0.017
Peaches, canned	0.009	0.002
Apricots, dried	0.206	0.036
Avocado	0.443	0.015
Raisins, seedless	0.230	0.154
Cereals/Grains		
Wheat bran	0.903	0.326
Shredded wheat, cereal	0.313	0.087
Rice, brown	0.237	0.055

(continued)

Table 5 *(continued)*

Food	Vitamin B$_6$ (mg/100 g)	Glycosylated vitamin B$_6$ (mg/100 g)
Cereals/Grains (continued)		
Rice, bran	3.515	0.153
Rice, white	0.076	0.015
Rice cereal, puffed	0.098	0.007
Rice cereal, fortified	3.635	0.382

n.d. = none detected.
Sources: Ref. 36 and Leklem and Hardin, unpublished.

IV. ABSORPTION AND BIOAVAILABILITY

The question of how much vitamin B$_6$ is biologically available (i.e, absorbed and utilizable) and factors that influence this is important in terms of estimating a dietary requirement. Before considering the factors that influence bioavailability, a brief description of absorption of the forms of vitamin B$_6$ is appropriate.

Absorption of the various forms of vitamin B$_6$ has been studied most extensively in animals, particularly rats. However, gastrointestinal absorption of pyridoxine has been examined with guinea pig jejunum preparations (56), intestine, cecum, and crop of the chicken (57), and intestine of the hamster (58).

In the rat, Middleton (58–60) and Henderson and co-workers (61) have conducted extensive research on intestinal absorpton of B$_6$ vitamers. The evidence to date indicates that pyridoxine and the other two major forms of vitamin B$_6$ are absorbed by a nonsaturable, passive process (61). Absorption of the phosphorylated forms can occur (62,63), but to a very limited extent. The phosphorylated forms disappear from the intestine via hydrolysis by alkaline phosphatase (60,63), and a significant part of this takes place intraluminally. Prior intake of vitamin B$_6$ in rats over a wide range (0.75–100 mg PH•HCl per kg diet) was found to have no affect on in vitro absorption of varying levels of PN•HCl (64). This study provides further support for passive absorption of B$_6$ vitamers. However, Middelton has recently questioned the concept of a nonsaturable process (65). Using an in vivo perfused intestinal segment model, he found there was a gradient of decreasing rates of uptake from the proximal to the distal end of the intestine and that there was a saturable component of uptake, especially in the duodenum.

The various forms of vitamin B$_6$ that are absorbed into the rat intestinal cell (intracellular) can be converted to other forms (i.e., PL to PLP, PN to PLP, and PM to PLP), but that which is ultimately transported to other organs via the circulation system primarily reflects the nonphosphorylated form originally absorbed (62,63). A similar pattern of uptake and metabolism has been observed in mice (66), however, in mice given PN, pyridoxal was the major form detected in the circulation. Portal blood was not examined. The liver was likely the primary organ that further metabolized the PN absorbed and released PL to the circulation.

Bioavailability of a nutrient from a given food is important to an organism in that it is the amount of a nutrient that is both absorbed and available to cells. The word *available* is key here in that the vitamin may not be needed by the cell and simply excreted or metabolized to a nonutilizable form such as 4-pyridoxic acid in the case of vitamin B_6.

Methods used to evaluate the bioavailability of nutrients such as vitamin B_6 include balance studies in which input and output are determined. A second approach is to measure an in vivo response such as growth after a state of deficiency has been created. The third type of study is the examination of blood levels of the nutrient or a metabolite of the nutrient over a specified period of time after a food is fed. The concentration of a metabolite, such as PLP, is then compared with concentrations after ingestion of graded amounts of the crystalline form of vitamin B_6. Gregory and Ink (67) and Leklem (68) have reviewed vitamin B_6 bioavailability.

One of the early studies which suggested a reduced availability of vitamin B_6 involved feeding canned combat rations which had been stored at elevated temperatures (69). Feeding diets containing 1.9 mg of total vitamin B_6 resulted in a marginal deficiency based on urinary excretion of tryptophan metabolites. Some 18 years later Nelson et al. observed that the vitamin B_6 in orange juice was incompletely absorbed by humans (70). These authors suggested that a low molecular weight form of vitamin B_6 was present in orange juice and responsible for the reduced availability. Kabir and co-workers (36) have subsequently found that approximately 50% of the vitamin B_6 present in orange juice is the pyridoxine $5'$-β-glucoside.

Leklem et al. conducted one of the first human studies which directly determined bioavailability of vitamin B_6 (71). In their study, nine men were fed either whole wheat bread, white bread enriched with pryidoxine (0.8 mg), or white bread plus a solution containing 0.8 mg of pyridoxine. After feeding each bread for a week, urinary vitamin B_6 and 4-pyridoxic and fecal vitamin B_6 excretion were measured to asses vitamin B_6 bioavailability. Urinary 4-pyridoxic acid excretion was reduced when whole wheat bread was fed compared to the other two test situations, and the vitamin B_6 from this bread was estimated to be 5–10% less available than the vitamin B_6 from the other two breads. While this relatively small difference in bioavailability may not be nutritionally significant by itself, in combination with other foods of low vitamin B_6 bioavailability, vitamin B_6 status may be compromised.

In other studies in humans, feeding 15 g of cooked wheat bran slightly reduced vitamin B_6 bioavailability (72). Using urinary vitamin B_6 as the sole criterion, Kies and co-workers estimated that 20 g of wheat, rice, or corn bran reduced vitamin B_6 availability 35–40% (73). Since various brans are good sources of vitamin B_6, it is not possible to determine if the vitamin B_6 in the bran itself was unavailable or if the bran may have been binding vitamin B_6 present in the remainder of the diet.

The bioavailability of vitamin B_6 from specific foods or groups of foods has been examined utilizing balance and blood levels (dose response) studies. Tarr et al. estimated a 71–79% bioavailability of vitamin B_6 from foods representing the "average" American diet (74). Using a triple lumen tube perfusion technique, Nelson et al. found that the vitamin B_6 from orange juice was only 50% as well absorbed as crystalline pyridoxine (75). In my laboratory, a study comparing bioavailability of vitamin B_6 from beef and soybeans showed that the vitamin B_6 in soybeans was 6–7% less available than the vitamin B_6 in beef (76). Also in our laboratory, Kabir et al. compared the vitamin B_6 bioavailability from tuna, whole wheat bread, and peanut butter (77). A balance approach was used in which one-half of the vitamin B_6 intake was from the respective food. Compared to the vitamin B_6 in tuna, the vitamin B_6 in whole wheat bread and peanut butter was 75 and 63% as available, respectively. The level of glycosylated vitamin B_6 in these foods was inversely correlated with vitamin B_6 bioavailability as based on urinary vitamin B_6 and 4-pyridoxic acid (78). More recently we have observed an inverse relationship between vitamin B_6 bioavailability as based on urinary 4-pyridoxic acid excretion and the glycosylated vitamin B_6 content of six foods (79). These foods and the respective availabilities were walnuts (78%), bananas (79%), tomato juice (25%), spinach (22%), orange juice (9%), and carrots (0%). While the glycosylated vitamin B_6 content of foods appears to be a significant contributor to bioavailability, the presence of other forms of vitamin B_6 and/or binding of specific forms of vitamin B_6 to other components in a food may also contribute to availability. The difference in bioavailability we observed for orange juice (9%) as compared with the 50% observed by Nelson et al. (75) is probably due to the different methods used to determine bioavailability.

V. INTERORGAN METABOLISM

Extensive work by Lumeng and Li and co-workers in rats (80) and dogs (81) has shown that the liver is the primary organ responsible for metabolism of vitamin B_6 and supplies the active form of vitamin B_6, PLP, to the circulation and other tissues. The primary interconversion of the B_6 vitamers is depicted in Figure 4. The three nonphosphoryalted forms are converted to their respective phosphorylated forms by a kinase enzyme

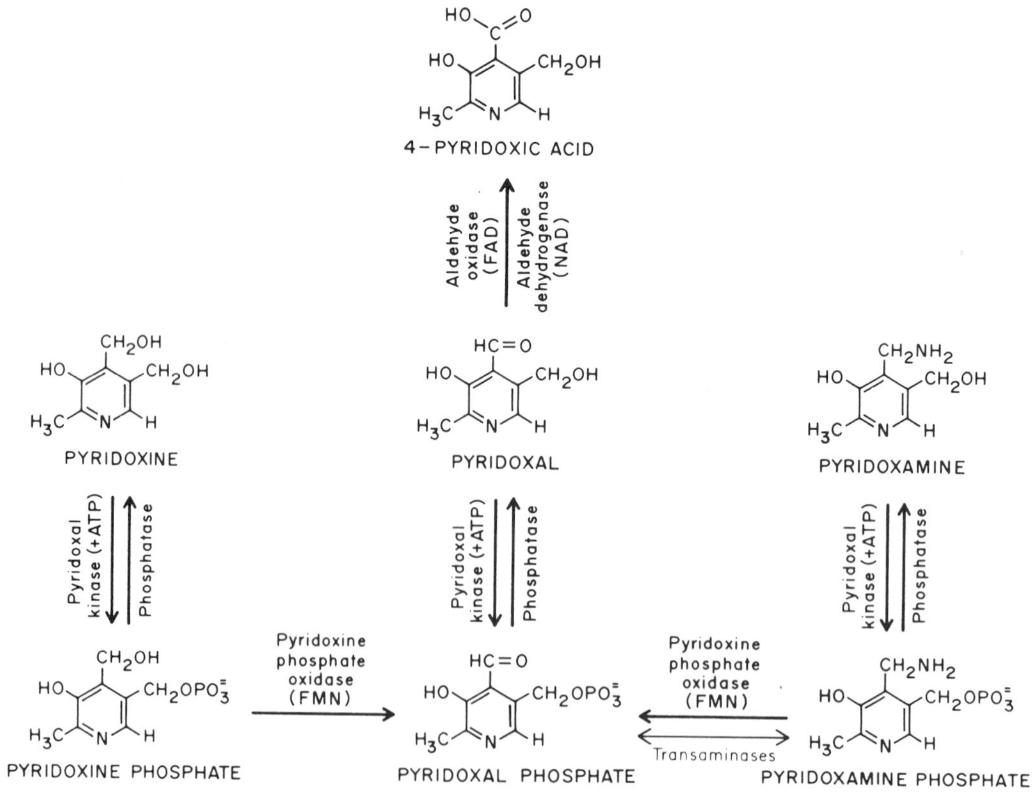

Figure 4 Metabolic interconversions of the B_6 vitamers.

(pyridoxine kinase EC2.7.1.35). Both ATP and zinc are involved in this conversion, with ATP serving as a source of the phosphate group. The two phosphorylated forms, pyridoxamine-5′-phosphate and pyridoxine-5′-phosphate, are converted to PLP via a flavin mononucleoticle (FMN) requiring oxidase (82).

Dephosphorylation of the 5′-phosphate compounds occurs by action of a phosphatase. This phosphatase is considered to be alkaline phosphatase (83) and is thought to be enzyme bound in the liver (84). PL arising from dephosphorylation or that taken up from the circulation can be converted to 4-pyridoxic acid by either an NAD-dependent dehydrogenase or a FAD-dependent aldehyde oxidase. As discussed below, in humans only aldehyde oxidase (pyridoxal oxidase) activity has been detected in human liver (85). The conversion of pyridoxal to 4-pyridoxic acid is an irreversible reaction. Thus, 4-pyridoxic acid is an end product of vitamin B$_6$ metabolism. A majority of ingested vitamin B$_6$ is converted to 4-pyridoxic acid (86–88).

The interconversion of vitamin B$_6$ vitamers in human liver has been extensively studied by Merrill et al. (85,89). While only five subjects were examined, this study provides the first detailed work in humans on the activities of enzymes involved in vitamin B$_6$ metabolism. The activities of pyridoxal kinase, pyridoxine (pyridoxamine) 5′-phosphate oxidase, PLP phosphatase, and pyridoxal oxidase are summarized in Table 6. These activities are optimal activities and, as Merrill et al. have pointed out, at the physiological pH of 7.0 pyridoxal phosphatase activity was less than 1% of the optimal activity at pH 9.0. Considering this, the kinase reaction would be favored and, hence, formation of PLP. The kinase enzyme is a zinc-requiring enzyme. The limiting enzyme in the vitamin B$_6$ pathway appears to be pyridoxine-5′-phosphate oxidase. Since this enzyme requires FMN (82), a reduced riboflavin status may affect the conversion of PN and PM to PLP. Unfortunately there are no in vivo studies in humans which have directly examined this relationship. Lakshmi and Bamji have reported that whole blood PLP in persons with oral lesions (presumably riboflavin deficiency) were normal, and supplemental riboflavin had no significant effect on these levels (90). In studies of red cell metabolism of vitamin B$_6$, Anderson and coworkers have shown that riboflavin increases the conversion rate of pyridoxine to PLP (91).

Another riboflavin-dependent (FAD) enzyme, aldehyde oxidase (pyridoxal oxidase), was suggested by Merrill et al. (85) to be the enzyme that converts pyridoxal to 4-pyridoxic acid. The activity of the aldehyde (pyridoxal) oxidase in humans appears to be sufficient so that PL which arises from hydrolysis of PLP or that which is taken up into liver would be readily converted to 4-pyridoxic acid. Such a mechanism may prevent large amounts of the highly reactive PLP from accumulating.

The PLP that is formed in liver (and other tissues) can bind via a Schiff base reaction with proteins. The binding of PLP to proteins may be the predominant factor influencing

Table 6 Activity of Human Liver Enzymes Involved in Vitamin B$_6$ Metabolism

Enzyme (activity)	Per mg protein	Per g liver
Pyridoxal kinase (nmol/min)	0.16 ± 0.05	11.2 ± 3.6
Pyridoxine-P-oxidase (pmol/min)	0.64 ± 0.22	47 ± 19
Pyridoxal-P-phosphatase (nmol/min)	4.0 ± 3.2	272 ± 183
Pyridoxal oxidase (nmol/min)	0.37 ± 0.24	28 ± 20

Source: Ref. 85.

tissue levels of PLP (84,92). This binding of PLP to proteins is thought to result in metabolic trapping PLP (vitamin B_6) in cells (80,84). PLP synthesized in liver cells is released and found bound to albumin. Whether the PLP is bound to albumin prior to release from the liver or released unbound and subsequently binds to albumin has not been determined.

The binding of PLP to albumin in the circulation serves to protect it from hydrolysis and allows for the delivery of PLP to other tissues. This delivery process of PLP to other tissues is thought to involve hydrolysis of PLP and subsequent uptake of PL into the cell. Hydrolysis occurs by action of phosphatases bound to cellular membranes. Other forms of vitamin B_6 are present in the circulation (plasma). Under fasting conditions, the two aldehyde forms comprise 70–90% of the total B_6 vitamers in plasma, with PLP making up 50–75% of the total (Table 7). The next most abundant forms are PN, PMP, and PM. Interestingly, pyridoxine-5'-phosphate is essentially absent in plasma.

Within the circulating fluid (primarily blood), the erythrocyte also appears to play an important role in the metabolism and transport of vitamin B_6. However, the extent of these roles remains controversial (5,95). Both PN and PL are rapidly taken up by a simple diffusion process (96). In the erythrocytes of humans, PL and PN are converted to PLP since both kinase and oxidase activity are present (96). The PLP formed can then be converted to PL by the action of phosphatase, however, this may not be quantitatively important because the phosphatase is considered to be membrane bound. Any role that the erythrocyte might play in transport of vitamin B_6 is complicated by the tight binding of both PLP and PL to hemoglobin (97,98). PL does not bind as tightly as PLP, and each is bound at distinct sites (99). In comparison to the binding to albumin, PL is bound more tightly to hemoglobin (5). As a result, the PL concentration in the erythrocyte is up to four to five times greater than that in plasma (100).

The PLP and PL in plasma as well as perhaps the PL in erythrocytes represent the major B_6 vitamers available to tissues. To a limited extent, PN would be available following a meal if the uptake was high enough and if the PN escaped metabolism in the liver. Another situation in which PN would be available is following ingestion of vitamin B_6 supplements (primarily as PN· HCl). While PN can be converted to PNP in most tissues, conversion to PLP does not take place in many tissues because the oxidase enzyme is absent (101). Since muscle tissue is not capable of converting PN or PM to PLP, pyridoxal is the only form that serves as a source of PLP.

Table 7 B_6 Vitamers in Plasma

	PLP	PL	PNP	PN	PMP	PM
			(nmol/l)			
Coburn ($n = 38$)[a]	57	23	0	19	8	2
	±26	±10		±33	±8	±2
Lumeng ($n = 6$)[b]	62	13	n.d.	32	3	6
	±11	± 4		± 7	±3	±1
Hollins ($n = 10$)[c]	61	5	n.d.	n.d.	n.d.	n.d.
	±34	± 9				

n.d. = none detected.
All data obtained by HPLC methods
[a]From Ref. 92.
[b]From Ref. 93.
[c]From Ref. 94.

A majority of the vitamin B$_6$ in muscle is present as PLP bound to glycogen phosphorylase (102). Coburn et al. calculated that approximately 66 and 69% of the total vitamin B$_6$ in muscle is present as PLP in males and females, respectively (103). Further, they estimated that the total vitamin B$_6$ pool in muscle was 850 and 900 μmol in males and females, respectively. This pool plus the pool of vitamin in other tissues and circulation would thus total about 1 mmol (1000 μmol). Previous estimates of total body pools have been made based on metabolism of a radioactive dose of pyridoxine (104,105). These pools ranged from 100 to 700 μmol.

The precise turnover time of these pools in humans in not known, however, Shane has estimated there are two pools, one with a rapid turnover of about 0.5 days and a second with a slower turnover of 25–33 days (105). Johansson et al. have also shown that the change in blood levels following administration of tritium-labeled pyridoxine was consistent with a two-compartment model (104). Johansson et al. further suggested that the slow turnover compartment was a storage compartment, but they did not determine the nature of this storage compartment. Figure 5 shows a semi-log plot of the decrease in plasma PLP concentration with time in 10 control females and 11 oral contraceptive users fed a diet low in vitamin B$_6$ (0.19 mg, 1.1 μmol) for 4 weeks (86). There was an initial rapid decline in plasma PLP concentration followed by a slower decrease. Extrapolation of the slope for the slow-decreasing portion of the curve for each of the two groups and determination t$_{1/2}$ of the plasma PLP revealed a value of 28 days for the control females and 46 days for the oral contraceptive users. The value for controls is consistent with the data of Shane (105). The longer t$_{1/2}$ for oral contraceptive users may reflect higher levels of enzymes with PLP bound to them (106).

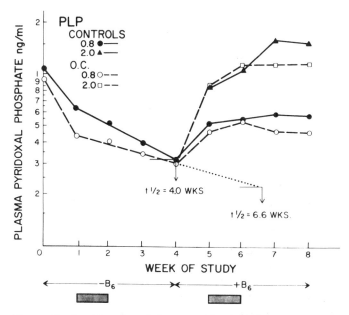

Figure 5 Semi-log plot of plasma pyridoxal-5'-phosphate concentration over 4 weeks of feeding a vitamin B$_6$–deficient diet and 4 weeks of repletion with pyridoxine in control subjects and oral contraceptive users. (From Ref. 86.)

Muscle has been suggested as a possible storage site for vitamin B_6. This is based in part on the vitamin B_6 content of muscle and the total muscle mass of animals. As previously mentioned, in muscle a majority of the vitamin B_6 is present as PLP bound to glycogen phosphorylase (102,103). In contrast, glycogen phosphorylase accounts for only about 10% of the vitamin B_6 content of liver (107). Black and co-workers examined the storage of vitamin B_6 in muscle by studying the activity of muscle glycogen phosphorylase (108). In their studies, Black et al. found that feeding rats a diet high in vitamin B_6 (70 g of vitamin B_6/kg of diet) resulted in a high vitamin B_6 content in muscle and a high glycogen phosphorylase content. This increase in content and enzyme level occurred in concert for 6 weeks whereas the level of alanine and aspartic aminotransferase increased for the first 2 weeks and then plateaued. In subsequent work (109), these same researchers found that muscle phosphorylase content (and thus vitamin B_6 content) decreased only when there was a caloric deficit and not necessarily with a deficiency of vitamin B_6. This observation of muscle not acting as a mobile reservoir during a vitamin B_6 deficiency was also observed in adult swine (110).

In humans, indirect evidence for muscle serving as a vitamin reservoir has come from my laboratory (111). We have observed an increase in plasma PLP concentration during and immediately after exercise (112,113). While some of this increase may be related to a decrease in plasma volume associated with strenuous exercise, a significant amount is not. Strenuous exercise results in a metabolic state of acute caloric deficit and increased need for gluconeogenesis. Thus, the increased circulating levels of PLP following exercise may reflect PLP released from muscle glycogen phosphorylase. Such a mechanism for this release would mean that either PLP must cross the muscle cell membrane or that PLP is hydrolyzed, PL released, and this PL rapidly converted to PLP in liver. Because phosphorylated compounds are thought not to easily cross membranes, the direct release of PLP is not considered likely by some. However, PLP formed in liver is released, and studies of uptake of phosphorylated B_6 vitamers have examined only uptake and not possible transport out of the cell. Further work in my laboratory has shown that in rats starved for 1–3 days there is an increased plasma PLP concentration and an increased PLP concentration in liver, spleen, and heart tissue (unpublished observations). Thus, both direct studies in animals and indirect evidence in humans suggest that vitamin B_6 is stored in muscle and released in times of decreased caloric intake and/or increased need for gluconeogenesis.

VI. ASSESSMENT OF STATUS

The assessment of vitamin B_6 status is central to an understanding of vitamin B_6 nutrition in humans. A variety of methods have been utilized to assess vitamin B_6 status. These methods are given in Table 8 and are divided into direct, indirect, and dietary methods (114,115). Direct indices of vitamin B_6 status are those in which one or more of the B_6 vitamers or the metabolite 4-pyridoxic acid are measured. These are usually measured in plasma, erythrocytes, or urine samples since tissue samples are not normally available. Indirect measures are those in which metabolites of metabolic pathways in which PLP is required for specific enzymes are measured, or in which activities of PLP dependent enzymes are determined. In this latter case an activity coefficient is often determined by measuring the enzyme activity in the presence and absence of excess PLP.

Dietary intake of vitamin B_6 itself is not sufficient to assess vitamin B_6 status, especially if only a few days of diet intake are obtained. In addition to the inherent problems in

Table 8 Methods for Assessing Vitamin B$_6$ Status and Suggested Values for Adequate Status

Index	Suggested value for adequate status
Direct	
Blood	
Plasma pyridoxal-5'-phosphate[a]	>30 nmol/L[a]
Plasma pyridoxal	NV
Plasma total vitamin B$_6$	>40 nmol/L
Erythrocyte pyridoxal-5'-phosphate	NV
Urine	
4-Pyridoxic acid	>3.0 mol/day
Total vitamin B$_6$	>0.5 mol/day
Indirect	
Blood	
Erythrocyte alanine aminotransferase	< 1.25[b]
Erythrocyte aspartic aminotransferase	< 1.80[b]
Urine	
2 g Tryptophan load test; xanthurenic acid	< 65 mol/day
3 g Methionine load test; cystathionine	<350 μmol/day
Oxalate excretion	NV
Diet intake	
Vitamin B$_6$ intake, weekly average	> 1.2-1.5 mg/day
Vitamin B$_6$: protein ratio	> 0.02
Pyridoxine-β-glucoside	NV
Other	
Electroencephalogram pattern	NV

[a]Reference values in this table are dependent on sex, age, and protein intake and represent lower limits.
[b]For each aminotransferase measure, the activity coefficient represents the ratio of the acitivity with added PLP to the activity without PLP added (143).
NV = no value established; limited data available, each laboratory should establish their own reference with an appropriate healthy control population.

obtaining accurate dietary intakes, the nutrient data bases used in determining vitamin B$_6$ content of diets are often incomplete with respect to values for vitamin B$_6$. Thus, reports of vitamin B$_6$ status based only on nutrient intake must be viewed with caution.

Plasma pyridoxal-5'-phosphate concentration is considered one of the better indicators of vitamin B$_6$ status (116). Lumeng et al. (93) have shown that plasma PLP concentration is a good indicator of tissue PLP levels in rats. In humans, plasma PLP concentration is significantly correlated with dietary vitamin B$_6$ intake (88). Table 9 contains mean plasma PLP values reported by several laboratories for males and females. These are selected references and drawn from reports where the sex of the subjects studied was clearly identified. The means reported range from 27 to 75 nmol/l for males and 26 to 93 nmol/l for females. These ranges should not necessarily be considered as normal ranges, since the values given in Table 9 reflect studies in which dietary intake was controlled and other studies in which dietary intake was not assessed. As discussed by Shultz and Leklem (88), dietary intake of both vitamin B$_6$ and protein influence the fasting plasma PLP concentration. Miller et al. (122) have shown that plasma PLP and total vitamin B$_6$ concentrations

Table 9 Selected Mean Plasma Pyridoxal-5-′ Concentrations Reported for Healthy Males and Females

Reference	No. subjects	Age (yr)	Diet[a]	PLP (nmol/l)	Method[b]
Males					
Wachstein, 1960 (117)	27	—[c]	—	35.2 ± 9.3	TDC
Chabner, 1970 (118)	17	20–34	SS,F	74.8 ± 22.2	TDC
	7	35–49	SS,F	63.9 ± 13.3	TDC
Rose, 1976 (119)	26	18–29	SS,NF	59.1 ± 28.9	TDC
	43	30–39	SS,NF	59.9 ± 29.2	
	82	40–49	SS,NF	53.4 ± 22.0	
	152	50–59	SS,NF	46.9 ± 21.7	
	59	60–69	SS,NF	49.4 ± 24.9	
	65	70–79	SS,NF	47.7 ± 26.1	
	24	80–90	SS,NF	31.1 ± 19.8	
Contractor, 1970 (120)	5	—	—	54.6 ± 11.7	FL
Wozenski, 1980 (87)	5	27 ± 3	SS,F	35 ± 14	TDC
Leklem, 1980 (71)	8	27 ± 4	SS,F	51.5 ± 14.1	TDC
			Met,(1.55),F	33.8 ± 11.2	
Shultz, 1981 (88)	35	38 ± 14	SS,(2.0 ± 8),F	51.9 ± 19.3	TDC
Shultz, 1982 (121)	4	22–35	Met,(1.60),F	59.9 ± 41.7	TDC
Leklem, 1983 (112)	7	16 ± 1	SS,F	47.6 ± 18.7	TDC
Lindberg, 1983 (72)	5	27 ± 6	Met,(1.60),F	43.3 ± 6.5	TDC
Kabir, 1983 (77)	9	25 ± 4	SS,F	81.5 ± 36.0	TDC
			Met,F	65.0 ± 23.3	
Miller, 1985 (122)	8	27 ± 4	Met 1,(1.6)LP,F	43.5 ± 19.4	TDC
			Met,(1.6)MP,F	33.7 ± 9.0	
			Met,(1.6)HP,F	27.9 ± 11.5	
Leklem, 1988 (123)	8	20–30	Met,(1.6)F	38.8 ± 10.9	TDC
Swift, 1986 (124)	9	57	SS,(1.9),F	45.5 ± 15.0	TDC
	5	60	SS,(1.5),F	39.2 ± 22.4	
Tarr, 1981 (74)	6	21–35	Met,(1.1),F	27.5 ± 2.7	TDC
			(2.3),F	55.0 ± 5.7	
			(2.7),F	114.5 ± 7.0	

Females	n	Age	Diet	Value ± SD	Method
Wachstein, 1960 (117)	20	—	—	34.0 ± 10.1	TDC
Chabner, 1970 (118)	12	20–34	SS,F	67.9 ± 14.6	TDC
	7	35–49	SS,F	46.1 ± 13.8	TDC
Reinken, 1974 (125)	29	—	SS,—	36.8 ± 8.9	TDC
Miller, 1975 (126)	11	20–29	SS,F	25.9 ± 15.4	TDC
Lumeng, 1974 (127)	77	29 ± 8	SS,NF	38.0 ± 17.0	TDC
Brown, 1975 (86)	6	22 ± 2	Met,(0.8),F	22.9 ± 13.9	TDC
	3	22 ± 2	Met,(1.8),F	60.7 ± 20.2	TDC
Brophy, 1975 (128)	4	20–34	SS,—	68.4	TDC
Cleary, 1975 (128)	58	20–34	SS,—	43.4	TDC
Prasad, 1975 (130)	?	—	SS,(1.19),—	51.8 ± 30.7	TDC
	?	—	SS,(1.02),—	46.5 ± 24.3	TDC
Shultz, 1982 (121)	4	24–32	SS,F	38.4 ± 15.8	TDC
Shultz, 1981 (88)	41	50 ± 14	SS,(1.6 ± 0.5),F	37.7 ± 14.7	TDC
Guilland, 1984 (131)	23	27	SS,(1.1),F	92.8 ± 7.3	LC/FL
	29	84	Met,(1.0),F	52.0 ± 4.1	
Lee, 1985 (132)	5	24 ± 3	SS,F	35.5 ± 14.8	TDC
	5	55 ± 4	SS,F	31.3 ± 13.3	
	5	24 ± 3	Met,(2.3),F	61.7 ± 25.6	
	5	55 ± 4	Met,(2.3),F	40.5 ± 12.2	
	5	24 ± 3	Met,(10.3),F	202 ± 45	
	5	55 ± 4	Met,(10.3),F	168 ± 38	
Driskell, 1986 (133)	41(C)[d]	12	SS,(1.23),F	48.1 ± 17.9	TDC
	32(C)	14	SS,(1.23),F	44.5 ± 15.8	
	23(C)	16	SS,(1.25),F	43.7 ± 15.3	
	32(B)	12	SS,(1.30),F	46.1 ± 15.8	
	39(B)	14	SS,(1.24),F	42.1 ± 15.8	
	19(B)	16	SS,(1.17),F	46.5 ± 13.9	
Ubbink, 1987 (134)	9	—	SS,F	31.7 ± 19.4	HPLC

[a]The notations for diet indicate if the blood samples were obtained from subjects who self-selected (SS) their diets or were receiving a controlled intake (Met) and the amount of vitamin B₆ consumed (value given as mg/day in parentheses), if known. F indicates the blood sample was collected after a fast of at least 8 hours, NF indicates nonfasting. LP, MP, HP refer to gm of protein as 0.5, 1.0, and 2.0 gm/kg body weight.

[b]Abbreviations for the methods used are TDC = tyrosine apodecarboxylase; HPLC = high performance liquid chromatography; FL = fluorometric.

[c]A dash indicates data was not given in the respective reference.

[d]C = Caucasian; B = black.

in males were inversely related to protein intake (see Table 9) in males fed protein intakes ranging from 0.5 to 2 g per kg per day. Similar studies in females are not available.

There are other factors that may influence plasma PLP and should be considered when using this index as a measure of vitamin B_6 status. These include the physiological variables of age (119,132,135), exercise (111), and pregnancy (127). Rose et al. determined the plasma PLP concentration in males ranging in age from 18 to 90 years (119). They observed a decrease in plasma PLP with age, especially after 40 years of age. However, one must keep in mind that the PLP concentration was determined 1–2 hours after a meal. The intake of vitamin B_6 may have influenced the data. Also, the carbohydrate intake could have resulted in a depressed plasma PLP concentration (111). Hamfelt has reviewed the effect of age on plasma PLP and observed that investigators in several countries (135) have seen decreased vitamin B_6 status with increasing age. The mechanism of this decrease remains to be determined. To date there is only one controlled metabolic study which has evaluated vitamin B_6 status in different age groups. Lee and Leklem (132) studied five women age 20–27 yr and eight women age 51–59 yr under conditions where they received a constant daily vitamin B_6 intake of 2.3 mg for 4 weeks followed by 3 weeks of 10.3 mg per day. Compared to the younger women, the older women had a lower mean plasma PLP, plasma and urinary total vitamin B_6, and a slightly higher urinary 4-PA excretion with the 2.3 mg intake. With supplementation the only significant difference was for urinary total vitamin B_6. Interestingly, there was no difference in urinary excretion of xanthurenic or kynurenic acid following a 2-g L-tryptophan load. Thus, while there may be age-related differences in vitamin B_6 metabolism, there is no significant age effect on functional activity of vitamin B_6 when intake is adequate. The effect of age on functional tests at lower intakes (0.5–1.2 mg; 25–60% of the RDA) remains to be determined.

Recently the use of plasma PLP as a status indicator has been questioned and the determination of plasma PL recommended. Others have also suggested that plasma PL may be an important indicator of status (136). Barnard et al. studied the vitamin B_6 status of pregnant females and nonpregnant controls and found that plasma PLP concentration was 50% lower in pregnant females, but the concentration of the total of PLP and PL was only slightly lower. When concentrations of PLP and PL were expressed on per gram albumin basis, there was no difference between groups. Unfortunately, urinary vitamin B_6 metabolites were not measured in this study. In contrast, in pregnant rats both plasma PLP and PL decreased, as did liver PLP, in comparison to nonpregnant control rats (137). These studies are in direct opposition to each other but do provide support for the need to determine several indices of vitamin B_6 status (31,88,116).

Urinary 4-pyridoxic acid excretion is considered a short-term indicator of vitamin B_6 status. In deficiency studies in males (138) and females (86), the decrease in urinary 4-PA paralleled the decrease in plasma PLP concentration. Table 10 lists values for urinary 4-PA and vitamin B_6 in males and females. As reflected in the studies in which dietary intake was assessed or known, 4-PA excretion amounts for about 40–60% of the intake. Because of the design of most studies and limited number of studies done with females compared to males, it is not possible to determine if there is a significant difference between males and females. The limited data in Table 11 suggest there is little difference. However, males consistently had higher plasma PLP and total vitamin B_6 concentrations as well as higher excretion of 4-PA and total vitamin B_6. Urinary total vitamin B_6 (all forms, including phosphorylated and glycosylated) excretion is not a sensitive indicator of vitamin B_6, except in situations where intake is very low (138).

Table 10 Urinary 4-Pyridoxic Acid and Vitamin B$_6$ Excretion in Males and Females

Reference	No. subjects	Age (yr)	Diet	4-PA (μmol/day)	UB6 (μmol/day)
Males					
Kelsay, 1968 (138)	5	20-25	Met(1.66 mg, P = 150)	5.51 ± 1.75	—
	6	18-35	(1.66 mg, P = 54)	4.80 ± 0.60 (50)[a]	—
Mikai-Devic, 1972 (139)	10	16-51		5.7 ± 1.4	—
Leklem, 1980 (71)	8	27 ± 4	Met(1.55)	4.04 ± 0.85 (44)	0.76 ± 0.17
Wozenski, 1980 (87)	5	27 ± 3	SS	5.4 ± 0.5	0.8 ± 0.1
Shultz, 1982 (121)	4	22-35	Met(1.6)	5.71 ± 1.08	—
Shultz, 1982 (88)	35	35 ± 14	SS(2.0 ± 0.8)	7.46 ± 4.34 (63)	0.92 ± 0.49
Lindberg, 1983 (72)	10	26 ± 4	SS	4.78 ± 1.40	0.81 ± 0.18
	10	26 ± 4	Met(1.60)	3.62 ± 0.59	0.76 ± 0.10
Kabir, 1983 (77)	9	25 ± 4	Met(1.55)	4.89 ± 1.10 (53)	1.05 ± 0.20
Dreon, 1986 (140)	6	28 ± 6	Met(4.2 ± 0.4)	11.15 ± 1.86 (45)	0.77 ± 0.14
Miller, 1985 (122)	8	27 ± 4	Met(1.60)	4.37 ± 0.89(LP)	0.71 ± 0.09
				3.58 ± 0.54(MP)	0.68 ± 0.15
				2.74 ± 0.71(HP)	
Females					
Mikai-Devic, 1972 (139)	15	18-47	SS	4.5 ± 0.9	
Contractor, 1970 (120)	26	—	SS	6.62 ± 4.6	
Reinken, 1974 (125)	29	25	SS	8.32 ± 1.30	
Adams, 1973 (140)	28	—	SS	3.9 ± 0.7	
Brown, 1975 (86)	6	22 ± 2	Met(0.82)	1.98 ± 0.81(41)	
	3	22 ± 2	Met(1.81)	6.03 ± 2.04(56)	
Donald, 1979 (141)	8	18-23	Met(1.54)	2.4 ± 0.1 (26)	0.33 ± 0.3
			(2.06)	3.78 ± 0.41(31)	
Shultz, 1981 (88)	41	50 ± 14	SS(1.6 ± 0.5)	5.57 ± 3.09 (59)	0.76 ± 0.24
Lee, 1985 (132)	5	24 ± 3	Met(2.3)	6.89 ± 0.55 (50)	1.12 ± 0.29
	5	55 ± 4	Met(2.3)	7.35 ± 0.80 (59)	0.89 ± 0.19
	5	24 ± 3	Met(10.3)	36.6 ± 1.4 (60)	6.89 ± 0.86
	5	55 ± 4	Met(10.3)	38.5 ± 4.7(63)	5.48 ± 1.26
Ubbink, 1987 (134)	9	—	SS	5.48 ± 2.93	

Abbreviations are as used in Table 9, except for 4-pyridoxic, which is 4-PA; urinary vitamin B$_6$, which is UB6.

[a]The number in parentheses refers to the percent of intake excreted as 4-PA.

Table 11 Plasma Pyridoxal-5′-Phosphate and Total Vitamin B_6 Concentration and Urinary 4-Pyridoxic Acid and Vitamin B_6 Excretion in Males and Females Consuming 2.2 mg Vitamin B_6

	PLP (nmol/l)	TB6 (nmol/l)	4-PA (μmol/day)	UB-6 (μmol/day)
Males (n = 4)	78.4 ± 27.0	86.2 ± 37.1	7.86 ± 0.74	0.92 ± 0.20
Females (n = 4)	58.5 ± 12.6	71.5 ± 15.8	7.02 ± 0.78	0.82 ± 0.19

Erythrocyte transaminase activity (alanine and aspartate) has been used to assess vitamin B_6 status in a variety of populations (119,131,133,142–148), including oral contraceptive users (88,146). Transaminase activity is considered a long-term indicator of vitamin B_6 status. Most often the transaminase activity has been measured in the presence and absence of excess PLP (143). Table 8 indicates suggested norms for activity coefficients for alanine and aspartate aminotransferase. While transaminase activity is used to assess status, there is not unanimous agreement, and some consider this measure to be less reliable than other indices of vitamin B_6 status (88,148). The long life of the erythrocyte and tight binding of PLP to hemoglobin may explain the lack of a consistent significant correlation between plasma PLP and transaminase activity or activity coefficient.

Urinary excretion of tryptophan metabolites following a tryptophan load, especially excretion of xanthurenic acid, has been one of the most widely used tests for assessing vitamin B_6 status (149,150). Table 8 gives a suggested normal value for xanthurenic acid excretion following a 2-g L-tryptophan load test. The use of the tryptophan load test for assessing vitamin B_6 status has been questioned (151,152), especially in disease states or in situations in which hormones may alter tryptophan metabolism independent of a direct effect on vitamin B_6 metabolism (153).

Other tests for status include the methionine load (154), oxalate excretion, and electroencephalogram tracings. These are less commonly used tests but under appropriate circumstances may provide useful information.

VII. FUNCTIONS

A. Immune System

The involvement of PLP in a multiplicity of enzymatic reactions (155) suggests that it would serve many functions in the body. Table 12 lists several of the known functions of PLP and the cellular systems (123) affected. PLP serves as a coenzyme for serine transhydroxymethylase (156), one of the key enzymes involved in 1-carbon metabolism. Alteration in 1-carbon metabolism can then lead to changes in nucleic acid synthesis. Such changes may be one of the keys to vitamin B_6 affecting immune function (157,158). Studies in animals have shown that a vitamin B_6 deficiency adversely affects lymphocyte production (159) and antibody response to antigens (158). Additional studies in animals support an effect of vitamin B_6 on cell mediated immunity (160). Miller et al. found that the immune system of 11 elderly females was impaired and treatment with 50 mg pyridoxine per day for two months improved their immune system as judged by lymphocyte response (161). However, in humans a diet-induced marginal vitamin B_6 status for 11 weeks was not found to significantly influence cellular or humoral immunity (162). These two studies differed in their experimental design. The study by van den Berg et al. (159) employed a diet

Table 12 Cellular Processes Affected by Pyridoxal-5'-Phosphate

Cellular process or enzyme	Function/System influenced
1-carbon metabolism, hormone modulation	Immune function
Glycogen phosphorylase, transamination	Gluconeogenesis
Tryptophan metabolism	Niacin formation
Heme synthesis, transamination, O$_2$ affinity	Red cell metabolism and formation
Neurotransmitter synthesis, lipid metabolism	Nervous system
Hormone modulation, binding of PLP to lysine on hormone receptor	Hormone modulation

marginally deficient in vitamin B$_6$ in young adults, that of Miller et al. (161) utilized a treatment of elderly with an excess of vitamin B$_6$. This excess intake may be necessary for increased activity of certain cell types of the immune system in the elderly. Further studies are needed to determine if an age difference in response exists.

B. Gluconeogenesis

Gluconeogenesis is key to maintaining an adequate supply of glucose during caloric deficit. Pyridoxal-5'-phosphate is involved in gluconeogenesis via its role as a coenzyme for trans-amination reactions (155) and for glycogen phosphorylase (102). In animals a deficiency of vitamin B$_6$ results in decreased activities of liver alanine and aspartate aminotransferase (163). However, in humans (females) a low intake of vitamin B$_6$ (0.2 mg per day) as compared to an adequate intake (1.8 mg per day) did not significantly influence fasting plasma glucose concentratiaons (164). Interestingly, the low vitamin B$_6$ intake was associated with impaired glucose tolerance.

Glycogen phosphorylase is also involved in maintaining adequate glucose supplies within liver and muscle and, in the case of liver, a source of glucose for adequate blood glucose levels. In rats a deficiency of vitamin B$_6$ has been shown to result in decreased activities of both liver (165) and muscle glycogen phosphorylase (102,109,165). Muscle appears to serve as a reservior for vitamin B$_6$ (102,109,110), but a deficiency of the vitamin does not result in mobilization of these stores. However, Black et al. (109) have shown that a caloric deficit does lead to decreased muscle phosphorylase content. These results suggest that the reservoir of vitamin B$_6$ (as PLP) is only utilized when there is a need for enhanced gluconeogenesis. In male mice the half-life of muscle glycogen phosphorylase has been shown to be approximately 12 days (166).

C. Erythrocyte Function

Vitamin B$_6$ has a further role in erythrocyte function and metabolism. The function of PLP as a coenzyme for transaminases in erythrocytes has been mentioned. In addition both PL and PLP bind to hemoglobin (96,98). The binding of PL to the alpha-chain of hemoglobin (167) increased the O$_2$ binding affinity (168), while the binding of PLP to the beta-chain of hemoglobin S or A lowers O$_2$ binding affinity (169). The effect of PLP and PL on O$_2$ binding may be important in sicle-cell anemia (170).

Pyridoxal-5'-phosphate serves as a cofactor for δ-aminolevulinic acid synthetase (171), the enzyme that catalyzes the condensation between glycine and succinyl-CoA to form δ-aminoleuvulinic acid. This latter compound is the initial precursor in heme synthesis (172). Therefore, vitamin B_6 plays a central role in erythropoiesis. A deficiency of vitamin B_6 in animals can lead to hypochromic, microcytic anemia. Further, in humans there are several reports of patients with pyridoxine-responsive anemia (173,174). However, not all patients with sideroblastic anemia (in which there is a defect in δ-aminolevulinic acid synthetase) respond to pyridoxine therapy (175).

D. Niacin Formation

One of the more extensive functions of vitamin B_6 that has been researched is its involvement in the conversion of tryptophan to niacin (150). This research is in part related to the use of the tryptophan load in evaluating vitamin B_6 status. While PLP functions in at least four enzymatic reactions in the complex tryptophan–niacin pathway (Fig.6), there is only one PLP-requiring reaction in the *direct* conversion of tryptophan to niacin. This step is the conversion of 3-hydroxykynurenine to 3-hydroxyanthranilic acid and is catalyzed by kynureninase. Leklem et al. have examined the effect of vitamin B_6 deficiency on the conversion of tryptophan to niacin (176). In this study the urinary excretion of N'-methylnicotinamide and N'-methyl-2-pyridone-5-carboxamide, two metabolites of niacin, was evaluated in women. After 4 weeks of a low vitamin B_6 diet, the total excretion of these two metabolites following a 2-g L-tryptophan load was approximately half that when subjects received 0.8–1.8 mg vitamin B_6 per day. This suggests that low vitamin B_6 has a moderate negative effect on niacin formation from tryptophan.

E. Nervous System

In addition to the effect of vitamin B_6 on tryptophan-to-niacin conversion, there is another tryptophan pathway which is vitamin B_6 dependent. The conversion of 5-hydroxytryptophan to 5-hydroxytryptamine is catalyzed by the PLP-dependent enzyme 5-hydroxytryptophan

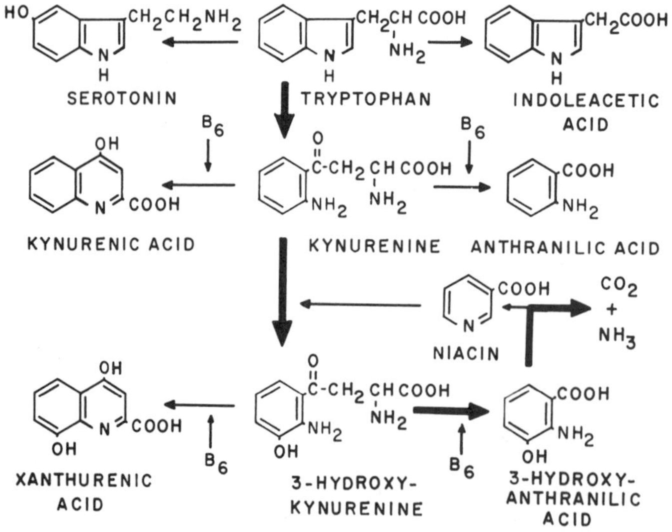

Figure 6 Tryptophan-niacin pathway, B_6 indicates the steps in the pathway in which pyridoxal-5′-phosphate functions as a coenzyme.

decarboxylase (177). Other neurotransmitters, taurine, dopamine, norepinephrine, histamine, and γ-aminobutyric acid, are also synthesized by PLP-dependent enzymes (177). The involvement of PLP in neurotransmitter formation and the observation that there are neurological abnormalities in human infants(178,179) and animals (177,180) deficient in vitamin B$_6$ provide support for a role of vitamin B$_6$ in nervous system function. Reviews on the relationship between the nervous system function and vitamin B$_6$ are available (177,182,183).

In infants fed a formula in which the vitamin B$_6$ was lost during processing, convulsions and abnormal EEG tracings were observed (178,183). Treatment of the infants with 100 mg of pyridoxine produced a rapid involvement in the EEG tracings. In these studies reported by Coursin, the protein content of the diet appeared to be correlated with the vitamin B$_6$ deficiency and the extent of symptoms. Other evidence for a role of vitamin B$_6$ comes from studies of pyridoxine-dependent seizures, which is an autosomal recessive disorder. Vitamin B$_6$ dependency, while a rare cause of convulsions, has been reported by several investigators (184–187). The convulsions occur during the neonatal period, and administration of 30–100 mg of pyridoxine are usually sufficient to prevent convulsions and correct abnormal EEG (187,188). However, there are atypical patients who present a slightly different clinical picture and course but are responsive to pyridoxine (189).

Vitamin B$_6$ deficiency in adults has also been reported to result in abnormal EEGs (190), especially in individuals on a high-protein (100 g per day) intake. These subjects were receiving a diet essentially devoid of vitamin B$_6$ (0.06) mg). In a separate study, Grabow and Linkswiler fed a high-protein diet (150 g) and 0.16 mg of vitamin B$_6$ for 21 days to 11 men (191). No abnormalities in EEGs were observed, nor were there changes in motor nerve conduction times in five subjects who had this measurement. While there were differences in the length of deficiency in these studies, which may explain the differences observed, it appears that long-term very low vitamin B$_6$ intakes of a vitamin B$_6$ dependency are necessary before abnormal EEGs are observed in humans.

A further aspect of the relationship of vitamin B$_6$ (as PLP) with the nervous system is the development of the brain under conditions of varying intakes of vitamin B$_6$. Kirksey and co-workers have conducted numerous well-designed studies in this area. These studies have utilized the rat model to examine the development of the brain, especially during the critical period when cells are undergoing rapid mitosis. Early experiments showed that dietary restriction of vitamin B$_6$ in the dams were associated with a decrease in alanine aminotransferase and glutamic acid decarboxylase activity and low brain weights of progeny (192). Alterations in fatty acid levels, especially those involved in myelination, were observed in the cerebellum and cerebrum of progeny of dams fed a low-(1.2 mg/kg diet) vitamin B$_6$ diet (193). Kurtz et al. have found a 30–50% decrease in cerebral sphingolipids of progeny of dams fed a vitamin B$_6$–deficient diet (194). In the progeny of dams fed graded levels of vitamin B$_6$, a decrease in the area of the neocortex and cerebellum as well as reduced molecular and granular layers of the cerebellum were noted (195). Myelination was reduced in the progeny of severely deficient dams (196). Noting in previous studies that Purkinje cells were dispersed from the usual nonocellular layer in progeny of severely vitamin B$_6$–deficient dams, Chang et al. (197) carried out further studies and found that a maternal vitamin B$_6$ deficiency interferes with normal development of Purkinje cells seen as reduced total length of Purkinje cell dendrites. At the biochemical level, a vitamin B$_6$ deficiency led to reduced GABA levels, which were associated with impaired function of the extrapyramidal motor system (198). Both Wasynczuk et al. (199) and Kurtz et al. (194) found that with vitamin B$_6$ deficiency amino acid levels were altered in specific regions of the brain. Glycine, leucine, isoleucine, valine, and cystathionine levels were elevated, while alanine and serine levels were reduced. More recent studies have shown that PLP levels in certain areas of the central nervous system are more dramatically affected by vitamin B_6 deficiency than others. Levels in the spinal cord and hypothalamus were less affected than the corpus striatum and cerebellum (200). These findings suggested a metabolic trapping in a caudal to rostral direction.

F. Lipid Metabolism

One of the more intriguing and controversial functions of vitamin B_6 is its role in lipid metabolism (201). Studies conducted some 50 years ago suggested a link between fat metabolism and vitamin B_6 (202). These studies showed a similarity (visual) in symptoms between a lack of essential fatty acids and a deficiency of vitamin B_6. Other early studies found that a vitamin B_6 deficiency in rats resulted in a decrease in body fats (203). Subsequent research showed that liver lipid levels were significantly lower in vitamin B_6–deficient vs. pair-fed rats (204). The changes were due mainly to lower trigylceride levels, while cholesterol levels were not different. In contrast, Abe and Kishino showed that rats fed a high-protein (70%), vitamin B_6–deficient diet developed fatty livers, and they suggested this was due to impaired lysosomal degradation of lipid (205). The synthesis of fat in vitamin B_6–deficient rats has been reported to be greater (206) or normal (207,208) or depressed (209). The differences observed may be related to the meal pattern of the animals (209).

The effect of vitamin B_6 deprivation on fatty acid metabolism has also received attention. A pyridoxine deficiency may impair the conversion of linoleic acid to arachidonic acid (210,211). Cunnane and co-workers (211) found that phospholipid levels of both linoleic and γ-linolenic acid were increased in vitamin B_6–deficient rats, but the level of arachidonic acid was decreased as compared to control levels in plasma, liver, and skin. They suggested that both linoleic desaturation and γ-linoleic acid elongation may be impaired by a vitamin B_6 deficiency. In one of the few studies of vitamin B_6 and fatty acid metabolism in humans, desoxypyridoxine was utilized to induce a vitamin B_6 deficiency (212). Xanthurenic acid excretion following a 10-g- D,L-tryptophan load indicated a moderate vitamin B_6–deficient state. Only minor changes in fatty acid levels in plasma and erthyrocytes were observed as a result of the deficiency produced. The pattern of fatty acids observed was interpreted by the authors to support the findings by Witten and Holman (210). Delmore and Lupien also observed a decreased proportion of arachidonic acid in liver phospholipids and an increased level of linoleic acid in vitamin B_6–deficient rats (213). They suggested that changes were based on the decrease in phosphatidylcholine via methylation of phosphoethanolamine. Support for this comes from the studies of Loo and Smith (214), in which it was found that a deficiency of vitamin B_6 resulted in decreased phospholipid methylation in the liver of rats. The level of S-adenosylmethionine (SAM) in livers of vitamin B_6–deficient rats were nearly five times higher than in livers of pair-fed animals. This change in SAM is secondary to the inhibition of the catabolism of homocysteine, a PLP-dependent process. Negative feedback of SAM on the conversion of phosphatidyl ethanolamine to phosphatidyl choline may thus explain the changes seen in fatty acid metabolism. This provides a plausible mechanism, since the primary metabolic steps in fatty acid metabolism do not involve nitrogen-containing substrates, a feature common to most PLP-dependent enzymatic reactions.

The change observed in arachidonic acid levels and the role it plays in cholesterol metabolism (215) may have clinical implications (216). The effect, if any, of vitamin B_6 on cholesterol metabolism remains controversial. The increase in plasma cholesterol in monkeys made vitamin B_6 deficient (217) provided much of the impetus for research relating vitamin B_6, cholesterol, and atherosclerosis. Studies by Lupien and co-workers have shown that the rate of incorporation of acetate ^{14}C into cholesterol was increased in vitamin B_6–deficient rats as compared to controls (218). However, the amount of cholesterol in plasma and liver of rats and other species has been reported to be increased, not changed, or even decreased (218–221). In humans a deficiency of vitamin B_6 did not result in a significant change in serum cholesterol (222). Significant positive correlation between plasma PLP and HDL cholesterol and negative correlations with total cholesterol and LDL cholesterol have been reported in monkeys fed atherogenic Western diets and a "prudent" Western diet (223). However, the diets fed the monkeys contained distinctly different amounts of vitamin B_6. The use of supplemental vitamin B_6 in reduction of blood cholesterol has not been definitively tested. Serfontein and Ubbink reported decreased serum cholesterol (0.8 mmol/l) in 34 subjects given a multivitamin containing 10 mg of pyridoxine (224). The reduction was mainly as LDL cholesterol. In another study, pyridoxine (50 mg/d) administration prevented the increase in serum cholesterol seen when disulfram was administered (225). Controlled trials of pyridoxine are needed to resolve the role of vitamin B_6 in modifying serum cholesterol levels.

The role of vitamin B_6 in lipid metabolism remains unclear. Evidence to date suggests a role of vitamin B_6 in modifying methionine metabolism and thus an indirect effect on phospholipid and fatty acid metabolism. This effect (214) and an effect of vitamin B_6 on carnitine synthesis (215) appear to be the primary effects of vitamin B_6 on lipid/fatty acid metabolism.

G. Hormone Modulation

A recently identified function of PLP is as a modulator of steroid action (227,228). PLP can be used as an effective tool in extracting steroid receptors from the nuclei of tissues on which the steroid acts (229). Under conditions of physiological concentrations of PLP, reversible reactions occur with receptors for estrogen (230), androgen (231), progesterone (232), and glucocorticoids (233). PLP reacts with a lysine residue on the steroid receptor. As a result of the Schiff base that is formed, there is inhibition of the binding of the steroid–receptor complex to DNA (227). Holley et al. found that when female rats were made vitamin B_6 deficient and injected with ^3H-estradiol, a greater amount of the isotope accumulated in the uterine tissues of the deficient animal compared to the tissue of control rats (234). Bunce and co-workers studied the dual effect of zinc and vitamin B_6 deficiency on estrogen uptake by the uterus (235). They found that there was an increased uptake of estrogen in both the vitamin B_6– and the zinc-deficient animals. A combined deficiency to the two nutrients resulted in an even greater retention of estrogen. The number of estrogen receptors was not altered by the deficiency of vitamin B_6. This study suggests there would be increased sensitivity of the uterus (or other end-target tissues) to steroids when vitamin B_6 status was abnormal.

As yet there is no direct evidence of any physiological significance for the interaction of PLP with steroid receptors. Sturman and Kremzner found enhanced activity of ornithine decarboxylase in testosterone-treated vitamin B_6–deficient animals as compared to control animals (236). DiSorbo and Litwack observed increased typrosine aminotransferase activity in hepatoma cells raised on a pyridoxine-deficient medium and treated with triamcinolone acetonide as compared to pyridoxine-sufficient cells treated with the same steroid (237). Whether this function of PLP has application in steroid-responsive cancers or in premenstrual syndrome remains to be determined.

VIII. REQUIREMENTS

Considering the numerous functions in which vitamin B_6 is involved, the assessent of the requirement for this vitamin becomes important. Recent publications have addressed the question of human requirements for vitamin B_6 (1,238). In addition, each of the last three RDA publications (239–241) have evaluated the requirements for vitamin B_6. While vitamin B_6 has been known for over 50 years, it has only been in the past 20 years that a requirement has been established in the United States. The requirements established for different age groups as well as adult males and females are summarized in Table 13. The 1989 RDA for vitamin B_6 reflect decreases for children, males, and females as compared to the 1974 and 1980 RDAs.

There are numerous factors that may contribute to the requirement for vitamin B_6. Several of these factors are listed in Table 14. Many of these have not been experimentally tested, while others have received greater attention and have been examined in more detail. Of dietary factors (Table 15) that influence requirement, the effect of protein intake (122,190,242) has received the greatest attention. Protein intake is known to influence plasma PLP and urinary 4-PA excretion in an inverse relationship (122). Amino acids resulting from a protein intake greater than needed for growth and maintenance are metabolized, and this process requires increased transaminase levels. Thus, there is a greater need for PLP in tissues. The net result is retention of PLP in tissues and less PLP in the circulation and less conversion to 4-PA. Because of the close relationship between protein and vitamin B_6, the requirement for vitamin B_6 has been expressed as a vitamin B_6-to-protein ratio (243). While bioavailability of vitamin B_6 has been examined in the context of factors which influence bioavailability and the % availability from specific foods

Table 13 Vitamin B_6 U.S. Recommended Dietary Allowances in mg

	Age (yr)	1974	1980	1989
Infants	0.0–0.5	0.3	0.3	0.3
	0.0–1.0	0.4	0.6	0.6
Children	1–3	0.6(0.026)	0.9(0.039)	1.0
	4–6	0.9(0.030)	1.3(0.034)	1.1
	7–10	1.2(0.033)	1.6(0.047)	1.4
Males	11–14	1.6(0.036)	1.8(0.040)	1.7
	15–18	2.0(0.037)	2.0(0.036)	2.0
	19–22	2.0(0.037)	2.2(0.039)	2.0
	23–50	2.0(0.036)	2.2(0.039)	2.0
	51+	2.0(0.036)	2.2(0.039)	2.0
Females	11–14	2.6(0.036)	1.8(0.039)	1.4
	15–18	2.0(0.043)	2.0(0.043)	1.5
	19–22	2.0(0.043)	2.0(0.045)	1.6
	23–50	2.0(0.043)	2.0(0.045)	1.6
	51+	2.0(0.043)	2.0(0.045)	1.6
Pregnant		2.5(0.033)	+0.6(0.035)	2.1
Lactating		2.5(0.033)	+0.5(0.039)	2.1

The values in parentheses indicate the respective vitamin B_6 to protein ratio, using the recommended protein intake for the respective age and sex group.
Source: Refs. 239–241 for respective years.

Table 14 Factors Affecting Vitamin B_6 Requirement

1. Dietary
   a. Physical structure of a food
   b. Forms of vitamin B_6 natural; those due to processing
   c. Binding of forms of vitamin B_6
2. Defect in delivery to tissues
   a. Impaired g.i. absorption
   b. Impaired transport-albumin, synthesis, and binding, phosphatase activity
3. Physiological/Biochemical
   a. Physical activity–increased loss, gluconeogenesis
   b. Protein-enzyme induction
   c. Increased catabolism/turnover–phosphatase activity, illness
   d. Impaired phosphorylation and/or interconversion, competing pathways, nutrient deficiencies, drugs
   e. Pregnancy—demand of fetus
   f. Growth—increased cell mass, repair
   g. Lactation—adequate levels in milk
   h. Excretion rate—urinary, sweat, menstrual loss
   i. Sex—differences in metabolism
   j. Age differences in metabolism
4. Genetic
   a. Apoenzyme defects—altered binding to apoenzyme
   b. Altered apoenzyme levels—biochemical individuality
5. Disease prevention/treatment
   a. Which? heart, cancer, diabetes, PMS, kidney, alcohol

examined (70–79), specific studies addressing the quantitative effect of bioavailability on requirements for vitamin B_6 have not been conducted in humans.

Of the factors listed in Table 14, pregnancy and lactation are the ones in which additional needs could be estimated from the total vitamin B_6 content of the fetus and vitamin B_6 content of human milk, respectively. While the former is not entirely feasible except in nonhuman primates, the latter is possible since the vitamin B_6 content of human milk has been determined. Table 16 lists values for the vitamin B_6 content of human milk which have been reported and shows the relationship with vitamin B_6 intake and the change in content over time of lactation. While a gradual increase in vitamin B_6 content of milk in the first several months of lactation has been obsered (250), a gradual decrease in content from 7 to 25 months of lactation has been reported (251). Intake of vitamin B_6 is reflected in milk vitamin B_6 concentration, especially at intakes above 5 mg per day.

As indicated, several of the factors of Table 14 have not been adequately studied to provide a quantitative estimation of their effect on requirements. Sex differences in

Table 15 Dietary Factors Influencing Vitamin B_6 Status/Requirements

Protein	Increased intake increases need (190,242)
Carbohydrate	Increased intake decreases plasma PLP concentration (111)
Bioavailability	Decreased bioavailability increases need (68)
Caloric intake	Decreased calories, increased 4-PA excretion

Table 16 Vitamin B_6 Content of Human Milk

References	No. of subjects[a]	Stage of lactation[b]	Vitamin B_6 intake[c] (mg)	Vitamin B_6 content[d] (μmol/l)
Thomas	6	5– 7 days	1.45	0.76
et al. (244)	7	5– 7 days	5.69	1.3
	6	43–45 days	0.84	1.21
	7	43–45 days	5.11	1.40
Roepke and	9	3 days	2.19	0.05
Kirksey (245)	42	3 days	7.65	0.10
	9	14 days	2.19	0.24
	38	14 days	7.65	0.33
Sneed et al. (246)	7	5– 7 days	1.52	0.72
	9	5– 7 days	5.33	1.46
	7	43–45 days	1.41	0.70
	9	43–45 days	5.21	1.42
Styslinger and	6	77 days	2.0	0.55
Kirksey (247)	6	77 days	4.4	1.13
	6	77 days	11.3	1.46
	6	77 days	21.1	2.44
Bamji et al. (248)	27	6–30 days	ND	0.12
	26	7–12 mo	ND	0.42
	18	18 mo	ND	0.37
Borschel	8	1– 6 mo	3.6	0.87–1.25
et al. (249)	9	1– 6 mo	14.0	2.21–3.16

[a]No. of subjects in which milk samples assayed.
[b]Days after birth.
[c]Intake of mother.
[d]1 μmol/l = 169 μg/l.
ND = not determined.

metabolism is one which has received surprisingly little attention. As indicated in Table 9, which lists plasma PLP values, there is a tendency for plasma PLP levels to be lower in females than males. Part of the difference is no doubt related to different intakes of vitamin B_6. A recent study (unpublished observations) in my laboratory indiates there may be a sex difference in metabolism. As shown in Table 11, plasma PLP and total vitamin B_6 as well as urinary 4-PA and total vitamin B_6 were consistently lower in females than males. The eight subjects were fed a diet containing 2.2 mg of vitamin B_6 for 3 weeks. While these sex differences were not statistically significant, the consistency of the difference and the fact that they were all being fed the same diet suggests there may be a metabolic difference in vitamin B_6 metabolism between males and females. Age differences in vitamin B_6 metabolism also have implications for requirements. There are several reports of decreased plasma PLP levels with age. Only one controlled metabolic study of age differences in vitamin B_6 metabolism has been conducted. Lee and Leklem (132) have shown that middle-aged women (mean age 53 yr) fed a constant diet (2.3 mg vitamin B_6) had significantly lower plasma PLP, plasma, and urinary total vitamin B_6 and slightly higher urinary 4-PA excretion than young women (mean age 24 yr). The implication of these findings for requirements remains to be determined.

Requirements for vitamin B$_6$ for infants and children are based on relatively few studies (252–254). In fact, no experimental studies have been conducted to directly determine requirements as related to protein intake. Bessey et al. (254) evaluated the amount of pyridoxine required to relieve convulsions in infants who had accidentally received a diet low in vitamin B$_6$. An intake of 0.26 mg was required. In some infants 1.0–1.4 mg vitamin B$_6$ was required to normalize urinary excretion of xanthurenic acid. Considering these results, there was a wide range of vitamin B$_6$ required (0.3–1.4 mg) by these infants. For children and adolescents there are no well-designed studies that have evaluated vitamin B$_6$ requirements. The only data available are for intakes of vitamin B$_6$ (255).

Vitamin B$_6$ requirements in adult males and females have been established from a combination of metabolic studies, vitamin B$_6$ intake data, and protein intake. The use of data on vitamin B$_6$ intake of populations in establishing a requirement is based on the assumption that the intake of a healthy population is indeed the amount necessary to maintain the health of that population. This assumption may be proper if the health and well-being have been adequately evaluated. In most studies this evaluation was not done. The intakes of vitamin B$_6$ for adult males and females as assessed in the 1985 and 1986 nationwide food consumption surveys (256,257) are listed in Tables 17 and 18. In general, women had intakes about 60% of the 1980 RDA, and men 80–115%.

Metabolic studies in males and females have been conducted to evaluate vitamin B$_6$ requirements (Table 19). A common feature of nearly all of these studies has been that they are depletion-repletion studies and often utilized semi-synthetic diets and doses of vitamin B$_6$ in a form considered to be essentially 100% available. These points should

Table 17 Protein and Vitamin B$_6$ Intake In Adult Men and Women[a]

Income level and age	Protein (g)		B$_6$		B$_6$/Protein	
	1977	1985	1977	1985	1977	1985
Women						
Under 131% poverty						
19–34	—	66.3	—	1.25	—	0.019
35–50	—	63.2	—	1.07	—	0.017
131–300% poverty						
19–34	—	66.3	—	1.26	—	0.019
35–50	—	64.9	—	1.23	—	0.019
Over 300% poverty						
19–34	—	66.2	—	1.39	—	0.021
34–50	—	64.0	—	1.30	—	0.020
Men						
Under 131% poverty						
19–34	113	98.5	1.93	1.61	0.017	0.016
34–40	108	128.8	1.75	2.25	0.016	0.018
131–300% poverty						
19–34	97.7	98.0	1.76	1.94	0.018	0.020
34–40	96.7	100.4	1.74	1.86	0.018	0.019
Over 300% poverty						
19–34	96.4	100.5	1.83	2.01	0.019	0.020
34–40	96.3	95.5	1.89	1.89	0.019	0.020

Source: Refs. 256, 257.

Table 18 Mean Intake of Vitamin B_6 Below the 1980 RDA, by Household Income Level and by Race

	Women	Men
	---percentage of RDA---	
Income level		
Under 131% of poverty	58	82
131–300% of poverty	61	87
Over 300% of poverty	66	89
Race		
White	63	118
Black	52	70
All	62	115

Sources: Ref. 257 for women, Ref. 256 for men.

be carefully considered when establishing recommendations for allowances. While some of these studies were not specifically designed to assess vitamin B_6 requirements, they have been used in estimating a requirement (239–241). A majority of these studies were conducted in young men and women. Requirements for older adults have been made based on extrapolation of data in these younger groups. The experimental tests used in the metabolic studies have been primarily the tryptophan load test and to a lesser extent urinary 4-PA excretion, aminotransferase activity, and plasma PLP concentration. The amount of tryptophan administered to subjects varied between studies. In the studies in both men and women, the protein content of the diets has varied over a wide range (30–150 g). These variations and others such as the types of foods, length of adjustment, deficiency and repletion periods, and the amount of vitamin B_6 in the depletion/repletion diets make it difficult to set specific vitamin B_6 requirements. As pointed out in a recent assessment of RDAs (267), better, well-controlled experiments specifically designed to evaluate vitamin B_6 requirements are needed. One feature of the metabolic studies by Canham et al. (190) and Miller et al. (242) has been an evaluation of the relationship between protein intake and vitamin B_6 need. The Dietary Standard for Canada, 1975 (243), suggests that a ratio of 0.02 mg of vitamin B_6 per gram of protein be used to set vitamin B_6 allowances. This suggested ratio was used, in part, to establish the 1980 U.S. RDA for vitamin B_6 (241).

IX. DISEASE AND TOXICITY

Several books (2,3,7) and reviews (6) have examined the relationship of specific diseases and vitamin B_6 nutrition in detail. There are numerous diseases or pathological conditions in which vitamin B_6 metabolism is altered. The primary indicator of an alteration in metabolism of vitamin B_6 has been in evaluation of tryptophan metabolism or the plasma PLP concentration. As previously discussed, the first of these is an indirect measure of status and the second is a direct measure. Further, using only PLP as a measure really begs the question as to whether vitamin B_6 metabolism is really altered. Conditions in which tryptophan metabolism has been shown to be altered and in which vitamin B_6 (pyridoxine) administration was used include asthma (268), diabetes (269), certain cancers (152), pellagra (270), and rheumatoid arthritis (271). Diseases and pathological conditions in which plasma PLP levels have been shown to be depressed include asthma (272),

Table 19 Studies in Which Vitamin B$_6$ Requirements Have Been Investigated

Ref.	No. of subjects	Sex	Age (yr)	Wt (kg)	B$_6$ (mg)	Diet protein	Energy (kcal)	Food types[c]	Adj	Duration[a] defic	Repletion	Tests[b]	Suggested requirements
Canham (190)	6	M	—	—	0 0	80 40	— —	SS SS	7(2)	28	14(10)	10g DL-Try,XA;SGOT; NMe; Urinary B-6	NS
Baker (258)	5	M			0.06	30		Liquid Formula	7(4)	49	(1.5)	10 g DL Try;XA; Urinary B-6; EEG	1.0
Harding (69)	6 9	M M	20-28	65-83	0.06 4.28 2.76 1.93	100 149 164 165	3800	SS A.R. (34) A.R. (100)	24 24 24	21		10g DL Try,XA	1.5 1.97-2.76
Canham (259)	—	M	—	—	0.34	100	3000	SS		—	8	5g-LTry,XA;EEG/EKG GPT (WB)	> 0.35;0.35 submarginal
Swan (260) Yess (261) Brown (262) Baysal (222)	6	M	24-35	61-82	0.16	100	2500-3000	SS	5-SSd	28-41	9-19(0.8 to 1.1)	5g L-Cysteine; 2g L-Try;TM, NMe,QA;PLP	NS NS
Miller (242)	5	M	21-25	63-73	0.16	54	2800-3700	SS	6(1.66)	33-40	7(0.76)	2g L-Try,TM;4-PA: Urinary B-6	NS(0.8)
Kelsay (138)	6	M	19-31	63-71	0.16	150	2800-3600	SS	18(1.66)	16	16(0.76)	2g L-Try, TM; EEG; 4PA; Urinary B-6; QA;NMe	
Cheslock (263)	7 1	F M	18-20 —	— —	0.41 0.50	26 36	2045 2724	Natural Natural	—	52	—	5g L-Try,XA,Blood B-6	>0.5
Aly (264)	5	F	21-31	—	1.3	81	—	Liquid/ Solid	6	—	—	2g L-Try,XA;Urinary B-6; Amino Acids	NS
Donald (265)	8	F	21-31	56	0.34	57	1300+	Natural	—	44	7(0.94) 3(1.54)	Urinary 4PA,B-6; E-B6;EGOT;Amino Acids	1.5
Shin (266)	5	F	23	49	0.16	109		SS	7(2.16)	14	14(2.16)	2g L-Try; TM; Urinary B-6; 3g L-Meth.	NS
Leklem (86,176)	10	F	22	60	0.19	78	1992	SS	4	28	28(0.83)	2g L-Try,TM;4PA;PLP; EGOT, EGPT; 3g Meth; NMe	>0.83

[a]Duration refers to length of any adjustment (Adj) period, deficiency (Defic) period, or repletion period given as days. Values in parentheses are mg of vitamin B$_6$ fed.

[b]Tests: Biochemical tests used to evaluate vitamin B$_6$ status. Abbreviations: XA, xanthurenic acid; SGOT, EGOT serum or erythrocyte glutamic oxalacetate transaminase; NMe, N-methyl-nicotinamide; EEG, electroencephalogram; EKG, electrocardiogram; GPT(WB), glutamic pyruvate transaminase in whole blood; TM, tryptophan metabolites; QA, quinolinic acid; PLP, pyridoxal-5'-phosphate; 4-PA,4-pyridoxic acid; Try, tryptophan; Meth, methionine.

[c]Food types; the types of foods used in the metabolic study. SS, semi-synthetic; AR, army ration stored at 34 or 100°F.
NS = none suggested by authors.

diabetes (273), renal disorders (274), alcoholism (275), heart disease (276), pregnancy (117,129,136,277), breast cancer (278), Hodgkins' disease (279), and sickle-cell anemia (170). Hypophosphatasia is an example of a condition in which plasma PLP levels are markedly elevated in some individuals (83). Relatively few of these studies have exhaustively evaluated vitamin B_6 metabolism.

Vitamin B_6 in the form of pyridoxine hydrochloride has been used as a therapeutic agent to treat a variety of disorders. A recent international conference on vitamin B_6 explored research in this area (7,115). Examples of disorders that have been treated with pyridoxine include Down's syndrome (280), autism (281), hyperoxaluria (282), gestational diabetes (283), premenstrual syndrome (284), carpal tunnel syndrome (285), depression (286), and diabetic neuropathy (287). It sould be emphasized that the extent to which pyridoxine was effective in treating these diseases or reducing symptoms has been variable. In addition, in the treatment of these diseases, the amount of pyridoxine given often varied as did the length of time over which the pyridoxine was given. These two variables as well as the important consideration of whether a double-blind placebo-controlled design was used are necessary considerations in evaluating the effectiveness of vitamin B_6 therapy (115).

A. Coronary Heart Disease

A relationship between vitamin B_6 and coronary heart disease can be viewed from both an etiological perspective and that of the effect of the disease state on vitamin B_6 metabolism. With respect to an etiological role, an altered sulfur amino acid metabolism has been suggested to result in vascular damage. A poor vitamin B_6 status can result in an increased circulating concentration of homocysteine (288). In the transulfuration pathway, serine and homocysteine condense to produce cystathionine. This reaction is catalyzed by the PLP-dependent enzyme, cystathionine β-synthase. In genetic disorders of this enzyme, homocysteine accumulates in the plasma (289). An increased incidence of arteriosclerosis has been associated with this enzyme defect (290). In addition, an elevated concentration of homocysteine has been observed in persons with ischemic heart disease (291). These observations support a role for methionine metabolites inducing vascular damage.

While some animal experiments have shown that rhesus monkeys made vitamin B_6–deficient results in atherosclerotic lesions (217,292), a subsequent experiment repeating this work did not reveal any pathological lesions (293). In humans at risk for coronary heart disease, a negative correlation between dietary vitamin B_6 and bound homocysteine has been observed (124). For some persons with homocystinuria, treatment with high doses of vitamin B_6 reduces the plasma concentration of homocysteine in certain patients but does not totally correct methionine metabolism (294), especially when there is an increased methionine intake. Thus, if vitamin B_6 therapy is to be successful in reducing vascular lesions, diet modification with a lowered methionine intake may be necessary. The extent to which supplemental vitamin B_6 intake (beyond normal dietary intakes) may reduce the risk for coronary heart disease is not known.

A second aspect of coronary heart disease is the relationship between the presence of the disease and vitamin B_6 status. Several recent studies have found that the plasma PLP concentration in persons with coronary heart disease are significantly lower (21–41 nmol/l) than healthy controls (32–46 nmol/l) (224,276,295,296). However, Vermaak et al. have found that the decrease in plasma PLP concentration is only seen in the acute phase of myocardial infarction (297). Unfortunately, other measures of vitamin B_6 status have not been evaluated in this disease. In one study (296), cardiac patients given vitamin B$_6$ supplements (amounts not given) resulted in plasma PLP levels well above normal. The effect of long-term vitamin B$_6$ therapy on recurrence of coronary artery disease has not been evaluated.

Elevated plasma cholesterol concentration has been strongly associated with an increased risk for coronary heart disease. As previously reviewed, vitamin B$_6$ may influence cholesterol metabolism. Serfontein and Ubbink (224) have found that use of a multivitamin supplement containing about 10 mg of pyridoxine for 22 weeks by hypercholesterolemic adult men resulted in a significant decrease in cholesterol levels, with most of the reduction due to a decreased level of LDL cholesterol. Smoking is an additional risk factor of coronary heart disease. Interestingly, smokers have decreased plasma levels of PLP (224,298). Evidence to date suggests a link between several risk factors for coronary heart disease and altered vitamin B$_6$ status and a potential beneficial effect of increased vitamin B$_6$ intake on cholesterol levels. Further well-controlled studies are needed before the therapeutic effect of vitamin B$_6$ can be evaluated for this disease.

B. Premenstrual Syndrome (PMS)

Premenstrual syndrome (PMS) is another clinical situation for which vitamin B$_6$ supplementation has been suggested (299). Estimates of 40% of women being affected by this syndrome have been made (300). Using a wide variety of parameters, no difference in vitamin B$_6$ status was observed in women with PMS compared to those not reporting symptoms (151,207,308). Nevertheless, beneficial effects of B$_6$ administration on at least some aspects of PMS have been reported.

Treatment of PMS with vitamin B$_6$ has been based in part on the studies of Adams et al. (301) in which PN was used to treat the depression observed in some women taking oral contraceptives. Of the several studies in which PN was used to treat PMS, three have been of the open type and four studies were double-blind placebo controlled. Open studies are prone to a placebo effect error, often as high as 40%. Of the well-controlled type, one study showed no effect of pyridoxine therapy (303), while three studies reported significant improvement in at least some of the symptoms associated with PMS. In one study 21 of 25 patients improved (304). The other study found that about 60% of the 48 women showed improvement with pyridoxine (200 mg/day) and 20% showed improvement with the placebo (305). The fourth study (306) reported involvement in some symptoms in the 55 women treated daily with 150 mg of pyridoxine. Brush (299) reported results of studies he has conducted using vitamin B$_6$ alone and vitamin B$_6$ plus magnesium. His data suggest that doses of 150–200 mg of vitamin B$_6$ are necessary before a significant positive effect is observed. In addition, the combination of vitamin B$_6$ plus magnesium appears to be beneficial. The complexity of PMS and the subjective nature of symptom reporting continue to result in contradictions and controversy in the lay and scientific literature. Nonetheless, vitamin B$_6$ appears to be useful in alleviating various PMS symptoms in some women, possibly those suffering from distinct subtypes of the syndrome. There may be a decrease in the availability of vitamin B$_6$ during PMS, possibly due to cell transport competition from fluctuating hormone concentrations. An increase in vitamin B$_6$ concentration could overcome competition and may explain the relief of symptoms seen in some women following high dose vitamin B$_6$ supplementation.

C. Sickle-Cell Anemia

Low levels (18 nmol/l) of plasma PLP have been reported in 16 persons with sickle-cell anemia (170). Treatment of five of these patients with 100 mg of pyridoxine hydrochloride per day for 2 months resulted in a reduction of severity, frequency, and duration of painful crises in these persons. The mechanism by which vitamin B_6 acts is not known, but it may be related to pyridoxal and PLP binding to hemoglobin.

D. Asthma

Depressed levels of plasma and erythrocyte PLP have also been reported in 15 persons with asthma (272). Of significance was the fact that all persons were receiving bronchodilators. Treatment of seven asthmatics with 100 mg of pyridoxine hydrochloride per day resulted in a reduction in the duration, occurrence, and severity of their asthmatic attacks. Subsequent work by one of these authors has not fully supported the earlier findings (309). Treatment of 15 asthmatics with vitamin B_6 did not result in a significant difference in symptom scores, medication usage, or pulmonary function tests as compared to placebo treatment. The depressed levels of plasma PLP in these asthmatics should also be evaluated in the context of research showing that theophylline and gentamicin lower plasma PLP levels (310).

E. Carpal Tunnel Syndrome

At least five placebo-controlled trials from four different laboratories have shown that administration of PN relieved the symptoms of carpal tunnel syndrome (pain and/or numbness in hands) (285,310a,310b). In one study no significant improvement was observed (310c). Since supplementation with vitamin B_6 well in excess of the RDA level was required for improvement (generally 50–150 mg) it would seem that individuals with this disorder either have a high metabolic demand or that the vitamin is active in some non-coenzyme role.

F. Drug–Vitamin B_6 Interaction

Treatment of persons with various drugs may also compromise vitamin B_6 status and hence result in an increased need for vitamin B_6. Table 20 lists several drugs and the effect these have on vitamin B_6. Bhagavan has reviewed these interactions in detail (311). A common feature of these drug interactions is the adverse effect they have on central nervous system function. In addition, many of these drugs react with PLP via a Schiff base formation. This reaction can then result in decreased levels of PLP in tissues, such as the brain, leading to a functional deficiency. In most cases supplemental vitamin B_6 reverses the adverse consequences of the drug. Oral contraceptives do not directly react with PLP, but do induce enzyme synthesis. Some of these enzymes are PLP dependent, and as a result PLP is metabolically trapped in tissues. This may then lead to a depressed plasma concentration of PLP (312). In addition, the synthetic estrogens specifically affect enzymes of the tryptophan–niacin pathway resulting in abnormal tryptophan metabolism (176). There may be a need for extra vitamin B_6 above the current RDA in a small proportion of women using oral contraceptives and consuming low levels of vitamin B_6. Any drug that interacts with the reactive molecule PLP in a Schiff base reaction should be considered a candidate for resultant adverse effects on vitamin B_6 status and a subsequent negative influence on central nervous system function.

Table 20 Drug–Vitamin B$_6$ Interactions

Drug or drug type	Examples	Mechanism of interaction
Hydrazines	Iproniazed, isonicotinyhydrazine hydralazine	React with pyridoxal and PLP to form a hydrazone
Antibiotic	Cycloserine	Reacts with PLP to form an oxime
L-DOPA	L-3,4-dihydroxyphenylalanine	Reacts with PLP to form tetrahydroquinoline derivatives
Chelator	Penicillamine	Reacts with PLP to form thiazolidine
Oral contraceptives	Ethinyl estradiol, mestranol	Increased enzyme levels in liver other tissues; retention of PLP
Alcohol	Ethanol	Increased catabolism of PLP, low plasma levels

G. Hazards of High Doses

With the therapeutic use of pyridoxine for various disorders and self-medication has come the potential problem of toxicity. Shaumburg et al. have identified several individuals who developed a peripheral neuropathy associated with chronic high-dose use of pyridoxine (313). Subsequent to this other reports of toxicity related to pyridoxine ingestion have been made (314,315). The minimal dose at which toxicity develops remains to be determined. Other toxicity symptoms have been identified. These symptoms and those reported by Schaumburg are listed in Table 21. These symptoms are relatively rare, and the use of pyridoxine doses of 2–250 mg per day for extended periods of time appears to be safe. (316).

X. SUMMARY

In the more than 50 years that vitamin B$_6$ has been known, a great deal of knowledge about its functional and metabolic characteristics has been gathered. The involvement of the active form of vitamin B$_6$, pyridoxal 5′-phosphate, in such a wide spectrum of enzymatic reactions is an indication of the importance of this vitamin. In addition to the involvement of PLP in amino acid metabolism and carbohydrate metabolism, its reactivity with proteins points to the diversity of this vitamin. Further research is needed about

Table 21 Toxicity Symptoms Reported to Be Associated with Chronic High Doses of Pyridoxine

Reference	Symptoms
Coleman et al. (280)	Motor and sensory neuropathy; vasicular dermatosis on regions of the skin exposed to sunshine.
Schaumburg (313)	Peripheral neuropathy; loss of limb reflexes; impaired touch sensation in limbs; unsteady gait, impaired or absent tendon reflexes; sensation of tingling that proceeds down neck and legs
Brush (298)	Dizziness; nausea; breast discomfort or tenderness
Bernstein (287)	Photosensitivity on exposure to sun

the factors controlling the metabolism of vitamin B_6 and determination of vitamin B_6 needs of specific population. With knowledge of the functional properties of vitamin B_6 and quantitation of the metabolism of vitamin B_6 under various physiological and nutritional conditions, the health and well-being of individuals, can be improved.

REFERENCES

1. J. E. Leklem and R. D. Reynolds, (eds.), *Methods in Vitamin B-6 Nutrition*, Plenum Press, New York, 1981.
2. G. P. Tryfiates, (ed.) *Vitamin B-6 Metabolism and Role in Growth*, Food and Nutrition Press, Westport, CN, 1980.
3. R. D. Reynolds and J. E. Leklem, (eds.), *Vitamin B-6: Its Role in Health and Disease*, A. R. Liss, New York, 1985.
4. D. Dolphin, R. Poulson, and O. Avramovic, (eds.), *Coenzymes and Cofactors*, Vol. 1. Vitamin B-6 pyridoxal phosphate, John Wiley and Sons, New York, 1986.
5. S. L. Ink and L. M. Henderson, Vitamin B-6 metabolism, *Ann. Rev. Nutr., 4*:445–470 (1984).
6. A. H. Merrill, Jr. and J. M. Henderson, Diseases associated with defects in vitamin B-6 metabolism or utilization, *Ann. Rev. Nutr. 7*:137–156 (1987).
7. J. E. Leklem and R. D. Reynolds (eds.), *Clinical and Physiological Applications of Vitamin B-6*, A. R. Liss, New York, 1988.
8. E. R. Gruberg and S. A. Raymond, *Beyond Cholesterol*, St. Martin's, New York, 1981.
9. P. Gyorgy, Vitamin B-2 and the pellagra-like dermatitis of rats, *Nature, 133*:448–449 (1934).
10. P. Gyorgy, Crystalline vitamin B-6, *J. Am. Chem. Soc., 60*:983–984 (1938).
11. S. Lepkovsky, Crystalline factor I, *Science, 87*:169–170 (1938).
12. R. Kuhn and Wendt, G. Über das antidermatitische Vitamin der Hefe. *Ber. Deut. Chem. Ges. 71B*:780–782 (1938).
13. J. C. Keresztesy and J. R. Stevens, Vitamin B-6. *Proc Soc. Exp. Biol. Med., 38*:64–65 (1938).
14. A. Ichiba and K. Michi, Isolation of vitamin B-6, *Soc. Papers Inst. Phys. Chem. Res.* (Tokyo), *34*:623–626 (1938).
15. S. A. Harris and K. Folkers, Synthesis of vitamin B-6, *J. Am. Chem. Soc., 61*:1245–1247 (1939).
16. R. Kuhn, K. Westphal, G. Wendt, and O. Westphal, Synthesis of adermin, *Natur-wissenschaften, 27*:469–470 (1939).
17. P. Gyorgy and R. E. Eckhardt, Vitamin B-6 and skin lesions in rats, *Nature 144*:512 (1939).
18. E. E. Snell, Vitamin B-6 analysis: some historical aspects. In: J. E. Leklem and R. D. Reynolds, (eds.), *Methods in Vitamin B-6 Nutrition*, Plenum, New York, 1981, pp. 1–19.
19. E. E. Snell, B. M. Guirard, and R. J. Williams. Occurrence in natural products of a physiologically active metabolite of pyridoxine, *J. Biol. Chem., 143*:519–530 (1942).
20. E. E. Snell, The vitamin B-6 group. I. Formation of additional members from pyridoxine and evidence concerning their structure, *J. Am. Chem. Soc., 66*:2082–2088 (1944).
21. E. E. Snell, The vitamin activities of pyridoxal and pyridoxamine, *J. Biol. Chem., 154*:313–314 (1944).
22. S. A. Harris, D. Heyl, and D. Folkers, The structure and synthesis of pyridoxamine and pyridoxal, *J. Biol. Chem., 154*:315–316; *J. Am. Chem. Soc., 66*:2089–2092 (1944).
23. IUPAC-IUB Commission on Biochemical Nomenclature. Nomenclature for vitamin B-6 and related compounds. *Eur. J. Biochem., 40*:325–327 (1973).
24. C. Y. W. Ang, Stability of three forms of vitamin B-6 to laboratory light conditions, *J. Assoc. Off. Anal. Chem., 62*:1170–1173 (1979).
25. C. A. Storvick, E. M. Benson, M. A. Edwards, and M. J. Woodring, Chemical and microbiological determination of vitamin B-6, *Methods Biochem. Anal., 12*:183–276 (1964).
26. S. A. Harris, E. E. Harris, and R. W. Bukrg, Pyridoxine. *Kirk-Othmer Encycl. Chem. Tech., 16*:806–824 (1968).

27. J. W. Bridges, D. S. Davies, and R. T. Williams. Fluorescence studies on some hydroxypyridines including compounds of the vitamin B-6 group, *Biochem. J.* 98:451–468 (1966).
28. W. E. Schaltenbrand, M. S. Kennedy, and S. P. Coburn, Low-ultraviolet "white" fluorescent lamps fail to protect pyridoxal phosphate from photolysis, *Clin. Chem.*, 33:631 (1987).
29. R. C. Hughes, W. T. Jenkins, and E. H. Fischer, The site of binding of pyridoxal-5'-phosphate to heart glutamic-aspartic transaminase, *Proc. Natl. Acad. Sci. USA*, 48:1615–1618 (1962).
30. Leussing, D. L. Model reactions, In: D. Dolphin, R. Poulson, O. Avramovic, eds. *Coenzymes and Cofactors*, Vol. 1. Vitamins B-6 pyridoxal phosphate, John Wiley and Sons, New York, 1986, pp. 69–115.
31. H. E. Sauberlich, Interaction of vitamin B-6 with other nutrients. In: R. D. Reynolds, J. E. Leklem, eds. *Vitamin B-6: Its Role in Health and Disease*, A. R. Liss, New York, 1985, pp. 193–217.
32. L. Atkin, A. S. Schultz, W. L. Williams, and C. N. Frey, Yeast microbiological methods for determination of vitamins-pyridoxine, *Ind. and Eng. Chem. Anal. Ed.* 15:141–144 (1943).
33. M. Polansky, Microbiological assay of vitamin B-6 in foods. In: J. E. Leklem and R. D. Reynolds, eds. *Methods in Vitamin B-6 Nutrition*, Plenum, New York, 1981, pp. 21–44.
34. M. L. Orr, *Pathothenic Acid, Vitamin B-6 and Vitamin B-12* in Foods. Home Economics Research Report No. 36, U.S. Dept. of Agriculture, Washington, D.C., 1969.
35. K. Yasumoto, H. Tsuji, K. Iwami, and H. Metsuda, Isolation from rice bran of a bound form of vitamin B-6 and its identification as 5'-0-(B.D.-glucopyranosyl) pyridoxine, *Agric. Biol. Chem.* 41:1061–1067 (1977).
36. H. Kabir, J. E. Leklem, and L. T. Miller, Measurement of glycosylated vitamin B-6 in foods, *J. Food Sci.*, 48:1422–1425 (1983).
37. Y. Suzuki, Y. Inada, and K. Uchida, β-Glucosylpyridoxines in germinating seeds cultured in the presence of pyridoxine, *Phytochemistry*, 25:2049–2051 (1986).
38. K. Tadera, T. Kaneko, and F. Yagi, Evidence for the occurrence and distribution of a new type of vitamin B-6 conjugate in plant foods, *Agric. Biol. Chem.*, 50:2933–2934 (1986).
39. K. Tadera, E. Mori, F. Yagi, A. Kobayashi, K. Imada, and M. Imabeppu, Isolation and structure of a minor metabolite of pyridoxine in seedlings of *Pisum sativum* L, *J. Nutr. Sci. Vitaminol.*, 31:403–408 (1985).
40. C. H. Lushbough, J. M. Weichman, and B. S. Schweigert, The retention of vitamin B-6 in meat during cooking, *J. Nutr.* 67:451–459 (1959).
41. F. W. Bernhart, E. D'Amato, and R. M. Tomarelli, The vitamin B-6 activity of heat-sterilized milk, *Arch. Biochem. Biophys.*, 88:267–269 (1960).
42. L. R. Richardson, S. Wilkes, and S. J. Ritchey. Comparitive vitamin B-6 activity of frozen, irradiated and heat-processed foods, *J. Nutr.*, 73:363–368 (1961).
43. H. N. Daoud, B. S. Luh, and M. W. Miller, Effect of blanching, EDTA and NaHSO₃ on color and vitamin B-6 retention in canned garbanzo beans, *J. Food Sci.*, 42:375–378 (1977).
44. J. Augustin, G. I. Marousek, L. A. Tholen, and B. Bertelli, Vitamin retention in cooked, chilled and reheated potatoes, *J. Food Sci.*, 45:814–816 (1980).
45. J. Augustin, G. I. Marousek, W. E. Artz, and B. G. Swanson, Retention of some water-soluble vitamins during home preparation of commercially frozen potato products, *J. Food Sci*, 46:1697–1700 (1981).
46. J. F. Gregory and J. R. Kirk, Assessment of roasting effects on vitamin B-6 stability and bioavailability in dehydrated food systems, *J. Food Sci.*, 43:1585–1589 (1978).
47. O. S. Abou-Fadel and L. T. Miller, Vitamin retention, color and texture in thermally processed green beans and Royal Ann cherries packed in pouches and cans, *J. Food Sci.*, 48:920–923 (1983).
48. C. Y. W. Ang, Comparison of sample storage methods of vitamin B-6 assay in broiler meats, *J. Food Sci.*, 47:336–337 (1981).
49. M. J. Woodring and C. A. Storvick, Vitamin B-6 in milk: review of literature, *J. Assoc. Off. Agric. Chem.*, 43:63–80 (1960).

50. J. T. Vanderslice, S. R. Brownlee, and M. E. Cortissoy, Liquid chromatographic determination of vitamin B-6 in foods, *J. Assoc. Off. Anal. Chem.*, *67*:999–1007 (1984).

51. E. DeRitter, Stability characteristics of vitamins in processed foods, *Food Tech.* (Jan): 48–51,54 (1976).

52. A. D. Perera, J. E. Leklem, and L. T. Miller, Stability of vitamin B-6 during bread making and storage of bread and flour, *Cereal Chem.*, *56*:577–580 (1979).

53. J. F. Gregory and J. R. Kirk. Interaction of pyridixoal and pyridoxal phosphate with peptides in a model food system during thermal processing, *J. Food Sci.*, *42*:1554–1561 (1977).

54. J. F. Gregory, Effects of ε-pyridoxyllysine bound to dietary protein on the vitamin B-6 status of rats, *J. Nutr.*, *110*:995–1005 (1980).

55. K. Tadera, M. Arima, S. Yoshino, F. Yagi, and A. Kobayashi, Conversion of pyridoxine into 6-hydroxypyridoxine by food components, especially ascorbic acid, *J. Nutr. Sci. Vitaminol.*, *32*:267–277 (1986).

56. S. Yoshida, K. Hayashi, and T. Kawasaki, Pyridoxine transport in brush border membrane vesicles of guinea pig jejunum, *J. Nutr. Sci. Vitaminol.*, *27*:311–317 (1981).

57. G. S. Heard and E. F. Annison, Gastrointestinal absorption of vitamin B-6 in the chicken (*Gallus domesticus*), *J. Nutr. 116*:107–120 (1986).

58. H. A. Serebro, H. M. Solomon, J. H. Johnson, and T. R. Henrix, The intestinal absorption of vitamin B-6 compounds by the rat and hamster, *Bull. Johns Hopkins Hosp.*, *119*:166–171 (1966).

59. H. M. Middleton, Uptake of pyridoxine hydrochloride by the rat jejunal mucosa in vitro, *J. Nutr.*, *107*:126–131 (1977).

60. H. M. Middleton, Characterization of pyridoxal 5'-phosphate disappearance from in vivo perfused segments of rat jejunum, *J. Nutr. 112*:269–275 (1982).

61. L. M. Henderson, Intestinal absorption of B-6 vitamers. In: R. D. Reynolds, and J. E. Leklem, eds., *Vitamin B-6 Its Role in Health and Disease*, A. R. Liss, New York, 1985, pp. 22–33.

62. H. Mehansho, M. W. Hamm, and L. M. Henderson, Transport and metabolism of pyridoxal and pyridoxal phosphate in the small intestine of the rat, *J. Nutr. 109*:1542–1551 (1979).

63. M. W. Hamm, H. Mehansho, and L. M. Henderson, Transport and metabolism of pyridoxamine and pyridoxamine phosphate in the small intestine of the rat, *J. Nutr.*, *109*:1552–1559 (1979).

64. D. A. Roth-Maier, P. M. Zinner, and M. Kirchgessner, Effect of varying dietary vitamin B-6 supply on intestinal absorption of vitamin B-6, *Internat. J. Vit. Nutr. Res.*, *52*:272–279 (1982).

65. H. M. Middleton, Uptake of pyridoxine by in vivo perfused segments of rat small intestine: a possible role for intracellular vitamin metabolism, *J. Nutr. 115*:1079–1088 (1985).

66. T. Sakurai, T. Asakura, and M. Matsuda, Transport and metabolism of pyridoxine and pyridoxal in mice, *J. Nutr. Sci. Vitaminol.*, *33*:11–19 (1987).

67. J. F. Gregory and S. L. Ink, The bioavailability of vitamin B-6. In: R. D. Reynolds and J. E. Leklem, eds. *Vitamin B-6: Its Role in Health and Disease*: A. R. Liss, New York, 1985, pp. 3–23.

68. J. E. Leklem, Bioavailability of vitamins: application of human nutrition. In: A. R. Dobernz, J. A. Milner, and B. S. Schweigert, eds., *Food and agricultural research opportunities to improve human nutrition*, University of Delaware, Newark, 1986, A56-A73.

69. R. S. Harding, I. S. Plough, and T. E. Friedemann, The effect of storage on the vitamin B-6 content of packaged army ration with a note on the human requirement for the vitamin, *J. Nutr.*, *68*:323–331 (1959).

70. E. W. Nelson, C. W. Burgin, and J. J. Cerda, Characterization of food binding of vitamin B-6 in orange juice, *J. Nutr. 107*:2128–2134 (1977).

71. J. E. Leklem, L. T. Miller, A. D. Perera, and D. E. Peffers, Bioavailability of vitamin B-6 from wheat bread in humans, *J. Nutr.*, *110*:1819–1828 (1980).

72. A. S. Lindberg, J. E. Leklem, and L. T. Miller, The effect of wheat bran on the bioavailability of vitamin B-6 in young men, *J. Nutr., 113*:2578–2586 (1983).

73. C. Kies, S. Kan, and H. M. Fox, Vitamin B-6 availability from wheat, rice, corn brans for humans, *Nutr. Repts. Int., 30*:483–491 (1984).

74. J. B. Tarr, T. Tamura, and E. L. R. Stokstad, Availability of vitamin B-6 and pantothenate in an aveage diet in man, *Am. J. Clin. Nutr., 34*:1328–1337 (1981).

75. E. W. Nelson, H. J. R. Lane, and J. J. Cerda, Comparative human intestinal bioavailability of vitamin B-6 from a synthetic and a natural source, *J. Nutr. 106*:1433–1437 (1976).

76. J. E. Leklem, T. D. Shultz, and L. T. Miller, Comparative bioavailability of vitamin B-6 from soybeans and beef, *Fed. Proc. 39*:558 (abst) (1980).

77. H. Kabir, J. E. Leklem, and L. T. Miller, Comparative vitamin B-6 bioavailability from tuna, whole wheat bread and peanut butter in humans, *J. Nutr., 113*:2412–2420 (1983).

78. H. Kabir, J. E. Leklem, and L. T. Miller, Relationship of the glycosylated vitamin B-6 content of foods of vitamin B-6 bioavailability in humans, *Nutr. Rept. Int. 28*:709–716 (1983).

79. N. D. Bills, J. E. Leklem, and L. T. Miller, Vitamin B-6 bioavailability in plant foods is inversely correlated with % glycosylated vitamin B-6, *Fed. Proc., 46*:1487 (abst.) (1987).

80. L. Lumeng, and T-K. Li, Mammalian vitamin B-6 metabolism: regulatory role of protein-binding and the hydrolysis of pyridoxal 5′-phosphate in storage and transport. In: G. P. Tryfiates, ed., *Vitamin B-6 Metabolism and Role in Growth*, Food and Nutrition Press, Westport, CT, 1980, pp. 27–51.

81. L. Lumeng, R. E. Brashear, and T-K. Li, Pyridoxal 5′-phosphate in plasma: source, protein binding, and cellular transport, *J. Lab. Clin. Med. 84*:334–343 (1974).

82. H. Wada, and E. E. Snell, The enzymatic oxidation of pyridoxine and pyridoxamine phosphates, *J. Biol. Chem. 236*:2089–2095 (1961).

83. S. P. Coburn and M. P. Whyte, Role of phosphatases in the regulation of vitamin B-6 metabolism in hypophosphatasia and other disorders, In: J.E. Leklem, and R. D. Reynolds, eds., *Clinical and Physiological Applications of Vitamin B-6*, A. R. Liss, New York, 1988, pp. 65–93.

84. T-K, Li, L. Lumeng, and R. L. Veitch, Regulation of pyridoxal 5′-phosphate metabolism in liver, *Biochem. Biophys. Res. Comm., 61*:627–634 (1974).

85. A. H. Merrill, J. M. Henderson, E. Wang, B. W. McDonald, and W. J. Millikan, Metabolism of vitamin B-6 by human liver, *J. Nutr., 114*:1664–1674 (1984).

86. R. R. Brown, D. P. Rose, J. E. Leklem, H. Linkswiler, and R. Anand, Urinary 4-pyridoxic acid, plasma pyridoxal phosphate and erythrocyte aminotransferase levels in oral contraceptive users receiving controlled intakes of vitamin B-6, *Am. J. Clin. Nutr., 28*:10–19 (1975).

87. J. R. Wozenski, J. E. Leklem, and L. T. Miller, The metabolism of small doses of vitamin B-6 in men, *J. Nutr. 110*:275–285 (1980).

88. T. D. Shultz and J. E. Leklem, Urinary 4-pyridoxic acid, urinary vitamin B-6 and plasma pyridoxal phosphate as measures of vitamin B-6 status and dietary intake of adults. In: J.E. Leklem and R. D. Reynolds, eds., *Methods in Vitamin B-6 Nutrition*, Plenum, New York, (1981), pp. 297–320.

89. A. H. Merrill, J. M. Henderson, E. Wang, M. A. Codner, B. Hollins, and W. J. Millikan, Activities of the hepatic enzymes of vitamin B-6 metabolism for patients with cirrhosis, *Am. J. Clin. Nutr., 44*:461–467 (1986).

90. A. V. Lakshmi and M. S. Bamji, Tissue pyridoxal phosphate concentration and pyridoxamine phosphate oxidase activity in riboflavin deficiency in rats and man, *Brit. J. Nutr., 32*:249–255 (1974).

91. G. M. Perry, B. B. Anderson, and N. Dodd, The effect of riboflavin on red-cell vitamin B-6 metabolism and globin synthesis, *Biomedicine 33*:36–38 (1980).

92. S. P. Coburn, and J. D. Mahuren, A versatile cation-exchange procedure for measuring the seven major forms of vitamin B-6 in biological samples, *Anal. Biochem., 129*:310–317 (1983).

93. L. Lumeng, T-K. Li, and A. Lui. The interorgan transport and metabolism of vitamin B-6. In: R. D. Reynolds and J. E. Leklem, eds., *Vitamin B-6: Its Role in Health and Disease* A. R. Liss, New York, 1985, pp. 35–54.

94. B. Hollins and J. M. Henderson, Analysis of B-6 vitamers in plasma by reversed-phase column liquid chromatography, *J.Chromatogr. 380*:67–75 (1986).

95. B. B. Anderson, Red-cell metabolism of vitamin B-6. In: G. P. Tryfiates, ed., *Vitamin B-6 Metabolism and Role in Growth*, Food and Nutrition Press, Westport, CT, 1980, pp. 53–83.

96. H. Mehansho and L. M. Henderson, Transport and accumulation of pyridoxine and pyridoxal by erthrocytes, *J. Biol. Chem., 255*:11901–11907 (1980).

97. M. L. Fonda and C. W. Harker, Metabolism of pyridoxine and protein binding of the metabolites in human erythrocytes, *Am. J. Clin. Nutr., 35*:1391–1399 (1982).

98. S. L. Ink, H. Mehansho, and L. M. Henderson, The binding of pyridoxal to hemoglobin, *J. Biol. Chem., 257*:4753–4757 (1982).

99. R. E. Benesch, S. Yung, T. Suzuki, C. Bauer, and R. Benesch, Pyridoxal compounds as specific reagents for the alpha and β N-termini of hemoglobin, *Proc. Natl. Acad. Sci. USA, 70*:2595–2599 (1973).

100. S. L. Ink and L. M. Henderson, Effect of binding to hemoglobin and albumin on pyridoxal transport and metabolism, *J. Biol. Chem., 259*:5833–5837 (1984).

101. B. M. Pogell, Enzymatic oxidation of pyridoxamine phosphate to pyridoxal phosphate in rabbit liver, *J. Biol. Chem., 232*:761–766 (1958).

102. E. G. Krebs and E. H. Fischer, Phosphorylase and related enzymes of glycogen metabolism. In: R. S. Harris, I. G. Wool, J. A. Lovaine, eds., *Vitamins and Hormones*, Vol 22, Academic Press, New York, 1964 , pp. 399–410.

103. S. P. Coburn, D. L. Lewis, W. J. Fink, and J. D. Mahuren, W. E. Schaltenbrand, and D. L. Costill, Estimation of human vitamin B-6 pools through muscle biopsies, *Am. J. Clin. Nutr., 48*:291–294, 1988.

104. S. Johansson, D. Lindstedt, U. Register, and L. Wadstrom, Studies on the metabolism of labeled pyridoxine in man, *Am. J. Clin. Nutr. 18*:185–196 (1966).

105. B. Shane, Vitamin B-6 and blood. In: Human Vitamin B-6 Requirements, Natl. Acad. Sci., Washington, D. C. 1978, pp. 111–128.

106. D. P. Rose, and R. R. Brown, The influence of sex and estrogens on liver kynureninase and kynurenine aminotransferase in the rat, *Biochem. Biophys. Acta., 184*:412–419 (1969).

107. L. Lumeng, M. P. Ryan, and T-K. Li, Validation of the diagnostic value of plasma pyridoxal 5'-phosphate measurements in vitamin B-6 nutrition of the rat, *J. Nutr., 108*:545–553 (1978).

108. A. L. Black, B. M. Guirard, and E. E. Snell, Increased muscle phosporylase in rats fed high levels of vitamin B-6, *J. Nutr., 107*:1962–1968 (1977).

109. A. L. Black, B. M. Guirard, and E. E. Snell, The behavior of muscle phosphorylase as a reservoir for vitamin B-6 in the rat, *J. Nutr., 108*:670–677 (1978).

110. L. E. Russell, P. J. Bechtel, and R. A. Easter, Effect of deficient and excess dietary vitamin B-6 on aminotransaminase and glycogen phosphorylase activity and pyridoxal phosphate content in two muscles from postpubertal gilts, *J. Nutr., 115*:1124–1135 (1985).

111. J. E. Leklem, Physical activity and vitamin B-6 metabolism in men and women: interrelationship with fuel needs. In: R. D. Reynolds and J. E Leklem, eds., *Vitamin B-6: Its Role and Health and Disease*, A. R. Liss, New York, 1985, pp. 221–241.

112. J. E. Leklem, and T. D. Shultz, Increased plasma pyridoxal 5'-phosphate and vitamin B-6 in male adolescents after a 4500-meter run, *Am. J. Clin. Nutr. 38*:541–548 (1983).

113. M. Manore, J. E. Leklem, and M. C. Walter, Vitamin B-6 metabolism as affected by exercise in trained and untrained women fed diets differing in carbohydrate and vitamin B-6 content, *Am. J. Clin. Nutr. 46*:995–1004 (1987).

114. H. E. Sauberlich, Vitamin B-6 status assessment: past and present. In: J. E. Leklem and R. D. Reynolds, eds., *Methods in Vitamin B-6 Nutrition*, Plenum Press, New York, 1981, pp. 203–240.

115. J. E. Leklem and R. D. Reynolds, Challenges and direction in the search for clinical applications of vitamin B-6. In: J. E. Leklem and R. D. Reynolds, eds., *Clinical and Physiological Applications of Vitamin B-6*, A. R. Liss, New York, 1988, pp. 437–454.

116. J. E. Leklem and R. D. Reynolds, Recommendations for status assessment of vitamin B-6. In: J. E. Leklem and R. D. Reynolds, eds., *Methods in Vitamin B-6 Nutrition*, Plenum Press, New York, 1981, pp. 389–392.

117. M. Wachstein, J. D. Kellner, and J. M. Orez, Pyridoxal phosphate in plasma and leukocytes of normal and pregnant subjects following B-6 load tests, *Proc. Soc. Exp. Biol. Med., 103*:350–353 (1960).

118. B. Chabner, and D. Livingston, A simple enzymic assay for pyridoxal phosphate, *Analyt. Biochem., 34*:413–423 (1970).

119. C. S. Rose, P. Gyorgy, M. Butler, R. Andres, A. H. Norris, N. W. Shock, J. Tobin, M. Brin, and H. Spiegel, Age differences in vitamin B-6 status of 617 men, *Am. J. Clin. Nutr., 29*:847–853 (1976).

120. S. F. Contractor and B. Shane, Blood and urine levels of vitamin B-6 in the mother and fetus before and after loading of the mother with vitamin B-6, *Am. J. Obstet, Gynecol., 107*:635–640 (1970).

121. T. D. Shultz, and J. E. Leklem, Effect of high dose ascorbic acid on vitamin B-6 metabolism, *Am. J. Clin. Nutr. 35*:1400–1407 (1982).

122. L. T. Miller, J. E. Leklem, and T. D. Shultz, The effect of dietary protein on the metabolism of vitamin B-6 in humans, *J. Nutr., 115*:1663–1672 (1985).

123. J. E. Leklem, Vitamin B-6 metabolism and function in humans. In: J. E. Leklem and R. D. Reynolds, eds., *Clinical and Physiological Applications of Vitamin B-6*, A. R. Liss, New York, pp. 1988, pp. 1–26.

124. M. E. Swift, and T. D. Shultz, Relationship of vitamins B-6 and B-12 to homocysteine levels: risk for coronary heart disease, *Nutr. Rep. Int., 34*:1–14 (1986).

125. L. Reinken and H. Gant. Vitamin B-6 nutrition in women with hyperemesis gravidarium during the first trimester of pregnancy, *Clin. Chem. Acta, 55*:101–102, (1974).

126. L. T. Miller, A. Johnson, E. M. Benson, and M. J. Woodring. Effect of oral contraceptives and pyridoxine on the metabolism of vitamin B-6 and on plasma tryptophan and α-amino nitrogen, *Am. J. Clin. Nutr., 28*:846–853 (1975).

127. L. Lumeng, R. E. Cleary, and T-K. Li, Effect of oral contraceptives on the plasma concentration of pyridoxal phosphate, *Am. J. Clin. Nutr., 27*:326–333 (1974).

128. M. H. Brophy and P. K. Siiteri, Pyridoxal phosphate and hypertensive disorders of pregnancy, *Am. J. Obstet. Gynecol. 121*:1075–1079 (1975).

129. R. E. Cleary, L. Lumeng, and T-K. Li, Maternal and fetal plasma levels of pyridoxal phosphate at term: adequacy of vitamin B-6 supplementation during pregnancy, *Am. J. Obstet. Gynecol., 121*:25–28 (1975).

130. A. S. Prasad, K-Y. Lei, D. Oberleas, K. S. Moghissi, and J. C. Stryker, Effect of oral contraceptive agents on nutrients: II Vitamins, *Am. J. Clin. Nutr., 28*:385–391 (1975).

131. J. C. Guilland, B. Berekski-Regung, B. Lequeu, D. Moreau, and J. Klepping, Evaluation of pyridoxine intake and pyridoxine status among aged institutionalized people, *Internat. J. Vit. Nutr. Res. 54*:185–193 (1984).

132. C. M. Lee, and J. E. Leklem, Differences in vitamin B-6 status indicator responses between young and middle-aged women fed constant diets with two levels of vitamin B-6, *Am. J. Clin. Nutr., 42*:226–234 (1985).

133. J. A. Driskell, and S. W. Moak, Plasma pyridoxal phosphate concentrations and coenzyme stimulation of erythrocyte alanine aminotransferase activities of white and black adolescent girls, *Am. J. Clin. Nutr. 43*:599–603 (1986).

134. J. B. Ubbink, W. J. Serfontein, P. J. Becker, and L. S. DeVilliers, The effect of different levels of oral pyridoxine supplementation on plasma pyridoxal 5'-phosphate and pyridoxal levels and urinary vitamin B-6 excretion, *Am. J. Clin. Nutr., 45*:75–85 (1987).

135. A. Hamfelt and L. Soderhjelm, Vitamin B-6 and aging. In: J. E. Leklem and R. D. Reynolds, eds., *Clinical and Physiological Applications of Vitamin B-6*, A. R. Liss, New York, 1988, pp. 95–107.

136. H.C. Barnard, J. J. deKock, W. J. H. Vermaak, and G. M. Potgieter, A new perspective in the assessment of vitamin B-6 nutritional status during pregnancy in humans, *J. Nutr.*, *117*:1303–1306 (1987).

137. H. van den Berg and J. J. P. Bogaards, Vitamin B-6 metabolism in the pregnant rats: effect of progesterone on the (re)distribution in maternal vitamin B-6 stores, *J. Nutr. 117*:1866–1874 (1987).

138. J. Kelsay, A. Baysal, and H. Linkswiler, Effect of vitamin B-6 depletion on the pyridoxal, pyridoxamine and pyridoxine content of the blood and urine of men, *J. Nutr.*, *94*:490–494 (1968).

139. D. Mikac-Devic and C. Tomanic, Determination of 4-pyridoxic acid in urine by a fluorimetric method, *Clin. Chim. Acta, 38*:235–238 (1972).

140. D. M. Dreon and G. E. Butterfield, Vitamin B-6 utilization in active and inactive young men, *Am. J. Clin. Nutr.*, *43*:816–824 (1986).

141. E. A. Donald and T. R. Bosse, The vitamin B-6 requirement in oral contraceptive users II. Assessment by tryptophan metabolites vitamin B-6 and pyridoxic acid levels in urine, *Am. J. Clin. Nutr. 32*:1024–1032 (1979).

142. W. J. H. Vermaak, H. C. Barnard, E. M. S. P. van Dalen, and G. M. Potgieter, Correlation between pyridoxal 5′-phosphate levels and percentage activation of aspartate aminotransferase enzyme in haemolysate and plasma drug in vitro incubation studies with different B-6 vitamers, *Enzyme 35*:215–224 (1986).

143. H. E. Sauberlich, J. E. Canham, E. M. Baker, N. Raica, and Y. F. Herman, Biochemical assessment of the nutritional status of vitamin B-6 in the human, *Am. J. Clin. Nutr.*, *25*:629–642 (1972).

144. L. Lumeng, R. E. Cleary, R. Wagner, P-L. Yu, and T-K. Li, Adequacy of vitamin B-6 supplementation during pregnancy: a prospective study, *Am. J. Clin Nutr.*, *29*:1376–1383 (1976).

145. J. A. Driskell, A. J. Clark, and S. W. Moak, Longitudinal assessment of vitamin B-6 status in Southern adolescent girls, *J. Am. Diet. Assoc.*, *87*:307–310 (1987).

146. B. Shane and S. F. Contractor, Assessment of vitamin B-6 status. Studies on pregnant women and oral contraceptive users, *Am. J. Clin. Nutr. 28*:739–747 (1975).

147. A. D. Cinnamon and J. R. Beaton, Biochemical assessment of vitamin B-6 status in man, *Am. J. Clin. Nutr.*, *23*:696–702 (1970).

148. A. Kirksey, K. Keaton, R. P. Abernathy, andd J. L. Greger, Vitamin B-6 nutritional status of a group of female adolescents, *Am. J. Clin. Nutr.*, *31*:946–954 (1978).

149. J. E. Leklem, Quantitative aspects of tryptophan metabolism in humans and other species: a review, *Am. J. Clin. Nutr.*, *24*:659–671 (1971).

150. R. R. Brown, The tryptophan load test as an index of vitamin B-6 nutrition. In: J. E. Leklem and R. D. Reynolds, eds., *Methods in Vitamin B-6 Nutrition*, Plenum Press, New York, 1985, pp. 321–340.

151. H. van den Berg, E. S. Louwerse, H. W. Bruinse, J. T. N. M., Thissen, and J. Schrijver, Vitamin B-6 status of women suffering from premenstrual syndrome, *Human Nutr.: Clin. Nutr., 40C*:441–450 (1986).

152. R. R. Brown, Possible role of vitamin B-6 in cancer prevention and treatment. In: J. E. Leklem and R. D. Reynolds, eds., *Clinical and Physiological Applications of Vitamin B-6*, A. R. Liss, New York, 1988, pp. 279–301.

153. D. A. Bender, Oestrogens and vitamin B-6, actions and interactions, *Wld. Rev. Nutr. Diet, 51*:140–188 (1987).

154. H. M. Linkswiler, Methionine metabolite excretion as affected by a vitamin B-6 deficiency. In: J. E. Leklem and R. D. Reynolds, eds., *Methods in Vitamin B-6 Nutrition*, Plenum Press, New York, 1981, pp. 373–381.

155. H. E. Sauberlich, Section IX. Biochemical systems and biochemical detection of deficiency. In: W. H. Sebrell and R. S. Harris, eds., *The Vitamins: Chemistry, Physiology, Pathology, Assay*, 2nd ed. vol. II, Academic Press, New York, 1968, pp. 44–80.

156. L. Schirch and W. T. Jenkins, Serine transhydroxymethylase, *J. Biol. Chem.*, *239*:3797–3800.

157. A. E. Axelrod and A. C. Trakatelles, Relationship of pyridoxine to immunological phenomen, *Vitamin Horm.*, *22*:591–607 (1964).

158. R. K. Chandra and S. Puri, Vitamin B-6 modulation of immune responses and infection. In: R. D. Reynolds and J. E. Leklem, eds., *Vitamin B-6: Its role in Health and Disease*, A. R. Liss, New York, 1985, pp. 163–175.

159. H. van den Berg, J. Mulder, S. Spanhaak, W. van Dokkum, and T. Ockhuizen, The influence of marginal vitamin B-6 status on immunological indicies. In: J. E. Leklem and R. D. Reynolds, eds., *Clinical and Physiological applications of Vitamin B-6* A. R. Liss, New York, 1988, pp. 147–155.

160. K. Cheslock and M. T. McCully, Response of human beings to a low-vitamin B-6 diet, *J. Nutr.*, *70*:507–513 (1960).

161. M. C. Talbott, L. T. Miller, and N. I. Kerkvliet, Pyridoxine supplementation: effect on lymphocyte responses in elderly persons, *Am. J. Clin. Nutr.*, *46*:659–664 (1987).

162. L. C. Robson and M. R. Schwarz, Vitamin B-6 deficiency and the lymphoid system. I. Effect of cellular immunity and in vitro incorporation of 3H-uridine by small lymphocytes, *Cell Immunol.*, *16*:135–144 (1975).

163. J. F. Angel, Gluconeogenesis in meal-fed, vitamin B-6 deficient rats, *J. Nutr.*, *110*:262–269 (1980).

164. D. P. Rose, J. E. Leklem, R. R. Brown, and H. M. Linkswiler, Effect of oral contraceptives and vitamin B-6 deficiency on carbohydrate metabolism, *Am. J. Clin. Nutr.*, *28*:872–878 (1975).

165. J. F. Angel and R. M. Mellor, Glycogenesis and gluconeogenesis in meal-fed pyridoxine-deprived rats, *Nutr. Rep. Int.*, *9*:97–107 (1974).

166. P. E. Butler, E. J. Cookson, and R. J. Beyon, The turnover and skeletal muscle gycogen phosphorylase studied using the cofactor, pyridoxal phosphate, as a specific label, *Biochim. Biophys. Acta*, *847*:316–323 (1985).

167. J. A. Kark, R. Bongiovanni, C. U. Hicks, G. Tarassof, J. S. Hannah, and G. Y. Yoshida, Modification of intracellular hemoglobin with pyridoxal and pyridoxal 5′-phosphate, *Blood Cells*, *8*:299–314 (1982).

168. R. Benesch, R. E. Benesch, R. Edalji, and T. Suzuki, 5′-Deoxypyridoxal as a potential anti-sickling agent, *Proc. Natl. Acad. Sci., USA*, *74*:1721–1723 (1977).

169. N. Maeda, K. Takahashi, K. Aono, and T. Shiga, Effect of pyridoxal 5′-phosphate on the oxygen affinity of human erythrocytes, *Br. J. Haematol*, *34*:501–509 (1976).

170. R. D. Reynolds and C. L. Natta. Vitamin B-6 and sickle cell anemia. In: R. D. Reynolds, J. E. Leklem, eds., *Vitamin B-6: Its Role and in Health and Disease*, A. R. Liss, New York, 1985, pp. 301–306.

171. G. Kikuchi, A. Kumar, and P. Talmage, The enzymatic synthesis of δ-aminolevulinic acid, *J. Biol. Chem.*, *233*:1214–1219 (1958).

172. S. S. Bottomley, Iron and vitamin B-6 metabolism in the sideroblastic anemias. In: Lindenbaum, ed., *Nutrition in Hematology*, Churchill Livingston, New York, 1983, pp. 203–223.

173. J. W. Harris, R. M. Wittington, R. Weisman, Jr., and D. L. Horrigan, Pyridoxine responsive anemia in the human adult, *Proc. Soc. Exp. Biol. Med.*, *91*:427–432 (1956).

174. D. L. Horrigan, and J. W. Harris, Pyridoxine responsive anemia in man, *Vitam. Horm.*, *26*:549–568 (1968).

175. A. V. O. Pasanen, M. Salmi, R. Tenhunen, and P. Vuopio, Haem synthesis during pyridoxine therapy in two families with different types of hereditary sideroblastic anemia, *Ann. Clin. Res.*, *14*:61–65 (1982).

176. J. E. Leklem, R. R. Brown, D. P. Rose, H. Linkswiler, and R. A. Arend, Metabolism of tryptophan and niacin in oral contraceptive users receiving controlled intakes of vitamin B-6, *Am. J. Clin. Nutr. 28*:146–156 (1975).

177. K. Dakshinamurti, Neurobiology of pyridoxine. In: H. H. Draper, ed., *Advances in Nutritional Research*, Vol. 4, Plenum Press, New York, 1982, pp. 143–179.

178. D. B. Coursin, Convulsive seizures in infants with pyridoxine-deficient diet, *J. Am. Med. Assoc., 154*:406–408 (1954).

179. C. J. Maloney and A. H. Parmalee, Convulsions in young infants as a result of pyridoxine deficiency, *J. Am. Med. Assoc. 154*:405–406 (1954).

180. M. G. Alton-Mackey and B. L. Walker. Graded levels of pyridoxine in the rat during gestation and the physical and neuromotor development of offspring, *Am. J. Clin. Nutr., 26*:420–428 (1973).

181. M. C. Stephens, V. Havlicek, and K. Dakshinamurti, Pyridoxine deficiency and development of the central nervous system in the rat, *J. Neurochem., 18*:2407–2416 (1971).

182. D. A. Bender, B vitamins in the nervous system, *Neurochem. Int., 6*:297–321 (1984).

183. D. B. Coursin, Vitamin B-6 and brain function in animals and man, *Ann. N.Y. Acad. Sci., 166*:7–15 (1969).

184. A. D. Hunt, J. Stokes, W. W. McCrory, and H. H. Stroud, Pyridoxine dependency: Report of a case of intractable convulsions in an infant controlled by pyridoxine, *Pediatrics, 13*:140–145 (1954).

185. C. R. Scriver, Vitamin B-6-dependency and infant convulsions, *Pediatrics 26*:62–74 (1960).

186. R. Garty, Z. Yonis, J. Braham, and K. Steinitz, Pyridoxine-dependent convulsions in an infant, *Arch. Dis. Child, 37*:21–24 (1962).

187. K. Iinuma, K. Narisawa, N. Yamauchi, T. Yoshida, and T. Mizuno, Pyridoxine dependent convulsion: effect of pyridoxine therapy on electroencephalograms, *Tokohu J. Exp. Med., 105*:19–26 (1971).

188. A. Baniker, M. Turner, and I. J. Hopkins, Pyridoxine dependent seizures-a wider clinical spectrum, *Arch. Dis. Child., 58*:415–418 (1983).

189. F. Goutieres, J. Aicardi, Atypical presentations of pyridoxine-dependent seizures: a treatable cause of intractable epilepsy in infants, *Ann. Neurol., 17*:117–120 (1985).

190. J. E. Canham, E. M. Baker, R. S. Harding, H. E. Sauberlich, and I. C. Plough, Dietary protein-its relationship to vitamin B-6 requirements and function, *Ann. N.Y. Acad. Sci., 166*:16–29 (1969).

191. J. D. Grabow and H. Linkswiler, Electroencephalographic and nerve-conduction studies in experimental vitamin B-6 deficiency in adults, *Am. J. Clin. Nutr., 22*:1429–1434 (1969).

192. J. E. Aycock, and A. Kirksey, Influence of different levels of dietary pyridoxine on certain parameters of developing and mature brains in rats, *J. Nutr. 106*:680–688 (1976).

193. M. R. Thomas, and A. Kirksey, A Postnatal patterns of fatty acids in brain of progeny for vitamin B-6 deficient rats before and after pyridoxine supplementation, *J. Nutr., 106*:1415–1420 (1976).

194. D. J. Kurtz, H. Levy, and J. N. Kanfer, Cerebral lipids and amino acids in the vitamin B-6 deficient suckling rat, *J. Nutr., 102*:291–298 (1972).

195. D. M. Morre, A. Kirksey, and G. D. Das, Effects of vitamin B-6 deficiency on the developing central nervous system of the rat. Gross measurements and cytoarchitectural alterations, *J. Nutr. 108*:1250–1259 (1978).

196. D. M. Morre, A. Kirksey, and G. D. Das, Effects of vitamin B-6 on the developing central nervous systems of the rat. Myelination, *J. Nutr., 108*:1260–1265 (1978).

197. S-J., Chang, A. Kirksey, and D. M. Morre, Effects of vitamin B-6 deficiency on morphological changes in dendritic trees of purkinje cells in developing cerebelum of rats, *J. Nutr., 111*:848–857 (1981).

198. A. Wasynczuk, A. Kirksey, and D. M. Morre, Effects of vitamin B-6 deficiency on specific regions of developing rat brain: the extrapyramidal motor system, *J. Nutr., 113*:746–754 (1983).

199. A. Wasynczuk, A. Kirksey, and D. M. Morre, Effect of maternal vitamin B-6 deficiency on specific regions of developing rat brain: amino acid metabolism, *J. Nutr., 113*:735–745 (1983).

200. S. Groziak, A. Kirksey, and B. Hamaker, Effect of maternal vitamin B-6 restriction on pyridoxal phosphate concentrations in developing regions of the central nervous system in rats, *J. Nutr., 114*:727–732 (1984).

201. J. F. Mueller, Vitamin B-6 in fat metabolism, *Vit. Horm., 22*:787–796 (1964).

202. T. W. Birch, The relations between vitamin B-6 and the unsaturated fatty acid factor, *J. Biol. Chem., 124*:775–793 (1938).

203. E. W. McHenry and G. Gauvin, The B vitamins and fat metabolism, I. Effects of thiamine, riboflavin and rice polish concentrate upon body fat, *J. Biol. Chem., 125*:653–660 (1938).

204. A. Audet and P. J. Lupien, Triglyceride metabolism in pyridoxine-deficient rats, *J. Nutr., 104*:91–100 (1974).

205. M. Abe and Y. Kishino, Pathogenesis of fatty liver in rats fed a high protein diet without pyridoxine *J. Nutr., 112*:205–210 (1982).

206. D. J. Sabo, R. P. Francesconi, and S. N. Gershoff, Effect of vitamin B-6 deficiency on tissue dehydrogenases and fat synthesis in rats, *J. Nutr., 101*:29–34 (1971).

207. H. S. R. Desikachar and E. W. McHenry. Some effects of vitamin B-6 deficiency on fat metabolism in the rat, *Biochem. J., 56*:544–547 (1954).

208. J. F. Angel, Lipogenesis by hepatic and adipose tissues from meal-fed pyridoxine-deprived rats, *Nutr. Rept. Int., 11*:369–378 (1975).

209. J.F. Angel and G-W. Song, Lipogenesis in pyridoxine-deficient nibbling and meal-fed rats, *Nutr. Rept. Int., 8*:393–403 (1973).

210. P.W. Witten, and R. T. Holman, Polyethenoid fatty acid metabolism, VI. Effect of pyridoxine on essential fatty acid conversions, *Arc. Biochem. Biophys., 41*:266–273 (1952).

211. S. C. Cunnane, M. S. Manku, and D. F. Horrobin, Accumulation of linoleic and α-linolenic acids in tissue lipids of pyridoxine-deficient rats, *J. Nutr., 114*:1754–1761 (1984).

212. J. F. Mueller, and J. M. Iacono, Effect of desoxypyridoxine-induced vitamin B-6 deficiency on polyunsaturated fatty acid metabolism in human beings, *Am. J. Clin. Nutr., 12*:358–367 (1963).

213. C. B. Delrome, and P. J. Lupien, The effect of vitamin B-6 deficiency on the fatty acid composition of the major phospholipids in the rat, *J. Nutr., 106*:169–180 (1976).

214. G. Loo and J. T. Smith. Effect of pyridoxine deficiency on phospholipid methylation in rat liver microsomes, *Lipids 21*:409–412 (1986).

215. S. C. Cunnane, M. S. Manku, and D. F. Horrobin, Effect of vitamin B-6 deficiency on essential fatty acid metabolism. In: R. D. Reynolds and J. E. Leklem, eds. *Vitamin B-6: Its Role in Health and Disease*, A. R. Liss, New York, 1985, pp. 447–451.

216. M. S. Chi. Vitamin B-6 in cholesterol metabolism, *Nutr. Res., 4*:359–362 (1984).

217. J. F. Rinehart and L. D. Greenberg, Vitamin B-6 deficiency in the rhesus monkey with particular reference to the occurrence of atherosclerosis, dental caries, and hepatic cirrhosis, *Am. J. Clin. Nutr., 4*:318–328 (1956).

218. P. J. Lupien, C. M. Hinse, and M. Avery, Cholesterol metabolism and vitamin B-6. I. Hepatic cholesterogenesis and pyridoxine deficiency, *Can. J. Biochem., 47*:631–635 (1969).

219. L. Swell, M. D. Law, P. E. Schools, Jr., and C. R. Treadwell, Tissue lipid fatty acid composition pyridoxine-deficient rats, *J. Nutr., 74*:148–156 (1961).

220. M. A. Williams, D. J. McIntosh, and I. Hincenbergs, Changes in fatty acid composition in liver lipid fractions of pyridoxine-deficient rats fed cholesterol, *J. Nutr., 88*:193–201 (1966).

221. T. Iwami, and M. Okada, Stimulation of cholesterol metabolism in pyridoxine-deficient rats, *J. Nutr. Sci. Vitaminol, 28*:77–84 (1982).

222. A. Baysal, B. A. Johnson, and H. Linkswiler. Vitamin B6 depletion in man: blood vitamin B-6, plasma pyridoxal-phosphate, serum cholesterol, serum transaminases and urinary vitamin B-6 and 4-pyridoxic acid, *J. Nutr., 89*:19–23 (1966).

223. J. E. Fincnam, M. Faber, M. J. Weight, D. Labadarious, J. J. F. Taljaard, J. G. Steytler, P. Jacobs, and D. Kritchevsky, Diets realistic for westernized people significantly effect lipoproteins, calcium, zinc, vitamin-C, vitamin-E, vitamin B-6 and hematology in vervet monkeys, *Atherosclerosis 66*:191–203 (1987).

224. W. J. Serfontein and J. B. Ubbink, Vitamin B-6 and myocardial infarction. In: J. E. Leklem and R. D. Reynolds, eds., Clinical and Physiological Applications of Vitamin B-6, A. R. Liss, New York, 1988, pp. 201–217.

225. L. F. Major, and P. F. Goyer, Effects of disulfiram and pyridoxine on serum cholesterol, *Ann. Int. Med., 88*:53–56 (1978).

226. Y-O. Cho, and J. E. Leklem, In vivo evidence of vitamin B-6 requirement in carnitine synthesis, *J. Nutr., 120*:258–265 (1990).

227. G. Litwack, A. Miller-Diener, D. M. DiSorbo, and T. J. Schmidt, Vitamin B-6 and the glucocorticoid receptor. In: R. D. Reynolds and J. E. Leklem, eds., *Vitamin B-6: Its Role in Health and Diseases*, A. R. Liss, New York, (1985), pp. 177–191.

228. J. A. Cidlowski, and J. W. Thanassi, Pyridoxal phosphate: a possible cofactor in steroid hormone action, *J. Steroid Biochem., 15*:11–16 (1981).

229. M. M. Compton and J. A. Cidlowski, Vitamin B-6 and glucocorticoid action, *Endocr. Rev. 7*:140–148 (1986).

230. T. G. Muldoon and J. A. Cidlowski, Specific modification of rat uterine estrogen receptor by pyridoxal 5'-phosphate, *J. Biol. Chem., 255*:3100–3107 (1980).

231. R. A. Hiipakka, and S. Liao, Effect of pyridoxal phosphate on the androgen receptor from rat prostate: Inhibition of receptor aggregation and receptor binding to nuclei and to DNA-cellulose, *J. Steroid Biochem., 13*:841–846 (1980).

232. H. Nishigori, V. K. Moudgil, and D. Taft, Inactivation of avian progesterone receptor binding to ATP-sepharose by pyridoxal 5'-phosphate, *Biochem. Biophys. Res. Comm., 80*:112–118 (1978).

233. D. M. DiSorbo, D. S. Phelps, V. S. Ohl, and G. Litwack, Pyridoxine deficiency influences the behavior of the glucocorticoid receptor complex, *J. Biol. Chem., 255*:3866–3870 (1980).

234. J. Holley, D. A. Bender, W. F. Coulson, and E. K. Symes, Effects of vitamin B-6 nutritional status on the uptake of (3H) oestradiol into the uterus, liver and hypothalamus of the rat, *J. Steroid. Biochem., 18*:161–165 (1983).

235. G. E. Bunce, and M. Vessal, Effect of zinc and/or pyridoxine deficiency upon oestrogen retention and oestrogen receptor distribution in the rat uterus, *J. Steroid. Biochem., 26*:303–308 (1987).

236. J. A. Sturman and L. T. Kremzner, Regulation of ornithine decarboxylase synthesis: effect of a nutritional deficiency of vitamin B-6, *Life Sci., 14*:977–983 (1974).

237. D. M. DiSorbo and G. Litwack, Changes in the intracellular levels of pyridoxal 5'-phosphate affect the induction of tyrosine aminotransferase by glucocorticoids, *Biochem. Biophys. Res. Comm., 99*:1203–1208 (1981).

238. *Human Vitamin B-6 Requirements*, National Acad. Sci. Natl. Res. Council, Washington, D. C., 1978.

239. Recommended Dietary Allowances, 8th ed., Natl. Acad. Sci.-Natl. Res. Council, Washington, D.C., 1974.

240. Recommended Dietary Allowances, 9th ed., Natl. Acad. Sci.-Natl. Res. Council, Washington, D. C., 1980.

241. Recommended Dietary Allowances, 10th ed., Natl. Acad. Sci.-Natl. Res. Council, Washington, D.C., 1989.

242. L. T. Miller, and H. Linkswiler, Effect of protein intake on the development of abnormal tryptophan metabolism by men during vitamin B-6 depletion, *J. Nutr., 93*:53–67 (1967).

243. Dietary Standard for Canada, Bureau of Nutritional Sciences, Dept. of Natl. Health and Welfare, Ottawa, Canada, 1975.

244. M. R. Thomas, J. Kawamoto, S. M. Sneed, and R. Eakin, The effects of vtamin C, vitamin B-6 and vitamin B-12 supplementation on the breast milk and maternal status of well-nourished women, *Am. J. Clin. Nutr.*, *32*:1679–1685 (1979).

245. J. L. Roepke and A. Kirksey. Vitamin B-6 nutriture during pregnancy and lactation 1. Vitamin B-6 intake levels of the vitamin in biological fluids, and condition of the infant at birth, *Am. J. Clin. Nutr.*, *32*:2249–2256 (1979).

246. S. M. Sneed, C. Zane, and M. R. Thomas, The effect of ascorbic acid, vitamin B-6, vitamin B-12, and folic acid supplementation on the breast milk and maternal nutritional status of low socioeconomic lactating women, *Am. J. Clin. Nutr.*, *34*:1338–1346 (1981).

247. L. Styslinger and A. Kirksey, Effects of different levels of vitamin B-6 supplementation on vitamin B-6 concentrations in human milk and vitamin B-6 intakes of breast fed infants, *Am. J. Clin. Nutr.*, *41*:21–31 (1985).

248. M. L. S. Bamji, K. Prema, C. M. Jacob, B. A. Ramalakshmi, and R. Madhavapeddi, Relationship between maternal vitamins B-2 and B-6 status and the levels of these vitamins, in milk at different stages of lactation, *Human Nutr.: Clin. Nutr.*, *40C*:119–124 (1986).

249. M. W. Borschel, A. Kirksey, and R. E. Hannemann, Effects of vitamin B-6 intake on nutriture and growth of young infants, *Am. J. Clin. Nutr.*, *43*:7–15 (1986).

250. M. B. Andon, M. P. Howard, P. B. Moser, and R. D. Reynolds, Nutritionally relevant supplementation of vitamin B-6 in lactating women: effect on plasma prolactin, *Pediat.* *76*:769–773 (1985).

251. M. V. Karra, S. A. Udipi, A. Kirksey, and J. L. B. Roepke, Changes in specific nutrients in breast milk during extended lactation, *Am. J. Clin. Nutr.*, *43*:495–503 (1986).

252. E. E. McCoy, Vitamin B-6 requirements of infants and children. Human vitamin B-6 requirements, Natl. Res. Council, Washington, D. C., (1978), pp. 257–271.

253. S. E. Snyderman, E. H. Holt, Jr., R. Carreters, and K. G. Jacobs, Pyridoxine deficiency in the human infant, *Am. J. Clin. Nutr.*, *1*:200–207 (1953).

254. O. A. Bessey, D. J. D. Adam, and A. E. Hansen, Intake of vitamin B-6 and infantile convulsions: A first approximation of requirements of pyridoxine in infants, *Pediatr.*, *20*:33–44 (1957).

255. S. J. Richey, F. S. Johnson, and M. K. Korslund, Vitamin B-6 requirement in the preadolescent and adolescent. Human vitamin B-6 requirements, Natl. Res. Council, Washington, D.C., 1978, pp. 257–271.

256. U.S. Department of Agriculture, Human Nutrition Information Service. 1985. *Nationwide Food Consumption Survey Continuing Survey of Food Intakes by Individuals: Men 12–50 years, 1 day*, U.S. Dept. Agric. Rpt. No. 85-3, 1985.

257. U.S. Department of Agriculture, Human Nutrition Information Service, 1986, *Nationwide Food Consumption Survey Continuing Survey of Food Intakes by Individuals: Women, 19–50 years and their children 1-5 years, 1 day*, U.S. Dept. Agric., Rpt. No. 86-1, 1987.

258. E. M. Baker, J. E. Canham, W. T. Nunes, H. E. Sauberlich, and M. E. McDowell, Vitamin B-6 requirement for adult men, *Am. J. Clin. Nutr.*, *15*:59–66 (1964).

259. J. E. Canham, E. M. Baker, N. Raica, Jr., and H. E. Sauberlich, Vitamin B-6 requirement of adult men. In: *Proc. Seventh Int. Congress Nutr.*, Hamburg 1966, Vol. 5, Physiology and biochemistry of food components, Pergamon Press, New York, 1967, pp. 555–562.

260. P. Swan, J. Wentworth, and H. Linkswiler, Vitamin B-6 depletion in man: urinary taurine and sulfate excretion and nitrogen balance, *J. Nutr.*, *84*:220–228 (1964).

261. N. Yess, J. M. Price, R. R. Brown, P. Swan, and H. Linkswiler, Vitamin B-6 depletion in man: urinary excretion of tryptophan metabolites, *J. Nutr.* *84*:229–236 (1964).

262. R. R. Brown, N. Yess, J. M. Price, H. Linkswiler, P. Swan, and L. V. Hankes, Vitamin B-6 depletion of man: urinary excretion of quinolinic acid and niacin metabolites, *J. Nutr.* *87*:419–423 (1965).

263. K. E. Cheslock, and M. T. McCully, Response of human beings to a low-vitamin B-6 diet, *J. Nutr.*, *70*:507–513 (1960).

264. H. E. Aly, E. A. Donald, and M. H. W. Simpson, Oral contraceptives and vitamin B-6 metabolism, *Am. J. Clin. Nutr. 24*:297–303 (1971).

265. E. A. Donald, L. D. McBean, M. H. W. Simpson, M. F. Sun, and H. E. Aly, Vitamin B-6 requirement of young adult women, *Am. J. Clin. Nutr., 24*:1028–1041 (1971).

266. H. K. Shin, and H. Linkswiler, Tryptophan and methionine metabolism of adult females as affected by vitamin B-6 deficiency, *J. Nutr., 104*:1348–1355 (1974).

267. Food and Nutrition Board - Natl. Res. Council, Recommended dietary allowances: scientific issues and process for the future, *J. Nutr. 116*:482–488 (1986).

268. P. J. Collip, S. Goldzier, N. Weiss, Y. Soleyman, and R. Snyder, Pyridoxine treatment of childhood bronchial asthma, *Ann. Allergy, 35*:93–97 (1975).

269. L. Musajo and C. A. Benassi, Aspects of disorders of the kynurenine pathway of tryptophan metabolism in man. In: H. Sobotka and C. P., Stewart, eds., *Advances in Clinical Chemistry*, Vol. 7, Academic Press, New York, 1964, 63–135.

270. L. V. Hankes, J. E. Leklem, R. R. Brown, and R. C. P. M. Mekel, Tryptophan metabolism of patients with pellagra: problem of vitamin B-6 enzyme activity and feedback control of tryptophan pyrrolase enzyme, *Am. J. Clin. Nutr., 24*:730–739 (1971).

271. J. H. Flinn, J. M. Price, N. Yess, and R. R. Brown, Excretion of tryptophan metabolites by patients with rheumatoid arthritis, *Arth. Rheumat. 7*:201–210 (1964).

272. R. D. Reynolds and C. L. Natta, Depressed plasma pyridoxal phosphate concentrations in adult asthmatics, *Am. J. Clin. Nutr., 41*:684–688 (1985).

273. C. B. Hollenbeck, J. E. Leklem, M. C. Riddle, and W. E. Connor, The composition and nutritional adequacy of subject-selected high carbohydrate, low fat diets in insulin-dependent diabetes mellitus, *Am. J. Clin. Nutr., 38*:41–51 (1983).

274. W. J. Stone, L. G. Warnock, and C. Wagner, Vitamin B-6 deficiency in uremia, *Am. J. Clin. Nutr., 28*:950–957 (1975).

275. L. Lumeng and T-K. Li, Vitamin B-6 metabolism chronic alcohol abuse. Pyridoxal phosphate levels in plasma and the effects of acetaldehyde on pyridoxal phosphate synthesis and degradation in human erythrocytes, *J. Clin. Invest., 53*:693–704 (1974).

276. W. J. Serfontein, J. B. Ubbink, L. S. DeVilliers, C. H. Rapley, and P. J. Becker, Plasma pyridoxal-5′-phosphate level as risk index for coronary artery disease, *Atherosclerosis, 55*:357–361 (1985).

377. A. Hamfelt and T. Tuvemo, Pyridoxal phosphate and folic acid concentration in blood and erythrocyte aspartate aminotransferase activity during pregnancy, *Clin. Chim. Acta, 41*:287–298 (1972).

278. C. Potera, D. P. Rose, and R. R. Brown, Vitamin B-6 deficiency in cancer patients, *Am J. Clin. Nutr., 30*:1677–1679 (1977).

279. V. T. Devita, B. A. Chabner, D. M. Livingston, and V. T. Oliverio, Anergy and tryptophan metabolism in Hodgkin's disease, *Am. J. Clin. Nutr., 24*:835–840 (1971).

280. M. Coleman, Studies of the administration of pyridoxine to children with Down's syndrome. In: J. E. Leklem and R. D. Reynolds, eds., *Clinical and Physiological Applications of Vitamin B-6*, A. R. Liss, New York, 1988, pp. 317–328.

281. C. Barthelemy, J. Martineau, N. Bruneau, J. P. Muh, G. Lelord, and E. Callaway, Clinical and biological effects of pyridoxine plus magnesium in autistic subjects. In: J. E. Leklem and R. D. Reynolds, eds., *Clinical and Physiological Applications of Vitamin B-6*, A. R. Liss, New York (1988), pp. 329–356.

282. R. W. E. Watts, Hyperoxaluria. In: J. E. Leklem and R. D. Reynolds, eds., *Clinical and Physiologial Aspects of Vitamin B-6*, A. R. Liss, New York, 1988, pp. 245–261.

283. H. J. T. Coelingh-Bennink and W. H. P. Schreurs, Improvement of oral glucose tolerance in gestational diabetes by pyridoxine, *Brit. Med. J., 3*:13–15 (1975).

284. J. B. Day, Clinical trials in the premenstrual syndrome, *Curr. Med. Res. Opin. 6*: (suppl. 5):40–45 (1979).

285. J. Ellis, K. Folkers, T. Watanabe, M. Kaji, S. Saji, J. W. Caldwell, C. A. Temple, and F. S. Wood. Clinical results of a cross-over treatment with pyridoxine and placebo of the carpal tunnel syndrome, *Am. J. Clin. Nutr., 32*:2040–2046 (1979).

286. P. W. Adams, V. Wynn, M. Seed, and J. Folkard, Vitamin B-6, depression and oral conception, *Lancet, ii*:516–517 (1974).

287. A. L. Bernstein and C. S. Lobitz, A clinical and electrophysiologic study of the treatment of painful diabetic neuropathies with pyridoxine. In: J. E. Leklem, R. D. Reynolds, eds., *Clinical and Physiological Applications and Vitamin B-6*, A. R. Liss, New York, 1988, pp. 415–423.

288. K. S. McCully, Homocysteine theory of arteriosclerosis development and current status, *Atherosclerosis Rev., 11*:157–246 (1983).

289. S. H. Mudd and H. L. Levy, Disorders of transsulfuration. In: J. B. Stanbury, et al., eds., *The Metabolic Basis of Inherited Disease*, McGraw-Hill, New York, 1983, pp. 522–559.

290. R. T. Wall, J. M. Harlan, L. A. Harker, et al. Homocysteine-induced endothelial cell injury in vitro: A model for the study of vascular injury, *Throm. Res., 18*:113–121 (1980).

291. A. J. Olszewski and W. B. Szostak, Homocysteine content of plasma proteins in ischemic heart disease, *Atherosclerosis 69*:109–113 (1988).

292. Pathogenesis of experimental arteriosclerosis in pyridoxine deficiency with notes on similarities to human arteriosclerosis, *Arch. Pathol., 51*:12–18 (1951).

293. K. Krishnaswarmy and S. B. Rao, Failure to produce atherosclerosis in Macca radiata on a high-methionine, high fat, pyridoxine-deficient diet, *Atherosclerosis, 27*:253–258 (1977).

294. G. H. Boers, A. G. H. Smals, et al. Pyridoxine treatment does not prevent homocystinemia after methionine loading in adult homocystinuria patients, *Metab., 32*:390–397 (1983).

295. A. M. Gressner and D. Sittel, Plasma pyridoxal 5′-phosphate concentrations in relation to apo-aminotransferase levels in normal, uraemic, and post-myocardial infarct sera, *J. Clin. Chem. Clin. Biochem., 23*:631–636 (1985).

296. W. J. H. Vermaak, H. C. Barnard, G. M. Potgieter, and J. D. Marx, Plasma pyridoxal-5′-phosphate levels in myocardial infarction, *S. Afr. Med. J. 70*:195–196 (1986).

297. W. J. H. Vermaak, H. C. Barnard, G. M. Potgieter, and H. du T. Theron, Vitamin B-6 and coronary artery disease. Epidemiological observations and case studies, *Atherosclerosis, 63*:235–238 (1987).

298. W. J. Serfontein, J. B. Ubbink, L. S. DeVilliers, and P. J. Becker, Depressed plasma pyridoxal-5′-phosphate levels in tobacco-smoking men, *Atherosclerosis, 59*:341–346 (1986).

299. M. G. Brush, Vitamin B-6 treatment of premenstrual syndrome. In: J. E. Leklem and R. D. Reynolds, eds., *Clinical and Physiological Applications of Vitamin B-6*, A. R. Liss, New York, 1988, pp. 363–379.

300. P. M. S. O'Brien, The premenstrual syndrome: A review of the present status of therapy, *Drugs, 24*:140–151 (1982).

301. P. W. Adams and D. P. Rose, et al. Effects of pyridoxine hydrochloride (vitamin B-6) upon depression associated with oral contraception, *Lancet, i*:897 (1973).

302. M. S. Biskind, Nutritional deficiency in the etiology of menorrhagia, metrorrhagia, cystic mastitis and premenstrual tension; treatment with vitamin B complex, *J. Clin. Endocrinol. Metab., 3*:227–234 (1943).

303. J. Stokes and J. Mendels, Pyridoxine and premenstrual tension, *Lancet, i*:1177–1178 (1972).

304. G. E. Abraham and J. T. Hargrove, Effect of vitamin B-6 on premenstrual symptomatology in women with premenstrual tension syndromes: a double blind crossover study, *Infertility, 3*:155–165 (1980).

305. W. Barr, Pyridoxine supplements in the premenstrual syndrome, *Practitioner, 228*:425–428(1984).

306. K. E. Kendall and P. P. Schurr, The effects of vitamin B-6 supplementation on premenstrual syndromes, *Obstet. Gynecol., 70*:145–149 (1987).

307. C. D. Ritchie and R. Singkamani, Plasma pyridoxal 5′-phosphate in women with the premenstrual syndrome, *Human Nutr. Clin. Nutr. 40C*:75–80 (1986).

308. M. Mira, P. M. Stewart, and S. F. Abraham, Vitamin and trace element status in premenstrual syndrome, *Am. J. Clin. Nutr.*, *47*:636–641 (1988).

309. R. A. Simon and R. D. Reynolds, Vitamin B-6 and asthma. In: J. E. Leklem and R. D. Reynolds, eds., *Clinical and Physiological Applications of Vitamin B-6*, A. R. Liss, New York, 1988, pp. 307–315.

310. R. C. Keniston and M. R. Weir, Aminophylline and gentamicin-2, *Am. J. Clin. Nutr.*, *43*:636–637 (1986) (letter).

310a. J. A. Driskell, R. L. Wesley and I. E. Hess, Effectiveness of pyridoxine hydrochloride treatment on carpal tunnel syndrome patients, *Nutrition Report International, 34*:1031–1040 (1986).

310b. M. L. Kasdan and C. James, Carpal tunnel syndrome and vitamin B-6, *Plast. Reconstructive Surgery, 79*:456–459 (1987).

310c. G. P. Smith, P. J. Rudge, and J. J. Peters, Biochemical studies of pyridoxal and pyridoxal phosphate status and therapeutic trial of pyridoxine in patients with carpal tunnel syndrome, *Ann. Neurology, 15*:104–107 (1984).

311. H. N. Bhagavan, Interaction between vitamin B-6 and drugs. In: R. D. Reynolds and J. E. Leklem, eds., *Vitamin B-6: Its Role in Health and Disease*, A. R. Liss, New York, 1985, pp. 401–415.

312. J. E. Leklem, Vitamin B-6 requirement and oral contraceptive use—a concern? *J. Nutr.*, *116*:475–477(1986).

313. H. Schaumburg, J. Kaplan, A. Windebank, N. Vick, S. Rasmus, D. Pleasure, and M. J. Brown, Sensory neuropathy from pyridoxine abuse: a new megavitamin syndrome, *New Engl. J. Med.*, *309*:445–448 (1983).

314. G. J. Parry and D. E. Bredesen, Sensory neuropathy with low-dose pyridoxine, *Neurol.*, *35*:1466–1468 (1985).

315. K. Dalton, M. J. T. Dalton, Characteristics of pyridoxine overdose neuropathy syndrome, *Acta. Neurol. Scand., 76*:81–11 (1987).

316. M. Cohen and A. Bendich, Safety of pyridoxine—a review of human and animal studies, *Toxicol. Letters, 34*:129–139 (1986).

10
Biotin

Jean-Pierre Bonjour
F. Hoffmann-La Roche, Ltd.
Basel, Switzerland

I. HISTORY

At the turn of the century, Wildiers discovered that certain strains of yeast required for their growth a factor found only in yeast and wort. He called this factor *bios*. Subsequent investigators recognized the complex nature of bios and were able to fractionate and identify different components: bios I was shown to be myoinositol, bios IIA to consist of β-alanine and pantothenic acid, and bios IIB to be identical with biotin, a substance isolated by Kögl and Tönnis in 1936 from egg yolk.

The detrimental effect of feeding high doses of raw egg white to animals was first observed by Bateman in 1916. These findings of dermatosis and loss of hair were confirmed in rats by Boas in 1927, who noted that the condition that she called egg white injury was cured by a "protective factor X" found in liver. Independently, György in 1931 also discovered this factor in liver and named it *vitamin H* (*Haut*, German for skin). Other names given to this factor were coenzyme R, protective factor against egg white injury, factor S, factor W, or vitamin B_w (1–3).

György and co-workers were able, in 1940, to show that their vitamin H–active liver fraction was also microbiologically active and that Kögl's biotin cured the skin lesions in animals caused by vitamin H deficiency. In 1940, they succeeded in isolating biotin from liver. The structure of biotin was established by Kögl and his group in Europe and by du Vigneaud and collaborators in the United States between 1940 and 1943. An isomeric α-biotin was postulated by Kögl to exist in egg yolk, whereas the biotin isolated from liver was called β-biotin. The structure of biotin as elucidated by du Vigneaud has been confirmed by Harris, who achieved its first chemical synthesis in 1945, whereas no such confirmation for the α form has yet appeared. Today, it is generally accepted that the α and β forms of biotin are identical (1).

II. CHEMISTRY

A. Isolation

Different natural sources have been used for the isolation of biotin as its methylester: egg yolk, beef liver, and milk.

From 1000 egg yolks it was isolated by extraction with acetone and precipitation with ethanol. Impurities were removed by several precipitations with lead acetate, mercuric chloride, and with phosphotungstic acid. The preparation with further purified by absorption on charcoal, esterification with methanolic hydrogen chloride, precipitation as reineckate, high vacuum distillation, and crystallization from a mixture of chloroform and light petroleum yielding 4 mg of a product with a melting point of 146–147 °C. A purer preparation obtained by means of molecular distillation had a melting point of 161–165 °C. Liver has to be autoclaved with acid, digested with papain, or hydrolyzed under high pressure prior to starting the isolation of biotin. Similar to the isolation from egg yolk, precipitation with phosphotungstic acid, esterification, and chromatography on activated aluminum oxide were used for purification. This procedure yielded a product with a melting point of 166–167 °C. Biotin was also similarly isolated from a crude milk concentrate (1–4).

B. Structure and Nomenclature

Kögl reported the correct empirical formula $C_{11}H_{18}O_3N_2S$ for biotin methylester in 1937, and this was confirmed by du Vigneaud in 1941. These two groups elucidated the structure of biotin. The approach by which the two groups found biotin to be a fusion of an imidazolidone ring with a tetrahydrothiophene ring bearing a valeric acid side chain has been extensively discussed (1–4). Kögl postulated that α-biotin from egg yolk contained an isovaleric acid side chain, whereas the biotin isolated from liver, with the valeric acid side chain, was called β-biotin (3). The differences in melting point and optical rotation seen by Kögl between these two compounds were probably due to impurities rather than to structural differences, especially as the biological activity of both α- and β-biotin were comparable for different microorganisms. Furthermore, the structure of β-biotin has been confirmed by synthesis, whereas no such confirmation for α-biotin has appeared. The complete structural determination established that chemically biotin is hexahydro-2-oxo-1H-thieno[3,4-d]imidazole-4-pentanoic acid (Fig. 1) and contains three asymmetric carbon atoms; hence, eight stereoisomers are possible. Of these, only D-biotin is biologically active. The absolute stereochemistry of D-biotin was established by x-ray crystallography and revealed that the imidazolidone and the tetrahydrothiophene rings are fused in the *cis* configuration, producing a boatlike structure. The ureido ring projects upward at an angle of 62° with respect to the plane formed by the four carbon atoms of the tetrahydrothiophene ring, and a second plane, made by the sulfur atom and carbon atoms 2 and 5, projects upward at an angle of 37.6°. The valeric side chain attached to C-2 of the sulfur ring is *cis* with respect to the ureido ring (5,6).

C. Structures of Important Analogs and Antagonists

All eight biotin isomers have been synthesized, but only D-biotin has been found to be biologically active (1,2,4). Other compounds bearing a structural relationship to biotin have been either chemically synthesized during the period of structural analysis or have been isolated from natural sources (4). Some of these compounds (Fig 2), such as oxybiotin

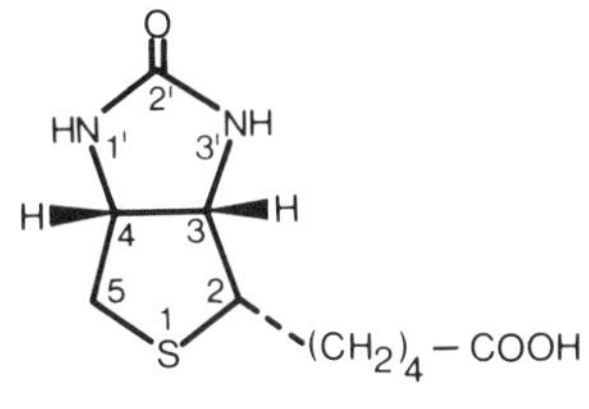

Figure 1 The absolute stereochemistry of D-biotin.

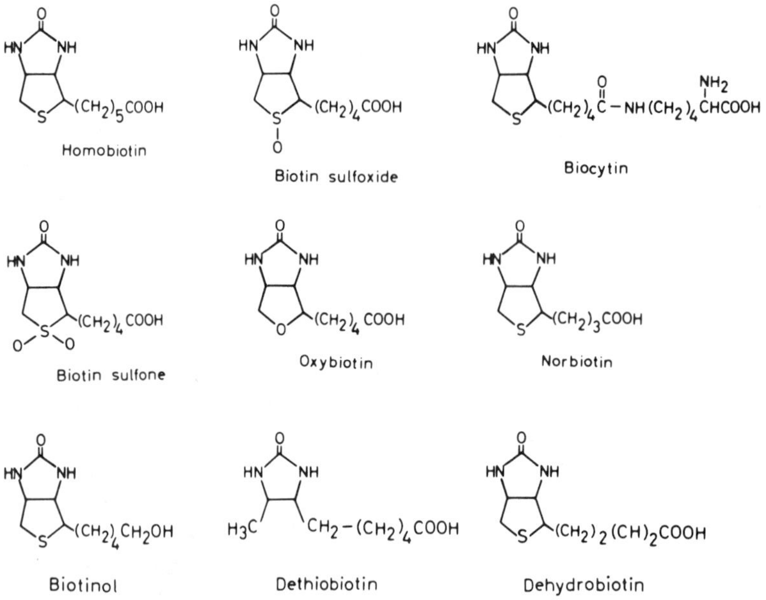

Figure 2 Biotin analogs.

or biotinol, can replace biotin in nutrition and in alleviating deficiency symptoms in animals, although with a lower activity. Biocytin, a bound form of biotin, is also biologically active in several species, including animals. This naturally occurring compound has been shown to be ϵ-N-biotinyl-L-lysine. Biocytin and free biotin are water-soluble dialyzable compounds. In contrast, biotin as it occurs in tissues and as it participates in various specific metabolic reactions is bound to proteins or peptides in an amide linkage to the amino group of a lysyl residue, as in biocytin. Dethiobiotin and biotin sulfoxide are inactive in animals but active in certain microbial species. Homologs of biotin with a shortened or elongated side chain, such as norbiotin or homobiotin, are potent antagonists of biotin, as is biotin sulfone, which can be formed by the oxidation of biotin (1,2,4,6). α-Dehydrobiotin (7) is one of the most potent biotin inhibitors uncovered to date; it is produced by a strain of *Saccharomyces lydicus*.

Besides these biotin analogs, other compounds exist that can bind biotin to form a stable complex, thus preventing the utilization of the vitamin by animals and/or microorganisms. Such a biotin-binding protein is streptavidin, which has been isolated from fermentation sources (8). The microorganism *Saccharomyces avidinii* produces, in addition to streptavidin, stravidin (9) and a third compound related to stravidin. All these structures can inactivate free biotin and apparently inhibit biotin synthesis in susceptible microorganisms. Another compound that strongly binds biotin is avidin, the protein component of egg white. Avidin is a glycoprotein with a molecular weight of about 70,000 daltons that possesses a tetrameric structure with identical subunits containing one biotin-binding site each. Not only free biotin is complexed by avidin but also compounds structurally related to biotin containing an intact ureido function in a *cis* configuration. Modifications of the tetrahydrothiophene ring and substitution of the carboxyl group have no effect on the binding with avidin, and therefore biocytin and enzyme-bound biotin are also complexed by avidin. The avidin–biotin complex is formed by a weak but specific affinity for ureido groups of the tryptophan residues that are located on the biotin-binding site of avidin. The complex is stable over a wide range of pH and is not degraded in the gastrointestinal tract. However, when administered intraperitoneally to rats, the [^{14}C] biotin–avidin complex can be dissociated as evidenced by the excretion of labeled biotin in the urine (2,4).

D. Synthesis

Since detailed discussions of biotin synthesis have been published (1,3,4) and recent developments have been reviewed (10), only a general outline is given here. The first total synthesis of biotin was achieved by Harris and co-workers between 1943 and 1945. In this synthesis cysteine was reacted with chloroacetic acid and the intermediate amino acid benzylated and methylated. After cyclization and decarboxylation, 4-benzamido-3-ketotetrahydrothiophene was obtained. Into this compound the valeric acid side chain was introduced using γ-carbomethoxybutyraldehyde. The keto group of this α,β-unsaturated compound was then converted to the amino group. Hydration and saponification resulted in 3,4-diamino-2-(4-carboxybutyl)tetrahydrothiophene, which after reaction with phosgene yielded the bicyclic compound having the structure of biotin.

A different approach to the total synthesis of biotin has been used by Grüsner in 1945 and Baker and associates in 1947. Both groups introduced the side chain, either partially (Grüssner) or totally (Baker) concurrently with the formation of the tetrahydrothiophene ring. Baker condensed the esters of 2-bromopimelic acid with the ester of ω-mercaptopropionic acid; cyclization of this triester led to 2-(4-carboxybutyl)-3-keto-4-tetrahydrothiophenecarboxylic acid; the selective degradation of the two nuclear carboxyl groups, without affecting the side chain carboxyl group, then yielded 3,4-diamino-2-(4-carboxybutyl)tetrahydrothiophene, which on treatment with phosgene gave biotin.

All these methods for the total synthesis of biotin have the great disadvantage that the steric configuration of biotin is salved only in the final steps of the synthesis or that special intermediates are introduced to obtain stereospecificity, thus using excessive time and materials. These shortcomings have been avoided in the synthesis developed by Goldberg and Sternbach in 1949 in the laboratories of Hoffmann-La Roche, in which the required all-*cis* configuration of the final product is predetermined by the choice of the starting material. This highly stereospecific multistep synthesis is not complicated by the formation of the other biotin isomers, epibiotin, allobiotin, and epiallobiotin, and it is the method by which biotin is synthesized commercially (11).

E. Chemical Properties

Biotin, hexahydro-2-oxo-1H-thieno[3,4-*d*]imidazole-4-pentanoic acid ($C_{10}H_{16}O_3N_2S$; molecular weight, 244.31 daltons), which crystallizes from water as fine long needles, melts with decomposition at 230–232 °C (uncorrected). Free biotin is soluble in dilute alkali and hot water, sparingly soluble in dilute acid, cold water ($\cong 0.82$ mmol/liter), and alcohol, and practically insoluble in most organic solvents. Its specific rotation $[\alpha]_D^{22}$ is + 92.0° (0.1 N NaOH; C = 0,3). Dry crystalline D-biotin is fairly stable to air, daylight, and heat; it is gradually destroyed by ultraviolet radiation. Aqueous solutions are relatively stable if weakly acid or weakly alkaline. In strongly acid and alkaline solutions the biological activity is destroyed by heating (1,2,4).

III. ANALYTICAL PROCEDURES

Many microorganisms require biotin as a growth factor, and several of these have been used in assays for biotin (1,4,12). Table 1 lists the most commonly used microorganisms for biotin assays together with the growth-promoting activity of some biotin analogs compared with that of D-biotin. All other biotin isomers, as well as protein-bound biotin, do not support the growth of microorganisms. Bound biotin is released from the test material by acidic hydrolysis with sulfuric acid or by digestion with papain. Unsaturated fatty acids interfere with the assay and have to be removed either by filtration or by ether extraction. The biotin content of test materials is determined by measuring the growth response of microorganisms after inoculation and incubation either turbidimetrically or titrimetrically and by comparison with standards of known biotin concentration.

Using the high affinity of avidin for the ureido group of biotin, an isotope dilution assay for biotin has been developed (13) that is sensitive in the 4–41 pmol range and that for feed (14) and animal liver samples (15) yields results comparable with those obtained by the *Lactobacillus plantarum* assay. Bound biotin has to be hydrolzyed (13,14) or digested with papain (15) in these assays. Recent advances in the understanding of biotin-responsive inborn errors of metabolism (see Sec. XI) have stimulated the interest in the accurate measurement of biotin concentrations in plasma and urine. Mostly radioligand assays have been developed, which can be characterized by the radiotracers used—[14C]biotin (13,14), [3H]biotin (15–18), 125I-labeled biotin derivatives (19–21), or 125I-labeled avidin (22)—or by the separation agents used—activated charcoal (15,19), nitrocellulose filters (16), bentonite (17), and solid-phase reagents (18,20,22). In addition, a radiometric-microbiological assay has been reported (23) which is based on the measurement of 14CO2 released during the metabolism of L-[14C]methionine in *Kloeckera brevis*. Also chemiluminescence energy transfer (24) and liquid chromatography with fluorimetric detetion (25) are used.

The activity of biotin-dependent enzymes is reduced in animals deficient in biotin (2). This finding has led to the development of methods for the assessment of biotin status based on the measurement of enzyme activity. Thus, the acetyl-CoA carboxylase-dependent

Table 1 Microorganisms Used for Biotin Assay and Activity of Biotin Analogs

Microorganism	Biotin analog activity in percentage of D-biotin						
	Methyl-ester	D-sul-foxide	Sulfone	Nor-biotin	Oxi-biotin	D-de-thiobiotin	Biocytin
Lactobacillus casei (ATCC 7469)	0	0	Inhibitors of utiliza-tion of biotin	40	0[a]	100
Lactobacillus plantarum (ATCC 8014)	—	100		50	0	0
Neurospora crassa	—	—		—	100	100
Ochromonas danica	—	—		—	0	100
Saccharomyces cerevisiae (ATCC 7754)	100	100		10–25	100	100

[a]Competitively inhibits utilization of biotin by this organism.

CO_2 fixation in chicken blood has been found to depend on the biotin status (26,27). The in vitro stimulation by biotin of acetyl-CoA carboxylase activity in liver of chicks can be used for estimation of biotin status, whereas in chicken blood no consistent results with the acetyl-CoA carboxylase activation test have as yet been obtained (27). Pyruvate carboxylase, another biotin-containing enzyme is also present in the blood of the domestic fowl and seems to be a more sensitive indicator for biotin status than is acetyl-CoA carboxylase (28). This enzyme has been used to assess biotin status by measuring its activity in the blood of chicken (28,29), and turkeys (29), either directly or by assaying the in vitro activity before and after addition of biotin in rat (30) and chicken (31) erythrocytes and in chicken liver (31).

Furthermore, colorimetric procedures based on the reaction of biotin with *p*-(dimethylamino)cinnamaldehyde, on the measurement of the absorbance of iodine formed during the oxidation of biotin to its sulfone with potassium iodate, or on the displacement of the dye, 4-hydroxyazobenzene-2′-carboxylic acid from avidin by biotin, as well as gas chromatographic and polarographic methods, have been developed for the assessment of biotin (2).

IV. BIOASSAY PROCEDURES

The biological estimation of biotin may be conducted with rats and chicks made biotin deficient by the use of special diets. Weanling rats of the same sex and weight (35–40 g) are fed a synthetic experimental diet in which raw egg white (fresh or dried) or avidin has been incorporated. The avidin prevents the utilization of biotin by forming an unabsorbable complex with the vitamin. After a depletion period of 6–7 weeks, the rats show a cessation of growth and specific symptoms of biotin deficiency. During 4 weeks, groups of rats then receive either graded amounts of test sample or pure synthetic biotin as the reference standard in two or more dilutions. The supplements are given by injection rather than by mouth to ensure its availability to the rats despite the presence of dietary avidin. The biotin content of the test sample can be calculated from the growth-response curves, sinc the weight gain is proportional to the logarithm of the biotin dose.

In the chicks, the same technique as in the rat is used for the biological assay of biotin. But since the chick requires much larger amounts of biotin than does the rat, a deficiency can be produced by a diet low in biotin alone without the aid of avidin. Without avidin, the test and standard vitamin supplements may be given orally with the diet (2,4).

V. CONTENT IN FOOD

A. Table of Food Content

Comprehensive compilations of available data on biotin content of foodstuffs have been published (32–35) and the values given in Table 2 are based on a compilation (32) of values given in literature. These tables show that biotin-containing foods are numerous, although the absolute amount of biotin present in even the richest dietary sources are low. Recently, the biotin content of breakfast cereals (36), of pasteurized milk and its regional and seasonal variation (37), and of baby milk formulae (38) have been determined using *L. plantarum* as test organism. Using radioassay methods, biotin contents of various foodstuffs (39), cereals (40), baby food (40), and infant food (41) have been reported.

Table 2 Biotin Contents of Food (Edible Portion)

Amount (pmol/100 g)	Meat, fish	Cereals	Fruits, vegetables	Miscellaneous
1680	—	—	—	Royal jelly
820	—	—	—	Brewer's yeast
520	Liver, lamb	—	—	—
410	Liver, pork	—	—	Food yeast, torula
393	Liver, beef	—	—	—
287	—	Soy flour, cooked	—	—
250	—	Soy beans, cooked	—	—
246	—	Rice bran, raw	—	—
238	—	Rice germ, raw	—	—
234	—	Rice polishings, raw	—	—
213	—	—	—	Egg, yolk
160	—	—	—	Peanut, butter
152	—	—	Walnuts, halves	—
139	—	—	Peanuts, roasted	—
131	—	—	—	Chocolate
127	—	Barley, whole cooked	—	—
111	—	—	Pecan, halves	—
98	Sardines, Pacific, canned	Oats, cooked	—	—
92	—	—	—	Egg, whole
86	—	Corn, yellow, cooked	Cowpeas, cooked or fresh	—
75	—	—	Split peas, cooked	—
74	Mackerel, Pacific, canned	—	Almonds	—
70	—	—	Cauliflower, buds fresh	—
66	—	Wheat, whole, cooked	Mushrooms, fresh	—
62	Salmon, canned	—	—	—
57	—	Wheat, bran, raw	—	—

Biotin				
54	—	—	Lentils, cooked	—
49	—	Rice, brown, cooked	—	—
46	Chicken, white meat	Rice, parboiled	Garbanzos, cooked	—
41	Chicken, dark meat	—	Lima beans, cooked	—
40	—	Flour, whole wheat	Peas, green, cooked	—
39	—	—	—	Molasses
37	Oysters, canned	—	—	—
36	Halibut, canned	—	—	—
33	Bacon, pork	Rice, converted, cooked	Mung bean, cooked	—
31	—	—	Mushrooms, canned, with liquid	—
30	—	—	—	Egg, white
28	—	Cornmeal, white	Spinach, fresh	—
27	—	—	Corn, fresh	—
25	Leg, lamb	—	—	—
24	—	—	Avocados, fresh, cubed	—
23	—	—	—	—
21	Loin, pork	Rice, white, refined, cooked	—	—
19	Ham, pork	—	Raisins, seedless	Milk, whole
18	—	—	Bananas	Cheese, processed
18	—	—	Potatoes, sweet, fresh	Milk, evaporated, reconstituted
16	—	—	Tomatoes, fresh / Strawberries, sweetened	—
15	—	—	Watermelon, diced	Cheddar, cheese
14	Rib roast, lean, beef	—	Onion, fresh	Milk, non-fat, reconstituted

(Continued)

Table 2 *Continued*

Amount (pmol/100 g)	Meat, fish	Cereals	Fruits, vegetables	Miscellaneous
13	—	—	Lettuce, fresh	—
12	Tuna, canned	—	Cantaloupe, diced	—
11	Round, beef	—	Grapefruit, small	—
10	—	—	Beet, fresh, green	—
			Carrots, grated, fresh	
9.8	—	—	Cabbage, fine shreds, fresh	—
9.4	—	—	Spinach, canned with liquid	—
9.0	—	—	Corn, canned, with liquid	—
8.6	—	—	Peas, green, canned with liquid	—
8.2	Chop, veal	—	—	—
7.8	—	Bread, whole wheat	Beets, diced, fresh	—
			Oranges, small	
7.4	—	—	Tomatoes, canned, with liquid	—

Biotin			
7.0	—	—	Asparagus, green, canned, with liquid; Peaches, sweetened, fresh
6.6	—	—	Grapes
6.1	—	—	Carrots, diced, canned, with liquid
5.3	—	Rice, ready to eat	Beans, green, string, canned, with liquid
4.5	—	Bread, white	—
4.1	—	Flour, white	Apples, fresh
3.7	—	—	Grapefruit, juice, canned; Orange, juice, canned
2.9	—	Hominy, grits, cooked	Grapefruit, juice, fresh
1.6	—	—	Apple, juice, fresh
1.2	—	—	Grape, juice, fresh; Orange, juice, fresh
0.8	—	—	Peaches, canned

B. Stability and Availability in Food

From Table 2 it can be seen that processing and preservation of food—e.g., milling of wheat or corn and canning of corn, carrots, spinach, or tomatoes—reduce its biotin content. In canned baby foods an approximately 15% reduction in biotin content after a 6-month storage has been observed (42).

Part of the dietary biotin exists in protein-bound form (2,43), which on digestion or acid hydrolysis yields biocytin. Only 10–80% of total biotin was found to be extractable with water, thus free biotin, in feedstuffs (44). In general, foodstuffs of plant origin have a greater free biotin content than foodstuffs of animal origin (44). Many of the microorganisms used for biotin assay can use biocytin for their growth (see Table 1). Biocytin binds also to avidin but is not cleaved to biotin by papain or by acid hydrolysis (45). The observed differences in the biotin content of foods depending on the treatment of samples and on the analytical method used (39,40) are probably due to the extent to which biocytin is estimated as biotin by the analytical methods used. Furthermore, when the bioavailability of biotin in cereals was tested in the animal growth tests, only part of the analytically determined biotin was found to be available to chickens (46), turkeys (47) and weaning pigs (48). Due to these difficulties in the estimation of the biotin content in food, the availability of biotin to mammals remains unclear.

VI. METABOLISM

A wide variety of microorganisms (4) are capable of synthesizing biotin, and the current knowledge in the field of biotin biogenesis has been reviewed (2,5,6,49,50). Most microorganisms capable of biosynthesizing the vitamin appear to utilize a pathway from pimelic acid through 7,8-substituted pelargonic acids and dithiobiotin prior to the incorporation of sulfur to form biotin. The means by which dithiobiotin is converted to biotin have not yet been established, but it undoubtedly involves more than one step. Also, the uptake and metabolism of biotin have been investigated by using a pseudomonad that can use the vitamin as sole source of C, N, S, and energy. McCormick (51) found that much of the carbon needed for growth of the microorganism is derived by successive β-oxidative cleavage of the valeric acid side chain to form the 2-carbon shorter bis-nor-biotin and then the 4-carbon shorter tetra-nor-biotin. The ureido ring can be cleaved between the N and bridgehead C opposite the side chain of the bis-nor-catabolite with oxidation at the bridgehead carbon. Most of the nitrogen is released by a second cleavage of the ureido compound to form urea (5,51). Degradation of the remaining thiolane ring fragments produce inorganic sulfur at different oxidation-reduction levels. Even earlier oxidation of the thioether sulfur of biotin leads to some formation of both D- and L-sulfoxide (51).

Dietary biotin exists free and bound (43,44). The protein-bound biotin is digested in the intestinal tract to biocytin. Only the enzyme biotinidase (EC 3.5.1.12), which has been detected in most mammalian tissues (43), catalyzes the hydrolysis of biocytin to form biotin and free lysine (52). Very little is known about the uptake of biotin by the intestine. It seems that some species have a passive diffusion transport mechanism for biotin, while others have an active transport mechanism (50). The transport of biotin was examined in different areas of the human small intestine and was found to be saturable in the presence of a Na+ gradient but was linear in the presence of a choline gradient. Transport of biotin by the Na+-dependent process was noted to be higher in the duodenum than the jejunum, which was in turn higher than that in the ileum, and it was concluded that the proximal part of the human small intestine was the site of maximum transport of biotin (53). In the plasma of chickens, two biotin-binding proteins have been detected, which appear to be functionally differentiated; one is probably involved in biotin distribution for general maintenance, the other is specifically involved in transport of biotin to the oocyte (54). There are indications that also in mammalian plasma part of the circulating biotin is bound to proteins (55) and recently a biotin-binding protein has been isolated from the serum of the pregnant rat (56). Biotinidase was found to be the only protein in human serum that exchanges with [^{3}H]($+$)-biotin, and thus biotinidase could be the major carrier of biotin in plasma, and as such functions in biotin transport (57). Very little is known about the catabolism of biotin. Most of the radioactivity of ureido carbonyl-labeled [^{14}C] biotin was found to be excreted in the urine of the rat and none was found in the feces or expired as CO_2. In addition to the recovered vitamin, several biotin metabolites, namely, the D- and L-sulfoxides, bis-*nor*-biotin and a neutral ketone, were isolated from the rat urine. The mammal does not seem to be able to degrade the ring system of biotin, as no labeled CO_2 or urea was found in these experiments (58,59). In the urine of healthy humans small amounts of biotin metabolites have also been detected, none of which were biotinsulfoxide or biotin sulfone (45). The catabolism of biotin-containing holocarboxylases can lead to biocytin, from which biotin can be liberated by biotinidase, leading to a endogenous recycling of biotin (55).

Any investigation into the metabolism of biotin in animals and humans is complicated by the fact that biotin-producing microorganisms exist in their intestinal tract distal to the cecum. Feed composition, sulfonamides, and the antibiotics were found to influence intestinal biotin synthesis in animals (60). Investigations in humans to assess the role of intestinal biotin synthesis were carried out by looking at the effect of diet, sulfonamides, or antibiotics on biotin metabolism, and it was found that, in general, the amount of biotin excreted in urine and feces together exceeds the total dietary intake, whereas the urinary excretion of biotin is usually lower than the intake (61). But these experiments were inconclusive in assessing the extent and significance of the intestinally synthesized biotin on the overall biotin turnover. Children with biotinidase deficiency (see Sec. XI.B), who cannot liberate biotin from biocytin, depend on pharmacological doses of free biotin for their survival. When biotin supplementation was stopped in three children with this biotin-responsive inborn error of metabolism, plasma biotin levels fell within 7 days below the detection limit (0.4 nmol/liter) and also the carboxylase activities rapidly declined and were about 25% of control values after 20 days. All children showed clinical and biochemical signs of a biotin deficiency (62). It can be concluded from these findings that the intestinally synthesized biotin is not sufficient to maintain normal biotin levels.

VII. BIOCHEMICAL FUNCTION

Biotin serves as a prosthetic group in a number of enzymes in which the biotin moiety functions as a mobile carboxyl carrier. The biotin prosthetic group is linked covalently to the ϵ-amino group of a lysyl residue of the biotin-dependent enzyme. The attachment of biotin to the protein, i.e., the formation of the holoenzyme from its apoenzyme, was found to be mediated by enzymes termed holoenzyme synthetases and to be dependent on ATP and Mg^{2+} ions. The holoenzyme synthetase reaction was postulated to occur in two steps: an activation of biotin by ATP to biotinyladenylate and a transfer of the biotinyl moiety to the apoenzyme to form the holoenzyme. Both partial reactions are presumably catalyzed by the same enzyme. Although this holoenzyme synthetase shows a high specificity for D-biotin, the specificity for the apoenzyme is rather broad, suggesting that the environment of the lysine residue to which the biotin is attached may be similar in the various apoenzymes (2,5,50).

The biotin-dependent enzymes can be divided into carboxylases, in which the carboxyl group is fixed on a substrate transferred froma donor to an acceptor, and into decarboxylases, in which a carboxyl group is removed from a donor as CO_2. The known biotin enzymes, the reactions they catalzye, and their biochemical functions are presented in Table 3. The overall reactions carried out by biotin-dependent enzymes can be subdivided into two discrete steps, which are coupled through a carboxybiotin–enzyme complex intermediate according to the following scheme:

$$HCO_3^- + ATP + biotin\text{-}enzyme \; \overset{Mg^{2+}}{\rightleftharpoons} \; CO_2^-\text{-}biotin\text{-}enzyme + ADP + P_i \quad (1a)$$

$$CO_2^-\text{-}biotin\text{-}enzyme + substrate \rightleftharpoons substrate\text{-}CO_2^- + biotin\text{-}enzyme \quad (1b)$$

$$\overline{HCO_3^- + ATP + substrate \rightleftharpoons substrate\text{-}CO_2^- + ATP + P_i} \quad (1)$$

In all carboxylase reactions, HCO_3^- is the carboxyl donor [Eq. (1a)] and is activated by ATP and Mg^{2+}, whereas in transcarboxylase reactions HCO_3^- and ATP are replaced by an acyl CoA as active CO_2 donor. With decarboxylases, partial reaction (1b) proceeds right to left, followed by the decomposition of the carboxylated biotin enzyme to yield CO_2. The nature of the carboxybiotin–enzyme complex was elucidated by Lynen and his co-workers in 1959 in a model system; the biologically reactive form of the CO_2 carrier is now known to be $1'$-N-carboxy-D-biotin (63).

All the biotin-dependent enzymes seem to follow a nonclassic, or "two-site," ping-pong mechanism. This implies that partial reactions (1a) and (1b) are performed by dissimilar subunits. The active site of a biotin enzyme consists of a carboxylase subsite that catalyzes the carboxylation of the biotinyl prosthetic group, of a carboxyl transferase subsite that catalyzes the transfer of the carboxyl group from the biotin to the substrate, and of the biotinyl-carrying site. The biotin prosthetic group is attached to this carrier protein by a flexible arm of 1.4 nm length, enabling biotin to oscillate back and forth between the carboxylase and transferase subsites. The mechanisms involved in the bond-making and the bond-breaking steps at these subsites are beginning to be understood. The current knowlege has been reviewed (64).

Even though the overall reactions catalyzed by biotin enzymes are very similar, a considerable variety has been noted in their quaternary structures. All enzymes studied thus far were oligomeric and varied in structural complexity from the relatively simple tetrameric pyruvate carboxylase of mammalian origin to the extreme case of transcarboxylase composed of 30 polypeptides (64). Furthermore, the functional components of an active site can be differently distributed among the constituent polypeptides of a given enzyme: there are biotin enzymes, such as the acetyl N1-C CoA carboxylase of *Escherichia coli*, that contain unifunctional subunits, and there are distinct protein components for the carboxylation subsite, the carboxyl carrier component, and the carboxyl transferase subsite. Other biotin enzymes contain two or even all three functional components needed to constitute an active site, on a single polypeptide (65). These various arrangements of the active site might represent various stages in the evolution of the enzyme system. However, tests by immunological procedures have not as yet provided support for this hypothesis, but a high degree of conservation in the amino acid sequence of the active

Table 3 Biotin-Dependent Enzymes

Enzyme	Reactions catalyzed	Biochemical role
I. Carboxylases		
Pyruvate carboxylase (EC 6.4.1.1)	Pyruvate → oxaloacetate	Gluconeogenesis, lipogenesis
Acetyl-CoA carboxylase (EC 6.4.1.2)	Acetyl CoA → malonyl CoA	Fatty acid biosynthesis
Propionyl-CoA carboxylase (EC 6.4.1.3)	Propionyl CoA → methylmalonyl CoA	Propinate metabolism
3-Methylcrotonyl-CoA carboxylase (EC 6.4.1.4)	3-Methylcrotonyl CoA → 3-methylglutaconyl CoA	Catabolism of leucine
Geranyl-CoA carboxylase (EC 6.4.1.5)	Geranyl CoA → carboxygeranyl CoA	Microbial catabolism of isoprenoid
Urea carboxylase (EC 6.3.4.6)	Urea → N-carboxyurea	Bacterial catabolism of urea in microbes that lack urease and grow on urea as sole source of nitrogen
II. Transcarboxylase		
Methylmalonyl-CoA carboxyltransferase (EC 2.1.3.1)	Methymalonyl CoA + pyruvate → oxaloacetate + propionyl CoA	Fermentation of certain carbohydrates to propionate in propionibacteria
III. Decarboxylases		
Methylmalonyl-CoA decarboxylase (EC 4.1.1.41)	Methylmalonyl CoA → propionyl CoA + CO_2	Last step in lactate fermentation in *Micrococcus lactilyticus*
Oxaloacetate decarboxylase (EC 4.1.1.3)	Oxaloacetate → pyruvate + CO_2	Inducible enzyme in *Aerobacter aerogenes* challenged to grow on citrate as carbon source

site could indicate that the biotin enzymes may have evolved at least in part from a common ancestor (64).

Of the biotin enzymes in Table 3, which have all been extensively reviewed by Moss and Lane (66), only the first four (EC 6.4.1.1 to EC 6.4.1.4) are present in human and animal tissues. The relevant aspects of these enzymes in biochemical nutrition, their metabolic functions, and their regulation have been extensively reviewed (2,6,67). Therefore, only a brief outline of the metabolic functions of these four enzymes is given here.

Pyruvate carboxylase, a mitochondrial enzyme, yields oxaloacetate from pyruvate; it has an absolute requirement for acetyl CoA, also synthesized and found in mitochondria. In combination with phosphoenolpyruvate carboxykinase (PEPCK), pyruvate carboxylase achieves the formation of phosphoenolpyruvate from three carbon precursors. This is a key reaction in gluconeogenesis by which glucose is formed from noncarbohydrate precursors, such as pyruvate, lactate, or gluconeogenic amino acids, especially alanine. Gluconeogenesis has portions located in separate subcellular sites: the oxaloacetate formed in the mitochondria has to be translocated into the cytosol, where the other enzymes of the gluconeogenic sequence are located. Since the mitochondrial membrane is not permeable to oxaloacetate and NADH, the translocation is achieved by a shuttle scheme in which oxaloacetate is reduced by NADH to malate under formation of NAD. Both products are transported to the cytosol and reconverted by malate dehydrogenase to oxaloacetate and NADH. Thus, this "dicarboxylic acid shuttle" enables both oxaloacetate and NADH to be transferred from the mitochondria to the cytosol (Fig. 3). Pyruvate carboxylase also has an important function in lipogenesis: although fatty acid synthesis takes place in the cytosol, the starting metabolite, acetyl CoA, is generated within the mitochondria, the membrane of which is not permeable to this compound. Acetyl CoA is condensed with oxaloacetate to citrate, which then passes the membrane. In the cytosol the citrate is broken down again into oxaloacetate and acetyl CoA. Thus, oxaloacetate is continuously removed from mitochondria and its replenishment is necessary to maintain normal citric acid cycle activity and citrate formation for lipogenesis. Pyruvate carboxylase fulfills this anaplerotic requirement.

Acetyl-CoA carboxylase, which depends on the presence of citrate for its activity and which is widely distributed in animals, plants, and microorganisms, catalyzes the carboxylation of acetyl CoA to malonyl CoA. This represents the first committed step in fatty acid synthesis. A cytosolic multienzyme complex, fatty acid synthetase, then accomplishes the synthesis of palmitate from malonyl CoA.

Propionyl-CoA carboxylase catalyzes the formation of methylmalonyl CoA from propionyl CoA. Methylmalonyl CoA is then converted to succinyl CoA, which through a series of reactions yields oxalacetate and then either glucose or CO_2 and water. Thus, propionate, which is produced in animal tissues as a result of oxidation of odd-numbered fatty acids, the degradation of branched-chain amino acids, of methionine and threonine, by fermentation in the ruminant, and by the gastrointestinal microflora, can be used for both energy derivation and glucose production.

3-Methylcrotonyl-CoA carboxylase plays a role in the catabolism of the ketogenic amino acid leucine. 3-Methylcrotonyl is formed as an intermediate and is converted to 3-methylglutaconyl CoA by the carboxylase. The latter is converted to 3-hydroxy-3-methylglutaconyl CoA, which then is cleaved to acetyl CoA and acetoacetate.

The activity of these carboxylases is dependent on the biotin status (see also Sec. III). The activity of hepatic pyruvate carboxylase increases in the growing chick with increasing

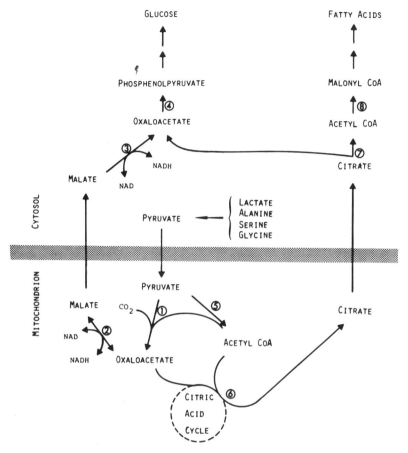

Figure 3 Gluconeogenesis and lipogenesis: (1) Pyruvate carboxylase; (2) mitochondrial malic dehydrogenase; (3) cytosolic malic dehydrogenase; (4) phosphoenolpyruvate carboxykinase; (5) pyruvate dehydrogenase complex; (6) citrate synthetase; (7) citrate cleavage enzyme; (8) acetyl-CoA carboxylase.

dietary biotin intake, whereas in rats and chicks fed a diet containing 20% egg white a progressive decrease in the hepatic activities of pyruvate and propionyl-CoA carboxylases and, to a lesser extent, of acetyl-CoA carboxylase, have been noted. These observations have also been found to hold true for other tissues containing biotin-dependent enzymes, such as kidney, brain, and heart, but the liver is the tissue most adversely affected. The activities of the biotin-dependent enzymes in the various tissues are rapidly restored on administration of the vitamin to the deficient animals. The rate of restoration of activities differs for the various tissues; it is fastest in kidney and brain and slower in liver and heart. This might be indicative of differences in the availability of the vitamin to the various tissues or of the rates at which the holoenzymes are synthesized (2). Also in healthy humans the administration of biotin for 5 days enhances the specific activities of leukocyte propionyl-CoA carboxylase, 3-methylcrotonyl-CoA carboxylase, and pyruvate carboxylase, whereas the specific activity of acetyl-CoA carboxylase was not affected. This increase occurred 10 days after the first administration of biotin and lasted for about one week (68). The administration of 4 μmol biotin in a child with biotinidase deficiency, in whom 3-methylcrotonyl-CoA carboxylase and propionyl-CoA carboxylase in lymphocytes were below 10% of normal, normalized carboxylase activity within 2 hours (62).

VIII. DEFICIENCY SIGNS

A. Animals

Biotin deficiency can easily be induced in most animals by inclusion of raw egg white in the diet or, in some, by feeding a purified biotin-free diet. After a certain time these animals cease to grow and start to develop characteristic pathological symptoms. These have been described in great detail (2,4,60,69), and therefore, only the main deficiency signs of the egg white injury are given in Table 4. Experimental work with biotin deficiency in animals found changes in the tissue fatty acid composition with an increase in the relative proportions of the 16-carbon fatty acids in the rat, pig, and chick (60,69); an increase in cholesterol synthesis in biotin deficiency; similarities in carbohydrate metabolism beween biotin-deficient and diabetic rats; an alteration of the need for and response to biotin by sex hormones; and interrelationships with other vitamins that may affect the metabolism and biotin requirement of animals (6,67,70).

As minute amounts of biotin are known to be adequate to support the body functions of animals, it was assumed that their requirements are covered by the natural biotin content of the feed and by the intestinal biosynthesis of this vitamin by the animal. In recent years, however, spontaneous outbreaks, under field conditions, of clinical biotin deficiency that respond to biotin treatment have occurred, although the microbiologically determined biotin content of the feed seemed adequate (60,69,71). Not only species with relatively high biotin requirements, such as turkeys, minks, foxes, and fish, were involved, but also chickens, pigs, and dogs. The lesions seen in these field outbreaks are similar to those produced under experimental conditions. Whether these outbreaks were due to the poor bioavailability of biotin in the feeds used or to the presence of sulfonamides, antibiotics, or other antimicrobial agents, of biotin antagonists, or of biotin-binding proteins in feed ingredients, is not known. Furthermore, biotin-responsive disease conditions were found that were not caused by a primary biotin deficiency or, at least, involve further etiological factors (60,69,71). This is the case for the fatty liver and kidney syndrome (FLKS) that had been causing heavy economic losses in commercial broiler flocks. FLKS was found to be due to a suboptimal biotin content in the rations coupled with certain nutritional and environmental stress factors. Although the symptoms of FLKS are not those of classic biotin deficiency, they can virtually be eliminated by supplementing the chick starter or the breeder rations with biotin. The "blue slime" disease in trout can also be prevented by adding biotin to the diet. Biotin supplementation was found to reduce the incidence and severity of claw lesions in pigs (72). Also in horses with weak hoof horn, supplementation with biotin improved the horn quality markedly (73).

B. Humans

In humans, the addition of raw egg white to a diet low in biotin provoked deficiency symptoms (2,4,6): four volunteers developed during the 3rd and 4th week a fine scaly desquamation of the skin without pruritus, which spontaneously disappeared; in the 7th week one of the volunteers developed maculosquamous dermatitis on the neck, hand, arms,

Table 4 Deficiency Signs in Animals

Animals	Signs
Rat	Reduction of food intake and decrease in growth rate; subsequently changes occur in the skin (seborrheic dermatitis), in advanced cases general exfoliative dermatitis and hyperkeratosis; hair (achromatrichia, alopecia, "spectable eye"), locomotion ("kangaroo gait"), and reproduction defects (abnormalities in the offspring and in severe cases resorption of fetuses or stillbirths)
Mouse	Similar to the rat: reduction in growth rate, changes in posture and gait, hypertonicity, and alopecia, but dermatitis only with moderate keratosis
Hamster	Loss of weight, abnormalities in movements, dry and scaly skin with only a moderate keratosis eventually complete alopecia
Guinea pig	Loss of weight, alopecia, and achromatrichia
Rabbit	Loss of weight, alopecia, and achromatrichia
Fur animals (mink, fox)	General dermatitis with hyperkeratosis; unsteady walk; "spectacle eye"; failure of normal pigmentation in the underfur ("turkey waste greying"); in severe cases "wet belly" can occur in males, which might not be due to biotin deficiency alone
Cat	Weight loss, accumulation of dried salivary, nasal, and lacrymal secretion, alopecia, scaly dermatitis, and achromatrichia
Dog	Not well investigated; a progressive ascending paralysis has been seen, but appears to be due primarily to potassium deficiency
Monkey	Severe dermatitis on face, feet, and hands; fur loses its color; watery eyes with incrustations on lids
Pig	Reduction in growth rate and food conversion efficiency; loss of hair; cracked skin with pustules and fissures; hyper- and parakeratosis; transverse fissures across the soft sole and cracks in the hard horn of the sole and the claw wall
Chicken and turkey	
Growing	Reduced growth rate, weight gain, and food conversion efficiency; disturbed and broken feathering; dermatitis with fissures on the undersurfaces of the feet; incrustations at the corners of beak; mainly in poults shortening of the metatarsal bones and perosis due to chondrodystrophy; "parrot beak" in chicks and poults
Adult	No deficiency symptoms; normal rate of egg production but reduced hatchability of fertile eggs; increased embryonic mortality and reduced viability after hatching
Fish	In salmonids, general listlessness, reduced swimming stamina, loss of appetite, then darkening of the skin, atrophy of muscles, and lesions in the colon; in eels, reduction in growth rate and abnormal swimming pose
Ruminants	No biotin deficiencies probable in adult animals because of their digestive systems; in calves, a progressive paralysis that is biotin and potassium responsive has been observed, but no classic biotin deficiency has been reported

and legs. During the 9th and 10th weeks all subjects showed fine brawny desquamation accompanied by mild depression and followed by extreme lassitude, somnolence, muscle pains, hyperesthesia, and localized parasthesias. After the 10th week anorexia occurred with occasional nausea. Slight anemia, a large increase in serum cholesterol, and a smaller increase in bile pigments were noted. The daily urinary excretion of biotin was reduced after 7–8 weeks to 14.3–30.3 nmol as compared with 120–210 nmol/day on a normal diet.

In infants under 6 months of age a self-limiting, benign skin eruption that is not eczematous or itchy can appear; the seborrheic dermatitis of infancy. Also, Leiner's disease, or erythroderma desquamativa, occurs in infancy and is probably a generalized and greatly intensified seborrheic dermatitis. The precise etiology of these infantile skin disorders is not known. As judged by the many reports (61) of a beneficial effect of biotin treatment, both seborrheic dermatitis and Leiner's disease could be the signs of a biotin deficiency in infants. This possibility is corroborated by the low circulating and excreted biotin levels found in both these conditions but not in cases of infantile eczema. Thus, in infants suffering from seborrheic dermatitis or Leiner's disease, mean urinary biotin excretions of 19.3 nmol/liter ($n = 10$) [normal mean level (74): 61.4 nmol/liter] and of 60.5 nmol/liter ($n = 4$) [normal (75): 126.4 nmol/liter] were found. The mean circulating biotin level in eight affected infants was 690 pmol/liter and in another seven infants, 869 pmol/liter, compared with a normal value of 1640 pmol/liter (74).

An erythematous rash was noted in patients with egg white injury (Sec. XI), in children with an inborn error of metabolism affecting the biotin-dependent enzymes (Sec. XI), and in children and adults on total parenteral nutrition (see Sec. XI). These findings seem to indicate that an erythematous exfoliative dermatitis is the first clinical sign of a biotin deficiency. Alopecia seen in the two children with egg white injury, in most infants with an inborn error of metabolism, and in many of the patients on total parenteral nutrition would then be at least in children, the expression of a long-lasting, severe biotin deficiency.

IX. METHODS OF NUTRITIONAL ASSESSMENT

For the evaluation of biotin nutritional status in humans, the circulatiang levels of the vitamin in whole blood, plasma, or serum and the urinary biotin excretion are employed. These levels are assessed mainly by the microbiological methods mentioned in Section III. Some urinary biotin excretion and circulating biotin levels are compiled in Tables 5 and 6, respectively. The great variation in the reported biotin values can be due, in both urine and blood, to the analytical method: the microorganisms used utilize biotin and its metabolites to different extents. Additionally, bound biotin in blood has to be liberated by papain digestion or by hydrolysis, and in urine, a dependency of the excretion levels on dietary intake has been noted (61). All these factors contribute to differences in urinary excretion and circulating biotin levels, but even so the great variations seen especially in the blood values are hard to explain. In feces, mean biotin levels of 474.8 ± 155.6 nmol per 24 hr with a range of 335.7–781.8 nmol per 24 hr using *Saccharomyces cerevisiae* as test organism and with *Lactobacillus casei* mean values of 544.4 nmol per 24 hr (range: 466.6–822.7 nmol per 24 hr) have been reported. Quite large day-to-day variations in fecal biotin excretion have been found, but excretion in feces is always greater than that in urine (61). From the available data (Tables 5 and 6), a biotin level in urine of approximately 160 nmol per 24 hr or 70 nmol/liter and a circulating level in blood, plasma, or serum of around 1500 pmol/liter seem to indicate an adequate supply of biotin for humans.

Table 5 Biotin in Urine of Healthy Subjects

	Biotin		Subjects	Assay	Reference
Low	Mean ± SD	High			
	nmol per 24 hr				
1.7	6.5	8.7	7 babies, 2–4 weeks old	S. cerevisiae	75
4.7	28	36.1	10 babies, 4–24 weeks old	S. cerevisiae	75
32.7	76 ± 35	167.8	31 adults	L. plantarum	76
	80 ± 71		119 adult males	O. danica	77
98.2	174 ± 56	331.5	20 adults	L. plantarum	78
57.3	187 ± 105	454.3	20 adults	S. cerevisiae	79
	nmol/liter				
13.4	26	38.9	7 babies, 2–4 weeks old	S. cerevisiae	75
12.3	61 ± 41	122.8	5 babies	S. cerevisiae	74
0	64 ± 70	163.7	24 babies, 1–7 days old	L. plantarum	80
49.1	70 ± 21	98.2	4 adults	L. plantarum	81
25.6	71 ± 45	155.5	12 adults	O. danica	82
57.3	81 ± 26	118.7	4 adults	N. crassa	81
19.4	126	290.8	10 babies, 4–24 weeks old	S. cerevisiae	75
31.9	147 ± 88	364.7	20 adults	S. cerevisiae	79

Table 6 Circulating Blood Levels

| Biotin (pmol/liter) | | | | | | | |
Low	Mean ± SD	High	Subjects	Source	Assay	Preparation	Reference
512.2	934 ± 385	1639.0	23 adult females	Plasma	Radiometric-microbiological		23
491.2	1054 ± 302	1725.3	25 adults	Blood	*L. plantarum*	Acidic	83
512.2	1065 ± 375	1704.9	15 adult males	Plasma	Radiometric-microbiological		23
660.0	1260 ± 500	3300.0	30 adults	Plasma	Protein-binding		19
601.7	1325 ± 465	2271.8	30 infants (2–27 months)	Blood	*L. plantarum*	Acidic	83
409.8	1393	3442.6	51 adults	Serum	Radioligand		21
	1557		632 children (10–13 years)	Blood	*O. danica*	Papain	84
1023.3	1576	2456.0	89 adults	Plasma	*L. plantarum*	Papain	61
818.7	1637 ± 737	2865.3	7 babies	Blood	*S. cerevisiae*	Basic	74
982.4	1719	3029.0	174 mothers at parturition	Blood	*O. danica*	Papain	85
1372.9	1893	3114.7	362 elderly	Blood	*O. danica*	Papain	86
881.1	1988	3073.7	600 adults	Blood	*O. danica*	Papain	87
1200.0	2410 ± 910	4300.0	20 adults	Serum	Chemiluminescence		24
818.7	2415	4093.3	76 females	Blood	*O. danica*	Papain	85
1170.0	242 ± 700	3850.0	15 adults	Plasma	Protein-binding		20
	2660 ± 979		118 males	Serum	*O. danica*	Papain	77
2149.0	3316	5878.0	68 neonates	Cord blood	*O. danica*	Papain	85
1637.3	4781 ± 2174	9005.3	25 infants (< 5 months)	Serum	*L. plantarum*	Acidic	88

X. NUTRITIONAL REQUIREMENTS

A. Animals

Assessment of the nutritional requirements for animals is complicated because of the enteric synthesis of the vitamin by microorganisms. These microorganisms are found in the lower part of the intestinal tract, a region in which absorption of nutrients is generally reduced. The intestinal flora, which also consists of biotin-requiring microorganisms, is, furthermore, influenced by the composition of the feed, and therefore, the amount of intestinally synthesized biotin may vary. Whether this biotin is at all available to the animal and, if so, how much it contributes to the total biotin requirement of the animal still has to be elucidated. The composition of the feed can also influence the determination of biotin requirements, as different bioavailabilities have been noted for the various feed components (Sec. V.B), and as no generally valid marker for biotin deficiency is yet available, a rather wide range of requirement data is found in the literature (2,4,60,71); these are compiled in Table 7.

B. Humans

Several factors complicate the assessment of nutritional requirement in man: the analytical determined biotin content in the diet can vary depending on the assay used, and not all of the determined biotin may be bioavailable. Second, biotin is synthesized, as in animals, by bacteria in the human intestine. The contribution of this intestinally synthesized biotin to the overall biotin supply is not yet determined, but studies in children with biotinidase deficiency showed that not enough free biotin was taken up from the intestine or ingested with the diet to maintain adequate circulating biotin levels (62). Furthermore, biotin can be recovered from the catabolismus of biotin-containing carboxylases by the action of biotinidase. This endogenous recyclization may be the reason it takes several months for clinical symptoms of a dietary biotin deficiency—skin changes and loss of hair—to appear. For the assessment of the nutritional requirements, not the clinical signs of a biotin deficiency, but other parameters such as the activity of biotin-dependent carboxylases or the excretion of abnormal organic acids should be used.

A recent evaluation of the available scientific knowledge on biotin has led the Food and Nutrition Board of the U.S. National Academy of Sciences (89) to establish for the first time estimated safe and adequate daily dietary intakes for biotin. These suggested daily biotin intakes are 0.15 μmol (35 μg) for infants up to 6 months and 0.2 μmol (50 μg) up to 1 year; for children 1–3 years old, 0.3 μmol (65 μg); for 4- to 6-year-old children, 0.35 μmol (85 μg); for 7- to 10-year-olds, 0.5 μmol (120 μg); and for older children and adults, 0.4–0.8 μmol (100–200 μg) biotin per day. This new development may stimulate authorities in other countries to stipulate dietary allowances for biotin, which up to now have only rarely been recommended (61).

XI. FACTORS THAT INFLUENCE VITAMIN STATUS AND IDENTIFICATION OF GROUPS AT GREATEST RISK OF DEFICIENCY

A. "Egg White Injury"

The excessive ingestion of raw eggs, which contain the biotin-binding glycoprotein avidin, led to symptoms of biotin deficiency. All patients (two adults, two children) developed

Table 7 Biotin Requirements in Animals

Animal	Requirement		Reference
	nmol/day	nmol/kg feed	
Rat	2–4		2, 4, 60
	8		2, 4, 60
		820	60
		1230	60
Mouse		330	2, 4
Mink		615–860	60
Cat		820	60
Dog		2050	60
Monkey	80		2, 4
Pig	410		2, 4
		245–985	60
		410–900	60
		450	60
		615–1025	71
Chicken			
Growing	3	290–410	2, 4
	4		2, 4
		370	60
		410–615	60
		738	71
Adult		615	60
	65	416, 820	71
Turkey			
Growing		790	60
		>850	60
		1025–1230	71
		1130–1330	60
		1165	60
		1845	60
Adult		615–820	71
		635	60
		820	60
		2255	60
Trout		2050	60
		2050–4100	60
		3280–4920	71
		4100–8200	60
		125–165 nmol/kg body weight	60

an exfoliative dermatitis, and the two boys also developed a total alopecia (61,90). One patient, in whom circulating and excretion levels were measured, had a biotin value in whole blood of 1000 pmol/liter and a daily urinary excretion of 34.4 nmol per 24 hr. Both these values are much lower than those given for normal individuals by the same authors (78). One of the boys excreted elevated amounts of 3-hydroxyisovalerate,

3-methylcrotonylglycine, 3-hydroxypropionate, and methylcitrate, indicating a deficiency of the biotin-dependent enzymes 3-methylcrotonyl-CoA and propionyl-CoA carboxylases, which were both found to be reduced in mixed leukocytes (90).

B. Inborn Errors of Metabolism

Some infants with organic acidemia and aciduria, the manifestations of a defect mainly in the degradative metabolism of branched-chain amino acids and the propionate-methylmalonate pathway, suffer from an inborn error of metabolism of the biotin-dependent carboxylases. The clinical presentation of such cases, the biochemical findings in blood and urine, the results of enzyme activity determinations, and the effect of biotin treatment have been extensively reviewed (50,91–93); only a brief outline will, therefore, be given here. Children suffering from an inborn error of biotin-dependent carboxylases can be divided into two groups, namely, those affected by an isolated defect in only one and those with a combined deficiency of the four biotin-dependent enzymes.

Isolated defects have been described for 3-methylcrontonyl-CoA carboxylase leading to 3-methylcrontonyl glycinuria, for propionyl-CoA carboxylase (propionic acidemia), and for pyruvate carboxylase (lactic acidosis), whereas only one doubtful case of an isolated defect has been reported for acetyl-CoA carboxylase (92). Clinically, affected children present similarly with poor feeding, persistent vomiting, muscular hypotonia, lack of responsiveness, lethargy and coma, often ketoacidosis, and in older children, developmental retardation, independently of which isolated enzyme is defective. Differential diagnosis can therefore only be established after extensive biochemical investigations in blood and urine, and of enzyme activities. It has been proposed (91) that the main diagnostic metabolites are 3-methylcrotonic acid and/or 3-methylcrotonlyglycine in urine for 3-methylcrotonyl glycinuria; methylcitric and 3-hydroxypropionic acid in urine and propionic acid in blood for propionic acidemia; lactic acid in blood and urine, ketoglutaric acid in urine, and pyruvic acid and alanine in blood for lactic acidosis. All these main metabolites as well as the activity of the biotin-dependent carboxylases have to be investigated in cases of a suspected inborn error of biotin-dependent carboxylases. From the results of all these measurements it can then unequivocally be determined which of the biotin-dependent carboxylases is defective. Furthermore, such extensive biochemical investigations allow the identification of cases with a combined deficiency which in the past have often been wrongly classified as suffering from an isolated deficiency.

Infants affected by a combined deficiency of the biotin-dependent carboxylases present clinically with the symptoms of organic acidemia and aciduria and most prominently also with skin rash and mostly alopecia. Biochemically each of the above-mentioned main abnormal metabolites of an isolated enzyme defect is found in the blood and urine of affected infants. Measurements of enzyme activities in fibroblasts cultivated in medium containing biotin only in the amounts provided by the fetal calf serum were noted to be reduced in some affected children and normal in others. This difference led to the detection of one form of combined or multiple carboxylase deficiency, the holocarboxylase synthetase deficiency (94). Holocarboxylase synthetase (EC 6.3.4.10) catalyzes in a two-step reaction that attachment of biotin to the ϵ-amino group of a lysine residue of an inactive apocarboxylase enzyme. The K_ms for biotin of holocarboxylase synthetase are elevated in patients with a holocarboxylase synthetase deficiency and were found to be three- to 70-fold the normal mean. The degree of elevation of K_m for biotin seems to correlate with the age of onset and with the amount of biotin required (up to 246 μmol/day) to alleviate the clinical symptoms and the metabolic abnormalities (92).

The genetic defect in patients with a multiple carboxylase deficiency in whom enzyme activity was normal in cultured fibroblasts was found to be a deficiency of biotinidase (95). Biotinidase (EC 3.5.1.12) is the only enzyme that catalyzes the cleavage of biocytin (biotinyl-ϵ-lysine) derived from bound biotin in food and from the catabolism of biotin-containing carboxylases. Thus, patients with biotinidase deficiency cannot utilize biocytin, which is excreted in their urine (18,20,45). They depend solely upon free biotin from food to maintain normal biotin levels. An assay for biotinidase activity has been adapted in a screening method for newborns, and from this study the incidence of biotinidase deficiency was estimated to be 1 in 41,000 births (96).

Initially it had been thought that biotin-responsive multiple carboxylase deficiency could be differentiated by the age of onset. But both in holocarboxylase synthetase deficiency and in biotinidase deficiency early- and late-onset cases can be found (92,93,95). The age of onset depends, thus, not on the genetic defect, but on the amount of total biotin (in holocarboxylase synthetase deficiency) or of free biotin (in biotinidase deficiency) available pre- and postnatally.

Patients deficient in biotinidase usually respond to 41 μmol of oral biotin per day, with reversion to normal of all the biochemical and clinical features of the disease (50,91–93) except for hearing loss and optic atrophy, which has been detected in some patients (92,97). As none of the patients with holocarboxylase synthetase deficiency have developed these neurosensory abnormalities, the long-term treatment with biotin can be ruled out as a cause (92).

In cases of an isolated defect in one of the biotin-dependent carboxylases biotin treatment has been claimed to be ineffective. Nevertheless, some patients with propionic acidemia, the isolated defect with the largest number of cases reported, seemed to benefit from a treatment with 41 μmol biotin daily (91) and it has been recommended (98) that all propionyl-CoA carboxylase-deficient patients be maintained on continuous biotin treatment.

Recently, an 8-year-old boy has been reported (99) with normal carboxylase activity in cultured fibroblast, but deficient activity in thrombocytes, excreting abnormal organic acids in urine. Biotinidase deficiency and holocarboxylase synthetase deficiency have been excluded, and only a very slow but definite biochemical response to biotin treatment has been found. The molecular mechanism behind this multiple carboxylase deficiency has not been elucidated.

C. Total Parenteral Nutrition

In a study of the biochemical and clinical status of adults on long-term total parenteral nutrition, low circulating biotin levels have been detected as biotin was not included in the infusion, but no clinical symptoms have been reported (100). Later a number of reports have appeared of children (55,101–103) and adults (55,104) with clinical signs of biotin deficiency: skin lesions and loss of hair. Biotin concentrations were found to be reduced (55,101,104) and in urine excretion of abnormal organic acids were noted (55,101,102). In some patients on total parenteral nutrition neurological changes have been described (55,101,104). Such mental changes have been seen in volunteers made biotin deficient (Sec. VIII.B), and irritability is often mentioned in children with an inborn error of biotin-dependent enzymes (91). On treatment with biotin, skin lesions healed, hair began to regrow, and the mental status improved in all patients on long-term parenteral nutrition. A daily supply of 0.25 nmol (60 μg) biotin for adults (105) and of 0.08 nmol (20 μg) for children (106) has been recommended to maintain normal plasma biotin levels in patients on long-term total parenteral nutrition.

Also in short-term total parenteral nutrition, supplementation of adult patients with 0.25 nmol (60 μg) biotin daily is required to maintain normal levels of biotin in urine (107,108).

D. Seborrheic Dermatitis of Infancy

As mentioned in Section VIII.B, lower amounts of biotin than in controls were found to circulate in the blood and to be excreted in the urine of childen with seborrheic dermatitis. Also, the beneficial effect of a biotin treatment in this disease indicated that seborrheic dermatitis could be a sign of a biotin deficiency in infants. The children with an inborn error of metabolism affecting all four biotin-dependent enzymes, the patients on long-term total parenteral nutrition without biotin, the two boys, and the two adults with egg white injury, and the volunteers on a biotin-deficient diet (61) all presented with dermatological problems. This indicates, then, that the seborrheic dermatitis of infancy is the clinical manifestation of a nutritional biotin deficiency, and thus a true biotin-deficiency symptom.

E. Sudden Infant Death Syndrome

The sudden infant death syndrome (SIDS), which accounts for one-third of deaths among children aged between 2 weeks and 1 year is, after accidents, the major cause of fatalities among children, but its cause is a mystery. It has been postulated (61) that there might be a connection between biotin and the etiology of SIDS. The median biotin levels in the livers of infants who died from SIDS between 1 and 52 weeks of life were significantly lower than those of infants who died from explicable causes (109). As the majority of these SIDS cases had been fed infant formulations, and as a considerable loss of biotin has been found to occur during the manufacture of certain infant formulations (109), some bottle-fed infants may be receiving a diet marginally deficient in biotin. This biotin insufficiency may leave the infant in a condition in which SIDS can be triggered by mild stress, such as an infection, a missed meal, or excessive heat or cold (109). This evidence that biotin deficiency is an important contributory factor in SIDS is circumstantial, but unequivocal proof will be difficult to provide.

F. Pregnancy and Lactation

A significantly lower ($p < 0.005$) mean blood biotin level was observed in pregnant women than in normal adults, which was found to fall progressively during gestation (83). Also, other investigators found reduced mean levels of biotin (1719 pmol/liter) in the plasma of pregnant women, especially in those taking no vitamin supplements (1473 pmol/liter) compared with nonpregnant females (2415 pmol/liter) (85). But no statistically significant differences in the mean circulating biotin levels between mothers giving birth to normal- or to low-birth-weight (<2500 g) babies or between the two groups of neonates, were seen (101). Maternal plasma biotin concentrations which at delivery were found to be 1332 ± 357 pmol/l ($n = 11$) decreased to 1000 ± 160 pmol/l ($n = 16$) in the first 6 days post partum and increased then to 1467 ± 262 pmol/l at 5–10 weeks post partum (111). Cord blood samples of 17 newborn infants showed a mean biotin concentration of 2381 ± 783 pmol/1; biotin levels in the newborn were always higher than in the mother (112). In general biotin levels in neonates, infants, and children were found to be higher (Table 6), whereas the urinary excretion of biotin in the first few months is lower (Table 5) than in adults. During the first 10 days post partum, biotin excretion in urine is lower than normal; the values from day 72 onward are in the normal range for adults (61).

Mature human milk contains an average of 16 nmol/liter biotin compared with 143 nmol/liter for cow's milk. For the first 4 days following parturition, the biotin level in human milk is too low to be measured, and for the next 5 days the levels varied widely between individuals (61). These older findings were recently confirmed: the biotin concentration in human milk was undetectable in most of 200 samples during the first 5 days after delivery. At and after 2 months of lactation the geometric mean concentration of biotin was 18.4 nmol/l with large intra- and interindividual variations (from undetectable to 111 nmol/l). Biotin concentration in milk was found to correlate positively with the plasma biotin concentration from 2 to 6 months of lactation. The mean biotin intake of the exclusively breast-fed infants varied accordingly from 15 to 18 nmol/day (range 0–41 nmol/day) at 4, 6, and 9 months of lactation (113).

G. Epileptics

In a study on the effect of a long-term treatment with antiepileptic drugs on the vitamin status, the plasma biotin levels were determined in 404 patients (114). The mean plasma biotin level determined microbiologically in 404 epileptics was 0.90 ± 0.29 nmol/l, which is significantly ($p < 0.0005$) lower than the 1.63 ± 0.49 nmol/l found in the 112 persons used as control group. Whereas only 4% of the controls had a biotin concentration of less than 1.05 nmol/l, 78% of the patients were below this value. Patients with a high average daily dose of anticonvulsants had a significantly ($p < 0.0025$) lower plasma biotin concentration than the patients with a low dose (114). Whereas no significant differences in mean plasma levels were seen in patients on monotherapy with primidone (0.90 ± 0.28 nmol/l; $n = 84$), carbamazepine (0.88 ± 0.24 nmol/l; $n = 54$), or phenytoin (0.94 ± 0.29 nmol/l; $n = 54$), mean biotin levels in patients treated with valproate alone were significantly higher (1.30 ± 0.63 nmol/l; $n = 36$). The urine of six epileptics and three volunteers was investigated for the occurrence of abnormal organic acids, and in four of the epileptic patients elevated concentrations of abnormal organic acids were detected. These patients had plasma biotin levels < 1.0 nmol/l. The other two epileptics, who were treated with valproate, had a plasma biotin level > 1.33 nmol/l and excreted no abnormal organic acids as did the three controls. Also, lactate levels in urine were significantly higher in the four epileptics not treated with valproate than in the other subjects. The mean plasma lactate level was significantly ($p < 0.05$) higher in 37 epileptics (1.32 ± 0.44 nmol/l) undergoing long-term treatment with a combination of drugs than in 16 controls (1.05 ± 0.32 nmol/l) (114). These findings indicate that a treatment with anticonvulsant drugs other than valproate is reducing circulating biotin levels and that this reduction leads to the excretion of abnormal organic acids as in patients with an inborn error of metabolism, with egg white injury, and as in patients on total parenteral nutrition. But no clinical symptoms of a biotin deficiency have been reported in epileptic patients (114).

It has been shown recently that phenobarbital, carbamazepine, and phenytoin displaced biotin bound to purified human biotinidase, whereas valproate did so only slightly (57). Another study demonstrated that carbamazepine and primidone are competitive inhibitors of biotin transport in human intestine and that the inhibitory effect appeared to be specific in nature and is directed toward the biotin transport system in the luminal membrane of the enterocyte (115).

H. Other Cases with Low Biotin Levels

In about 15% of alcoholics a circulating plasma level of less than 140 pmol/liter was found, whereas only 1% of a randomly selected hospital population had such a low circulating level. Furthermore, alcoholics were found to have reduced biotin concentrations in the liver; cirrhotics had levels 80% of normal, and those with fatty liver less than 20% (61).

Patients with partial gastrectomy or other causes of achlorhydria had significantly ($p < 0.001$) lower mean urinary biotin excretion values (25.8 $\pm$ 11.2 and 33.6 $\pm$ 20.2 nmol per 24 hr, respectively) than controls (76.6 $\pm$ 34.6 nmol per 24 hr), whereas partially gastrectomized patients with acid gastric secretion had lowered means of 50.8 $\pm$ 29.3 nmol per 24 hr, and those with peptic ulcers, 55.7 $\pm$ 31.1 nmol per 24 hr; these values are not statistically different from normal (76).

In nine children with burns and scalds a significantly lower ($p < 0.01$) mean plasma biotin level of 721 $\pm$ 347 pmol/liter as compared with control children (mean: 1260 $\pm$ 380 pmol/liter) was found. But there did not appear to be any correlation between the extent of the injury and the blood level; the low levels might be due to increased requirements for tissue repair (116).

Eight of 16 (108) and 12 of 29 (107) surgical patients were found to excrete abnormally low biotin levels. Also, mean plasma biotin levels were lower in 94 patients before operation than in controls (117). On admission to hospital, lower plasma biotin levels than in controls were found in 23 patients with inflammatory bowel disease (118) and in 15 patients with Crohn's disease (119).

The elderly (mean: 1351 pmol/liter; $n = 12$) and athletes (mean: 1228 pmol/liter; $n = 10$) showed a significantly lower ($p < 0.01$ and $p < 0.001$, respectively) plasma biotin level than controls (mean: 1576 pmol/liter; $n = 89$) (61). No depression of the mean biotin level was noted in 362 elderly whether institutionalized or not (86). Nevertheless, these findings indicate that there are groups in the population with low circulating biotin levels, but the clinical significance of such a low level in humans is not yet clear.

XII. EFFICACY OF PHARMACOLOGICAL DOSES

A treatment with 20.5 μmol biotin daily for 10 days either orally or intramuscularly healed the skin lesions in about 90% of infants with seborrheic dermatitis of Leiner's disease (61). In the two adults with egg white injury, all symptoms of biotin deficiency cleared when they received a well-balanced diet and additional vitamins, containing in one case 0.82 μmol biotin (61). The boys received 8.2–16.4 μmol or 4.1 μmol biotin daily parenterally or orally, and not only did the skin manifestations disappear but also the hair started to grow (61,90). On biotin treatment most of the abnormal metabolites in urine disappeared, and the propionyl-CoA carboxylase activity returned to normal (90).

In patients with a biotin-responsive inborn error of metabolism (see Sec. XI.B), a dramatic biochemical and clinical improvement is usually seen on oral treatment with 41 μmol biotin daily. Some patients with holocarboxylase synthetase deficiency, although clinically well when given 41 μmol biotin per day, had small amounts of urinary metabolites or reduced activities of carboxylase, which became normal when the dose was increased (92). For maintenance therapy in patients with a biotin-responsive inborn error of metabolism, the daily dose of biotin might be reduced, but the exact dose of biotin required for each child has to be carefully established. Daily biotin treatment might also be beneficial to patients with an isolated defect of a biotin-dependent carboxylase by increasing residual enzyme activity (98) and thus reducing the metabolic block.

Nine patients undergoing chronic hemodialysis for over 2 years and suffering from encephalopathy (dialysis dementia) and peripheral neuropathy were given daily 41 μmol biotin in three doses. Within 3 months a marked improvement of the neurological disorders were noted in all patients (120). But when plasma biotin levels were determined in 88 patients undergoing chronic hemodialysis treatment using a radioligand assay (21), higher than normal levels were found (2.05–12.3 nmol/l; normal range: 0.41–3.28 nmol/l) (121). Also, when plasma biotin levels were measured microbiologically, higher mean concentrations were noted in 10 hemodialysis patients (9.02 $\pm$ 1.64 nmol/l) than in 10 healthy controls (1.64 $\pm$ 0.41 nmol/l) (122). Treatment with 24.6 μmol biotin daily for 11 weeks significantly increased hematocrit values but did not change the dry skin in these patients.

Biotin has been shown to be effective in reducing claw lesions in pigs (72) and in improving the horn quality in horses (73). Biotin has recently been found to be effective in the treatment of brittle fingernails, which are frequently seen particularly in women. Out of 71 patients treated with a daily oral dose of 10.2 μmol (2.5 mg) biotin, 45 patients (43 females) could finally be evaluated. Of these 41 showed a definite improvement with firmer and harder fingernails after an average treatment of 5.5 $\pm$ 2.3 months. In the remaining four patients the effect was questionable, but none of the patients considered the treatment altogether ineffective. Eleven of the 45 patients mentioned a reduced loss of hair or a strengthening of the hair (123).

Also in an 18-month-old boy with uncombable hair syndrome and seborrheic dermatitis, treatment with 1.2 μmol (0.3 mg) biotin three times a day cleared the scaling of the scalp, and the hair began to regrow. After 4 months of treatment, hair fragility and abnormal hair loss were no longer a problem; it was more pliable and could be combed for the first time (124).

Oral biotin in amounts of 41 μmol daily during 8–12 weeks or of 61.5 μmol daily for 6–8 weeks has been used with good success in the treatment of acne, of seborrheic eczema, and of defluvium capillorum (125). The use of a topical cream once daily and a shampoo three times weekly containing 0.25–1.0% biotin has been effective in reducing and controlling excessive hair loss in male pattern alopecia (126), and also the intravenous administration of 2.05 μmol biotin together with 2.4 mmol panthenol three times weekly for 6 weeks has been found useful in the treatment of chronic alopecia (127). These claims, however, need further confirmation by controlled clinical trials.

Table 8   Acute Toxicity, LD_{50} (mmol/kg Body Weight)

Species	Mode of administration		
	Oral	IV	IP
Mouse		> 4.1	
Rat	> 1.45		> 0.12
Cat			> 0.001

Table 9 Subchronic and Chronic Toxicity, LD_{50} (μmol/kg Body Weight)

Species	Mode of administration			Duration (days)
	Oral	SC	IV	
Rat	> 1450			10
Rabbit	> 0.82	>0.82		102
Rabbit		> 0.41		180
Rabbit			> 0.41	30
Dog			> 6.15	10
Piglet	> 0.41			122

XIII. HAZARDS OF HIGH DOSES

Biotin is generally accepted as well tolerated by humans and by various laboratory animals without any side effects, even at high doses. The results of acute, subchronic, and chronic toxicity studies are given in Tables 8 and 9 (128). Intravenous administration of high doses of biotin in biotin-dependent experimental animals has no effect on the heart rate, blood pressure, circulation, respiration, or gastric secretion. A single oral dose does not influence the metabolic turnover or renal function; repeated oral doses appear to lower the metabolic rate (4,128). Prolonged administration of biotin in rabbits (1.6 μmol/day) seems to prevent the formation of cholesterol-induced arteriosclerotic plaques in the aorta, although the cholesterol level in the plasma is not affected. In rats suffering from experimentally induced diabetes, administration of biotin increases the activity of hepatic glucokinase (128).

Only Paul and his co-workers (129) found abnormal effects on the reproductive performance of female rats when injecting subcutaneously 20.5 or 41 μmol per 100 g body weight biotin, in 0.1 N NaOH. The dose of biotin applied to a 200 g rat represents at least 5000 or 10,000 times the daily requirement of a rat (Table 7). But even with these high doses of biotin, Mittelholzer found no influence on the reproductive performance in the female rat (130). In humans, no adverse effects of a biotin treatment in seborrheic dermatitis of infancy, the egg white injury, in inborn errors of metabolism, or in the treatment of alopecia have been reported on administration of up to 41 μmol biotin daily either orally or intramuscularly for periods exceeding 6 months (61,125). Also, no side effects were reported during the intravenous application of 20.5 μmol biotin three times weekly for 6 weeks (127).

REFERENCES

1. P. György and F.- W. Zilliken, in *Fermente, Hormone, Vitamine*, 3rd Ed., Vol. 31., R. Amman and W. Dirscherl (Eds.), Georg Thieme Verlag, Stuttgart, 1974, p. 766.
2. P. N. Achuta Murthy and S. P. Mistry, *Prog. Food Nutr. Sci.*, 2:405 (1977).
3. F. A. Robinson, in *The Vitamin Co-Factors of Enzyme Systems*, Pergamon Press, Oxford, 1966, p. 497.
4. P. György and B. W. Langer, Jr., in *The Vitamins*, 2nd Ed., Vol. 2, W. H. Sebrell, Jr., and R. S. Harris (Eds.), Academic Press, New York, 1968, p. 261.
5. M. A. Eisenberg, in *Metabolic Pathways*, 3rd Ed., Vol. VII, D. M. Greenberg (Ed.), Academic Press, New York, 1975, p. 27.
6. S. P. Mystry and K. Dakshinamurti, *Vitam. Horm.*, 22:1 (1964).

7. L. J. Hanaka, L. M. Reineke, and D. G. Martin, *J. Bacteriol.*, *100*:42 (1969).

8. L. Chaiet and F. J. Wolf, *Arch. Biochem. Biophys.*, *106*:1 (1964).

9. K. H. Baggaley, B. Blessington, C. P. Falshaw, and W. D. Ollis, *J. Chem. Soc. Chem. Commun.*, *101* (1969).

10. A. Marquet, Pure Appl. Chem., 49:183 (1977).

11. L. H. Sternbach, in *Comprehensive Biochemistry*, Vol. II, M. Florkin and E. G. Stotz (Eds.), Elsevier, New York, 1963, p. 67.

12. H. Baker and H. Sobotka, *Adv. Clin. Chem.*, *5*:173 (1962).

13. K. Dakshinamurti, A. D. Landman, L. Ramamurti, and R. J. Constable, *Anal. Biochem.*, *61*:225 (1974).

14. R. L. Hood, *J. Sci. Food Agric.*, *26*:1847 (1975).

15. R. Rettenmaier, *Anal. Chim. Acta, 113*:107 (1980).

16. R. S. Sanghri, R. M. Lemons, H. Baker, and J. G. Thoene, *Clin. Chim. Acta, 124*:85 (1982).

17. R. P. Bhullar, S. H. Lie, and K. Dakshinamurti, *Ann. N.Y. Acad. Sci., 447*:122 (1985).

18. T. Suormala, E. R. Baumgartner, J. Bausch, W. Holick, and H. Wick, *Clin. Chim. Acta. 177*:253 (1988).

19. T. Horsburgh and D. Gompertz, *Clin. Chim. Acta, 82*:215 (1978).

20. P. W. Chan and K. Bartlett, *Clin. Chim. Acta, 159*:185 (1986).

21. E. Livaniou, G. R. Evangeliatos, and D. S. Ithakissions, *Clin. Chem., 33*:1983 (1987).

22. D. M. Mock and D. B. DuBois, *Anal. Biochem., 153*:272 (1986).

23. T. R. Guilarte, *Nutrit. Rep. Int., 31*:1155 (1985).

24. E. J. Williams and A. K. Campbell, *Anal. Biochem., 155*:249 (1986).

25. K. Hayakawa and J. Oizumi, *J. Chromatog., 413*:247 (1987).

26. D. Glatzle and M. Frigg, *Biochem. Biophys. Res. Commun., 66*:368 (1975).

27. D. Glatzle, M. Frigg, and F. Weber, *Acta Vitaminol. Enzymol., 1*:11 (1979).

28. D. W. Bannister and C. C. Whitehead, *Int. J. Biochem., 7*:619 (1976).

29. C. C. Whitehead and D. W. Bannister, *Br. J. Nutr., 39*:547 (1978).

30. R. Bitsch, A. Dersi, and D. Hötzel, *Klin. Wochenschr., 55*:145 (1977).

31. D. Glatzle, M. Frigg, and F. Weber, *Acta Vitaminol. Enzymol., 1*:19 (1979).

32. M. G. Hardinge and H. Crooks, *J. Am. Diet. Assoc., 38*:240 (1961).

33. A. A. Paul and D. A. T. Southgate in McCance and Widdowson's, *The Composition of Foods*, 4th ed., Elsevier, Amsterdam, New York, Oxford, 1978.

34. J. Wilson and K. Lorenz, *Fd. Chem., 4*:115 (1979).

35. S. W. Sauci, W. Fachmann, and H. Kraut, *Food Composition and Nutrition Tables 1981/82*, Wissenschaftliche Verlagsgesellschaft m.b.H. Stuttgart, 1981.

36. K. Hoppner and B. Lampi, *Nutrit. Rep. Int., 28*:793 (1983).

37. K. J. Scott, D. R. Bishop, A. Zecholko, J. D. Edwards-Webb, P. J. Zackson, and D. Scuffam, *J. Dairy Res., 51*:37 (1984).

38. K. J. Scott and D. R. Bishop, *J. Dairy Res., 52*:521 (1985).

39. R. Bitsch, I. Salz, and D. Hötzel, *Dtsch. Lebensmittel Rundschau, 82*:80 (1986).

40. T. R. Guilarte, *Nutrit. Rep. Int., 32*:837 (1985).

41. R. L. Hood, *Nutrit. Rep. Int., 36*:1039 (1987).

42. R. Karlin and C. Foisy, *Int. J. Vit. Nutr. Res., 42*:545 (1972).

43. J. Pipsa, *Ann. Med. Exp. Biol. Fenn., 43*: Suppl. 5:5 (1965).

44. J. M. Schreiner, *Ann. N.Y. Acad. Sci., 447*:420 (1985).

45. J. P. Bonjour, J. Bausch, T. Suormala, and E. R. Baumgartner, *Internat. J. Vit. Nutr. Res., 54*:223 (1984).

46. M. Frigg, *Poult. Sci., 55*:2310 (1976).

47. R. Misir and R. Blair, *Poult. Sci., 67*:1274 (1988).

48. R. Misir and R. Blair, *Can. J. Anim. Sci., 68*:523 (1988).

49. D. B. McCormick and L. D. Wright, in *Comprehensive Biochemistry*, Vol. 21, M. Florkin and E. G. Stotz (Eds.), Elsevier, Amsterdam, 1971, p. 81.

50. F. A. Hommes, *Wld. Rev. Nutr. Diet.*, *48*:34 (1986).
51. D. B. McCormick, *Nutr. Rev.*, *33*:97 (1975).
52. D. V. Craft, N. H. Gross, N. Chandramouli, and H. G. Wood, *Biochemistry, 24*:2471 (1985).
53. H. M. Said, R. Redha, and W. Nylander, *Gastroenterology, 95*:1312 (1988).
54. H. B. White and C. C. Whitehead, *Biochem. J., 241*:677 (1987).
55. J. P. Bonjour, *Ann. N.Y. Acad. Sci., 447*:97 (1985).
56. P. B. Seshagiri and P. R. Adiga, *Biochem. Biophys. Acta, 916*:474 (1987).
57. J. Chauhan and K. Dakshinamurti, *Biochem. J., 256*:265 (1988).
58. H. M. Lee, N. E. McCall, L. D. Wright, and D. B. McCormick, *Proc. Soc. Exp. Biol. Med., 142*:642 (1973).
59. H. M. Lee, L. D. Wright, and D. B. McCormick, *J. Nutr., 102*:1453 (1972).
60. L. Völker, *Uebers. Tierernährg., 5*:185 (1977).
61. J. P. Bonjour, *Int. J. Vit. Nutr. Res., 47*:107 (1977).
62. E. R. Baumgartner, T. Suormala, H. Wick, J. Bausch, and J. P. Bonjour, *Ann. N.Y. Acad. Sci., 447*:272 (1985).
63. H. G. Wood, *Trends Biochem. Sci., 1*:4 (1976).
64. H. G. Wood and R. E. Barden, *Annu. Rev. Biochem., 46*:385 (1977).
65. M. Obermayer and F. Lynen, *Trends Biochem. Sci., 1*:169 (1976).
66. J. Moss and D. Lane, *Adv. Enzymol., 35*:321 (1971).
67. T. Terroine, *Vitam. Horm., 18*:1 (1966).
68. J. H. Stirk, K. G. M. M. Alberti, and K. Bartlett, *Biochem. Soc. Trans. 11*:185 (1983).
69. C. C. Whitehead, in *Handbook Series in Nutrition and Food*, Section E, Vol. II, M. Rechcigl (Ed.), CRC Press, West Palm Beach, Florida, 1978, p. 65.
70. D. Balnave, *Am. J. Clin. Nutr., 30*:1408 (1977).
71. C. C. Whitehead, *Biotin in Animal Nutrition*, F. Hoffmann-La Roche Ltd, ISBN 3-906507-02-5, 1988.
72. E. T. Kornegay, *Ann. N.Y. Acad. Sci., 447*:112 (1985).
73. N. Comben, R. J. ClarK, and D. J. B. Sutherland, *Vet. Rec., 115*:642 (1984).
74. J. Svejcar and J. Homoka, *Ann. Pediatr., 174*:175 (1950).
75. H. Berger, *Int. Z. Vitaminforsch., 22*:190 (1950).
76. T. Markkanen, *Acta. Med. Scand. (Suppl.), 169*:360 (1960).
77. M. W. Marshall, J. T. Judd, and H. Baker, *Nutr. Res., 5*:801 (1985).
78. C. M. Baugh, J. H. Malone, and C. E. Butterworth, *Am. J. Clin. Nutr., 21*:173 (1968).
79. T. W. Oppel, *Am. J. Med. Sci., 204*:856 (1942).
80. B. M. Hamil, M. N. Coryell, C. Roderuck, M. Kaucher, E. M. Moyer, M. E. Harris, and H. H. Williams, *Am. J. Dis. Child., 74*:434 (1947).
81. L. D. Wright, E. L. Cresson, and G. A. Driscoll, *Proc. Soc. Exp. Biol. Med., 91*:248 (1956).
82. H. Baker, O. Frank, V. B. Matovitch, I. Pasher, A. Aaronson, S. H. Hutner, and H. Sobotka, *Anal. Biochem., 3*:31 (1962).
83. H. N. Bhagavan and D. B. Coursin, *Am. J. Clin. Nutr., 20*:903 (1967).
84. H. Baker, O. Frank, S. Feingold, G. Christakis, and H. Ziffer, *Am. J. Clin. Nutr., 20*:850 (1967).
85. H. Baker, O. Frank, A D. Thomson, A. Langer, E. D. Munves, B., De Angelis, and A. Kaminetzky, *Am. J. Clin. Nutr., 28*:56 (1975).
86. H. Baker, O. Frank, I. S. Thind, S. P. Jaslow, and D. B. Louria, *J. Am. Geriat. Soc., 27*:444 (1979).
87. H. Baker, *Ann. N.Y. Acad. Sci., 447*:129 (1985).
88. A. Nisenson and L. Sherwin, *J. Pediatr., 69*:134 (1966).
89. Food and Nutrition Board, *Recommended Dietary Allowances*, 9th Ed., National Academy of Sciences, Washington, D.C., 1980.
90. L. Sweetman, L. Suhr, H. Baker, R. M. Peterson, and W. L. Nyhan, *Pediatrics, 68*:553 (1981).

91. J. P. Bonjour, *World Rev. Nutr. Diet, 38*:1 (1981).

92. L. Sweetman and W. L. Nyhan, *Ann. Rev. Nutr., 6*:317 (1986).

93. W. L. Nyhan, *Int. J. Biochem., 20*:363 (1988).

94. L. Sweetman, B. J. Burri, and W. L. Nyhan, *Ann. N.Y. Acad. Sci., 477*:288 (1985).

95. B. Wolf, G. S. Heard, J. R. Secor McVoy, and R. E. Grier, *Ann. N.Y. Acad. Sci., 477*:252 (1985).

96. B. Wolf, G. S. Heard, L. G. Jefferson, V. K. Proud, W. E. Nance, and K. A. Weissbecker, *N. Engl. J. Med., 313*:16 (1985).

97. H. J. Wastell, K. Bartlett, G. Dale, and A. Shein, *Arch. Dis. Child., 63*:1244 (1988).

98. B. Wolf, *J. Pediatr., 97*:964 (1980).

99. E. Holme, C.-E. Jacobson, and B. Kristiansson, *J. Inter. Metab. Dis., 11*:270 (1988).

100. K. N. Jeejeeboy, B. Langer, G. Tsallas, R. C. Chu, A. Kuksis, and G. H. Anderson, *Gastroenterology, 71*:943 (1976).

101. D. M. Mock, D. L. Baswell, H. Baker, R. T. Holman, L. Sweetman, *Ann. N.Y. Acad. Sci., 447*:314 (1985).

102. P. Lagier, P. Bimar, S. Sériat-Gautier, J. M. Dejode, T. Brun, and J. Bimar, *Nouv. Presse Méd., 16*:1795 (1987).

103. H. Kadowaki, M. Ouchi, M. Kaga, T. Motegi, Y. Yamagakawa, H. Hayukawa, G. Hashimoto, and K. Furuya, *JPEN, 11*:322 (1987).

104. S. Matsusue, S. Kashihara, H. Takeda, and S. Koizumi, *JPEN, 9*:760 (1985).

105. M. E. Shils, H. Baker, and O. Frank, *JPEN, 9*:179 (1985).

106. M. C. Moore, H. L. Greene, B. Philipps, L. Franck, R. J. Shulman, J. E. Murrell, and M. E. Arent, *Pediatrics, 77*:530 (1986).

107. G. E. Nichoalds, R. W. Luther, T. R. Sykes, J. M. Kinney, D. H. Elwyn, and S. Beling, *JPEN, 6*:577 (1982).

108. D. T. Dempsey, J. L. Mullen, J. L. Rombcan, L. O. Crosby, J. L. Obrlander, L. S. Knox, and G Melnik, *JPEN, 11*:229 (1987).

109. G. S. Heard, R. L. Hood, and A. R. Johnson, *Med. J. Aust., 2*:305 (1983).

110. H. Baker, I. S. Thind, O. Frank, B. De Angelis, H. Caterini, and D. B. Louria, *Am. J. Obstet. Gynecol., 129*:521 (1977).

111. L. Dostalova, *Ann. Nutr. Metab. 28*:385 (1984).

112. L. Dostalova, *Dev. Pharmacol. Ther. 4*, Suppl. *1*:45 (1982).

113. L. Salmenperä, J. Perheentupa, J. P. Pisa, and M. A. Siimes, *Internat. J. Vit. Nutr. Res., 55*:281 (1985).

114. K. H. Krause, J. P. Bonjour, P. Berlit, and W. Kochen, *Ann. N.Y. Acad. Sci., 447*:297 (1985).

115. H. M. Said, R. Redha, and W. Nylander, *Am. J. Clin. Nutr. 49*:127 (1989).

116. G. B. Barlow, J. A. Dickerson, and A. W. Wilkinson, *J. Clin. Pathol., 29*:58 (1976).

117. S. Ogoshi, H. Sato, T. Muto, Y. Itokawa, T. Kobayashi, and K. Okuda, *J. Nutr. Sci. Vitaminol., 31*:7 (1985).

118. X. Xiol, E. Cabré, A. Abad-Lacruz, F. Gonzalez-Huix, A. Gil, R. Rufer, M. Esteve, C. Dolz, G. Brubacher, and M. A. Gasull, *Clin. Nutr., 6*: (Spec. Suppl.) 36 (1987).

119. F. Gonzales-Huix, A. Abad-Lacruz, A. Gil, M. Esteve, E. Cabré, R. Rufer, X. Xiol, G. Brubacher, and M. A. Gasull, *Clin. Nutr., 6*: (Spec. Suppl.) 70 (1987).

120. H. Yatzidis, D. Koutsicos, B. Agroyannis, C. Papastephanidis, M. Francos-Plemenos, and Z. Delatola, *Nephron, 36*:183 (1984).

121. E. Livanion, G. P. Evangelatos, D. S. Ithakissios, H. Yatzidis, and D. C. Koutsicos, *Nephron, 46*:331 (1987).

122. K. Ono and S. Doi, *Kidney Internat., 28*:348 (1985).

123. G. L. Floersheim, *Z. Hautkr., 64*:41 (1988).

124. W. B. Shelley and E. D. Shelley, *J. Am. Acad. Dermatol., 13*:97 (1985).

125. J. Bonnet and A. Florens, *Gaz. Méd. France, 76*:1201 (1969).

126. E. Settel, *Drug Cosm. Ind., 122*:34 (1977).

127. A. Dupré, J. Lassère, B. Christol, J. L. Bonafé, H. Rumeau, N. Arbarel, S. Corberand, N. Périole, and A. M. Sorbara, *Rev. Med. Toulouse, 13*:675 (1977).
128. W. F. Körner and J. Völlm, in *Klinische Pharmakologie und Pharmakotherapie*, H. P. Kuemerle, E. R. Garrett, and K. H. Spitzy (Eds.), Urban & Schwarzenberg, München, 1976, p. 381.
129. P. K. Paul, in *Handbook Series in Nutrition and Food*, Section E, Vol. I, M. Rechcigl (Ed.), CRC Press, West Palm Beach, Florida, 1978, p. 47.
130. E. Mittelholzer, *Int. J. Vit. Nutr. Res., 46*:33 (1976).

11
Pantothenic Acid

Hazel Metz Fox†
University of Nebraska
Lincoln, Nebraska

†Deceased.

I. HISTORY

Pantothenic acid, a water-soluble vitamin of the B complex, was discovered in 1933 by Williams (1). Tissue extracts from a variety of biological materials provided a growth factor for yeast; the growth factor was identified as "pantothenic acid," derived from the Green word *pantos*, meaning everywhere. Pantothenic acid was established as the growth-promoting factor for lactic acid bacteria, which are used as assay organisms for the vitamin (2). During early research, Jukes (3) and Woolley et al. (4) independently indentified the "antidermatitis factor" in chicks and the "liver filtrate factor" in rats, factors later proved to be identical with pantothenic acid.

II. CHEMISTRY

Pantothenic acid was isolated from liver; the free acid is a pale yellow viscous oil easily destroyed by alkali and acid but stable in neutral solutions.

The vitamin, synthesized by condensing butyrolactone with the ester of β-alanine, is comprised of β-alanine and a dihydroxy acid known as pantoic acid (5). The complete structure of the molecule is N-(2,4-dihydroxy-3,3-dimethyl-1-oxobutyl)β-alanine (6) (Fig. 1). Pantothenic acid produced commercially is a synthetic, white crystalline calcium salt, calcium pantothenate. Panthenol, the corresponding alcohol, is more easily absorbed and is converted to the acid in vivo (7). Some microorganisms are able to synthesize the vitamin in the rumen of cattle and sheep (8). Although the exact mechanism is not fully understood, it appears that organisms that synthesize pantothenic acid condense β-alanine with dihydroxybutyric acid or its lactone (9).

Various derivatives and analogs of pantothenic acid have been synthesized and their antagonistic action studied. ω-Methylpantothenic acid is the most common antagonist of pantothenic acid used to produce a deficiency of the vitamin in humans (10). Other antivitamins include pantoyltaurine and phenylpantothenate (11,12). Nishizawa and Matsuzaki (13) administered homopantothenic acid to the chick and observed a decrease of liver coenzyme A, a swelling of the gallbladder, suppression of weight, and other signs of pantothenic acid deficiency. D,L-pantothenic acid was shown to have one-half of the biological activity of d(+)pantothenic acid for chicks (14). Administration of 1(−)pantothenic acid resulted in depressed growth of mice and rats and in decreased liver cholesterol and triglycerides in rats. The adverse effects were reversed by d(+) pantothenic acid (15). Rats started dying of 1(−)pantothenic acid feeding after 20 days and after 6 days when either cholesterol or cholic acid was given in addition to the diet containing 1(−)pantothenic acid (16). These same investigators reported that 1(−)pantothenic acid inhibited the growth of *Lactobacillus arabinosus*, but not that of *Saccharomyces cerevisiae*. Recently, antimetabolites of the vitamin containing alkyl or aryl ureido and carbamate components in

PANTOTHENIC ACID

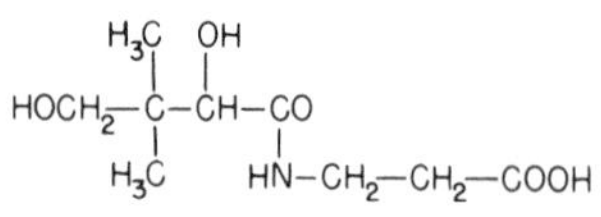

Figure 1 Pantothenic acid. (From Ref. 6).

the β-alanyl portion of the amide part of the molecule have been synthesized (17). These analogs are known to inhibit the growth of lactic acid bacteria and are antagonists of the vitamin.

III. ANALYTICAL AND BIOASSAY PROCEDURES

The pantothenic acid content of various substances has been analyzed by microbiological assay, animal bioassay, radioimmunoassay, and chemical methods. The earliest microbiological assays employed the yeast *Saccharomyces cerevisiae*. The essay lacked specificity because this species of yeast actually produced its own supply of pantothenate. Pennington and Williams (18) developed an assay method for pantothenic acid using *Lactobacillus casei* as the test organism. Strong et al. (19) reported that, although *L. casei* could be used successfully, it was more difficult to use than *Lactobacillus plantarum* (formerly *Lactobacillus arabinosus*). Other successful methods of estimating the vitamin microbiologically use the test organisms *Lactobacillus bulgaricus* and *Proteus morganii* (20). More recently, *Pediococcus acidilacti* has been suggested as an effective test organism for microbiological assay of the vitamin (21).

Chick bioassays have been used extensively in the past to determine the pantothenic acid content of food (22). Chick bioassay methods have been reported to yield higher pantothenic acid values than microbiological assays for the same foods suggesting that some pantothenic acid-containing compounds may be available to chicks that are not utilized by microorganisms (23). Curative assay methods using chicks are still practical because of the availability and low cost of chicks.

Radioimmunoassay, first introduced by Yalow and Berson (24), is a sensitive method for determining the concentration of substances present in small amounts in biological fluids. Radioimmunoassay made possible the specificity necessary to quantitate concentrations of hormones, drugs, and vitamins (25). Blood pantothenic acid levels have been determined by radioimmunoassay (26). After treatment with alkaline phosphatase and liver extract, the pantothenic acid content of whole blood analyzed by radioimmunoassay compared favorably to that determined by microbiological assay with *L. plantarum*.

Voight and Eitenmiller (27) describe the use of a liquid scintillation technique for microbial vitamin analysis. In this method the sample is incubated in a medium containing ^{14}C. $^{14}CO_2$ released from the reaction is trapped with 2-phenylethylamine and is used to measure thiamine, pyridoxine, and pantothenic acid.

The complex nature of natural products has deterred the development of chemical methods for assay of pantothenic acid. A method for determining pantothenic acid in foods was described by Tesmer et al. (28). Pantoyl lactone formed by acid hydrolysis of free and bound pantothenic acid is quantitatively measured by gas chromatography. Results obtained by this method compared favorably with results from accepted microbiological procedures (29). Prosser and Sheppard (30) developed a chemical procedure for determining pantothenates and pantothenol in multivitamin preparations using gas-liquid chromatography.

Although calcium pantothenate is widely used in multivitamin preparations, due to its interaction with other vitamins and the effects of storage, it has been difficult to analyze the calcium pantothenate content. In the past, colorimetric and fluorometric assay procedures have been employed (31). An automated fluorometric assay technique was recently reported (32) to be successful in hydrolytic cleavage of pantothenic acid to yield β-alanine and a salt of pantoic acid. β-Alanine, a component of calcium pantothenate, must be removed from the sample to make the assay specific for calcium pantothenate. Fluorescence intensity of the product corresponds to the concentration of β-alanine and to the original concentration of calcium pantothenate in the sample. Concentrations of from 0.1 to 20.0 mg calcium pantothenic acid per 100 ml were reported.

IV. CONTENT OF FOOD

Pantothenic acid occurs in both the bound and free forms in food. It is necessary to liberate the pantothenic acid from its bound form by enzymatic hydrolysis prior to microbiological analysis. Much of the data on pantothenic acid content of food has been obtained with the use of simpler enzyme preparations, such as mylase-P, papain, clarase, and takadiastase (33). Using the double-enzyme preparation, combined treatment with intestinal phosphatase and pigeon liver extract, Zook et al. (34) released free pantothenic acid from its bound forms. Orr (33) reported the pantothenic acid content of a number of foods using the double-enzyme treatment. Recently, the pantothenic acid content of 75 processed and cooked foods analyzed by radioimmunoassay was reported by Walsh et al. (35).

Another type of enzyme treatment, hydrolysis with papain and diastase, was reported satisfactory for release of pantothenic acid (36). Following this treatment, growth of *L. arabinosus* was measured potentiometrically.

Pantothenic acid is widely distributed in foods: heart, yeast, brain, avocado, meat, broccoli, bran, and molasses are excellent sources (Table 1). Estimates of pantothenic acid intakes have varied widely. A typical American diet is reported to contain approximately 4.9 mg pantothenic acid per 2500 kcal (37). Chung et al. (38) analyzed a series of typical American meals for levels of pantothenic acid and concluded that American

Table 1 Pantothenic Acid Content in Food (100 g Edible Portion)

Food groups	Pantothenic acid (mg)
Avocados, raw	1.070
Beef, raw	.620
Brains	2.600
Broccoli, raw	1.170
Cashew nuts	1.300
Eggs, whole	1.600
Egg, yolk	4.400
Heart, raw	2.500
Kidneys, raw	3.850
Lentils, dry	1.360
Liver, raw	7.700
Milk, dry	3.600
Peanuts, raw	2.800
Rice, brown	1.100
Soybeans, raw	1.700
Tongue, raw	2.000
Bran, 100%	2.900
Yeast, baker's	11.000

Source: Ref. 33.

diets provided between 10 and 20 mg pantothenic acid daily. Fox and Linkswiler (39) calculated pantothenic acid intakes of eight women on self-selected diets and reported a mean intake of 6.7 mg/day with a range from 3.4 to 10.3 mg. Generally, pantothenic intakes reported from recent studies are lower than those reported in the 1960s or earlier. Thus, Kathman (40) calculated pantothenic acid intakes for adults and adolescents from 4-day dietary records and found intakes for adults ranged from 1.3 to 16.9 mg, with a mean of 5.4 mg daily. Intakes of adolescents ranged from 4.0 to 7.9 mg per day, with a mean of 5.5 mg. Similarly, pantothenic acid intakes from self-selected diets reported by Lin (41) ranged from 2.6 to 7.0 mg, with a mean of 4.7 mg. The average American diet has recently been estimated from U.S.D.A. food-consumption data to contain 5.8 mg (2) and the average British diet from the National Survey of 1979, 5.1 mg of pantothenic acid daily (43). Pantothenic acid intakes may be underestimated using food composition tables since values for many food items are lacking. Black et al. (44) reported that pantothenic acid was underestimated by 11.5% when values were calculated using British food composition tables. The recent generally low reported pantothenic intakes may also be attributed to lower caloric intake. Mareschi et al. (45) reported that French diets providing 2500 kcal furnished 80% and those providing 1500 kcal, 50% or less of the pantothenic acid allowance. Similar findings were reported by Walsh et al. (46), who analyzed meals consumed in a Utah nursing home and found a mean daily pantothenic acid intake of 3.75 mg and a mean daily energy intake of 1688 kcal.

Pantothenic acid has been reported to be fairly stable during ordinary cooking and storage. In recent years there has been some concern that the vitamin may be destroyed during food processing. Pantothenic acid is stable at high temperatures when the pH is between 5 and 7 (47). At pH values above 7 or below 5, pantothenic acid is unstable at high temperatures.

The effect of sterilization and storage on the pantothenic acid content of canned foods has been studied, with losses as great as 50% reported (48). Losses of pantothenic acid during processing of food have been shown by Schroeder (49), who suggested enrichment of refined flours, sugars, and fats with pantothenic acid. Walsh et al. (35) also reported a relatively low pantothenic acid content in many highly processed foods, including products made from refined grains, fruit products, and fat- or cereal-extended meats and fish. Pasteurization does not affect pantothenic acid in milk, which may be due to the neutral pH of milk (50).

The availability of pantothenic acid from a mixed diet representative of the average American diet was assessed by comparing the urinary excretion of the vitamin by healthy male volunteers consuming the vitamin in the food with those provided the vitamin in purified form. Using the method availability of pantothenate ranged from 40 to 61% with a mean of 50% (42). Southern and Baker (51,52) compared growth of chickens fed food sources or purified pantothenic acid and reported that approximate bioavailable pantothenic acid in maize, barley, sorghum, wheat, and dehulled soya bean meal was 81, 173, 54, 75, and 164%, respectively. Barley and soya bean meal stimulate growth apart from their contribution of pantothenic acid, accounting for the high bioavailability estimates for these foods.

V. METABOLISM

The importance of pantothenic acid in human nutrition remained in question until coenzyme A (Fig. 2) was found to be its primary biochemically active form (53). The

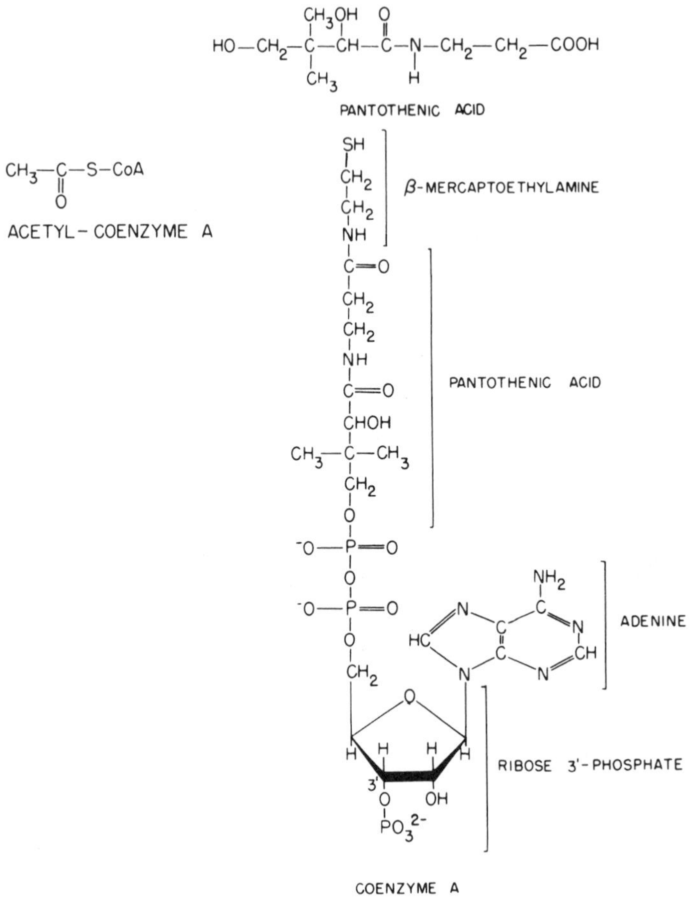

Figure 2 Coenzyme A. (From Ref. 171.)

primary role of pantothenic acid in metabolism is related to its incorporation into coenzyme A and acyl carrier protein.

As part of coenzyme A, pantothenic acid takes part in acetyl transfers and serves as either a hydrogen donor or acceptor (Fig. 3). Acetyl coenzyme A occupies a primary position in the transfer of other acyl groups in intermediary metabolism (54) (Fig. 2). Coenzyme A functions as a carrier of acyl groups in enzymatic reactions involved in the synthesis of fatty acids cholesterol, and sterols; the oxidation of fatty acids; pyruvate, and ketoglutarate; and in biological acetylations.

Various pathways have been proposed for the conversion of pantothenic acid to coenzyme A (55,56) (Fig. 4). The accepted pathway at present involves conversion of pantothenate to 4'-phosphopantothenic acid to 4'-phosphopantothenylcysteine to 4'-phosphopantotheine to dephosphocoenzyme A to coenzyme A (57). Robishaw et al. (58,59) reported that the primary site of control of coenzyme A synthesis is isolated perfused rat hearts was the pantothenate kinase–catalyzed reaction, the first intracellular step in the conversion of pantothenic acid to coenzyme A. The rate of this reaction was

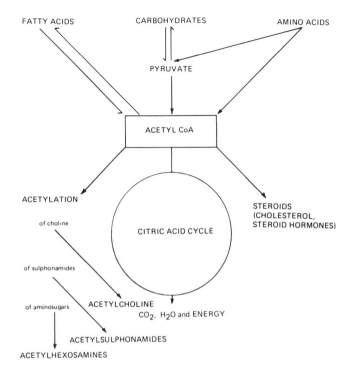

Figure 3 Acetylation reactions. (From Ref. 54.)

inhibited by including glucose, pyruvate, fatty acids, or β-hydroxybutyrate in the perfusate. Insulin also inhibited the reaction in the presence of glucose.

A new form of pantothenic acid has been isolated from a growth-stimulating factor using the test organism *Pediococcus cerevisiae*. The growth factor was analyzed chromatographically and determined to be 4'-O-(-D-glucopyranosyl)-D-pantothenic acid (60). Although the function of this new form of pantothenic acid is unknown, it may be involved in the transport and/or storage of pantothenic acid.

VI. BIOCHEMICAL FUNCTION

A protein-like enzyme that replaces coenzyme A during the building of the carbon chain in synthesis of fatty acids has been recognized (61). Acyl carrier protein (ACP) was isolated from pigeon-liver fatty acid synthetase and functions as a coenzyme in fatty acid synthesis (62). ACP is a protein with a sulfhydryl group covalently attached to acetyl, malonyl, and intermediate-chain acyl groups. The sulfhydryl group at the binding site of the ACP was identified as a cysteine residue (63). Analysis of ACP revealed the sulfhydryl-containing residue of ACP to be thioethanolamine. ACP contains 1 mole of β-alanine. The discovery of thioethanolamine and β-alanine residues suggested that both ACP and coenzyme A have similar acyl-binding sites. Later identification of 4'-phosphopantotheine as the prosthetic group of acyl carrier protein, bound to ACP through a phosphodiester linkage to a serine residue of ACP, confirmed that ACP and coenzyme A had the same binding site (Fig. 5).

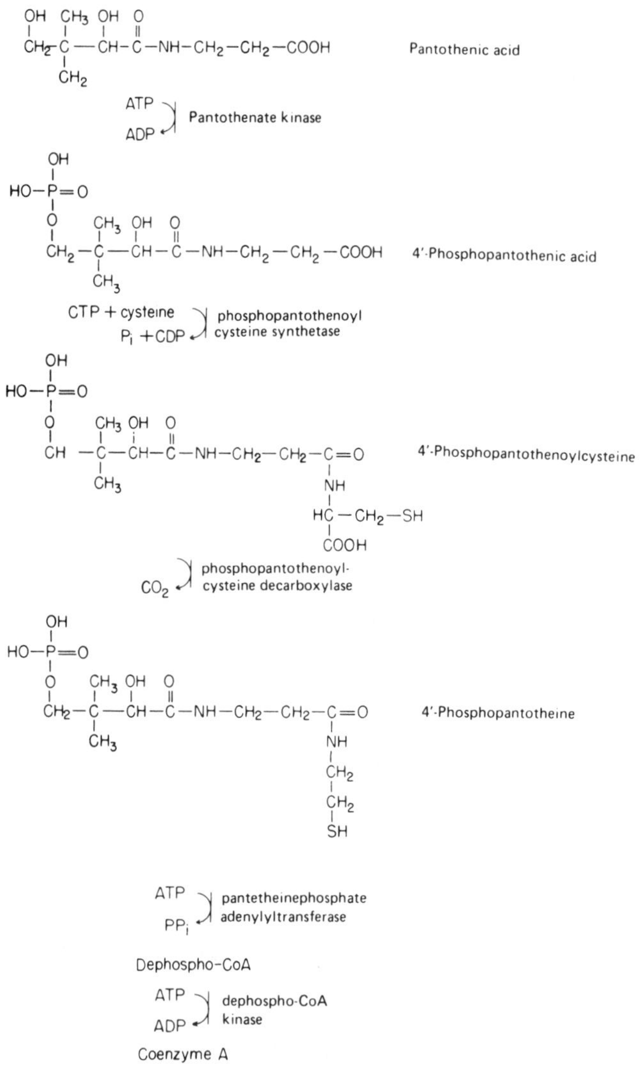

Figure 4 Pathway for conversion of pantothenic acid to coenzyme A. (From Ref. 171.)

The isolation and identification of 4'-phosphopantothenic acid and 4'-phosphopantotheine by its enzymatic conversion to coenzyme A further established this structure to be the same as 4'-phosphopantotheine in coenzyme A. This may account for the existence of the non–coenzyme A, protein-bound pantothenic acid content of the cell (62). One study reported the highest percentage of pantothenic acid was bound in tissue as coenzyme A, followed next by 4'-phosphopantotheine (possibly ACP), with small amounts of free pantothenic acid remaining (64). Examination of the organs of rats revealed that, next to the liver, the adrenal gland contained the highest concentration of the coenzyme, suggesting a close relationship between pantothenic acid level and adrenal cortex function (55). Coenzyme A tissue concentrations were maintained at normal levels in rats fed a pantothenic acid–deficient diet even though growth was depressed and pantothenic acid content of

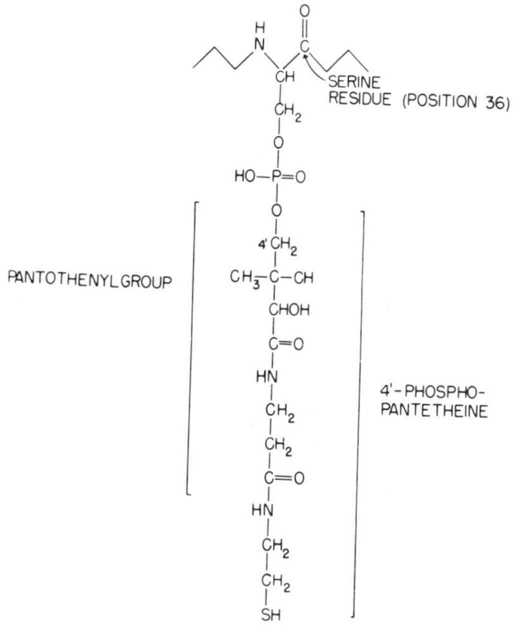

Figure 5 Binding site for coenzyme A and acetyl carrier protein. (From Ref. 63.)

heart, kidney, gastrocnemius, and testes was reduced more than 90%, and that of liver, 70% (65).

A correlation apparently exists between the amount of coenzyme A present in the liver and its ability to synthesize lipids. This relationship was demonstrated when liver slices from pantothenic acid–deficient rats and control rats were analyzed for labeled cholesterol and fatty acids. As the level of coenzyme A decreased in the liver, lipid synthesis decreased, suggesting that the coenzyme A level present in the liver is a limiting factor for the manufacture of fatty acids and steroids (54). In liver slices from deficient and sufficient rats, Carter and Hockaday (66) observed that pantothenic acid–deficient livers took up significantly less oxygen and produced significantly fewer ketone bodies when octanoate was added. Decrease in total body fat and ^{14}C acetate incorporation into body fat accompanied a reduction in hepatic coenzyme A and acetyl coenzyme A in chicks fed a diet deficient in pantothenic acid for 4 weeks (67).

Coenzyme A concentration of livers of rats fed a balanced diet or a pantothenic acid–deficient diet increased in response to clofibrate, a hypolipidemic acid, suggesting that the body attempts to compensate for a reduction of lipid levels by garnering its lipid-synthesizing metabolites (68). Environmental temperature has also been shown to influence coenzyme A synthesis. Exposure to a temperature of 6 °C increased the incorporation of labeled and total pantothenic acid into the livers of rats, primarily due to an increase in free coenzyme A (69).

Srinivasan and Belavady (70) found that male rats deprived of pantothenic acid for 6 weeks had lower levels of glycogen, pantothenic acid, coenzyme A, and hexosediphosphatase in the liver. An increased activity of glucose-6-phosphatase and a decreased incorporation of [^{14}C]alanine into blood glucose was reported in pantothenic acid–deficient rats. Mahboob (71) observed less phosphatidylcholine and more lysolecithin in phospholipids from rats deprived of pantothenic acid. Liver content of the coenzyme A precursors, 4'-phosphopantotheine and dephospho coenzyme A, decreased more rapidly and to a greater extent than did coenzyme A in weanling rats fed pantothenic acid–deficient diets (72). The relative stability of the hepatocyte coenzyme A pool was attributed to the cystosol ability to deposit the vitamin in the form of pantothenate–protein complexes.

Pantothenic acid is found in whole blood, plasma, serum, and red blood cells. The majority of the vitamin exists in the red blood cells as coenzyme A (73), and the serum reportedly contains no coenzyme A but does contain free pantothenic acid. Levels of pantothenic acid in the red blood cells are higher than levels of pantothenic acid in the plasma, and also red cells are more affected by dietary pantothenic acid.

In pantothenic acid–deficient rats, serum protein levels were severly depressed, but control animals maintained normal levels (55). The decrease in the level of serum protein may have been due to cellular failure of the liver to secrete newly synthesized proteins (74). Lederer et al. (75) reported that pantothenic acid–deprived rats failed to develop primary serum titers comparable to those in control rats, suggesting an impairment in antibody synthesis.

VII. DEFICIENCY SIGNS

A. Animals

A deficiency of pantothenic acid has been clearly defined in many animals, though the deficiency symptoms vary from species to species. Pantothenic acid deficiency in rats results in achromotrichia, scaly dermatitis, alopecia, and poryphyrin-caked whiskers (76). Kazuko et al. (77) reported that protoporphyrine IX is the compound that accumulates on the whiskers of rats deficient in pantothenic acid. Retardation of growth, adrenal necrosis, and congenital malformations in offspring of pantothenic acid–deficient rats have also been shown (78).

Chicks fed a pantothenic acid–deficient diet developed lesions at the corners of the mouth, swollen eyelids, hemorrhagic cracks on the feet, and listlessness (79). Other deficiency symptoms include retarded growth, poor feathering and hatchability, paralysis, fatty degeneration of the liver, and lymphoid cell necrosis in the thymus (80). Pantothenic acid deficiency adversely affected reproductive capacity of white Leghorn cockerols (81). Feeding a diet deficient in pantothenic acid resulted in 100% mortality of young Embden geese (82).

Dogs developed fatty livers, mottled thymus with pigmented spots, convulsions, nervous symptoms, and gastrointestinal tract disorders (83). Pigs fed a diet deficient in pantothenic acid grew slowly and developed a "goose-stepping" gate (84). Female hogs fed low pantothenic acid diets developed fatty livers, enlarged adrenal glands, intramuscular hemorrhage, dilation of the heart, diminution of the ovaries, and improper development of the uterus (85). Reproduction was adversely affected in female mink fed inadequate pantothenic acid resulting in a lower congestion rate (86) and reduced litter size (87).

Channel catfish fingerlings deprived of pantothenic acid developed gill lesions (88), anorexia, clubbed gills, anemia, eroded skins, and also experienced weight loss and a high mortality rate (89).

B. Humans

In humans, deficiencies of pantothenic acid have not been observed except in cases of severe malnutrition (10). A deficiency of the vitamin was reported to cause "burning feet syndrome" during World War II among prisoners in Japan and the Philippines (90). Symptoms included abnormal skin sensations of the feet and lower legs, which were increased by warmth and lessened by cold. Administration of large doses of calcium pantothenate improved the ability of the subjects to withstand stress (91).

A pantothenic acid deficiency has been observed in humans fed a pantothenic acid–deficient diet and the antagonist ω-methylpantothenic acid (92–93). The subjects developed a burning sensation in the feet, vomiting, depression, fatigue, insomnia, tenderness in the heels, and muscular weakness. In addition there was a reported change in glucose tolerance, a decrease in eosinopenic response to ACTH, increased sensitivity to insulin and loss of antibody production (10). Administration of large doses of pantothenic acid reversed the symptoms. A more recent study reported subjects fed an unsupplemented diet during a 9-week observation period appeared listless and complained of fatigue. However, no signs of clinical symptoms of pantothenic acid deficiency were observed (94).

VIII. STUDIES OF URINARY EXCRETION

In an effort to measure the metabolic responses of adult humans receiving varying amounts of pantothenic acid, Fox and Linkswiler (39) examined the intake of pantothenic acid in relationship to urinary excretions of women on controlled diets providing 2.8, 7.8, and 12.8 mg of pantothenic acid daily. Pantothenic acid excretion responded to changes in intake. Urinary pantothenic acid levels for women on the low pantothenic acid diet, 2.8 mg daily, exceeded the intake level, suggesting that either the body stores were being lost or synthesis was occurring. Raising the pantothenic acid intake level to 7.8–12.8 mg daily resulted in an increase in urinary pantothenic acid; however, at this dietary level excretion never exceeded intake. In comparing these results with the pantothenic acid intake of subjects on self-selected diets (6.7 mg/day), a daily intake of 7–8 mg was suggested for tissue maintenance. In the same laboratory, human adult subjects fed a low pantothenic acid diet and the same diet supplemented with 10 mg pantothenic acid were studied by Fry et al. (94). Mean daily urinary pantothenic acid excretion levels fell from approximately 3 to 0.8 mg in six male subjects fed the unsupplemented pantothenic acid diet for 63 days and increased from approximately 4 to 5.8 mg in four subjects fed the diet supplemented with 10 mg over the same time period. In two recent studies, urinary pantothenic acid excretion has been reported in relation to intake. Mean excretion increased from 2.3 to 3.9 mg daily as intake was raised from 5 to 10 mg (95). Higher excretions, 9.7 and 36.2 mg, were reported on 17 and 117 mg intakes, respectively (41,96). That the body conserves pantothenic acid was demonstrated by Karnitz et al. (97). Using isolated perfused rat kidneys, they found that at normal physiological plasma concentrations, pantothenic acid filtered by the kidney tubules were actively reabsorbed; only at high plasma levels was pantothenic acid secreted by the tubules.

Pregnant teenagers may require more pantothenic acid than adult pregnant women. A clinical study (98) of a small group of pregnant, nonpregnant, and postpartum teenage girls indicated from urinary excretion and dietary records that inadequate amounts of pantothenic acid were being consumed. The mean calculated intake of pantothenic acid was 4.7 mg/day. Urinary excretion of the vitamin was reported lower than the normal range.

Few studies have reported pathothenic acid excretion levels of preadolescent and adolescent children. Pace et al. (99) studied the dietary intake of pantothenic acid of children aged 7–9 years. Urinary excretions averaged 2.85/mg/day for 11 girls. Kerrey et al. (100) determined the nutritional status of preschool children from different socioeconomic backgrounds and reported higher urinary excretions for the higher than for the lower socioeconomic group. Kathman (40) reported a mean urinary pantothenic acid excretion of adolescents consuming self-selected diets of 5.5 mg/day with a range of 4.02–7.93/mg/day. Eissenstat et al. (101) reported that dietary intake of pantothenic acid of 63 adolescents was highly correlated with urinary excretion.

Hotzel et al. (102) examined 164 young humans and found urinary excretion ranged from 0.5 to 2.0 mg/day. Pantothenic acid excretions of elderly institutionalized and non-institutionalized males and females were reported by Srinivasan et al. (103). Pantothenic acid excretion of institutionalized subjects was 7.5 mg/g creatinine and of noninstitutionalized 5.0 mg/g creatinine. Excretion was higher for persons taking pantothenic acid supplements. The average pantothenic acid intake of these subjects was 5.9 mg/day.

Like urine, the pantothenic acid content of human milk reflects the pantothenic acid content of the diet. Johnson et al. (104) reported a correlation of 0.62 between dietary pantothenic acid and milk content. Song et al. (105) also reported that the vitamin content of milk from mothers who delivered at term was significantly correlated with circulating pantothenic acid and with dietary intake and urinary excretion of the mothers. These workers reported pantothenate content of preterm milk was significantly higher than that of term milk and no change in content with the progress of nursing in either group. Two other groups of investigators (106,107) reported that pantothenic acid content increased progressively over several weeks after parturition and no differences between the content of preterm and term milk.

IX. STUDIES OF BLOOD LEVELS

Free and total (free and bound) pantothenic acid content of whole blood and serum has been reported (Table 2). Total pantothenic acid blood levels below 100 μg/dl may be indicative of low levels of pantothenic acid in the diet (108). The total pantothenic acid content of whole blood for men of different age groups ranged from 94.0 to 117.4 μg/dl, and for women, from 87.1 to 109.6 μg/dl (109). The concentration of free pantothenic acid reported in pregnant, postpartum, and nonpregnant subjects was 8, 8, and 6 μg/dl blood, respectively (98). Total blood pantothenic acid values for the same groups were 103, 112, and 183 μg/dl blood. Ishiguro et al. (109) reported similar blood pantothenic acid values for pregnant women. Srinivasan and Belavady (70) indicated that the concentration of pantothenic acid in the blood of pregnant adult women was not significantly different from nonpregnant controls, but the concentration in infant cord blood was significantly higher than in maternal blood.

Total pantothenic acid levels in serum of adolescent subjects on self-selected diets have been reported (40); mean serum pantothenic acid for the adolescent group was 26.1 μg/dl. Pantothenic acid intake and serum pantothenic acid levels were correlated for adolescents. In the same laboratory, no correlation was found between intake and serum levels, 21.1 μg/dl, for adults on self-selected diets. Eissenstat et al. reported higher blood levels for adolescent females, 41.2 μg/dl. and males, 34.5 μg/dl, even though 49% of the females and 15% of the males consumed less than 4 mg/day of pantothenic acid (101). Serum pantothenic acid appears to be less sensitive to dietary pantothenic acid than

Table 2 Blood Pantothenic Values

Subjects	Pantothenic acid intake (mg/day)	Whole blood (μg/dl)		Serum (μg/dl)		Reference
		Free	Total	Free	Total	
5 Nonpregnant girls	3.3	6.0	112.0	—	—	98
14 Postpartum girls	4.1	8.0	183.00	—	—	98
17 Pregnant girls	4.7	8.0	103.00	—	—	98
11 Adolescents	5.5	—	—	—	26.1	40
Adolescent females		—	41.2	—	—	101
Adolescent males		—	34.5	—	—	101
23 Adults	5.4	—	—	—	21.1	40
12–24 Adults	4.7–30	—	—	8.2	—	110
2 Villagers (washed rice)		—	—	12.7	—	110
3 Villagers (wheat, flour, rice, potatoes)		—	—	15.7	—	110
Adult males	—	—	—	—	94.0–117.4	109
Adult females	—	—	—	—	87.1–109.6	109
9 Adult males	6.91	—	196.0	—	—	94
3 Adult males	—	—	—	—	—	95
5 Adult females	4.8	—	—	—	21.9	95
8 Adult females	9.8	—	—	—	23.4	95
65 Noninstitutionalized men and women over 65			53.7			103
25 Institutionalized men and women over 65			61.5			103
9 Adult females	17	—	—	—	26.4	41
8 Adult females	107	—	—	—	45.5	41

urinary excretion but does respond to extreme differences in intake (96). Thus, serum levels of 21.9 and 23.4 μg/dl were reported for subjects fed 5 and 10 mg pantothenic acid, respectively (98), and 26.4 and 45.5 μg/dl for those fed 17 and 107 mg, respectively (41).

Low levels of pantothenic acid in blood may be related to inadequate or low dietary intakes of the vitamin. Koyangi et al. (110) studied the effect of diet on pantothenic acid content of blood serum of villagers in Japan. Mean values in two villages, where rice was the main dietary component, were 8.2 and 12.7 μg/dl serum. In three other villages, where people consumed wheat flour, potatoes, and vegetables along with rice, mean serum values reported were 15.7 and 16.0 μg/dl serum.

Blood pantothenic acid values were determined in elderly subjects by Wyse and Hansen (26). Dietary pantothenic acid values did not correlate with blood values, but when a dietary supplement of pantothenic acid was given, blood pantothenic acid content increased significantly. A more recent study from his laboratory (103) reported mean whole blood pantothenic acid concentrations of 53.7 μg/dl for noninstitutionalized and 61.5 μg/dl for institutionalized persons 65 years or older.

Conenzyme A activity in blood has been determined by the sulfanilamide acetylation tests (111), and this may be a successful method of assessing the nutritional status of pantothenic acid. Elestad et al. (111) reported that, despite normal levels of free and bound pantothenic acid in blood and colonic mucosa, coenzyme A was significantly lower in colonic mucosa from patients with chronic ulcerative colitis.

X. NUTRITIONAL REQUIREMENTS

Due to the wide distribution of pantothenic acid in foods and the lack of conclusive evidence of quantitative need, no daily dietary allowance of the vitamin for humans has been established. Estimates of dietary intakes in the United States of the human adult population range between 5 and 20 mg/day (38). Based on dietary intakes, several researchers have made recommendations for daily intakes. Krehl (112) recommended a daily intake of 10–15 mg pantothenic acid as desirable intake for adults. Pace et al. (99) reported that diets that met the other nutritional needs of children 7–9 years of age contain 4–5 mg pantothenic acid per day. Telegdy-Kovats and Szorady (113) reviewed the literature and suggested an appropriate intake for infants to be 1.7–4.7 mg/day.

The Food and Nutrition Board of the National Research Council (114) proposed in the 1980 Revised Recommended Dietary Allowances a provisional allowance for pantothenic acid of 4–7 mg/day. A provisional allowance is less precise than a recommended intake. Further research is needed to establish the relationship of pantothenic acid intake to urinary excretion and blood pantothenic acid levels to provide suitable measures for evaluating pantothenic acid nutritional status.

XI. FACTORS THAT INFLUENCE VITAMIN STATUS
A. Fat Content of Diet

Pigs fed a pantothenic acid–deficient, high-fat diet failed to gain weight, exhibited a lower feed efficiency ratio, and developed deficiency symptoms more quickly than those fed diets low in fat (115). Feeding a high-fat diet resulted in significantly less liver coenzyme A and lower proportions of phospholipids regardless of pantothenic acid nutrition (116). A reduction in acyl coenzyme A was suggested as the reason for changes in lipid metabolism (117).

Disturbances of cholesterol metabolism are closely linked with impaired fat metabolism in a pantothenic acid deficiency. When fed a diet with 1% added cholesterol, pantothenic acid–deficient animals have higher liver fat and higher serum cholesterol than deficient animals not receiving cholesterol. Nevertheless, liver fat and cholesterol were lower than that found in animals receiving a normal diet with added cholesterol (118).

B. Effect of Dietary Protein

A possible sparing action of protein for pantothenic acid has been reported. Nelson and Evans (119) found that rats deficient in pantothenic acid fed a high-protein diet excreted more pantothenic acid and had accelerated growth and survival rates in comparison with rats fed a low-protein, low-pantothenic acid diet. The superiority of the high-protein diet may be due to the decreased level of dietary carbohydrate, which would presumably require coenzyme A for metabolism. Similar results were observed in rats in an experiment by Tao and Fox (120). Three levels of protein and three levels of panthothenic acid were administered. Significant growth improvements and an increase in pantothenic acid excretion occurred with increasing protein levels when the diet contained low or medium levels of pantothenic acid. A decrease in the urinary excretion level of pantothenic acid was found in rats fed the high–pantothenic acid diet. High levels of protein in the diet may promote better utilization of the vitamin in synthesis of coenzyme A. This sparing action of protein on pantothenic acid was also seen in pigs. Luecke et al. (121) fed pigs a low-protein diet and observed a significant improvement in growth rate when pantothenic acid was added to the diet. In comparison, growth rates of pigs on a high-protein diet were not significantly improved when additional amounts of pantothenic acid were added to the diet.

The nitrogen balance of adult men and women fed controlled diets providing limited amounts of protein (4.5, 5.5, or 6.5 g nitrogen daily) was affected by the addition of niacin or pantothenic acid supplements to the diet. Nitrogen retention increased with increased nitrogen intake. Nitrogen loss tended to decrease with the niacin supplements. Pantothenic acid had an adverse effect when added to the 4.5 g nitrogen diet but a positive effect when added to the 6.5 g nitrogen diet (122). Protein nutrition of six dry breakfast cereals for rats was also shown to be influenced by the niacin and pantothenic acid contents of the diet (123).

It has been suggested that the influence of protein on pantothenic acid metabolism is due to its methionine content. Increasing the level of methionine in the diet of rats deficient in pantothenic acid increased lymphotic production, growth, and survival. Methionine may induce a more efficient conversion of pantothenic acid to coenzyme A. Coenzyme A levels were lowered in pantothenic acid–, methionine-deprived rats (124).

C. Interrelationship with Other Vitamins

A sparing effect of vitamin B_{12} on pantothenic acid has been suggested (125). The pantothenic acid requirement for growth, survival, and prevention of dermatitis in chicks was estimated as 2 mg per 100 g diet when a vitamin B_{12}–deficient diet was fed. Addition of B_{12} to the diet decreased the free pantothenic acid level in the liver, indicating that vitamin B_{12} may aid in the conversion of free pantothenic acid into coenzyme A. Conversely, in rats deprived of vitamin B_{12} and fed levels of pantothenic acid, the level of vitamin B_{12} in the liver decreased (126). When large doses of vitamin B_{12} were administered to pantothenic acid–deficient rats, survival rates increased, indicating a sparing effect on pantothenic acid. Attempts to elucidate the mechanism of pantothenic acid–B_{12} interaction indicate that B_{12} reduces disulfide bonds (S—S) to the sulfhydryl (SH) state, the active part of the coenzyme A molecule. Therefore, in the absence of vitamin B_{12} coenzyme A production is decreased and fat metabolism impaired (126). Human subjects excreted less pantothenic acid when vitamin B_{12} and pantothenic acid were supplemented in the diet than when pantothenic acid alone was added (127).

1. Ascorbic Acid

Pantothenic acid may be necessary for efficient utilization of ascorbic acid. Decreased levels of ascorbic acid in blood serum were reported in guinea pigs fed ω-methylpantothenic acid (128).

Large amounts of ascorbic acid have been shown to delay the onset of pantothenic acid deficiency. Rats fed pantothenic acid–deficient diets supplemented with either ascorbic acid or pantothenic acid experienced improved reproductive performance in comparison to those fed control diets (129). One indication of improved performance was higher birth weight for animals fed ascorbic acid or pantothenic acid supplements. In addition, ascorbic acid lessened the severity of pantothenic acid deficiency symptoms. Barboriak and Krehl (130) found that ascorbic acid improved weight gains and suppressed deficiency in rats fed a pantothenic acid–deficient diet.

Ascorbic acid or pantothenic acid each inhibited the hemolysis of isolated red blood cells caused by photosensitive-inducing substances, but only a combination of ascorbic acid and pantothenic acid was effective in increasing the survival time of intact male mice given hemotoporphyrin, photosensitive inducing agent (131).

2. Biotin and Folic Acid, Vitamin B_6 and Niacin

Biotin and folic acid were found necessary for pantothenic acid utilization by the rat (132). Excretion of other vitamins has been reported to increase both under conditions of pantothenic acid deficiency and pantothenic acid excess. Thus, urinary B excretion of weanling mice and rats fed a pantothenic acid–deficient diet increased (133) as did the urinary niacin excretion of adolescent boys and girls fed a 100 mg per day pantothenic acid supplement (134).

3. Vitamin A

Vitamin A has been reported to influence the pantothenic acid status of early weaned pigs (135). Free pantothenic acid content of pig livers declined progressively as amount of vitamin A supplement increased (135).

D. Interrelationship with Minerals

Latymer and others reported that high levels of copper supplementation increased the pantothenic acid requirements of chicks (136) and pigs (137,138). Severe signs of pantothenic acid deficiency and reduced levels of liver coenzyme A occurred in copper-supplemented chicks fed marginal or low levels of pantothenic acid. Copper supplementation, while not producing symptoms of pantothenic acid deficiency, reduced weight gain and feed intake of pigs fed whitefish meal but not of pigs fed soybean meal. Livers of pig fed soybean meal had higher levels of both free and bound pantothenic acid compared to those fed whitefish meal. When maize oil was added to the diets, copper supplementation reduced weight gain and feed intake of pigs fed soybean meal as well as those fed whitefish meal, presumably because some pantothenic acid destruction occurred in the presence of maize oil (138).

E. Groups at Greatest Risk of Deficiency

Nutritional deficiencies associated with alcoholism are often attributed to dietary inadequacies of protein and the water-soluble vitamins, particularly the B-complex vitamins. Ethanol causes a decrease in the amount of pantothenic acid in tissues, resulting in an increase in serum levels of pantothenic acid (139). Tao and Fox (140) suggested that pantothenic acid utilization is impaired in cases of alcoholism. Increasing dietary pantothenic acid led initially to increased levels of urinary pantothenic acid in patients fed balanced diets. The urinary pantothenic acid level, however, decreased as nutrients were replenished in the tissues of the patients. These results were confirmed by Moiseenok et al. (141), who reported that pantothenic acid excretion of alcoholic patients was increased in comparison with controls following administration of 200 mg of pantothenic acid by mouth of muscle. These investigators also found that the level of coenzyme A and metabolites of pantothenate increased within 24 hours in the leukocytes of both alcoholic and healthy persons given 100 mg pantothenate or 126 mg pantotheine (142). Pantotheine was more effective than pantothenic acid in inducing this change, presumably because fewer steps are required for conversion to coenzyme A. In the same laboratory coenzyme A activity of liver was found to decrease markedly when rats were given rations providing 5–15% of ethanol for 8 months (143). Another group that may experience an increased need for pantothenic acid are oral contraceptive users. Blood and urinary pantothenic acid levels were lower for contraceptive users than nonusers consuming self-selected diets containing about 5 mg pantothenic acid, but no difference was observed between the two groups after a period of time when they both received a 10 mg supplement (144). The authors, however, interpreted the findings as indicating no difference between oral contraceptive users and nonusers in utilization of pantothenic acid when intake and period of menstrual cycle were equalized.

1. Diabetes

Pantothenic acid deficiency in humans has been found to lead to lowered blood sugar levels and an increased sensitivity to insulin (145). Hypoglycemia induced by mice by exposure of high temperature and humidity was improved by pantothenic acid and other substances that affect adrenal function (146). Urinary pantothenic acid excretion is high in patients with diabetes mellitus and in alloxan-diabetic rats (147). In an earlier study, Mookeryia and Sadhur (148) found that alloxan-diabetic rats receiving excess pantothenate excreted less acetoacetate than the diabetic group receiving no pantothenate. Further evidence of altered pantothenic acid metabolissm was obtained in alloxan-diabetic rats who had increased levels of pantothenic acid in heart, kidneys, brain, and pancreas and decreased levels in muscles (149).

In a recent study, diabetes and food deprivation were found to increase pantothenic acid intake, decrease muscle concentration, and increase liver concentration in rats, suggesting hormonal control of pantothenic acid metabolism (150). Urinary pantothenic acid decreased under these conditions, further indicating a regulatory mechanism to conserve pantothenic acid. Further study by the same group of investigators (151) indicated that coenzyme A levels were elevated in hearts from diabetic and fasting animals. Insulin strongly inhibited, in vitro, pantothenate kinase, the enzyme involved in the first step in the pathway of coenzyme synthesis, suggesting that the increased coenzyme A in diabetic and fasting animals results from the decreased circulating level of insulin.

2. Adrenal Function

The effects of pantothenic acid deficiency on acetylation capacity and corticosterone biosynthesis have been studied. In rats fed a diet deficient in pantothenic acid, corticosterone output by the adrenals was lower than for pair-fed rats receiving 10 mg pantothenic acid per 100 g diet (152). The reduction in output of corticosterone in rats fed the deficient diet was reversed by injection of pantothenic acid. Large doses of adrenocorticotropic hormone prevented the deleterious effects of ω-methylpantothenic acid.

ω-Methylpantothenic acid may interfere with the formation of coenzyme A and thus have a pharmacological action in the destruction of normal adrenal tissue. Pietrzik et al. (153) noted rats fed the antagonist ω-methylpantothenic acid showed reduced acetylation capacity. Fidanza et al. (154) reported that concentrations of cortisone, corticosteroned, and deoxycorticosterone increased in male rat adrenal glands in response to intramuscular injections of large doses of sodium pantothenate.

3. Digestive Function

Conditions in the digestive tract may alter the need for pantothenic acid. Adolescent boys and girls fed 10 or 20 g of either cellulose or hemicellulose had lower levels of serum pantothenic acid than when a similar diet was fed without fiber supplements (155). The intestinal flora may also influence the utilization of pantothenic acid. Urinary pantothenic acid increased in 12 older humans who consumed alternately 24 oz plain milk or sweet acidophilus milk for 28 days. The higher excretion due to the higher intake was greater for plain milk than the fermented product, suggesting that some of the vitamin may have been used by the microorganisms (156). Latymer and Coates (157) reported that microorganisms present in the digestive tract may increase the need for pantothenic acid. More pantothenic acid was required by conventional than by germ-free chicks to achieve the same body weight and freedom from signs of deficiency. Patients with chronic ulcerative or granulomatous colitis are likely to develop a deficiency of pantothenic acid. The activity of coenzyme A in colonic mucosa in 20 patients was estimated by the acetylation of sulfanilamide (158). Compared to normal activity in mucosa, coenzyme A activity was low in patients with chronic ulcerative or granulomatous colitis. The authors indicated that the conversion of free to bound pantothenic acid is blocked in conditions of diseased mucosa. In a study of Moiseenok and Nenesova (159), patients with ulcers excreted less bound and free pantothenic acid than normal control subjects, suggesting a deficiency of the vitamin in ulcer patients. The addition of pantothenic acid to the diet of the ulcer patients corrected this clinical condition.

Shibata et al. (160) reported that coenzyme A is hydrolyzed to pantetheine and pantothenate in the intestinal lumen and is absorbed by simple diffusion into the blood. In sheep absorption was shown to be proportional to the amount of pantothenic acid present in the small intestine also suggesting a passive mechanism (161). At low concentrations of pantothenic acid, absorption against a concentration gradient may occur as was demonstrated by Fenstermacher and Rose (162) in rat and chick intestines, a process they describe as sodium-dependent, secondary active transport.

XII. SAFETY

Although pantothenic acid toxicity has not been reported in humans, Unna and Gleslin (163) found calcium pantothenate acutely toxic for mice and rats. The LD_{50} dose in milligrams per kilogram body weight has been reported as 10.0, 2.7, 0.92, and 0.91 for mice and greater than 10.0, 3.4, 0.82, and 0.83 for rats fed calcium pantothenate.

XIII. EFFICACY OF PHARMACOLOGICAL DOSES

Pantothenic acid reportedly shows no pharmacological effects when administered to laboratory animals or humans. Dexpanthenol, the alcohol synthetically derived from D-pantothenic acid, has been given in large parenteral doses (250–500 mg) to adults and reported to increase gastrointestinal peristalsis by stimulating acetylation of choline to acetylcholine (164); however, the effectiveness of dexpanthenol has not been established. The alcohol has also been applied topically to alleviate itching and improve minor skin irritations. Again, the clinical significance of the drug has not been proven. Recent work suggests that pantothenic acid may accelerate wound healing in rabbits by increasing the fibroblast content of scar tissue (165,166). The effectiveness of pantothenic acid in prevention and treatment of arthritis has been evaluated both in experimental and clinical studies. Thus, pantothenate and some of its derivatives decreased swelling intensity of joints in experimental animals given 30 mg/kg prior to induction of the arthritis, but no effect was seen when pantothenic acid was given during the developmental stage of the disease (167). In a clinical trial large doses of calcium pantothenate (at least 500 mg/day) for 8 weeks showed no benefit over placebo treatment on the course of development of rheumatoid arthritis but the vitamin treatment was effective in reducing the duration of morning stiffness, degree of disability, and severity of pain (168). Although pantothenic acid has been prescribed for streptomycin therapy, neurotoxicity, salicylate toxicity, gray hair, alopecia, catarrhal respiratory disorders, osteoarthritis, diabetic neuropathy, and psychiatric states and as a counteractive agent against thyroid therapy in cretins, it has not been proven to have any of these therapeutic uses.

A reported beneficial effect of pantothenic acid with possible therapeutic implications is a protective effect against radiation sickness (169). Adult male rats were fed milk and either raw or boiled eggs, with or without pantothenic acid supplements, before and after irradiation. A survival rate of 75% in rats not given pantothenic acid was decreased somewhat when raw eggs were given but increased to about 86% when boiled eggs were fed.

REFERENCES

1. R. J. Williams, C. M. Lyman, G. H. Goodyear, J. H. Truesdail, and D. Holiday, *J. Am. Chem. Soc., 55*:2912 (1933).
2. E. E. Snell, F. M. Strong, and W. H. Peterson, *J. Am. Chem. Soc., 60*:6825 (1938).
3. T. H. Jukes, *J. Am. Chem. Soc., 61*:975 (1939).
4. D. H. Woolley, H. A. Waisman, and C. A. Elvehjem, *J. Biol. Chem., 129*:673 (1939).
5. R. J. Williams and R. T. Major, *Science, 91*:246 (1940).
6. Nomenclature Policy, *J. Nutr.,* 109 (1979).
7. J. Marks, in *The Vitamins in Health and Disease*, Churchill, London, 1968.
8. W. H. Peterson and M. S. Peterson, *Bacteriol. Rev., 9*:49 (1945).
9. H. R. Rosenberg, in *Chemistry and Physiology of the Vitamins*, Interscience, New York, 1945.
10. R. E. Hodges, M. A. Ohlson, and W. B. Bean, *J. Clin. Invest., 37*:1642 (1958).
11. H. McIlwain, *Biochem. J.,* 36–417 (1942).
12. D. W. Woolley and M. L. Collyer, *J. Biol. Chem.,* 159–263 (1945).
13. Y. Nishizawa and F. Matsuzaki, *J. Vitamin., 15*:8 (1969).

14. F. E. Staten, P. A. Anderson, D. H. Baker, and P. C. Harrison, *Poultry Sci.*, *59*:1664 (1980).
15. S. Kimura, Y. Furukawa, J. Waksasuzi, Y. Ishihara,, and A. Nakayana, *J. Nutr. Sci. Vitaminol.*, *26*:113 (1980).
16. Y. Furukawa, M. Saijo, K. Tani, and S. Kimura, *Tohuku J. Agr. Res.*, *36*(3/4):155 (1986).
17. D. R. Sargent, G. C. Clifton, S. R. Bryant, and C. G. Skinner, *Texas Rep. Biol. Med.*, *33*(3):433 (1976).
18. D. Pennington and R. J. Williams, *J. Biol. Chem.*, *135*:213 (1940).
19. F. M. Strong, R. E. Truney, and A. Earle, *Ind. Eng. Chem. Anal.*, *13*:566 (1941).
20. R. S. Goodhart and M. E. Shils, *Modern Nutrition in Health and Disease Dietotherapy*, 5th Ed., Lea and Febiger, Philadelphia, 1973, pp. 302–309.
21. O. Solberg, I. K. Hegna, and O. G. Clausen, *J. Appl. Bacteriol.* *39*:119 (1975).
22. T. H. Jukes, *J. Nutr.*, *21*:193 (1941).
23. E. A. Latymer and M. E. Coates, *Brit. J. Nutr.*, *47*:131 (1982).
24. R. S. Yalow and S. A. Berson, in *Principles of Competitive Protein Binding Assays*, Odell & Daughaday (Eds.), J. P. Lippincott, Philadelphia, 19781, p. 1.
25. J. C. Travis, in *Fundamentals of RIA and Other Ligand Assays, A Programmed Test*, Radioassay Publishers, Division of Scientific Newsletters, Inc., 1979.
26. B. W. Wyse and R. G. Hansen, *Fed Proc.*, *36*:1169 (1977).
27. M. N. Voight and R. R. Eitenmiller, *J. Food Sci.*, *44*:1780 (1979).
28. E. Tesmer, J. Leinert and D. Hotzel, *Nahrung*, *24*:697 (1980).
29. J. Davidek, J. Velisek, J. Cerna, and R. Davidek, *J. Micronutrient Anal.*, *1*:39 (1985).
30. A. Prosser and A. J. Sheppard, *J. Pharm. Sci.*, *58*:718 (1969).
31. R. Crokaert, *Bull. Soc. Chem. Biol.*, *31*:903 (1949).
32. R. B. Roy and A. Buccafuri, *J. Assoc. Off. Anal. Chem.*, *61*(3):720 (1978).
33. M. L. Orr, Home Econ. Res. Div., Agric. Res. Serv., USDA, Washington, D. C., 1969.
34. E. G. Zook, M. J. MacArthur, and E. W. Toepfer, USDA Handbook No. 97, U.S. Government Printing Office, Washington, D. C. 1956.
35. J. H. Walsh, B. W. Wyse, and R. G. Hansen, *J. Am. Diet. Assoc.*, *78*:140 (1981).
36. M. E. Sanchez Peinado, N. Sanchez Garcia, and M. R. Pascual Anderson, *Vol. Centro Nacional Alim. Nutr.*, *3/4*:5 (1981).
37. V. H. Cheldelin and R. R. Williams, *J. Nutr.*, *26*:417 (1943).
38. A. S. M. Chung, W. N. Pearson, W. J. Darby, O. N. Miller, and G. A. Goldsmith, *Am. J. Clin. Nutr.*, *9*:573 (1961).
39. H. M. Fox and H. Linkswiler, *J. Nutr.*, *75*:451 (1961).
40. J. V. Kathman and C. Kies, *Nutr. Res.*, *4*:245 (1984).
41. M. Lin, M. S. Thesis, University of Nebraska, Lincoln, Nebraska, 1981.
42. J. B. Tarr, T. Tamura, and E L. R. Stokstad, *Am. J. Clin. Nutr.*, *34*:1328 (1981).
43. N. L. Bull and D. H. Buss, *Human Nutr.: Applied Nutr.*, *36a*:190 (1982).
44. A. E. Black, A. A. Paul and C. Hall. *Human Nutr.: Applied Nutr.*, *39*:19 (1985).
45. J. P. Mareshi, F. Cousin, D. De La Villeon, and B. G. Brubacher, *Ann. Nutr. Metab.*, *28*:11 (1984).
46. J. H. Walsh, B. W. Wyse, and R. G. Hansen, *Ann. Nutr. Metab.*, *25*:178 (1981).
47. R. L. Pike and M. O. Brown, *Nutrition: An Integrated Approach*, 2nd Ed., John Wiley and Sons, New York, 1975.
48. E. W. Hellendoorm, A. P. Degrott, L. P. Van Der Myll Dekker, P. Slump, and J. L. Williams, *J. Am. Diet. Assoc.*, *58*:434 (1971).
49. H. A. Schroeder, *Am. J. Clin. Nutr.*, *24*:562 (1971).
50. J. Causret, *Ann. Nutr. Alim.*, *25*:313 (1971).
51. L. L. Southern and D. H. Baker, *J. Anim. Sci.*, *59*:1663 (1981).
52. L. L. Southern and D. H. Baker, *J. Anim. Sci.*, *53*:403 (1981).
53. F. Lipman, N. O. Kaplan, G. O. Novelli, L. C. Tuttle, and B. M. Gruraid, *J. Biol. Chem.*, *167*:869 (1947).

54. H. P. Klein and F. Lipman, *J. Biol. Chem.*, *203*:95 (1953).
55. D. G. Novelli, *Physiol. Rev.*, *33*:523 (1953).
56. Y. Shigeta and M. Shichiri, *J. Vitamin.*, *12*:186 (1966).
57. G. W. E. Plaut, C. M. Smith, and W. L. Alworth, *Annu. Rev.*, *Biochem.*, *43*:899 (1974).
58. J. D. Robishaw, D. Berkich, and J. R. Neely, *J. Biol. Chem.*, *257*:10967 (1982).
59. J. D. Robishaw and J. R. Neely, *Am. J. Physiol.*, *246* (4 Part 2):H 532 (1984).
60. M. Eto and A. Nakagawa, *Inst. Brew* (London), 81:232 (1975).
61. E. L. Pugh and S. J. Wakil, *J. Biol. Chem.*, *240*:4727 (1965).
62. A. A. Qureshi, F. A Lornitzo, and J. W. Porter, *Biochem. Biophys. Res. Commun.*, *60*:158 (1974).
63. P. W. Majerus, A. W. Alberts, and P. R. Vagelos, *J. Biol. Chem.*, 240–4723 (1965).
64. F. Sauer, E. L. Pugh, S. J. Wakil, R. Delaney, and R. L. Hill, *Proc. Natl., Acad., Sci. USA*, *52*:1360 (1964).
65. D. K. Reibel, B. W. Wyse, D. A. Berkich, and J. R. Neely, *J. Nutr.*, *112*:1144 (1982).
66. C. W. Carter and T. D. R. Hockaday, *Biochem. J.*, *84*:275 (1962).
67. M. A. Cupo and W. E. Donaldson, *Nutr. Rep. Int.*, *33*:147 (1986).
68. V. M. Sheibak and A. G. Moiseenok, *Khim-Farm ZH*, *17*:778 (1983).
69. M. Tsujikawa and S. Kimura, *Tohuku J. Exper. Med.*, *133*:457 (1981).
70. V. Srinivasan and B. Belavady, *Indian J. Biochem. Biophys.*, *13*:387 (1976).
71. S. Mahboob, *Nutr. Metab.*, *19*:91 (1975).
72. A. G. Moiseenok, W. M. Sheibak, and V. A. Gurinovich, *Int. J. Vitamin Nutr. Res.*, *57*:71 (1987).
73. M. Hatano, *J. Vitamin.*, *8*:134 (1962).
74. A. E. Axelrod, B. B. Carter, R. H. McCoy, and R. Geisinger, *Proc. Soc. Exp. Biol. Med.*, *66*:137 (1947).
75. H. Lederer, M. Kumar, and A. E. Axelrod, *J. Nutr.*, *105*:107 (1975).
76. L. M. Henderson, J. M. McIntire, H. A. Waisman, and C. A. Elvehjem, J. Nutr., 23:47 (1942).
77. E. Kazuko, N. Kubato, T. Nishigaki, and M. Kikutani, *Chem. Pharm Bull.*, *23*:1 (1975).
78. M. M. Nelson, F. Van Nouheys, and H. M. Evans, *J. Nutr.*, *34*:189 (1947).
79. D. M. Hegsted, J. J. Oelson, R. C. Mills, C. A. Elvehjem, and E. B. Hart, *J. Nutr.*, 20–599 (1940).
80. C. L. Gries and M. L. Scott, *J. Nutr.*, *102*:1269 (1972).
81. M. P. Goeger and G. H. Arscott, *Nutr. Rep. Int.*, *30*:1193 (1984).
82. J. A. Serafin, *Poultry Sci.*, *60*:1910 (1981).
83. A. E. Schaefer, J. M. McKubbin, and C. A. Elvehjem, *J. Biol. Chem.*, *143*:321 (1942).
84. E. H. Hughs, *J. Agric. Res.*, *64*:185 (1942).
85. D. E. Ullrey, D. E. Becker, S. W. Terrill, and R. A. Notzold, *J. Nutr.*, *9*:573 (1961).
86. M. Skrivan, L. Stolc, J. Plistilova and J. Plistil, *Biol. a Chem. Zivocisne Vyroby-Veterinaria*, *15*:213 (1979).
87. M. Skrivan, L. Stolc and K. Vorisek, *Biol. a Chem. Zivocisne Vyroby-Veterinaria*, *15*:207 (1979).
88. R. P. Wilson and P. R. Bowser, *J. Nutr. 113*:2124 (1983).
89. T. Murai and J. W. Andrews, *J. Nutr.*, *109*:1140 (1979).
90. M. Glusman, *Am. J. Med.*, *3*:211 (1947).
91. E. P., Ralli, in *Nutrition Under Climatic Stress*, Symposium Advisory Board on Quartermaster Research and Development, Committee on Foods, NAS-NRC, Washington, D. C., 1954.
92. W. B. Bean and R. E. Hodges, *Proc. Soc. Exp. Biol. Med.*, *86*:693 (1954).
93. R. Lubin, K. A. Daum, and W. B. Bean, *Am. J. Clin. Nutr.*, *4*:420.
94. P. C. Fry, H. M. Fox, and H. G. Tao, *J. Nutr. Sci. Vitamino.*, *22*:339 (1976).
95. Z. Foss, M.S. Thesis, University of Nebraska, Lincoln, Nebraska, 1981.

96. C. Kies, C. Wishart, M. McGee, Z. Foss, L. C. Yang, J. Quillian, and H. M. Fox, *Fed. Proc., 41*(3):276 (1982).

97. L. M. Karmitz, C. J. Gross and L. M. Henderson, *Biochem. Biophys. Acta., 769*:486 (1984).

98. S. H. Cohenour and D. H. Calloway, *Am. J. Clin. Nutr., 25*:512 (1972).

99. J. K. Pace, L. B. Stier, D. D. Taylor and P. S. Goodman, *J. Nutr., 74*:345 (1961).

100. E. Kerrey, S. Crispin, H. M. Fox and C. Kies, *Am. J. Clin. Nutr. 21*:1274 (1968).

101. B. R. Eissenstat, B. W. Wyse and R. G. Hansen, *Am. J. Clin. Nutr., 44*:931 (1986).

102. D. Hotzel, C. Hesse, and K. Pietrzik, in *Proceeding of the X International Congress of Nutrition.*, Vol. 39, 1975.

103. V. Srinivasan, N. Christensen, B. W. Wyse, and R. G. Hansen. *Am. J. Clin. Nutr., 34*:1736 (1981).

104. L. Johnston, L. Vaughan, and H. M. Fox, *Am. J. Clin. Nutr., 34*:2205 (1981).

105. W. O. Song, G. M. Chan, B. W. Wyse, and R. G. *Am. J. Clin. Nutr., 40*:317 (1984).

106. J. E. Ford, A. Zechalko, J. Murphy, and O. G. Brooke, *Arch. Dis. Child, 58*:367 (1983).

107. A. M. Bijur and M. M. Kumbhat, *Ind. Ped., 24*:33 (1987).

108. H. E. Sauberlich and J. H. Skala, *Laboratory Tests for the Assessment of Nutritional Status*, CRC Press, Cleveland, Ohio, 1974, p. 88.

109. K. Ishiguro, S. Kobayashi, and S. Kaneta, *Tohoku J. Exp. Med., 74*:65 (1961).

110. T. Koyangi, S. Hareyama, S. Kikuchi, and T. Kimura, *Tohoku J., Exp. Med., 88*:93 (1966).

111. J. J. Elestad, R A. Nelson, M. A. Adson, and W. M. Palmer, *Fed. Proc., 29*:820 (1970).

112. W. A. Krehl, *Nutr. Rev., II*:225 (1953).

113. M. Telegdy-Kovats and I. Szorady, *Nutr. Abstr. Rev., 38*:449 (1968).

114. Food and Nutrition Board, 1980 Revised Recommended Dietary Allowances, *J. Am. Diet. Assoc., 75*:625 (1979).

115. R. F. Sewell, D. G. Price, and M. C. Thomas, *Fed. Proc.*, 21–468 (1962).

116. M. A. Williams, L. C. Chu, D. J. McIntosh, and I. Hincenbergs, *J. Nutr., 94*:377 (1968).

117. Y. Furukawa and S. Kimura, *J. Vitam., 18*:213 (1972).

118. R. R. Guehring, L. S. Hurley, and A. F. Morgan, *J. Biol. Chem., 197*:485 (1952).

119. M. M. Nelson and H. M. Evans, *Proc. Soc. Exp. Biol. Med., 60*:319 (1945).

120. H. G. Tao and H. M. Fox, *Nutr. Rep. Int., 14*:97 (1976).

121. R. W. Luecke, J. A. Hoefer, and F. Thorp, Jr., *J. Anim. Sci., 11*:138 (1952).

122. B. Unver, C. Kies, and H. M. Fox, *Nutr. Rep. Int., 23*:841 (1981).

123. C. Kies and A. T. H. Chan, *Nutr. Rep. Int., 22*:239 (1980).

124. J. S. Dinning, R. Neatrour, and P. L. Day, *J. Nutr., 56*:431 (1955).

125. H. Yacowitz, L. C. Norris, and G. F. Heuse, *J. Biol. Chem., 192*:141 (1951).

126. K. Okuda, E. B. McCollum, J. M. Hsu, and B. F. Chow, *Proc. Soc. Exp. Biol. Med., 111*:300 (1962).

127. M. Perryman, M.S. Thesis, University of Nebraska, Lincoln, Nebraska, 1977.

128. C. Pudelkewicz and C. Roderuck, *J. Nutr., 70*:348 (1960).

129. G. Everson, L. Northrop, N. Y. Chung, and R. Getty, *J. Nutr., 54*:305 (1954).

130. J. J. Barboriak and W. A. Krehl, *J. Nutr., 63*:601 (1957).

131. S. Kimura and Y. Takahoshi, *J. Nutr. Sci., Vitaminol., 27*:521 (1981).

132. L. D. Wright and A. D. Welch, *Science, 97*:426 (1943).

133. M. T. Huang and C. Kries, *Nutr. Rep. Int., 23*:9 (1981).

134. J. F. Clarke and C. Kies, *Nutr. Rep. Int., 31*:1271 (1985).

135. M. V. Sorokin, *Brokhimii Pitaniya Sel'skohoyaistvennykh Zhivotnykh, 3*:44 (1984).

136. E. A. Latymer and M. E. Coates, *British J. Nutr. 45*:431 (1981).

137. E. A. Latymer, M. E. Coates, R. J. Pittman, J. Thomas, and K. G. Mitchell, *Livest. Prod. Sci., 9*:591 (1982).

138. E. A. Latymer, G. Mitchell, M. E. Coates, H. D. Keol, J. Thomas and S. C. Woodley, *Livest. Prod. Sci., 12*:265 (1985).

139. C. M. Leevy and H. Baker, *Arch. Environ. Health, 7*:453 (1963).

140. H. G. Tao and H. M. Fox, *J. Vitam.*, *22*:333 (1976).
141. A. G. Moiseenok, E. A. Tsverbaum and M. A. Rybaldo, *Voprosy Meditsinshoi Khinmu*, *27*:780 (1981).
142. A. G. Moiseenok, A. A. Tsverbaum, and M. A. Rybalko, *Khim-Farm ZH*, *15*:24 (1981).
143. A. H. Maisyayunak, A. A. Tsverbaum, and M. A. Rybalko, *Vyest Akad. Navuk BSSR. Syer. Biyal Navuk*, *0*(5):68 (1980).
144. C. M. Lewis and J. C. King, *Am. J. Clin. Nutr.*, *33*:382 (1980).
145. W. B. Bean, R. E. Hodges, and K. Daum, *J. Clin. Invest.*, *84*:1973, (1955).
146. T. Kameyama, T. Nabeshima, and H. Nagata, *Res. Commun. Chem. Pathol. Pharmacol.*, *32*:261 (1981).
147. M. Hatano, R. E. Hodges, R. C., Evans, R. F. Hagemann, D. B. Leeper, W. B. Bean, and W. A. Krehl, *Am. J. Clin. Nutr.*, *20*:960 (1967).
148. S. Mookeryia and D. P. Sadhur, *Biochem. J.*, *64*:6 (1956).
149. A. P. Martsinchyk, S. N. Amal'anchykp and A. G. Maisyaenak, *Vest. Akad. Novuk BSSR. Biyal. Novuk*, *3*:80 (1982).
150. D. K. Reibel, B. W. Wyse, D. A. Berkich, W. M. Palko, and J. R. Neely, *Am. J. Physiol.*, *240*(6):E 597 (1981).
151. D. K. Reibel, B. W. Wyse, D. A. Berkich, and J. R. Neely, *Am. J. Physiol.*, *240*(6):H 606 (1981).
152. A. D. Goodman, *Endocrinology*, *66*:420 (1960).
153. K. Pietrzik, C. Hesse, and D. Hotzel, *Int. J. Vitam. Nutr. Res.*, *45*:251 (1975).
154. A. Fidanza, C. Bruno, A. De Cicco, S. Floridi, and L. Martoneli, *Boll. Soc. Ital. Biol. Sper.*, *54*:2248 (1978).
155. S. Trimbo, J. Kathman, C. Kies, and H. M. Fox, *Fed. Proc.*, *38* (31):556 (1979).
156. J. A. Mathison, C. Kies, H. M. Fox, and K. Shahani, *Fed. Proc.*, *38*(3I):556 (1979).
157. E. A. Latymer and M. E. Coates, *Brit. J. Nutr.*, *45*:441 (1981).
158. J. J. Ellestad-Sayed, R. A. Nelson, M. A. Adson, W. M. Palmer, and E. H. Soule, *Am. J. Clin. Nutr.*, *29*:133 (1976).
159. A. G. Moiseenok and N. K. Nenesova, *Vestn. Akad. Nauk, BSSR Biyal. Navuk*, *1*:103 (1976).
160. K. Shibata, C. J. Gross and L. M. Henderson, *J. Nutr.*, *113*:2107 (1983).
161. H. J. Finlayson and R. C. Seeley, *J. Sci. Food Agri.*, *34*:417 (1983).
162. D. K. Fenstermacher and R. C. Rose, *Am. J. Physiol.*, *250*(2 Part 1):6155 (1986).
163. K. Unna and J. C. Greslin, *J. Pharmacol. Exp. Ther.*, *73*:85 (1941).
164. American Society of Hospital Pharmacists, Inc., *88*:8 (1979).
165. J. F. Grenier, M. Aprahamian, C. Genot, and A. Dentinger, *Acta Vita. et Enzy*, *4*:81 (1982).
166. M. Aprahamian, A. Dentinger, C. Stoch-Damge, J. C. Kouassi, and J. F. Grenier, *Am. J. Clin. Nutr.*, *41*:578 (1985).
167. A. G. Moiseenok, V. I. Astrauskas, A. Gurinovich, V. M. Sheibak, P. S. Prom', T. I. Khomick, N. K. Denislovo, V. I. Gunar, and V. M. Kopelvich, *Khim-Farm ZH*, *15*–176 (1981).
168. U. K. General Practitioner Research Group, *Pract.*, *224*:208 (1980).
169. N. D. Egarova and S. R. Perepelkin, *Gig. Santit.*, *10*:24 (1979).
170. A. H. Lehninger, *Biochemistry*, 2nd Ed., Worth Publishers, New York, 1975.

12
Folic Acid

Tom Brody
University of Hawaii at Manoa
Honolulu, Hawaii

The abbreviations used are: PteGlu$_n$, oligo- or poly-γ-L-glutamyl derivatives of folic acid, where n indicates the total number of glutamyl residues; PteGlu, pteroylglutamic acid, folic acid; MTX, methotrexate, amethopterin, 4-desoxy-4-amino-[N-10]methylpteroylglutamic acid; T-synthase, thymidylate synthase; FPGS, folate polyglutamate synthase; AdoMet, S-adenosyl-methionine; 5-FU, 5-fluorouracil.

I. HISTORY

Antianemia factors, animal growth factors, and lactic acid bacteria growth factors were discovered during the 1930s. Liver, yeast, and spinach proved to be good sources of these factors. Because of the relative ease in performing bacterial growth assays, the bacterial growth factors were extensively purified from liver and yeast and crystallized. Eventually it was determined that the various antianemia and growth factors all had a common structure, and they were named *folates*. Folic acid (Fig. 1) was identified and synthesized in 1946 using techniques previously used to study other pteridines, such as butterfly pigments.

How were the biochemical uses of folates first determined? Studies with bacteria revealed that purines or thymine could partly replace the nutritional requirements for folate or for *p*-aminobenzoic acid (PABA). Similarly, the inhibition of bacterial growth by folate analogues could be overcome by adding purines or thymine to the bacterial growth medium.

Studies with [^{14}C]formate and [^{14}C]formaldehyde disclosed the role of folate in transferring 1-carbon units. For example, [^{14}C]formate was incorporated into specific positions of the purine ring in studies of animals. This incorporation could be diminished with folate antagonists. In studies with liver extracts, it was shown that tetrahydrofolate stimulated the incorporation of [^{14}C]formaldehyde into the amino acid serine.

Folate polyglutamates (Fig. 1), discovered at about the same time as folate monoglutamate, was found to be the major intracellular form of the vitamin. The polyglutamate has the "property" of supporting animal growth but not bacterial growth. The monoglutamate supports growth of both. The value of the poly-γ-L-glutamyl chain was not recognized until the 1960s and 1970s, when it was determined that the folate polyglutamates were often the preferred substrates for enzymes and appeared to be more active metabolically in cells and better retained in cells than folate monoglutamates.

During the 1950s two drugs, methotrexate and 5-fluorouracil, were found to be useful in cancer chemotherapy. Both of these drugs are powerful inhibitors of folate-requiring enzymes and are now widely used in medicine.

In 1969, Blakley's book on folic acid and pteridines was published (1). This comprehensive and irreplaceable book is a valuable source of background information and references.

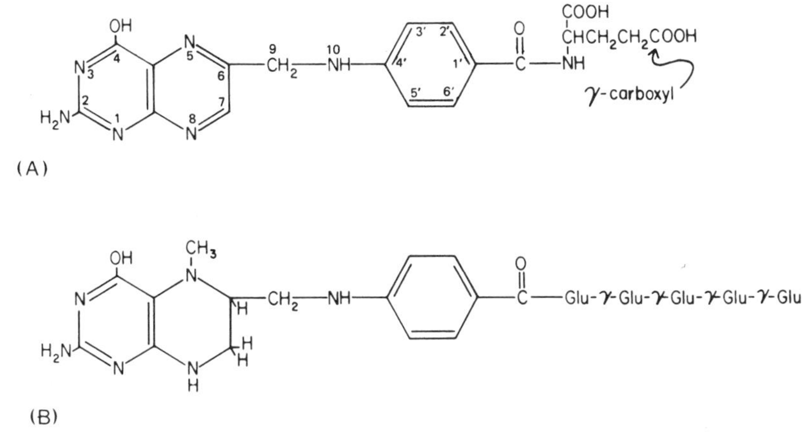

Figure 1 Structure of folic acid and of 5-methyl-tetrahydrofolate pentaglutamate. Although folic acid is not a naturally occurring biochemical, it is readily transported and reduced to the natural forms of the vitamin by animals and by some lactic acid bacteria. 5-Methyl-H$_4$PteGlu$_5$ is the methylated derivative of tetrahydrofolate pentaglutamate.

II. CHEMISTRY

A. Isolation

Folates in natural sources should be extracted and isolated under conditions that preserve the oligo-γ-glutamyl chain and the reductive state of the folate. For maximal recovery of intact folates, the biological sample may be minced, then heated for 5–10 min in a boiling water bath in the presence of antioxidants to denature folate-metabolizing enzymes, such as γ-glutamyl hydrolase, as well as folate-binding proteins. The boiled sample should then be cooled and homogenized (2). Suitable antioxidants for preserving reduced folates are 0.2 M 2-mercaptoethanol or 1.0% sodium ascorbate. One might be cautioned that heating folates in ascorbate alone may alter the folates themselves, though this should not be a problem where sulfhydryl agents are also present (3).

Although folates covalently bound to macromolecules have not yet been discovered, heat treatment may be needed to release folates bound to such components as folate-binding proteins (4, 162, 287), membranes (5), and viruses (6). The selective absorption to charcoal and solvent extractions were originally used to purify folates. These have given way to ionic exchange column chromatography, molecular sieve column chromatography, and high-pressure liquid chromatography.

B. Structure and Nomenclature

Folic acid (PteGlu, 2-amino-4-hydroxy-6-methyleneaminobenzoyl-L-glutamic acid pteridine) is composed of a pteridine moiety linked through a methylene group at the C-6 position to a p-aminobenzoylglutamate group (see Fig. 1). Natural folates occur in the reduced, 7,8-dihydro- and 5,6,7,8-tetrahydro- forms. Folates bearing one 1-carbon units are 5-methyl-, 10-formyl-, 5-formyl-, 5,10-methenyl-, 5,10-methylene-, and 5-formimino-tetrahydrofolate. Folates in nature occur as pteroyloligo-γ-L-glutamates (PteGlu$_n$) of from one to nine or more glutamates long. The subscript "n" indicates the total number of glutamate residues. "Folate" is a generic term for the above compounds.

C. Analog and Antagonists

A great variety of folate analogs have been prepared, mainly for the purposes of anticancer and antimicrobial therapy. Dihydrofolate reductase is the usual target of these drugs. Methotrexate is an analog of folic acid and is widely used in cancer chemotherapy (7). The drug binds extremely tightly to dihydrofolate reductase. The x-ray structure of the complex of enzyme and methotrexate has been determined (8). Dihydrofolate reductase is also inhibited by 10-formyl-PteGlu (9), trimethoprim (10), and pyrimethamine. The latter two compounds are used to treat malaria and other protozoal diseases. Analogs not usually thought of as analogs are the unnatural isomers of tetrahydrofolates, where the asymmetric center is at C-6. These may inhibit folate-requiring enzymes (11,12). Folate analogs containing peptides or amino acids other than glutamate have been made (13,14,86). Folates have been covalently bound to protein (6) and to agarose (15,16) for the purposes of antibody production and affinity chromatography, respectively.

Sulfonamides, though not folate analogues, are analogs of the folate biosynthetic intermediate, p-aminobenzoic acid (17), and are widely used as antibacterial agents. Folate analogs have been prepared and used to determine the mechanism of folate-requiring enzymes (18).

D. Synthesis

Folic acid was first synthesized by Lederle Laboratories by the condensation of triamino-6-hydroxypyrimidine, dibromopropionaldehyde, and *p*-aminobenzoylglutamic acid (19). Folic acid and pterins in general have been synthesized by the method of Taylor et al. (20). This method uses 2-amino-3-cyano-5-chloromethylpyrazine as a key intermediate and avoids a contaminating isomer formed in earlier procedures. The L-glutamyl group of folic acid may racemize in the above method, and a strategy for avoiding this problem has been suggested (21).

Pteroyloligo-L-γ-glutamates (folate polyglutamates) were synthesized by the Lederle group (22) and by Meienhofer et al. (23), as well as by Baugh et al. (13), who used the solid phase method.

Folic acid can be reduced to the dihydro- form (24). Folic acid can be formylated (25) followed by reduction to 10-formyl-H_4PteGlu (26) and reduced further to 5-methyl-H_4PteGlu (27). The natural isomers of reduced folates can be made by means of reduction with purified dihydrofolate reductase or by formylation with formyltetrahydrofolate synthetase.

E. Chemical Properties

Folic acid is yellow, has a molecular weight of 441.4, and is slightly soluble in water in the acid form but quite soluble in the salt form. Tetrahydrofolates in solutions are sensitive to oxygen, light, and pH extremes, and can break down to *p*-aminobenzoylglutamic acid and dihydroxanthopterin, pterin-6-carboxaldehyde, or pterin-6-carboxylic acid (28). An oxidation product of 5-methyl-H_4PteGlu is 5-methyl-H_2PteGlu (29). When acidified, 10-formyl- and 5-formylH_4PteGlu isomerize to the relatively oxygen stable folate, 5,10-methenyl-H_4Pteclu (30). When neutralized, the 5,10-methenyl-H_4PteGlu isomerizes to 10-formyl-H_4PteClu, one of the less stable folate compounds. The formyl group can be removed under anaerobic conditions (25). 5-Formimino-H_4PteGlu, although stable to oxygen, is readily hydrolyzed with the production of ammonia (31). Formaldehyde condenses reversibly with H_4PteGlu to form 5,10-methylene-H_4PteGlu (32). The concentration of this folate can be maintained only when excess formaldehyde is in the solution. 5,10-Methylene-H_4PteGlu is stable at pH 9.5 but is in somewhat rapid equilibrium with formaldehyde at neutral and lower pH (33). This equilibrium can be disturbed by the reaction of thiols with formaldehyde (32) and, perhaps, of thiols with H_4PteGlu (34).

III. ANALYTICAL PROCEDURES

The method used to identify folates depends on whether one needs to know the identities of the 1-carbon unit and reductive state of the cofactor, the length of the oligoglutamyl chain of the folate, or both. The methods to be used also will depend on the suspected heterogeneity of the unknown folates. If the unknown folates are a mixture of several major and minor forms, the compounds may first be fractionated on an anion exchange chromatograph column, such as diethylaminoethylcellulose (DEAE-cellulose) using a salt gradient (35) prior to analysis of the 1-carbon unit and polyglutamate chain length of each folate.

After the initial fractionation on DEAE-cellulose, the unknown folates eluting in the peak tubes can be treated with purified γ-glutamyl hydrolase for 30 min under N_2 followed by chromatography on a column of Sephadex G-25 to determine if the folate is in the

10-formyl-, 5-formyl-, 5-methyl-, or tetrahydro- form. Alternatively, the γ-glutamyl hydrolase–treated folate can be chromatographed on DEAE-cellulose, a medium capable of resolving dihydrofolates from the other forms. After identification of the reductive state and 1-carbon unit, the unknown folate (not treated with γ-glutamyl hydrolase) can be analyzed with the column of Sephadex G-25 to determine the oligo-γ-glutamyl chain length. Blue dextran, as well as a $PteGlu_n$ standard, should be co-chromatographed with the unknown folate (36).

The length of the chain can also be determined by cleaving the folate with zinc dust in acid/gelatin yielding the corresponding p-aminobenzoyloligoglutamate. The chain length of the latter compound can be assessed by direct chromatography of the $PABA\text{-}Glu_n$ (39) or after conversion of $PABA\text{-}Glu_n$ to the azo dye derivatives (40,41). The elution positions of the $PABA\text{-}Glu_n$ can be determined by radioactivity, where the parent folate was radioactive, by absorption after conversion of the $PABA\text{-}Glu_n$ to the azo dye, or by microbiological assay (58). Although $H_4PteGlu_n$ cleaves spontaneously in acid (or with prolonged acid treatment where 2-mercaptoethanol is present) and $PteGlu_n$ is cleaved rapidly with zinc dust in acid/gelatin, special protocols are used for cleavage of the other forms of folate, as pointed out by Shane and by Eto and Krumdieck. Another method of folate polyglutamate analysis involves conversion of all forms to 5-methyl-$H_4PteGlu_n$ followed by chromatography (42).

Superior separation of the various folate monoglutamates can be achieved by high-pressure liquid chromatography (3,43). HPLC has not yet been used for the routine analysis of intact (noncleaved) tissue folates.

Folates can be detected by microbiological assays (see Sec. IV), absorption spectra (1), fluorescent spectra (37), or by cleavage to $PABA\text{-}Glu_n$ followed by conversion to the azo dye (38).

IV. BIOASSAY PROCEDURES

The folate content of natural sources, as well as that in fractions recovered after chromatographic procedures, can be reliably measured by the method of microbiological assay. The hydrolysis of the oligo-γ-glutamyl chain by treatment with γ-glutamyl hydrolase is required to support a maximal growth response of the test microorganism (44). The method involving treatment with γ-glutamyl hydrolase followed by assay with *Lactobacillus casei* has been called an assay for "total folates." The amount of 5-methyl-tetrahydrofolates can be assessed by substracting the value obtained with *Streptococcus faecalis* from that obtained with *L. casei*, where the sample was treated with γ-glutamyl hydrolase prior to adding to the growth medium of both test microorganisms. *L. casei* does respond but *S. faecalis* does not to 5-methyl-$H_4PteGlu$.

The growth of *L. casei* or of *S. faecalis* on folate polyglutamates tends to be somewhat impaired compared to that with folate monoglutamate, the effect being stronger with *S. faecalis* as the test organism (285). This effect can be used to obtain an inaccurate and underestimated, though sometimes useful, measure of the amount of folate polyglutamates in a particular sample. In this case, one uses the test bacterium to determine the available folates in samples treated and not treated with γ-glutamyl hydrolase.

Another lactic acid bacterium, *Pediococcus cerevisiae*, does not respond to nonreduced folate, i.e., PteGlu, or to 5-methyl-$H_4PteGlu$. This property can be useful when assaying chromatographic fractions where it is desirable to avoid a response to huge amounts of synthetic standard marker folate polyglutamates.

Recent work has emphasized that the growth medium used for microbiological assays should be acidic and not higher than pH 6.2 (45). The "folic acid casei medium" available from the DIFCO Company yields beautiful results, where near linear standard curves range from an absorbance at 600 nm of 0.10 to over 1.5. The folate free blank may have an A_{600} under 0.05. The final volume of each assay may be 1.5 ml, with an incubation time of 18–22 hr at 37°.

V. CONTENT IN FOOD

A. Food Content Tables

The folate content of the following foods has been measured: milk (46–49), juices (48,50,51), vegetables (48,51–55), wheat and bread (48,51,56), soybeans (51,55), and organ meats (51,57,58). The folate content of a large variety of foods was measured by Hoppner et al. (59). Hurdle et al. (60), Santini et al. (61), and Hoppner and colleagues (62,63) for baby foods and for TV dinners.

When using food tables, attention should be given to the manner in which the test food was prepared, i.e., cooked or raw. Food folates may be lost in cooking water (52) and may be destroyed by cooking (52,60). Generally, fruits and meat, except organ meats, are poor sources of folate. Vegetables such as broccoli and spinach are good sources. The origin of most of the folate in bread is the yeast (56). The folate content per gram wet weight of some foods is given in Table 1. Some differences are apparent in similar food sources. These could arise from methodological differences, such as using different regions of the folate standard curve for determining the food folate value, or from actual differences in food folate. The food folate values listed in many early publications are not accurate or useful because antioxidants were not included in the microbiological assays.

B. Stability and Availability in Foods

Losses of food folate (20–75%) occur by extraction of the folate into the cooking water (52) and by destruction of highly oxygen-labile folates. All folate forms except $PteGlu_n$ and 5-formyl-$H_4PteGlu_n$ are highly labile (65). In aerobic conditions, destruction of most folates was significant with heating at 100°C for 10 min (65) or at 23°C for 1 hr for $H_4PteGlu$ (66), or at 23°C for 100 hr for 5-methyl-$H_4PteGlu$ and 10-formyl-H_4 PteGlu (66). Reduced folates are probably more stable when inside food because of the relatively anaerobic conditions and because the folates are protected from the light.

The availability of food folates may range from 30 to 80% that of PteGlu. This was found to be the case for folates extracted from yeast (67) and folates in the presence of certain foods, such as yeast or cabbage (51). Synthetic PteGlu in cooked food may be absorbed at a lesser rate than PteGlu administered in water (68). These rates were determined from increases in serum folates levels in people presaturated with folic acid prior to test doses (68). Stronger data on the biological availability of folic acid are those (69,70) showing that synthetic folic acid in cooked food was 55% as available as folic acid in tablet form, as determined by changes in red blood cell folate content. The test foods used by Colman et al. (68–70) were maize, rice, and bread. Certain foods such as cabbage and legumes contain conjugase inhibitors, which can decrease the availability of folate polyglutamates.

Table 1 Folate Content in Foods

Food	Total folate (μg/g wet weight)	Reference
Fresh bovine milk	0.05–0.12	46
Cooked liver	10.7	51
Raw liver	1.41	59
Banana	0.28	51
Hard-boiled egg yolk	1.4	51
Raw cabbage	0.30	52
Boiled cabbage (water discarded)	0.16	52
Raw broccoli	1.69	52
Boiled broccoli (water discarded)	0.65	52
Broccoli	0.91	64
Raw ground chuck	0.08	59
Canned tuna	0.15	59
Cheddar cheese	0.20	59
Whole wheat bread	0.54	59
Raw applies	0.06	59
Tomatoes	0.06	59
Tomatoes, canned	0.43	64
Oranges	0.24	59
Frozen orange juice, reconstituted	2.2	64
Concentrated frozen orange juice	1.4	51
Avocados	0.36	59

VI. METABOLISM

A. Absorption

Dietary folates are predominantly pteroylpolyglutamate derivatives. The process of vitamin absorption requires the hydrolysis to monoglutamyl derivatives prior to transport across the intestinal mucosa. Absorption of orally administered folate mono- and polyglutamates was followed by measuring the appearance of vitamin appearing in the mesenteric vein (71) or in the urine (72). The monoglutamate was absorbed at a greater rate, and with both derivatives, the monoglutamate was the only form detected in the bloodstream. In other experiments, the polyglutamate was absorbed at the same rate as the monoglutamate (51).

"Conjugase" is the trivial name of enzymes that hydrolyze folate polyglutamates to the monoglutamyl forms. The enzyme has not been detected in the lumen but can exist as a membrane-bound enzyme, possibly with the active site facing the lumen. This membrane-bound enzyme is an exopeptidase. It has been purified from the human brush border (73), but it may be absent from other sources such as the rat and monkey (74). The intestines, as well as the liver, contain a lysosomal conjugase. Although the relationship between the membrane-bound and lysosomal enzymes is not clear, it seems likely that the steps of folate absorption differ in different species.

Intestinal folate absorption occurs in the jejunum and has been measured via oral administration of vitamin or with jejunal perfusion, tied-off intestinal segments, everted gut sacs, or brush border membrane vesicles. Transport is maximal at pH 5–6 with a rather sharp pH optimum. Folic acid (PteGlu), reduced folates, and MTX can be transported, but it is not clear if one or more transport systems are employed (75).

During passage across the mucosa, reduced folates become converted to 5-methyl-H_4-PteGlu (76). With oral doses of PteGlu, some reduction and methylation occurs in the intestines, though most of this form of the vitamin appears in the blood as PteGlu. During passage through the liver, immediate conversion of the PteGlu to 5-methyl-H_4PteGlu occurs, with release of much of the converted vitamin back to the bloodstream (77,78). With large oral doses of PteGlu, substantial amounts of the vitamin are recovered, unchanged, in the urine.

A fraction of the folates absorbed by the liver may be secreted in the bile, where they occur as nonmethyl folates and as 5-methyl-H_4PteGlu (76). The bile folates may be reabsorbed through the intestines in a proposed enterophepatic cycle (79).

B. Transport

Folic acid, MTX, and naturally occurring folates may share a common transport system in mammalian cells (80). Other studies indicated separate systems for folic acid (81), a compound not normally found in nature, and for MTX as well (82). The K_t value for PteGlu ranges from 70 to 400 μM, while those for MTX, 5-methyl-H_4PteGlu, and 5-formyl-H_4PteGlu are lower and range from 0.2 to 10 μM.

Transport may occur by an anion exchange mechanism, where anion gradients may serve as an energy source for uptake (83). Folate transport may be partially dependent on sodium ions in the cell medium (84). Both high and low affinity 5-methyl-H_4PteGlu transport systems have been detected. Further complicating features include multiple efflux routes (85). Although an understanding of MTX and folate transport is of value in the control of folate metabolism, as during chemotherapy, a definitive picture has yet to emerge.

C. Tissue Deposition and Storage

Folates in cells and tissues occur almost exclusively as folate oligo-γ-glutamates. Every type of cell or organ is likely to contain a unique profile of these folate polyglutamates. For example, *Clostridium* contains the triglutamate (88), *S. faecalis* the tetra- and pentaglutamate (42). *L. casei* the octa- and nonaglutamate (42), and *Corynebacterium* the tetraglutamate (89). Cultured human cells may contain folate, hexa-, hepta-, and octaglutamates (90). In all cases the folates occur in the reduced forms, i.e., as tetrahydro-, 5-methyl-tetrahydro-, 10-formyl-tetrahydro-, 5,10-methylene-tetrahydro-, or dihydrofolates.

Livers from rats raised on a normal diet contain mainly H_4PteGlu$_5$ (44% of total), with smaller amounts of 5-methyl-H_4-PteGlu$_5$ (19%), 10-formyl-H_4PteGlu$_5$ (13%), H_4PteGlu$_6$ (13%), 10-formyl-H_4PteGlu$_6$ (4%), and 5-methyl-H_4PteGlu$_6$ (2%). Livers from rats raised on a methionine-deficient diet contained more equivalent amounts of folate penta- and hexaglutamates; H_4PteGlu$_5$ (31%), 5-methyl-H_4PteGlu$_5$ (13%), 10-formyl-H_4-PteGlu$_5$ (10%), H_4PteGlu$_6$ (31%), 5-methyl-H_4PteGlu$_6$ (9%), and 10-formyl-H_4PteGlu$_6$ (11%) (182). Generally, where the cellular level of tetrahydrofolate has been diminished, as during a folate deficiency, a methionine deficiency, or by feeding cultured cells 5-methyl-H_4PteGlu$_3$, the cells or animals tends to accumulate longer chain length folates. These trends may be a reflection of the substrate specificity of folate polyglutamate synthetase (86).

A number of folate-binding proteins have been studied, though the functions of the bound folate are unclear (162,287). These proteins have been purified from milk, serum, and cerebrospinal fluid. It has been speculated that the milk protein can prevent utilization of the vitamin in milk by enteric bacteria. Folate-binding activity is more readily detected in serum from folate-deficient patients than in normal people, indicating that the folate-binding protein is physiologically responsive (91). Possibly, the $H_4PteGlu_5$-binding proteins in mitochondria (181) prevent the immediate utilization of the folate in 1-carbon metabolism. A clear and vital function is known for cobalamin-binding proteins, for example, but not for folate-binding proteins.

D. Metabolism

Folic acid metabolism involves the reduction of the pterin ring to the tetrahydro-form, the elongation of the glutamyl chain, and the acquisition of 1-carbon units at the N-5 or N-10 positions. These 1-carbon units can be at the oxidation levels of formate, formaldehyde, or methanol. The metabolic roles of the folate coenzymes are to serve as acceptors or donors of 1-carbon units in a variety of reactions.

E. Excretion

The daily dietary intake of folate in humans has been estimated to range from 90 to 2300 μg, with the minimal daily requirement being 50μg. The daily urinary excretion of intact folates, however, is only between 1 and 12 μg, representing only a small fraction of the intake. Fecal folate levels are quite high, sometimes much higher than the estimated intake, presumably because of production by the gut microflora.

A major urinary excretory product of folate appears to be N-acetyl-*p*-aminobenzoylglutamate (92). This compound probably arises after cleavage of the labile C9–C10 bond of reduced folates, yielding *p*-aminobenzoylglutamate and pteridines, such as 6-hydroxymethylpterin (93).

VII. BIOCHEMICAL FUNCTION

Folates are used as cofactors and serve as acceptors and donors of 1-carbon units in a variety of reactions involved in amino acid and nucleotide metabolism. The 1-carbon units can be at the oxidation levels of methanol, formaldehyde, and formate but not carbon dioxide. These reactions, known as 1-carbon metabolism, are shown in Figure 2, which emphasizes the cyclical nature of folate metabolism.

It should be apparent that some folate-requiring enzymes are used for biosynthetic purposes, whereas others are used only for interconversion of the various forms of the vitamin. The folate molecule does not remain enzyme bound, but acts rather as a cosubstrate. The regulation or disturbance of any one of the reactions in Figure 2, particularly of those turning over rapidly, would be expected to have a profound affect on the activities of the other reactions.

A. Dihydrofolate Reductase

Dihydrofolate reductase (E.C.1.5.1.3) catalyzes the reduction of dihydrofolates and of nonreduced folates as follows:

$$H_2PteGlu \ (PteGlu) + NADPH + H^+ \ \text{------} \ H_4PteGlu \ (H_2PteGlu) + NADP^+ \quad (1)$$

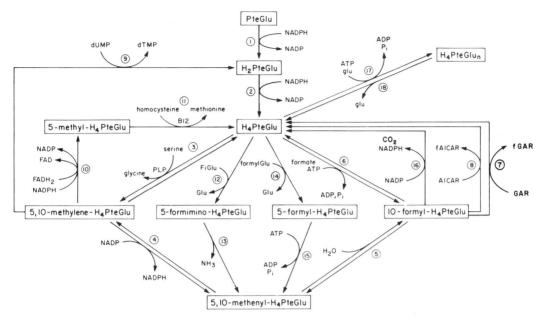

Figure 2 Folate-mediated reactions of 1-carbon metabolism. The numbers refer to reactions catalyzed by the following enzymes: (1) dihydrofolate reductase, (2) dihydrofolate reductase, (3) serine hydroxymethyltransferase, (4) 5,10-methylene-tetrahydrofolate dehydrogenase, (5) 5,10-methenyl-tetrahydrofolate cyclohydrolase, (6) 10-formyl-tetrahydrofolate synthetase, (7) glycinamide ribonucleotide transformylase, (8) aminoimidazole carboxamide ribonucleotide transformylase, (9) thymidylate synthase, (10) 5,10-methylene-tetrahydrofolate reductase, (11) methionine synthetase, (12) tetrahydrofolate formiminotransferase, (13) formiminotetrahydrofolate cyclohydrolase, (14) glutamate transformylase, (15) 5-formyl-tetrahydrofolate isomerase, (16) 10-formyl-tetrahydrofolate dehydrogenase, (17) folate polyglutamate synthetase, and (18) γ-glutamyl hydrolase. In mammals, reactions 12 and 13 are catalyzed by a single bifunctional enzyme, and reactions 4,5, and 6 are catalyzed by a trifunctional enzyme. dUMP, Deoxyuridine monophosphate; dTMP, deoxythymidine monophosphate (thymidine monophosphate); PLP, pyridoxal phosphate; FIGLU, formiminoglutamic acid; fAICAR, formyl-aminoimidazole carboxyamide ribonucleotide; AICAR, aminomidazole carboxamide ribonucleotide; GAR, glycinamide ribonucleotide; fGAR, formyl-glycinamide ribonucleotide; and B_{12}, vitamin B_{12} (cobalamin).

PteGlu is a poorer substrate than H_2PteGlu, and activity with PteGlu shows an acidic pH optimum. The activity with PteGlu is essential for utilizing the synthetic form of the vitamin, folic acid (PteGlu). The enzyme is the smallest in 1-carbon metabolism (MW 22,000) and is unusual because the activity with H_2PteGlu shows both acidic and neutral pH maxima and because the activity with H_2PteGlu can be stimulated markedly with salts and urea. The enzyme is the target of the anticancer drug methotrexate (MTX). MTX binds extremely tightly to the active site. MTX treatment provokes the buildup of the substrate of the enzyme H_2PteGlu. H_2PteGlu itself is not used in any other folate-requiring reaction. With the concomitant depletion of the tetrahydrofolates, other reactions in 1-carbon metabolism are impeded, notably that of T-synthase, and the cancer cell dies.

The concentration of H_2PteGlu reductase can increase in cells during exposure of MTX, leading to the development of clinical resistance to MTX with a variety of tumors. A mechanism of drug resistance is the amplification of genes coding for the enzyme, where the genes can be extra-chromosomal or on the chromosome (94). The specificity of the enzyme increases somewhat during the S phase of the cell cycle (95).

B. Serine Hydroxymethyltransferase

Serine hydroxymethyltransferase (E.C.2.1.2.1) catalyzes the transfer of formaldehyde, derived from serine, to H_4PteGlu as follows:

$$\text{L-Serine} + H_4\text{PteGlu} \overset{\text{PLP}}{\rightleftharpoons} 5,10\text{-methylene-}H_4\text{PteGlu} + \text{glycine} + H_2O \qquad (3)$$

The enzyme contains bound pyridoxal phosphate. The β-carbon of serine is the major source of 1-carbon units used in folate metabolism. The reaction, which is freely reversible, is also a major pathway of serine catabolism (250). A variable amount (5–50%) of the enzyme may be located in the mitochondria (97,163,164,251). Experiments with mutant cells lacking the mitochondrial enzyme (and half of the cytoplasmic enzyme) suggest that the mitochondrial enzyme is needed for protein synthesis, for converting glycine to serine, and for the oxidation of [3-^{14}C]serine to ^{14}C-CO_2 (163,250).

The enzyme can function, though poorly, in the complete absence of the folate cosubstrate (246). Serine hydroxymethyltransferase can catalyze the cleavage of allothreonine to glycine. Surprisingly, allothreonine can satisfy the glycine requirement of some cultured cells (164). Allothreonine has a unique use. It can be used as a probe for enzyme activity when one wants to eliminate the uncertainty due to variable tissue folate levels (164) or when one wants to detect the cytosolic form of the enzyme and not the mitochondrial form (266).

Schirch and Ropp (96) found that the enzyme can bind 5-methyl-H_4PteGlu (not a substrate) and glycine to form a complex. This complex can be enhanced by folate polyglutamates (97). These results are provocative, as the concentration of free glycine in the liver is high enough to support the formation of this complex in vivo (274). It is not clear at this time if this complex would have any secondary effects on 1-carbon metabolism.

C. 5,10-Methylene-Tetrahydrofolate Dehydrogenase

5,10-Methylene-H_4PteGlu dehydrogenase (E.C.1.5.1.5) catalyzes the reversible interconversion of folate 1-carbon units at the oxidation levels of formaldehyde and formate as follows:

$$5,10\text{-Methylene-}H_4\text{PteGlu} + \text{NADP}^+ \rightleftharpoons 5,10\text{-methenyl-}H_4\text{PteGlu}^+ + \text{NADPH} \qquad (4)$$

The enzyme plays a central role in 1-carbon metabolism as it occurs by a branching point where 1-carbon units can be used for the biosynthesis of methionine, thymidylate, or purines.

10-Formyl-H_4PteGlu synthetase, 5,10-methenyl-H_4PteGlu cyclohydrolase, and 5,10-methylene-H_4PteGlu dehydrogenase activities are associated with a single polypeptide chain in eukaryotes (98,99). The synthetase reaction is stimulated by potassium or ammonium ions but not by sodium ions. The complex of the above three activities has been called the "trifunctional enzyme" as well as "C_1-tetrahydrofolate synthase."

While monofunctional in some bacteria such as formate fixers (100), 5,10-methylene-H_4PteGlu dehydrogenase is bifunctional in others, containing 5,10-methenyl-H_4PteGlu cyclohydrolase.

An NAD-dependent 5,10-methylene-H_4PteGlu dehydrogenase was discovered by Scrimgeour and Huennekens (101). It is found in cultured mammalian and developmental cells of normal tissues, but not in normal liver (102). Mg^{2+} or Mn^{2+} is required for the NAD-dependent enzyme but not for the NADP-dependent enzyme. A unique function of the NAD-dependent enzyme is not known. This enzyme is not trifunctional, but bifunctional, and contains the cyclohydrolase.

D. 5,10-Methenyl-Tetrahydrofolate Cyclohydrolase

5,10-Methenyl-H_4PteGlu cyclohydrolase (E.C.3.5.4.9) catalyzes the reversible interconversion of folates at the oxidation level of formate as follows:

$$10\text{-Formyl-}H_4\text{PteGlu} \rightleftharpoons 5,10\text{-methenyl-}H_4\text{PteGlu} + H_2O \tag{5}$$

The cyclization of 10-formyl-H_4PteGlu to 5,10-methenyl-H_4PteGlu occurs nonenzymatically below pH 6, whereas ring opening occurs spontaneously at higher pH values. The cyclohydrolase is part of a trifunctional enzyme in eukaryotic cells.

E. 10-Formyl-Tetrahydrofolate Synthetase

10-Formyl-H_4PteGlu synthetase (E.C.6.3.4.3) catalyzes the entry of formate into the 1-carbon pool as follows:

$$H_4\text{PteGlu} + HCOOH + ATP \rightleftharpoons 10\text{-formyl-}H_4\text{PteGlu} + ADP + P_i \tag{6}$$

The enzyme is part of a trifunctional enzyme in eukaryotic cells, as mentioned earlier. The trifunctional enzyme is highest in liver and kidney (275).

F. Glycinamide Ribonucleotide and 5-Amino-4-Imidazolecarboxamide Ribonucleotide Transformylase

The C-8 and C-2 positions of the purine ring are derived from the 1-carbon pool in reactions catalyzed by glycinamide ribonucleotide (GAR) transformylase (E.C.2.1.2.2) and aminoimidazolecarboxamide ribonucleotide (AICAR) transformylase (E.C.2.1.2.3), as follows:

$$10\text{-Formyl-}H_4\text{PteGlu} + GAR \longrightarrow \text{formyl-GAR} + H_4\text{PteGlu} \tag{7}$$
$$10\text{-Formyl-}H_4\text{PteGlu} + AICAR \rightleftharpoons \text{formyl-AICAR} + H_4\text{PteGlu} \tag{8}$$

GAR transformylase catalyzes the third step in purine biosynthesis. The glycine moiety of the growing purine nucleotide (GAR) receives the formyl group from the 10-formyl-H_4PteGlu. It might be noted that in this, as well as in other folate reactions, the actual substrate in vivo normally is the folate polyglutamate.

Although reaction 7 has been thought to require 5,10-methenyl-H_4PteGlu, the ability to utilize this compound as a substrate was shown to arise from the association of GAR transformylase with the trifunctional enzyme (12), which converts 5,10-methenyl-H_4PteGlu to 10-formyl-H_4PteGlu. Furthermore, the inability to use 10-formyl-H_4PteGlu in assays of GAR transformylase arose from inhibition by the unnatural isomer of 10-formyl-H_4PteGlu present in the assay mixtures (12,103).

The hexaglutamate cofactor works slightly better than folates of other chain lengths for the chicken liver enzyme (104).

GAR transformylase is possibly part of a multifunctional protein that catalyzes two other steps in the purine biosynthetic pathway (105). Dissection of the enzyme by chymotrypsin was used to provide evidence for its multifunctional nature. The for-miminotransferase/cyclodeaminase has also been dissected by limited proteolysis with chymotrypsin, as described in Section VII.L (106).

AICAR transformylase catalyzes the penultimate step in purine biosynthesis. Potassium ions are required for activity (107). The reaction is pulled in the forward direction by ring closure of formyl-AICAR to form IMP. The ring closure is catalyzed by inosinicase, which co-purifies with AICAR transformylase, though the claim that both activities are catalyzed by the same protein has not been proven (108).

Aminoimidazolecarboxamide (AIC) is excreted in elevated amounts by animals and humans with a deficiency in folate or vitamin B_{12} (109). In fact, AIC was discovered because it accumulated when bacteria were treated with folate antagonists (110).

It might be noted that purine biosynthesis was elucidated in early experiments where pigeons fed radioactive formate incorporated this tracer into the 2 and 8 positions of uric acid, a purine (111). There has recently been some interest in the conversion of AICAR to small amounts of AICAR 5'-triphosphate (112,113).

Although folates are used as cofactors in purine biosynthesis, it is interesting to note that a purine (guanosine) is the biochemical precursor of folate.

G. Thymidylate Synthase

Thymidylate synthase (E.C.2.1.1.45) catalyzes the conversion of dUMP to dTMP, where the donated 1-carbon unit is at the oxidation level of formaldehyde:

$$5,10\text{-Methylene-}H_4\text{PteGlu} + \text{dUMP} \longrightarrow \text{dTMP} + H_2\text{PteGlu} \qquad (9)$$

The reaction is unique among folate-requiring reactions, as the folate is used as a reductant and transfers a hydride from the 6-position. The enzyme's activity is quite low, except during growth, as in fetal tissues, regenerating tissues, or in cancer. There is some evidence that the enzyme resides in a complex, with DNA polymerase, on the DNA replication fork. The above reaction is believed to be rate-limiting for growth and the enzyme is the target of the drug 5-fluorouracil (5FU).

5-Fluoro-deoxyuridylate, in the presence of 5,10-methylene-H_4PteGlu, forms a tight complex, covalent in some cases, with the enzyme and completely inhibits it. The complex is stable to urea (114) and dodecylsulfate (115) but may be dissociated by heat (116) or with dUMP (117).

5FU is widely used for cancer chemotherapy. It is converted in vivo to 5-fluoro-deoxyuridylate, which is a suicide inhibitor of thymidylate synthase. The above in vivo metabolite also becomes incorporated into RNA. Although this incorporation is believed to have some chemotherapeutic value, its actual importance remains unclear. Recent clinical studies suggest that MTX treatment followed by 5FU treatment may be useful (118).

Until recently, it has not been too clear how the anticancer drugs MTX and 5FU kill cells, rather than simply result in an arrest of cell growth. Goulian et al. (119) and Ayusawa et al. (120) demonstrated that blocking thymidylate synthase in vivo results in the accumulation of dUTP. The dUTP, which normally is not found, becomes incorporated into DNA. The sites containing the incorporated dU are then cleaved by enzymes. The resulting DNA breakage may be how antifolates kill cells.

H. 5,10-Methylene-Tetrahydrofolate Reductase

5,10-Methylene-H_4PteGlu reductase (E.C.1.1.1.68) catalyzes the conversion of 1-carbon units at the oxidation level of formaldehyde to that of methanol as follows:

5,10,Methylene-H_4PteGlu + FADH$_2$ + NADPH + H$^+$ $\longrightarrow$
5-methyl-H_4PteGlu + FAD + NADP$^+$ (10)

The enzyme is a flavoprotein and utilizes NADPH more effectively than NADH. Although reversible, the reaction strongly favors the formation of 5-methyl-H_4PteGlu such that it is essentially irreversible under physiological conditions. The 5-methyl-H_4PteGlu is used exclusively for the regeneration of methionine from homocysteine. 5-Methyl-H_4PteGlu is not known to donate its methyl group in any other biochemical reaction. Although methionine is used for protein synthesis, 5-methyl-H_4PteGlu is used to regenerate the methionine used, in the form of S-adenosyl-methionine (AdoMet), in biological methylation reactions. AdoMet is a feedback inhibitor of 5,10-methylene-H_4PteGlu reductase (121). The enzyme is also inhibited by H_2PteGlu$_n$, where a dependence on the polyglutamate chain length was noted (122).

I. 5-Formyl-Tetrahydrofolate Cyclohydrolase

Although 5-formyl-H_4PteGlu is not known to be required in any folate-dependent pathway, it is used pharmacologically as a source of reduced folate, as it is more stable than other forms of reduced folate. To participate in 1-carbon metabolism, the 5-formyl-H_4PteGlu must be metabolized to 5,10-methenyl-H_4PteGlu in a reaction catalyzed by 5-formyl-H_4PteGlu cyclohydrolase (E.C.6.3.3.a) as follows:

5-formyl-H_4PteGlu + ATP $\xrightarrow[Mg^{2+}]{}$ 5,10-methenyl-H_4PteGlu + ADP + P$_i$ (15)

J. Methionine Synthetase

Methionine synthetase (E.C.2.1.1.13) catalyzes the transfer of the methyl group of 5-methyl-H_4PteGlu to homocysteine, generating methionine:

5-Methyl-H_4PteGlu + homocysteine $\xrightarrow[AdoMet]{B_{12}}$ H_4PteGlu + methionine (11)

The enzyme contains tightly bound cobalamin, which is methylated by the folate substrate followed by transfer of the methyl group to homocysteine. This is the only reaction known for the metabolism of 5-methyl-H_4PteGlu with the consequent regeneration of H_4PteGlu. As discussed elsewhere, defects in this enzyme arising from genetics, a vitamin B_{12} deficiency, or from prolonged exposure to nitrous oxide gas lead to the accumulation of cellular folates in the 5-methyl-H_4PteGlu form.

Methionine synthetase is unique among cobalamin-containing enzymes as the cobalamin functions in a "superreduced" state (123). AdoMet is also a cofactor required by the enzyme. It is not used during each turnover of the enzyme but is thought to be involved in the remethylation of the cobalamin, should it revert from the superreduced state to a more oxidized state. Methionine synthetase is also unique as it loses activity upon prolonged exposure to the widely used anesthetic nitrous oxide (124).

Finally, it might be noted that the use of vitamin B_{12} as a standard component in the assay of the enzyme can lead to confusion. The added B_{12} does not function as a cofactor, but as part of a nonenzymatic reducing system (125). A reducing system, thought to act in vivo, has been isolated (178).

K. Formiminotransferase

The formiminotransferase (E.C.2.1.2.5) catalyzes one of the final steps in histidine catabolism. The forminino group of formiminoglutamate is transferred to $H_4PteGlu$ as follows:

$$\text{Formiminoglutamate} + H_4PteGlu \longrightarrow \text{glutamate} + \text{5-formimino-}H_4PteGlu \quad (12)$$

Thus, histidine can be a source of 1-carbon units, where the 1-carbon is at the oxidation state of formate. The enzyme is cytosolic. With a deficiency in folate or vitamin B_{12}, the above reaction is impaired. This results in increased urinary formiminoglutamic acid.

L. 5-Formimino-Tetrahydrofolate Cyclohydrolase

The 5-formimino-$H_4PteGlu$ formed by reaction 12 is deaminated in a reaction catalyzed by the cyclodeaminase (E.C.4.3.1.4) as follows:

$$\text{5-Formimino-}H_4PteGlu \rightleftharpoons \text{5,10-methenyl-}H_4PteGlu + NH_4^+ \quad (13)$$

Reactions 12 and 13 are catalyzed to a single protein in mammals, though separate proteins are used in bacteria. Tabor and Wyngarden discovered that reactions 12 and 13 can be selectively inactivated, illustrating the independence of the active sites in the mammalian enzyme (106). MacKenzie and Baugh (126,252) elegantly demonstrated the phenomenon of channeling. When the folate polyglutamate is used as the substrate, the vitamin remains bound to the enzyme during catalysis of the sequential reactions 12 and 13. This permits rapid formation of the final product and prevents accumulation of the formiminofolate, a compound of no known use. However, when folate monoglutamate is used as the substrate, the formiminofolate dissociates prior to engaging in reaction 13. Thus, the polyglutamate tail or chain is essential for channeling of the folate through the two-step reaction.

An unusual property of the polyglutamate chain was noted for another enzyme, thymidylate synthase. Here, there is a reversal in the order of substrate binding with an increase in the chain length of the polyglutamate substrate (127).

The formiminotransferase also catalyzes the deformylation of N-formyl-glutamate (128), a reaction initially reported in 1957 (129).

M. Methionyl-tRNA Transformylase

10-Formyl-$H_4PteGlu$: Methionyl-tRNA$_f^{met}$ transformylase catalyzes the transfer of a formyl group to methionyl-tRNA$_f^{met}$ as follows:

$$\text{10-Formyl-}H_4PteGlu + \text{methionyl-tRNA}_f^{met} \xrightarrow[Mg^{2+}]{} H_4PteGlu +$$
$$\text{N-formyl-methionyl-tRNA}_f^{met} \quad (14)$$

Protein biosynthesis in mitochondria (130), chloroplasts (131), and bacteria (132) is initiated by a special type of transfer RNA, N-formyl-methionyl-tRNA$_f^{met}$. The formylation of the methionine residue bound to the tRNA requires a folate cofactor and is catalyzed by an enzyme of $M_r = 25000-38000$. In mammals, the effect of a folate deficiency on the activity of this enzyme is not known. In certain bacteria, the requirement for the above folate-dependent reaction can be overidden during a folate deficiency (133).

N. Glycine Cleavage System

The glycine cleavage system is located in the mitochondria and catalyzes the following reaction:

$$\text{Glycine} + \text{H}_4\text{PteGlu} + \text{NAD}^+ \longrightarrow 5,10\text{-methylene-H}_4\text{PteGlu} +$$
$$\text{NH}_3 + \text{CO}_2 + \text{NADH} + \text{H}^+$$

The glycine cleavage system is composed of four weakly associated proteins, P, T, L, and H, where protein T catalyzes the folate-dependent step (134). The reaction is started by the P protein, which contains pyridoxal phosphate. When isolated in the absence of the other proteins, it can slowly catalyze the exchange of the glycine carboxyl with CO_2 (135). H protein contains reduced lipoic acid and accepts the aminomethylene moiety initially produced. T protein then catalyzes the breakdown of the lipoic acid–bound aminomethylene group and transfers the methylene to H_4PteGlu, yielding 5,10-methylene-H_4PteGlu and releasing ammonia. L protein is a lipoamide dehydrogenase and reoxidizes the lipoic acid. Thus, the 2-C of glycine is the carbon that enters 1-carbon metabolism.

Glycine decarboxylation by perfused rat livers can be inhibited by β-hydroxybutyrate, suggesting that the glycine cleavage system is sensitive to the ratio of mitochondrial NADH/NAD^+ (136). The glycine cleavage system from bacterial sources was characterized in the 1960s by R. D. Sagers and others.

The compartmentation of folate metabolism was strikingly illustrated in a recent experiment from G. Weber's laboratory. Nonradioactive glycine was shown not to compete with, i.e., inhibit, the labeling of purines by radioactive formate (270). This means that the transfer of the 2-carbon to H_4folate forming 5,10-methenyl-H_4folate and then 10-formyl-H_4folate occurs in a different compartment (mitochondria) than that where the transfer of formate to H_4folate forming 10-formyl-H_4folate occurs (cytosol).

O. 10-Formyl-Tetrahydrofolate Dehydrogenase

10-Formyl-H_4PteGlu dehydrogenase (E.C.1.5.1.6) catalyzes the following reaction:

$$\text{10-Formyl-H}_4\text{PteGlu} + \text{NADP}^+ + \text{H}_2\text{O} \longrightarrow \text{H}_4\text{PteGlu} + \text{CO}_2 \text{ NADPH} + \text{H}^+ \quad (16)$$

The enzyme has an absolute requirement for NADP, rather than NAD, has a K_m for $(-)$10-formyl-H_4PteGlu$_1$ of 8 μM, is inhibited by the product $(-)$H$_4$PteGlu$_1$ with a K_i of about 1 μM, and has a M_r of about 320,000 (137). The enzyme shows only a slight preference for $(\pm)$10-formyl-H_4PteGlu$_3$ over the other folate polyglutamate substrates (138). The dehydrogenase reaction probably is used to eliminate excess 1-carbon units from the folate pool formed during the catabolism of histidine, tryptophan, glycine, serine, or formate. Using radioactive vehicles to introduce ^{14}C-1-carbon units into cellular folates, the ^{14}C-CO_2 released can be detected in the breath gases. The enzyme also catalyzes a weak hydrolase reaction resulting in the conversion of 10-formyl-H_4PteGlu to H_4PteGlu and formic acid (253).

P. Folate Polyglutamate Synthetase

The immediate product of folate biosynthesis in bacteria and plants is H_2PteGlu$_1$. In mammals, dietary folates are converted to folate monoglutamates during digestion and absorption. On the other hand, the intracellular form of the vitamin in all organisms examined to date is folate polyglutamate. Folate polyglutamate synthetase (FPGS) catalyzes the biosynthesis of the following reaction:

$$H_4PteGlu_n + ATP + glutamate \longrightarrow H_4PteGlu_{n+1} + ADP + P_i \qquad (17)$$

The peptide bond occurs in an oligo-γ-glutamyl linkage. Recently, however, a mixed folate oligoglutamyl peptide was reported in some bacterial cells, namely, pteroyltri-γ-glutamylpenta-α-glutamate (139).

The mammalian enzyme functions maximally at an alkaline pH, has a M_r of about 65000, and prefers $H_4PteGlu$, $H_2PteGlu$, or 10-formyl-$H_4PteGlu$ rather than PteGlu, 5,10-methylene-$H_4PteGlu$, or 5-methyl-$H_4PteGlu$ as the monoglutamyl substrate (254). The poor utilization of 5-methyl-$H_4PteGlu_1$ explains the defects in folate metabolism occurring during a deficiency in vitamin B_{12}, where serum folates (from the diet) entering cells as 5-methyl-$H_4PteGlu_1$ are forced to remain as the poorly polyglutamatable 5-methyl-$H_4PteGlu_1$ (86). The hog liver enzyme has an absolute requirement for thiols and for a monovalent cation such as K^+. The K_m for the co-substrate glutamate is extremely sensitive to pH.

FPGS from *Corynebacteria* prefers $H_4PteGlu_1$ as the monoglutamate substrate, whereas 5,10-methylene-$H_4PteGlu_2$ appears to be the preferred diglutamate substrate (140). This property of FPGS may constitute a mechanism for the fine tuning of folate metabolism.

Bacterial FPGS functions at an alkaline pH, as does the mammalian enzyme, but it is a bifunctional protein and contains $H_2PteGlu$ synthetase. $H_2PteGlu$ synthetase catalyzes the final set in the folate biosynthetic pathway (141).

Tracer [^{3}H]folic acid is converted to [^{3}H]folate polyglutamates in bacterial and mammalian cells. Polyglutamation of the longer chain length compounds is impaired when large amounts of folic acid are included in the rat diet or in the bacterial growth medium. Conversely, greater proportions of the longer chain length folates accumulate in the cell when small amounts of folic acid are used. The same sort of phenomenon is observed in vitro when high or low concentrations of folate monoglutamate substrate are incubated with purified FPGS.

Methotrexate, as well as its metabolite 7-hydroxy-MTX, are polyglutamated inside the cell (142). The polyglutamation of MTX can enhance its retention in cells and hence is desirable in cancer cells, though not in normal cells. Tumor cells that are especially sensitive to MTX appear to have an enhanced ability to form MTX polyglutamates (143).

Q. γ-Glutamylhydrolase

Conjugase is the trivial name for a group for γ-glutamylhydrolases that cleave folate polyglutamates to shorter chain length compounds, such as folate monoglutamates. Intestinal conjugases digest dietary folate polyglutamates to the absorbable monoglutamyl form. The pancreatic conjugase operates at an alkaline pH and cleaves $PteGlu_n$ to $PteGlu_2$ (chicken enzyme) or $PteGlu_1$ (rat enzyme) (144). The enzyme seems not to be excreted into the intestines and its function is not clear. The liver enzyme seems to be located in the lysosomes (145), and while its function is also not clear, it may hydrolyze useless breakdown products of folates cleaved at the labile C9–N10 bond.

Conjugase is distinguished by the fact that it recognizes γ-glutamyl peptide bonds. There is little specificity for the pteridine moiety. Chicken intestines contains a soluble endopeptidic conjugase catalyzing:

$$PteGlu_7 \longrightarrow PteGlu_2 + oligo\text{-}\gamma\text{-}Glu_5$$

as well as an exopeptidic conjugase that cleaves $PteGlu_2$ to PteGlu and Glu (146). Rat intestines contain a soluble endopeptidase catalyzing the hydrolysis of $PteGlu_7$ to PteGlu plus oligo-γ-Glu$_6$ (147). As mentioned in Section VI, the membrane-bound intestinal conjugase is an exopeptidase. The liver enzyme prefers to cleave longer chain length folates, with a tendency to endo- over exohydrolytic action (148). Some conjugases may be zinc metalloenzymes.

Folate transpeptidase catalyzes the exchange of a [^{14}C]amino acid, such as [^{14}C]glutamate or [^{14}C]methionine, for the oligo-γ-glutamyl chain, yielding PteGlu-[^{14}C]amino acid (149). Folate transpeptidase is probably identical to conjugase (149–151). This suggestion is not surprising as other transpeptidases, such as γ-glutamyltranspeptidase, catalyze both hydrolytic and transpeptidic reactions. the enzyme also catalyzes the ligation of folate monoglutamate with an amino acid (149). This reaction is to be expected as it has been known for many decades that peptidases readily catalyze peptide bond synthesis under specific conditions.

R. Dimethylglycine and Monomethylglycine Dehydrogenase

Folate may be a cofactor for dimethylglycine and monomethylglycine (sarcosine) dehydrogenase. These enzymes catalyze the following reactions, respectively:

Dimethylglycine + FAD + H$_4$PteGlu → monomethylglycine + FADH$_2$ +
 5,10-methylene-H$_4$PteGlu

Monomethylglycine + FAD + H$_4$PteGlu → glycine + FADH$_2$ +
 5,10-methylene-H$_4$PteGlu

These mitochondrial enzymes are used in the catabolism of choline to glycine. Both contain a covalently bound flavin cofactor, as well as noncovalently bound tetrahydrofolate (267). The enzymes can function at a maximal rate in the absence of the folate (152). However, the H$_4$folate effectively traps the formaldehyde product and thus minimizes the accumulation of this potentially toxic compound in the cell (268).

S. Regulation of 1-Carbon Metabolism

The following discussion largely applies to folate polyglutamates rather than to folate monoglutamates. This is because the monoglutamate is the transport form of the vitamin and comprises only a small fraction of the tissue folates, whereas the polyglutamate is the intracellular form.

Folates carry a 1-carbon unit, such as a methylene, methenyl, or methyl group. Generally, the primary source of the 1-carbon unit is the 3-carbon of serine (153,270). Hence, the activity of serine transhydroxymethylase in the conversion of H$_4$folate to 5,10-methylene-H$_4$folate is of primary importance in maintaining the availability of "activated" 1-carbon units. 5,10-Methylene-H$_4$folate is a substrate of T-synthase, an enzyme of vital importance to growing cells. This folate can be reduced to 5-methyl-H$_4$folate for use in methionine biosynthesis, or it can be oxidized to 10-formyl-H$_4$PteGlu, which is used in two steps of the purine biosynthetic pathway.

Folates are used for catabolic pathways as well as for anabolic reactions. For example, folate-dependent enzymes are used for the degradation of purines by purine-fermenting bacteria, as studied by J. C. Rabinowitz and co-workers during the 1960s.

Histidine catabolism requires folate in the tetrahydro- form, H$_4$PteGlu. The ring 2-carbon of this amino acid can be incorporated into the 1-carbon pool and then discharged as carbon dioxide. A large fraction of an "overdose" of histidine can be broken down within a few hours by a folate-dependent pathway (87).

The general status of folate metabolism inside a living animal or cells can be assessed by measuring the conversion of radioactive nutrients to $[^{14}C]CO_2$. Formic acid (154), serine (155), and glycine can be catabolized by tetrahydrofolate-dependent pathways to yield CO_2, among other products. The measurement of $[^{14}C]CO_2$ arising from the catabolism of [ring-2-^{14}C]histidine is highly specific and dependent on the availability of tetrahydrofolate in the cell, and thus represents a unique tool for probing changes in folate regulation in animals. The oxidation of the other nutrients, such as formate or serine, are only partially dependent on the availability of tetrahydrofolate.

Formic acid can enter the 1-carbon pool (reaction 6). Formic acid can thus compete with the 3-carbon of serine (reaction 3) for being utilized for purine biosynthesis, for example (156,270). Entry of formic acid into the 1-carbon pool occurs in tryptophan catabolism (157) as well as during methanol catabolism (158).

Other innovative methods for assessing the rate folate-dependent reactions in vivo include following the transfer of tritium from 5-formyl-[6-^{3}H]H$_4$folate to thymidylate (159) or following the release of tritium into water from [5-^{3}H]deoxyuridine (160).

Methionine biosynthesis in mammals seems to be controlled as follows (161). With an increase in tissue methionine, as during excessive dietary intake, there may be an increase in tissue AdoMet (247). AdoMet is a feedback inhibitor of 5,10-methylene-H$_4$PteGlu reductase. An increased inhibition would curb the production of 5-methyl-H$_4$folates, hence resulting in a slower turnover of methionine synthase and less production of methionine. This mode of feedback inhibition is relaxed during a methionine deficiency.

Defects in methionine synthase, such as that occurring during a deficiency in vitamin B$_{12}$, result in a decreased production of methionine and thus of AdoMet as well. This leads to a relaxation of the normal, partial inhibition of 5,10-methylene-H$_4$PteGlu reductase. The unfortunate consequence of this is that cellular folates are forced to accumulate in the 5-methyl- form at the expense of the tetrahydro-form. The end result of an inhibition of methionine synthase is the impairment of reactions dependent on the availability of tetrahydro- folates: 1) the biosynthesis of thymidylate and purines—compounds essential for growth; 2) the activity of folate polyglutamate synthase—an activity that is vital to continuing growth; and 3) the catabolism of histidine and formate. The catabolism of glycine is probably not impaired as this takes place in the mitochondria, apparently away from the cytosolic methionine synthase.

Methylfolate metabolism appears to be restricted to the cytosol and to be absent or minimal in the mitochondria (282). The activities of 5,10-methylene-H$_4$PteGlu reductase (283) and methionine synthetase (282) are quite low in rat liver mitochondria. Disturbances in folate metabolism arising during short-term treatment with nitrous oxide probably do not affect the mitochondria. One study, however, reported changes in the mitochondria during a vitamin B$_{12}$ deficiency (284).

The rate of turnover of the 1-carbon unit was studied using folate labeled in the 1-carbon group and in the vitamin itself, i.e., 5-[^{14}C]methyl-H$_4$[^{3}H]PteGlu (159) and 5-[^{14}C]formyl-H$_4$[^{3}H] PteGlu (269). Both studies involved cultured mammalian cells and revealed that the labeled 1-carbon group was rapidly transferred to cellular metabolites, leaving folates containing the tritium label only.

Following a period of metabolism, the 5-[^{14}C]methyl-H$_4$[^{3}H]PteGlu was recovered as 5-[nonradioactive]methyl-H$_4$[^{3}H]PteGlu, indicating that methionine synthase represented a rate-limiting step in 1-carbon metabolism (159). Following a period of metabolism, the 5-[^{14}C]formyl-H$_4$[^{3}H]PteGlu was recovered as 10-[nonradioactive]formyl-H$_4$[^{3}H]PteGlu, indicating that purine biosynthetic reactions represented rate-limiting steps in 1-carbon metabolism (269).

Mitochondria uniquely contain the glycine cleavage system, the "folate binding proteins" dimethyl- and monomethyl glycine dehydrogenases (163,181), a unique isozyme of serine hydroxymethyltransferase (163,164), and methionyl-tRNA transformylase. It is known that mitochondria also contain the trifunctional enzyme (165). The identity of the folates in this organelle and the relation between cytoplasmic and mitochondrial folates remains poorly defined. Preliminary work suggests that different subcellular fractions of the brain, for example, contain different types of folate polyglutamates (166).

The activity of T-synthase can increase dramatically during cell growth, i.e., after a partial hepatectomy (168) or in cell culture (169). The enzyme dramatically decreases in activity in the transition between the fetal stage and early infancy (249). T-Synthase has been reported to be cytoplasmic (271) and nuclear (167,171).

Recent studies revealed that T-synthetase and $H_2PteGlu$ reductase form a weak complex involved in DNA synthesis in bacterial (170), and perhaps in mammalian (171) cells. The nature of this complex has not be established conclusively, but it is thought to enhance the concentration of dTTP near the replication fork.

T-synthetase and $H_2PteGlu$ reductase activities reside on a single bifunctional protein in protozoa (172,173).

T. Folate Polyglutamates and Regulation of 1-Carbon Metabolism

Folate monoglutamates can be used in vivo in the catalysis of 1-carbon metabolism, as shown with cultured cells (159). Normally however, folate polyglutamates are the only detectable intracellular folate. The folate polyglutamates are as effective as, and in many cases considerably more effective than, the monoglutamates as substrates for purified enzymes. Cultured mammalian cell mutants lacking in FPGS are auxotrophic for glycine, adenine, and thymidine (174). This nutritional requirement for products of 1-carbon metabolism can be overcome if the cells are supplied with very high levels of folate monoglutamate. The interpretation is that polyglutamation promotes the concentration of and retention of the vitamin in the cell—concentration to levels much higher than normally supplied by the medium. In addition, once inside the cell, the polyglutamyl forms appear to be dramatically more active than the monoglutamyl forms in supporting metabolism, as determined with growing bacteria (175).

Aside from one report (176) there is little to indicate the folate polyglutamates regulate metabolic pathways in a stimulatory fashion. A variety of studies suggest that folate polyglutamates can regulate in an inhibitory manner. Kisliuk et al. (177) and Matthews and Baugh (122) demonstrated that dihydrofolate polyglutamates can inhibit the activities of T-synthase and 5,10-methylene-$H_4PteGlu$ reductase, respectively. Increases in cellular $H_2PteGlu_n$ can be provided by MTX treatment (179). The increased $H_2PteGlu_n$, which can inhibit AICAR transformylase with a K_i of about 3 μM, may contribute indirectly but importantly to the chemotherapeutic action of MTX (273).

Methionine is the most toxic amino acid. The liver uses special enzymatic machinery to limit methionine's toxic effects. The methyl groups from excess methionine can be funneled off by conversion to AdoMet followed by transfer to glycine, yielding monomethylglycine (sarcosine) (274). The conversion of glycine to monomethylglycine is catalyzed by glycine N-methyltransferase. Along with being used for monomethylglycine formation, AdoMet inhibits the activity of 5,10-methylene-$H_4PteGlu$ reductase, resulting in decreases in 5-methyl-H_4folates, as mentioned earlier.

There is some thought that decreases in cellular 5-methyl-H$_4$folate polyglutamate can directly activate glycine N-methyltransferase, thus speeding the detoxification of methionine (180). It is expected that the abovementioned mechanisms work in reverse during times of a methionine deficiency.

The toxic effects of excess methionine may also be limited by genetically controlled increases in glycine-N-methyltransferase (272) and decreases in methionine synthase (247).

There is some indication that folate penta- and hexaglutamates can work differently from each other in vivo. This is based on folate identification data showing that the shorter chain length compounds may occur as the 5-methyl- form, whereas the longer chain length folates may occur in the 10-formyl- form (40) or in the tetrahydro- form (58,87).

VIII. DEFICIENCY SIGNS

The author recently completed a review of the folate requirements and deficiency signs in a variety of animals (286).

A. Animals

1. Chickens

Folate deficiency in the chick results in reduced growth rate, anemia, and impaired feather growth (183).

2. Guinea Pigs

Dietary folate deficiency in the guinea pig results in decreases in plasma and red blood cell folates, leukopenia, growth failure, and death. Thenen (184) demonstrated that when a sulfa drug was included in the folate-deficient diet, the above symptoms worsened and animals lost hair and had diarrhea. The hematocrit dropped with the folate-deficient diet but only when sulfa drugs were used.

3. Rats

Rats do not develop signs of a folate deficiency with a folate-free purified diet, unless a sulfa drug or folate antagonist is added. Although leukopenia develops universally in rats fed folate-free sulfa drug–containing diets, anemia occurs less frequently. The following studies used folate-free diets containing sulfa drugs. Hautvast and Barnes (185) observed rapid drops in white blood cell and granulocyte counts. Kodicek and Carpenter (186) also described drops in white blood cell counts and demonstrated slow decreases in red blood cell counts and eventually anemia.

Nelson and Evans (187) raised prospective mothers on folate-deficient diets containing sulfa drug for 0–3 months. With the longer times mothers resorbed implantations and produced dead young and smaller litters. Thenen (188) raised prospective mothers on folate-deficient diets with and without sulfa drug for 7 weeks. Whole blood and liver folates were quite low in both dams and fetuses, especially where the sulfa drug diet had been used.

B. Humans

The sequence of signs in the development of folate deficiency in humans is as follows. Serum folate falls below normal after 3 weeks of folate deprivation. After 7 weeks there is an increase in the average number of lobes of the nuclei of the neutrophils (hypersegmentation). Red blood cell folates gradually fall and reach subnormal levels after 4 months of folate deprivation. At about 4.5 months the bone marrow becomes megaloblastic and anemia occurs (189). Lesions throughout the intestinal tract may occur, with the severe interruption of folate metabolism during chemotherapy with MTX (190).

IX. METHODS OF NUTRITIONAL ASSESSMENT

A number of biochemical tests can be used to assess folate status (191). The most useful are those which measure directly the folate levels in serum and red cells. Less commonly utilized are tests which measure folate function, such as excretion of formimioglutamic acid excretion and the suppression of [^{3}H]thymidine incorporation into DNA by added deocyuridine.

It should be stressed that, although these tests can indicate a functional folate deficiency, they do not necessarily pinpoint the reason for the deficiency. For instance, vitamin B_{12} deficiency causes a functional folate deficiency that cannot be distinguished by these tests from an actual folate deficiency, unless specific tests for vitamin B_{12} status are also carried out.

A. Assay of Folate Derivatives in Serum

The measurement of serum or plasma folate levels has been used extensively as an index of folate status in humans. 5-Methyl-H$_4$PteGlu is the main folate in serum. The levels of this compound have usually been measured by microbiological assay using *L. casei* as the test organism. Other bacteria such as *S. faecalis* or *P. cerevisiae* are not suitable for the assay of serum folates as they do not respond to 5-methyl-H$_4$PteGlu. Serum folate levels of less than 3 ng/ml indicate a folate deficiency, levels of 3–6 ng/ml a marginal deficiency, and levels above 6 ng/ml adequate folate status. One problem in interpreting serum folate values is that they reflect recent dietary intake, and a vitamin deficiency can be ascribed only where serum folate remains low over a period of time.

Radioassay procedures for the measurement of serum folate have been developed and radioassay kits are used extensively in clinical laboratories. These competitive protein-binding assays are similar to perform than microbiological assays and are not affected by antibiotics, which give false low values in microbiological assays. However, the affinities of different folate monoglutamates for the binding proteins vary considerably, making this assay method useful only for those tissues in which one form of folate predominates, i.e., serum or plasma (192). In addition, serum folate values obtained by using the different commercially available kits fluctuate considerably. Because of this, no absolute values can be given to indicate folate deficiency. Each laboratory has to define its own lower limits based on a large number of sample assays from a representative population of normal subjects.

In measurement of serum folate levels by both microbiological and radioassay methods, great care must be taken to prevent hemolysis of the samples, as red cell levels of folate are considerably higher than serum levels.

B. Assay of Red Cell Folates

Red cell folate levels reflect the body folate stores at the time of red cell formation and hence reflect a more accurate and less variable index of folate status than plasma folate levels.

Folates in the red cell are polyglutamate derivatives and must be hydrolyzed to monoglutamates prior to their assay by microbiological or radioassay techniques. As practically all the whole blood folate is located in the red cell, this is usually accomplished by lysing whole blood and allowing plasma conjugase to hydrolyze the polyglutamate derivatives. As in the assay of serum folates, it is essential to protect the vitamin with reducing agents, such as ascorbate. Red blood cell folate levels of less than 140 ng/ml packed cells, measured by microbiological assay, indicate folate deficiency, levels of 140–160 ng/ml suggest marginal status, and levels above 160 ng/ml indicate normal folate status.

C. Histidine Load Test

Formiminoglutamic acid, a product of histidine catabolism, is degraded to glutamate, NH_3 and CO_2 by folate-dependent reactions. During a folate deficiency formiminoglutamate excretion in the urine is elevated. Excretion is particularly high following an oral dose of L-histidine (11 g) (193). Although this test is sensitive to a folate deficiency and is used in scientific studies, it is affected by other diseases and generally is not used for diagnostic purposes.

D. Deoxyuridine Suppression Test

Labeled thymidine incorporation into the NDA of bone marrow cells is reduced in the presence of deoxyuridine due to the conversion of dUMP to dTMP, and the consequent competition between labeled and unlabeled dTTP (194). The extent of the competition is a measure of T-synthetase activity, which depends on the level of functional folate in the cell. Under conditions of low cellular folate, the conversion of dU to dTMP is reduced and the suppression of labeled dT incorporation into DNA is reduced. This test, known as the dU suppression test, can distinguish between folate and vitamin B_{12} deficiency as, in the former case, addition of any folate to the medium increases the suppression rate. In the case of a vitamin B_{12} deficiency, addition of methylcobalamin or any folate (with the exception of 5-methyl-H_4PteGlu) increases the suppression. Although this test has been used experimentally, it has not found widespread usage, partly because of the difficulty in obtaining marrow cells from patients on a routine basis. Attempts to extend this test to other cells, such as lymphocytes, have met with mixed success.

X. NUTRITIONAL REQUIREMENTS

A. Animals

1. Chickens

Luckey et al. (195) determined that the folic acid requirement for chicks was about 0.25 mg folic acid/kg diet in the absence of sulfa drug and about 1.0 mg folic acid/kg diet with the drug. Criteria for reponses were growth, hemoglobin, hematocrit, and feathering. In another study the folate requirement for chicks was found to be 1 mg folate/kg diet using purified folate polyglutamate (vitamin B_c) as the source of vitamin (196). This folate level gave the same hematological responses as diets containing higher levels of folate and nearly the same responses as with a crude, unpurified diet.

2. Guinea Pigs

The folate requirement for the guinea pig is 6 mg folic acid/kg diet. Reid et al. (197) fed 2-day-old guinea pig diets containing 10 graded levels of folic acid. Although 3 mg folic acid/kg diet was adequate for maximal growth and red blood cell counts, hematocrit, and hemoglobin, 6 mg/kg was needed for maximal leukocyte counts.

3. Rats

The vitamin requirement for the rat may be between 5 and 20 μg/day as determined by giving folate supplements to severely folate-deficient animals (198). The rats had been maintained on semipurified diets containing sulfa drugs. The criteria for the requirement were recoveries of normal leukocyte counts and normal growth rates and lack of alopecia and spleen infarcts. As the food intake was stated to be about 5 g/day, the folate requirement may be between 1 and 4 mg folic acid/kg diet.

A more accurate estimation of an animal's requirement for folate can be made where sulfasuxidine is included in the diet. This sulfa drug prevents the growth of gut bacteria that normally provide the host with some of the vitamin. The prolonged use of sulfa drugs in animal experiments may lead to certain pathological conditions such as urinary tract stones (199).

B. Humans

1. Adult

The recommended dietary allowance for the adult male is 200 μg per day (210). The minimal requirement may be about 50 μg/day, as determined by the amount of synthetic PteGlu needed to maintain serum folate levels in three normal subjects (200). The experimental subjects were fed supplements of PteGlu (25–100 μg/day) and diets virtually free of the vitamin for 7 weeks. Only in the subject receiving 25 μg did the serum folate fall below 5 ng/ml. In another study with women, subjects were fed a folate-deficient diet (10 μg/day) for 4 weeks. Feeding the subjects 300 μg of food folate, following the period of depletion, supported a rise and restoration of plasma folate levels (281). It was concluded that the minimal requirement for women is 200–300 μg of food folate per day.

Herbert (201) recommended that 100 μg of PteGlu per day (oral or intramuscular) be given in therapeutic trials of subjects suspected of a deficiency. Although this value was derived from studies of hospital patients, it helps to define the requirement for healthy adults.

2. Pregnancy

The folate requirement in pregnancy is about 350 μg/day, as determined in studies of pregnant women supplemented with PteGlu. In pregnancy, increasing dietary folic acid by supplements of from 0 to 125–355 μg/day oral PteGlu were associated with drops in the frequency of postpartum megaloblastic anemia of from 1.4% to 0.7–0.3%, respectively. No further benefit was found with 530 μg/day, as determined by peripheral blood appearance. The food folate intake was estimated as less than 50 μg/day for the majority of the pregnant women (202,203). Similarly, other workers found that the frequency of prepartum megaloblastosis dropped from 13 to 5% when diets were supplemented with 100 μg PteGlu, as determined by marrow appearance. The average food folate intake was determined to be 675 μg/day. None of the women became anemic (204,205). Most of the women in the above studies received iron supplements.

3. Lactation

In lactation, folate supplements may be needed only when lactation is lengthy and the diet during pregnancy had been low in folate. In lactating Bantu women, deterioration of folate metabolism was prevented by folate supplements (5 mg/day, oral PteGlu). This was determined by serum folate, folic acid clearance from blood, and urinary formiminoglutamic acid (206). The actual minimal folate requirement in lactating women is lower and may be 200–300 μg/day (207).

4. Infant Folate Requirement

The folate requirement for infants may be about 5 μg/kg body weight per day (25–50 μg/day). This is based on the observation that a small group of healthy infants fed 5 μg PteGlu per kg body weight per day grew at a faster rate than those fed 3.5 or 4.3 μg/kg per day. The values for hemoglobin and for red blood cell folate were generally not different for the groups fed 3.6 μg and 5 μg (208).

The folate requirement might be expected to be about 20 μg of food folate per day, as determined by the total folate provided per day by human milk from lactating mothers (209).

Twice the stated requirement may actually be needed where the requirement had been determined with supplements of synthetic PteGlu, where the actual source of folate is to be food folate. For example, in experiments conducted by Willoughby (202) and Herbert (200), folate supplements were in the form of PteGlu and not food folate. The suggestion is based on findings that food folates (reduced folate polyglutamates) may be about half as available as PteGlu administered in water.

XI. FACTORS THAT INFLUENCE VITAMIN STATUS

Dietary folate deficiency megaloblastic anemia may occur in about one third of all pregnant women worldwide. Nutritional megaloblastic anemia is associated more with a folate deficiency than a vitamin B_{12} deficiency. Folate requirements are increased in a variety of conditions, such as pregnancy, lactation, and infancy. These are best defined by cases of folate deficiency megaloblastic anemia that fail to respond to small doses of PteGlu (50–100 μg) but do respond to larger doses of the vitamin.

A. Pregnancy and Lactation

An increased incidence of folate deficiency and megaloblastic anemia has been reported during pregnancy and the puerperium with an incidence of 3–5% in developed countries (212). The primary source of this deficiency is the increased nutritional need due to the growth of the fetus. The anemia of pregnancy may be associated with a high frequency of a folate deficiency, as determined in a study from Florida (276). The anemia presented as hematocrit values below the accepted norm for pregnancy, and the folate deficiency was indicated by low red blood cell folates.

A variety of trials have been conducted concerning the benefit of folate and iron supplements to the mother and infant (277). Some of these trials showed a benefit. Most did not. Folate or iron deficiency anemia continues to be a problem in a fraction of the general population. Supplements should be given to women identified on an individual basis as being deficient and to groups of women identified as being at risk, such as those described in the Florida study. Although the megaloblastic anemia of pregnancy may be common in Africa, Southeast Asia, and South America, nationwide programs of folate supplementation may result in a situation where cases of anemia are restricted to victims of pernicious anemia (278).

The association of abruptio placentae, a complication of pregnancy, with a folate deficiency has been controversial, as data from different studies have been conflicting (279).

B. Age

In the first month after birth, the infant may exhibit a drop in blood folate levels. The folate requirement of the infant is higher than that of the adult on a unit body weight basis, reflecting the rapid growth rate of the infant. There has been some concern about the megaloblastic anemia responding to folic acid in low birth weight infants. There is no reason, however, to supplement all low birth weight infants with folic acid (280). Infants should not be raised on goat milk, as this milk is folate deficient and may result in anemia in the infant.

The low-income elderly and institutionalized elderly are a group that may be at risk for folate deficiency (213). The risk reflects an inadequate diet rather than an increased requirement for the vitamin.

C. Drugs

1. Folate Antagonists

Folate antagonists are used to kill cancer cells and to treat infections. The most widely used drug is MTX, which inhibits $H_2PteGlu$ reductase. Another very common drug is 5FU (see Sec. VII.G). MTX is toxic and can lead to a functional folate deficiency and anemia. With signs of liver damage (serum transaminase) or neurological damage (seizures) its use should be interrupted and a large rescue doses of 5-formyl-H_4PteGlu may be given. 5FU is not a very toxic drug.

MTX is used to treat a variety of neoplasms, such as choriocarcinoma and cancer of the head and neck (211). A "rescue dose" of 5-formyl-H_4PteGlu follows the MTX dose. A recent report described the use of MTX to treat childhood acute lymphocytic leukemia (255). Although low doses of MTX have been used here, higher and more effective doses are possible where the high dose is followed by the large rescue dose (30 mg of 5-formyl-H_4PteGlu/square meter). The mechanism of action of the rescue dose is not fully understood.

Pneumonia due to protozoal infections is the most common source of mortality in AIDS patients (256). Therapy of the pneumonia may include large doses of folate (20 mg of 5-formyl-H_4PteGlu/square meter). The protozoan does not take up the folate, and hence the folate rescues the patient from the antifolate drug but does not rescue the protozoan.

Recently there has been a renewed interest in the treatment of rheumatoid arthritis by MTX (214). Here, as with the treatment of cancer and other diseases such as psoriasis, the patient should be monitored for anemia and other forms of MTX toxicity.

2. Anticonvulsants

A small percentage of epileptics treated with diphenylhydantoin develop a folate deficiency and anemia (215,240). Studies with mice (216) and humans (217) suggest that increased folate excretion may be a contributing factor. Large doses of folic acid (5–30 mg/day) have been used to reverse the hematological signs of folate deficiency (237), though the folic acid may exacerbate the seizures in certain patients.

It has been claimed that supplementing folate-deficient epileptics with oral PteGlu (3 × 5 mg/day) is associated with improvements in the mental state, but with increases in epileptic seizures (241). These claims were not supported by other studies (242). One should be prepared to discontinue folic acid therapy when the seizures appear to be aggravated by the vitamin.

3. Ethanol

Low serum folates are commonly encountered in alcoholics, largely because of poor nutritional habits. Chronic alcoholism is probably the major cause of folate deficiency in the United States. An antifolate effect of ethanol was shown in studies of humans (218). Megaloblastic anemia could be induced with a low-folate diet after 6–10 weeks, whereas the inclusion of alcohol with this diet provoked anemia at an earlier time, 2–3 weeks (218).

4. Other Drugs

Oral contraceptive use has been associated with the development of a folate deficiency (219). In some cases this rare association may be due mainly to other factors, whereas in others it may have nothing to do with the oral contraceptive use (220).

D. Disease

1. Hemolytic Anemias

Megaloblastic anemia due to a folate deficiency is associated with various hemolytic diseases. With increased damage to red blood cells there is increased cell division in the bone marrow, and it is thought the increased cell division provokes a greater requirement for folate.

2. Malabsorption

Diseases associated with general malabsorption by the gut, such as celiac sprue and tropical sprue, result in a folate deficiency. Folate deficiency can also occur in Crohn's disease and ulcerative colitis because of the malabsorption (221). Congential disorders associated with folate malabsorption have been reported, implying a specific transport system for the vitamin (222). The resulting deficiency can be relieved by large oral doses of the vitamin (40–100 mg).

3. Malignant Diseases

The anticancer drug MTX provokes a functional deficiency in folate in the cancer cell as well as in the host (see Sec. XI.C). In some neoplastic diseases, particularly cancer of the head and neck, the illness itself seems to provoke a folate deficiency (248). Folate metabolism may be altered in the cancer cell. 6-Hydroxymethylpterin is excreted in elevated amounts in the urine of cancer patients (93).

Megaloblastic anemia is a sign of a severe deficiency of folate, of course. But megaloblastic features have also been found in cervical cells, as during pernicious anemia or with steroid oral contraceptives (234). Cervical cells that are dysplasiac (precancerous) also have megaloblastic features. The group from the University of Alabama postulated that these cells may have developed some sort of deficiency in the vitamin. Supplements of folic acid (10 mg/day) seemed to provoke a trend toward normal cytological features and halt the progression toward carcinoma (235). Cervical smears provided suggestive data, whereas the examination of biopsies yielded more dramatic results. Cervical dysplasia may or may not be associated with oral contraceptive use (236).

Because of the interesting results from the cervical study, the Alabama group studied the effect of folate supplements on another precancerous cell type, atypical bronchial squamous metaplasia of smokers. They found that the metaplasia improved in a fraction of the smokers taking folate (10 mg/day) when compared to those taking the placebo (257).

E. Genetics

A number of inborn errors of folate metabolism have been described (258). These include patients with defective absorption affecting both the intestines and the central nervous system and patients with lowered levels of various folate-dependent enzymes. All these defects lead to an increased folate requirement and, with the possible exception of for-miminotransferase deficiency, to mental retardation.

A deficiency in 5,10-methylene-H_4PteGlu reductase is distinguishable from the homocystinuria observed in a deficiency of cystathionine synthetase, in that plasma methionine levels are not elevated (223).

Freeman et al. (229) described a psychiatric patient with homocysteinuria and low 5,10-methylene-H_4PteGlu reductase. This patient seemed to require large doses of folic acid (20 mg/day). Other patients with similar biochemical symptoms but perhaps different diseases were not helped by the folic acid (230).

Santiago-Borrero et al. (231) described a patient with defective intestinal absorption of folate who responded hematologically to the injected folic acid (15 mg every 3 weeks). It is possible that smaller doses could have been effective. Similarly, Lanzkowsky et al. (232) found a patient with defective folate absorption who responded to injections of folic acid (0.25 mg/day) or oral folic acid (40 mg/day). but not to smaller doses of folic acid (0.25 mg/day).

Tauro et al. (233) described two patients with megaloblastosis and lowered H_2PteGlu reductase. The megaloblastosis disappeared with injections of large amounts of 5-formyl-H_3PteGlu (3 mg/day), but not with injections of PteGlu.

Neural tube defects (NTD) are rare, fortunately, but are one of the more common congenital malformations. There has been some association of NTD with lower social classes and with low levels of vitamins in the pregnant mother's serum. Mothers with a previous NTD birth are at risk for repeated NTD births, and studies on mothers with prior NTD births revealed that folate (259) or multivitamin (260,261) supplements seemed to prevent NTD in subsequent births. The results from these three studies on preventing repeated NTD births seen quite striking and are difficult to ignore. Although folate or multivitamin supplements may be useful, a study by J. M. Scott's group revealed that there may be no association between folate deficiency and NTD (262).

Fragile X syndrome is commonly associated with mental retardation. As discussed in Section VII.G, the anticancer drugs MTX and FU may introduce multiple breaks in DNA. Also, simply growing cultured cells in the absence of folate and thymine results in chromosomal breaks, and these breaks occur at distinct sites (263). Where the cells (lymphocytes) are taken from a person with "fragile X syndrome" and then cultured without folate or thymine, a break occurs at a unique site called Xq27 (264). Efforts to find some sort of defect in folate metabolism in these retarded subjects have not been successful.

F. Vitamin B$_{12}$ Deficiency

Symptoms of a folate deficiency can occur in pernicious anemia or with a nutritional vitamin B$_{12}$ deficiency (224). The megaloblastic anemia of B$_{12}$ deficiency may be due to impaired utilization of cellular folates as well as to poor retention of folates from the diet (Sec. VII.S). Decreased activity of the vitamin B$_{12}$-requiring enzyme, methionine synthetase, leads to the accumulation of trapping of tissue folates in the 5-methyl- form, a form which has no use except for regenerating methionine.

G. Other Nutrients

A dietary iron deficiency may provoke symptoms of a folate deficiency (225,226). Normal serum and red cell folates may occur during a folate deficiency where there is also a more severe iron deficiency. The vitamin deficiency may be reflected by low tissue folate or by an abnormal dU supression test (227). Recent studies indicate that milk folates may drop where the mother is fed an iron-deficient diet, though it is not clear if other components of the milk drop as well (265).

XII. EFFICACY OF PHARMACOLOGICAL DOSES

Supplements of over 0.4 mg/day are considered to be pharmacological doses. Since these large doses may be difficult to consume in the form of food sources, folate pills may be preferred. Pharmacological doses are most commonly used in the "rescue dose" during cancer chemotherapy. Larges doses may also be used in nutritional deficiencies where the patient is expected to take the supplement only sporadically. However, it might be added that most of the excess folate may be lost in the urine.

Neurological symptoms of folate deficiency are rarely encountered but have been documented (228). Large doses of folic acid (10 mg/day) may eliminate a group of associated problems, namely restless legs, tired legs, and stocking and glove-type hypoesthesia. Hematological signs of folate deficiency generally were not severe.

XIII. HAZARDS OF HIGH DOSES

Folic acid is not very toxic. In adults no adverse effects were noted after 400 mg/day for 5 months or after 10 mg/day for 5 years (243). The acute toxicity (LD$_{50}$) is about 500 mg/kg body weight for rats and rabbits (238). Chronic doses of 10–75 mg PteGlu/kg body weight (intraperitoneal) can injure the kidneys, probably because of precipitation of the PteGlu at acidic pH (244,245).

Folic acid (5 mg/day) can delay and prevent the hematological relapses in patients with pernicious anemia (238). However, folic acid cannot prevent the irreversible neurological lesions of a vitamin B$_{12}$ deficiency or of pernicious anemia (238,239). The danger here is that the folate supplements can obscure the diagnosis of the B$_{12}$ deficiency; they can prevent anemia while permitting neurological damage.

REFERENCES

1. R. L. Blakley, in *The Biochemistry of Folic Acid and Related Pteridines, Frontiers of Biology*, Vol. 13, A Neuberger and E. L. Tatum (Eds.) North-Holland, Amsterdam, 1969.
2. O. D. Bird, V. M. McGlohon, and J. W. Vaitkus, *Can. J. Microbiol., 15*:465 (1969).

3. S. D. Wilson and D. W. Horne, *Analyt. Biochem.*, *142*:529 (1984).

4. T. Markkanen, S. Virtanen, P. Himanen, and R. Pajula, *Acta Haematol.*, *48*:213 (1972).

5. G. B. Henderson, E. M. Zevely, and F. M. Huennekens, *J. Biol. Chem.*, *252*:3760 (1977).

6. L. M. Kozloff, M. Lute, and L. K. Crosby, *J. Virol.*, *16*:1391 (1975).

7. M. C. Li, R. Hertz, and D. M. Bergenstal, *New Engl. J. Med.*, *259*:66 (1958).

8. D. A. Mathews, R. A. Alden, J. Y. Bolin, D. J. Filman, S. T. Freer, R. Hamlin, W. Hol, R. L. Kisliuk, E. J. Pastore, L. T. Plante, N. Xuong, and J. Kraut, *J. Biol. Chem.*, *253*:6946 (1978).

9. M. Friedkin, L. T. Plante, E. J. Crawford, and M. Crumm, *J. Biol. Chem.*, *250*:5614 (1975).

10. J. Burchanall and G. Hitchings, *Mol. Pharmacol.*, *1*:216 (1965).

11. R. L. Kisliuk, Y. Gaumont, and C. M. Baugh, *J. Biol. Chem.*, *259*:4100 (1974).

12. G. K. Smith, P. A. Benkovic, and S. J. Benkovic, *Biochemistry*, *20*:4034 (1981).

13. C. M. Baugh, J. Stevens, and C. Krumdieck, *Biochim. Biophys. Acta*, *212*:116 (1970).

14. B. L. Hutchings, J. H. Mowat, J. J. Olesen, E. L. R. Stokstad, J. H. Boothe, C. W. Waller, R. B. Angier, J. Semb, and Y. Subbarow, *J. Biol. Chem.*, *170*:323 (1947).

15. M. N. Williams, M. Poe, N. J. Greenfield, J. M. Hirshfield, and K. Hoogstein, *J. Biol. Chem.*, *248*:6375 (1973).

16. A. Lockshin, R. G. Moran, and P. V. Danenberg, *Proc. Natl. Acad. Si., USA*, *76*:750 (1979).

17. G. M. Brown, *J. Biol. Chem.*, *237*:536 (1962).

18. W. P. Bullard, L. J. Farina, P. R. Farina, and S. J. Benkovic, *J. Am. Chem. Soc.*, *96*:7295 (1974).

19. C. W. Waller, B. L. Hutchings, J. H. Mowat, E. L. R. Stokstad, J. H. Boothe, R. B. Angier, J. Semb, Y. Subbarow, D. B. Cosulich, M. J. Fahrenbach, M. E. Hultquist, E. Kuh, E. H. Northey, D. R. Seeger, J. P. Sickels, and J. M. Smith, *J. Am. Chem. Soc.*, *70*:19 (1948).

20. E. C. Taylor, R. Portnoy, D. Hochstetter, and T. Kobayashi, *J. Org. Chem.*, *40*:2347 (1975).

21. H. Mautner and Y. Kim, *J. Org. Chem.*, *40*:3447 (1975).

22. J. H. Boothe, J. H. Mowat, B. L. Hutchings, R. B. Angier, C. W. Waller, E. L. R. Stokstad, J. Semb, A. L. Gazzola, and Y. Subbarow, *J. Am. Chem. Soc.*, *70*:1099 (1948).

23. J. Meienhofer, P. M. Jacobs, H. A. Godwin, and I. H. Rosenberg, *J. Org. Chem.*, *35*:4137 (1970).

24. R. L. Blakley, *Nature* (Lond.), *188*:231 (1960).

25. B. Roth, M. E. Hultquist, M. J. Fahrenbach, D. B. Cosulich, H. P. Broquist, J. A. Brokman, J. M. Smith, R. P. Parker, E. L. R. Stokstad, and T. H. Jukes, *J. Am. Chem. Soc.*, *74*:3247 (1952).

26. R. L. Blakley, *Biochem. J.*, *65*:331 (1957).

27. I. Chanarin and J. Perry, *Biochem. J.*, *105*:633 (1967).

28. D. Chippel and K. G. Scrimgeour, *Can. J. Biochem.*, *48*:999 (1970).

29. G. Gapski, J. Whiteley, and F. M. Huennekens, *Biochemistry*, *10*:2930 (1971).

30. P. B. Rowe and G. P. Lewis, *Biochemistry*, *12*:1962 (1973).

31. J. C. Rabinowitz and W. E. Pricer, *J. Am. Chem. Soc.*, *78*:5702 (1956).

32. R. G. Kallen and W. P. Jencks, *J. Biol. Chem.*, *241*:5851 (1966).

33. M. J. Osborn, P. T. Talbert, and F. M. Huennekens *J. Am. Chem. Soc.*, *82*:4921 (1960).

34. S. F. Zakrzewski, *J. Biol. Chem.*, *241*:2957 (1966).

35. P. F. Nixon and J. R. Bertino, *Methods Enzymol.*, *18*:661 (1971).

36. Y. S. Shin, K. U. Buehring, and E. L. R. Stokstad, *J. Biol. Chem.*, *247*:7266 (1972).

37. K. Uyeda and J. C. Rabinowitz, *Analyt. Biochem.*, *6*:100 (1963).

38. B. L. Hutchings, E. L. R. Stokstad, J. H. Boothe, J. H. Mowat, C. W. Waller, R. B. Angier, J. Semb, and Y. Subbarow, *J. Biol. Chem.*, *168*:705 (1947).

39. B. Shane, *Am. J. Clin. Nutr.*, *35*:599 (1982).

40. I. Eto and C. L. Krumdieck, *Analyt. Biochem.*, *120*:323 (1982).

41. T. Brody, B. Shane, and E. L. R. Stokstad, *Analyt. Biochem.*, *92*:501 (1979).

42. K. U. Buehring, T. Tamura, and E. L. R. Stokstad, *J. Biol. Chem.*, *249*:1081 (1974).

43. S. A. Kashani and B. A. Cooper, *Analyt. Biochem.*, *146*:40 (1985).
44. O. D. Bird, M. V. McGlohon, and J. W. Vaitkus, *Analyt. Biochem.*, *12*:18 (1965).
45. A. J. A. Wright and D. R. Phillips, *Brit. J. Nutr.*, *53*:569 (1985).
46. F. M. Dong and S. M. Oace, J. Agric. Food Chem., 23:534 (1975).
47. Y. S. Shin, E. S. Kim, J. E. Watson, and E. L. R. Stokstad, *Can. J. Biochem.*, *53*:338 (1975).
48. S. Butterfield and D. H. Calloway, *J. Am. Diet. Assoc.*, *60*:310 (1972).
49. Y. Matoth, A. Pinkas, and C. Sroka, *Am. J. Clin. Nutr.*, *16*:356 (1965).
50. F. M. Dong and S. M. Oace, *J. Am. Diet. Assoc.*, *62*:162 (1973).
51. T. Tamura and E. L. R. Stokstad, *Br. J. Haematol.*, *25*:513 (1973).
52. J. Leichter, V. P. Switzer, and A. F. Landymore, *Nutr. Rep. Int.*, *18*:475 (1978).
53. J. Leichter, A. F., Landymore, and C. Krumdieck, *Am. J. Clin. Nutr.*, *32*:92 (1979).
54. J. R. Wagner, K. Batra, and E. L. R. Stokstad, *Can. J. Biochem.*, *55*:865 (1977).
55. C. Chan, Y. S. Shin, and E. L. R. Stokstad, *Can. J. Biochem.*, *51*:1617 (1973).
56. P. M. Keagy, E. L. R. Stokstad, and D. A. Fellers, *Cereal Chem.*, *52*:348 (1975).
57. Y. S. Shin, K. U. Buehring, and E. L. R. Stokstad, *Arch. Biochem. Biophys.* *163*:211 (1974).
58. T. Brody, Y. S. Shin, and E. L. R. Stokstad, *J. Neurochem.*, *27*:409 (1976).
59. K. Hoppner, B. Lampi, and D. E. Perrin, *Can. Inst. Food. Sci. Technol. J.*, *5*:60 (1972).
60. A. D. Hurdle, D. Barton, and I. Searles *Am. J. Clin. Nutr.*, *21*:1202 (1968).
61. R. Santini, C. Brewster, and C. E. Butterworth, *Am. J. Clin. Nutr.*, *14*:205 (1964).
62. K. Hoppner, *J. Inst. Can. Tech. Alim.*, *4*:51 (1971).
63. K. Hoppner, B. Lampi, and D. E. Perrin, *J. Am. Diet. Assoc.*, *63*:536 (1973).
64. M. F. Chen, J. W. Hill, and P. A. McIntyre, *J. Nutr.*, *113*:2192 (1983).
65. R. G. Cooper, T. Chen, and M. A. King, *J. Am. Diet. Assoc.*, *73*:406 (1978).
66. J. O'Broin, I. Temperley, J. Brown, and J. M. Scott, *Am. J. Clin. Nutr.*, *28*:438 (1975).
67. N. Grossowicz, M. Rachmilewitz, and G. Itzak, *Proc. Soc. Exp. Biol. Med.*, *150*:77 (1975).
68. N. Colman, R. Green, and J. Metz, *Am. J. Clin. Nutr.*, *28*:459 (1975).
69. N. Colman, M. Barker, R. Green, and J. Metz, *Am. J. Clin. Nutr.*, *27*:339 (1974).
70. N. Colman, J. Larsen, M. Barker, E. Barker, R. Green, and J. Metz, *Am. J. Clin. Nutr.*, *28*:465 (1975).
71. C. M. Baugh, C. L. Krumdieck, H. J. Baker, and C. E. Butterworth, *J. Clin. Invest.*, *50*:2009 (1971).
72. C. H. Halsted, C. M. Baugh, and C. E. Butterworth, *Gastroenterol.*, *68*:261 (1975).
73. C. J. Chandler, T. T. Y. Wang, and C. H. Halsted, *J. Biol. Chem.*, *261*:928 (1986).
74. T. T. Y. Wang, A. M. Reisenauer, and C. H. Halsted, *J. Nutr.*, *115*:814 (1985).
75. J. Selhub and I. H. Rosenberg, *J. Biol. Chem.*, *256*:4489 (1981).
76. R. F. Pratt and B. A. Cooper, *J. Clin. Invest.*, *50*:455 (1971).
77. H. Dencker, M. Jägerstaad, and A.-K. Westesson, *Acta Hepato-Gastroenterol.*, *23*:140 (1976).
78. J. Kiil, M. Jägerstaad, and L. Elsborg, *Internat. J. Vit. Res.*, *49*:296 (1979).
79. S. E. Steinberg, C. L. Campbell, and R. S. Hillman, *J. Clin. Invest.*, *64*:83 (1979).
80. G. B. Henderson, M. R. Suresh, K. S. Vitols, and F. M. Huennekens *Cancer Res.*, *46*:1639 (1986).
81. C.-H. Yang, M. Dembo, and F. M. Sirotnak, *J. Membrane Biol.*, *75*:11 (1983).
82. J. Galivan, *Arch. Biochem. Biophys.*, *206*:113 (1981).
83. C.-H. Yang, F. M. Sirotnak, and M. Dembo, *J. Membrane Biol.*, *79*:285 (1984).
84. D. W. Horne, W. Y. Briggs, and C. Wagner, *J. Biol. Chem.*, *253*:3529 (1978).
85. G. B. Henderson, J. M. Tsuji, and H. P. Kumar, *Cancer Res.*, *46*:1633 (1986).
86. J. D. Cook, D. J. Cichowicz,, S. George, A. Lawler, and B. Shane, *Biochemistry*, *26*:530 (1987).
87. T. Brody, J. E. Watson, and E. L. R. Stokstad, *Biochemistry*, *21*:276 (1982).
88. J. C. Rabinowitz and R. H. Himes, *Fed. Proc., Fed. Am. Soc. Exp. Biol.*, *19*:963 (1960).
89. B. Shane, *J. Biol. Chem.*, *255*:5649 (1980).
90. S. K. Foo, R. M. McSloy, C. Rousseau, and B. Shane, *J. Nutr.*, *112*:1600 (1982).

91. N. Colman and V. Herbert, *Ann. Rev. Med., 31*,433 (1980).

92. M. Murphy, M. Keating, P. Boyle, D. G. Weir, and J. M. Scott, *Biochem. Biophys. Res. Commun., 71*:1017 (1976).

93. B. Stea, P. S. Backlund, P. B. Berkey, A. K. Cho, B. C. Halpern, R. M. Halpern, and R. A. Smith, *Cancer Res., 38*:2378 (1978).

94. R. T. Schimke, *Cell, 37*:705 (1984).

95. B. D. Mariani, D. L. Slate, and R. T. Schimke, *Proc. Natl. Acad., Sci. USA, 78*:4985 (1981).

96. L. Schirch and M. Ropp, *Biochemistry, 6*:253 (1967).

97. R. G. Matthews, J. Ross, C. M. Baugh, J. D. Cook, and L. Davis, *Biochemistry, 21*:1230 (1982).

98. J. L. Paukert, L. D. 'Ari Straus, and J. C. Rabinowitz, *J. Biol. Chem., 251*:5104 (1976).

99. L. U. L. Tan, E. J. Drury, R. E. MacKenzie, *J. Biol. Chem., 252*:1117 (1977).

100. L. G. Ljungdahl, *J. Biol. Chem., 259*:3499 (1984).

101. K. G. Scrimgeour and F. M. Huennekens, *Biochem. Biophys. Res. Commun., 2*:230 (1960).

102. N. R. Meija and R. E. MacKenzie, *J. Biol. Chem., 260*:14616 (1985).

103. G. K. Smith, W. T. Mueller, P. A. Benkovic, and S. J. Benkovic, *Biochemistry, 20*:1241 (1981).

104. V. T. Chan and J. E. Baggott, *Biochim. Biophys. Acta, 702*:99 (1982).

105. S. C. Daubner, J. L. Schrimsher, F. J. Schendel, M. Young, S. Henikoff, D. Patterson, J. Stubbe, and S. J. Benkovic, *Biochemistry, 24*:7059 (1985).

106. H. Tabor and L. Wyngarden, *J. Biol. Chem., 234*:1830 (1959).

107. J. E. Baggott and C. L. Krumdieck, *Biochemistry, 18*:1036 (1979).

108. W. T. Mueller and S. J. Benkovic, *Biochemistry, 20*:337 (1981).

109. S. M. Oace, K. Tarczy- Hornoch, and E. L. R. Stokstad, *J. Nutr., 95*:445 (1968).

110. W. Shive, W. W. Ackermann, M. Gordon, M. E. Getzendaner, and R. E. Eakin, *J. Am. Chem. Soc., 69*:725 (1947).

111. J. C. Sonne, J. M. Buchanan, and A. M. Delluva, *J. Biol. Chem., 173*:69 (1948).

112. B. R. Bochner and B. N. Ames, Cell, 29:929 (1982).

113. R. L. Sabina, D. Patterson, and E. W. Holmes, *J. Biol. Chem., 260*:6107 (1985).

114. D. V. Santi and C. S. McHenry, *Proc. Natl. Acad. Sci., USA, 69*:1855 (1972).

115. P. V. Danenberg, R. J. Langenbach, and C. Heidelberger, *Biochemistry, 13*:926 (1974).

116. W. L. Washtien and D. V. Santi, *Cancer Res., 39*:3397 (1979).

117. P. V. Danenberg and K. D. Danenberg, *Biochemistry, 17*:4018 (1978).

118. J. R. Bertino, *Seminars in Oncology, 10*(Suppl. 2):1 (1983).

119. M. Goulian, B. Bleile, and B. Y. Tseng, *Proc. Natl. Acad. Sci. USA, 77*:1956 (1980).

120. D. Ayusawa, K. Shimizu, H. Koyama, K. Takeishi, and T. Seno, *J. Biol. Chem., 258*:12448 (1983).

121. C. Kutzbach and E. L. R. Stokstad, *Biochim. Biophys. Acta, 250*:459 (1971).

122. R. G. Matthews and C. M. Baugh, *Biochemistry, 19*:2040 (1980).

123. K. Fujii and F. M. Huennekens, in *Biochemical Aspects of Nutrition, Proceedings of the First Congress of the Federation of Asian and Oceanic Biochemists*, K. Yagi (Ed.), University Park Press, Baltimore, 1979, p. 173.

124. D. D. Koblin, J. E. Watson, J. E. Deady, E. L. R. Stokstad, and E. I. Eger, *Anesthesiology, 54*:318 (1981).

125. J. L. Peel, *J. Biol. Chem., 237*:263 (1962).

126. R. E. MacKenzie and C. M. Baugh, *Biochim. Biophys. Acta, 611*:187 (1980).

127. Y.-Z. Lu, P. D. Aiello, and R. G. Matthews, *Biochemistry, 23*:6870 (1984).

128. L. C. Bortoluzzi and R. E. MacKenzie, *Can. J. Biochem., 61*:248 (1983).

129. M. Silverman, J. C. Keresztesy, C. J. Koval, and R. C. Gardiner, *J. Biol. Chem., 226*:83 (1957).

130. R. Bianchetti, G. Lucchini, P. Crosti, and P. Tortora, *J. Biol. Chem., 252*:2519 (1977).

131. P. Crosti, A. Gambini, G. Lucchini, and R. Bianchetti, *Biochim. Biophys. Acta,* 477:356 (1977).
132. K. Marcker, *J. Mol. Biol.,* 14:63 (1965).
133. A. S. Delk and J. C. Rabinowitz, *Nature,* 252:106 (1974).
134. K. Okamura-Ikeda, K. Fujiwara, and Y. Motokawa, *J. Biol. Chem.,* 257:135 (1982).
135. K. Hiraga and G. Kikuchi, *J. Biol. Chem.,* 255:11664 (1980).
136. R. K. Hampson, M. K. Taylor, and M. S. Olson, *J. Biol. Chem.* 259:1180 (1984).
137. C. Kutzbach and E. L. R. Stokstad, *Methods Enzymol.,* Part B, 18:793 (1971).
138. I. Eto, *Fed. Proc., Fed. Am. Soc. Exp. Biol.,* 45:820 (1986).
139. R. Ferone, M. H. Hanlon, S. C. Singer, and D. F. Hunt, *J. Biol. Chem.,* 26:16356 (1986).
140. D. J. Cichowicz, S. K. Foo, and B. Shane, *Mol. Cell. Biochem.,* 39:209 (1981).
141. A. L. Bognar, C. Osborne, B. Shane, S. C. Singer, and R. Ferone, *J. Biol. Chem.,* 260:5625 (1985).
142. G. Fabre, I. Fabre, L. H. Matherly, J.-P. Cano, and I. D. Goldman, *J. Biol. Chem.,* 259:5066 (1984).
143. L. H. Matherly, C. K. Barlowe, and I. D. Goldman, *Cancer Res.,* 46:588 (1986).
144. M. Jägerstad, K. Lindstrand, and A.-K. Westesson, *Scand. J. Gastroenterol.,* 7:593 (1972).
145. Y. S. Shin, C. Chan, A. Vidal, T. Brody, and E. L. R. Stokstad, *Biochem. Biophys. Acta,* 444:794 (1976).
146. P. K. Saini and I. H. Rosenberg, *J. Biol. Chem.,* 249:5131 (1974).
147. B. Elsenhans, O. Ahmad, and I. H. Rosenberg, *J. Biol. Chem.,* 259:6364 (1984).
148. M. Silink, R. Reddel, M. Bethel, and P. B. Rowe, *J. Biol. Chem.,* 250:5982 (1975).
149. T. Brody and E. L. R. Stokstad, *J. Biol. Chem.,* 257:14271 (1982).
150. T. Brody and E. L. R. Stokstad, *Methods Enzymol.,* 122:367 (1986).
151. P. J. Vickers, R. Di Cecco, Z. B. Pristupa, and K. G. Scrimgeour, in *Chemistry and Biology of Pteridines 1986,* B. A. Cooper and V. M. Whitehead (Eds.), Walter de Gruyter, New York, 1986, pp. 933–936.
152. R. J. Cook and C. Wagner, *Methods Enzymol.,* 122:Part G:255 (1986).
153. I. K. Dev and R. J. Harvey, *Adv Enz. Reg.,* 13:99 (1974).
154. F. Chiao and E. L. R. Stokstad, *Biochim. Biophys. Acta,* 497:225 (1977).
155. A. J. Vidal and E. L. R. Stokstad, *Biochim. Biophys. Acta,* 399:228 (1975).
156. P. B. Rowe, D. Sauer, D. Fahey, G. Craig, and E. McCairns, *Arch. Biochem. Biophys.,* 236:277 (1985).
157. J. C. Rabinowitz and H. Tabor, *J. Biol. Chem.,* 233:252 (1958).
158. K. A. Black, J. T. Eells, P. E. Noker, C. A. Hawtrey, and T. R. Tephly, *Proc. Natl. Acad. Sci. USA,* 82:3854 (1985).
159. P. F. Nixon, G. Slutsky, and A. Nahas, and J. R. Bertino, *J. Biol. Chem.,* 248:5932 (1973).
160. J. Galivan, J. Inglese, J. J. McGuire, Z. Nimec, and J. C. Coward, *Proc. Nat. Acad. Sci. USA,* 82:2598 (1985).
161. B. Shane, J. E. Watson, and E. L. R. Stokstad, *Biochim. Biophys. Acta.,* 497:241 (1977).
162. C. Wagner, *Ann. Rev. Nutr.,* 2:229 (1982).
163. L. A. Chasin, A. Feldman, M. Konstam, and G. Urlaub, *Proc. Nat. Acad. Sci. USA,* 71:718 (1974).
164. R. T. Taylor and M. L. Hanna, *Arch. Biochem. Biophys.,* 217:609 (1982).
165. K. W. Shannon and J. C. Rabinowitz, *J. Biol. Chem.,* 261:12266 (1986).
166. T. Brody, B. Shane, and E. L. R. Stokstad, *Fed. Proc., Fed. Am. Soc. Exp. Biol.,* 34:905 (1975).
167. S. S. Brown, G. E. Neal, and D. C. Williams, *Biochem. J.,* 97:34c (1965).
168. R. Labow, C. F. Maley, and F. Maley, *Cancer Res.,* 29:366 (1969).
169. E. Cadman and R. Heimer, *Cancer Res.,* 46:1195 (1986).
170. J. R. Allen, G. W. Lasser, D. A. Goldman, J. W. Booth, and C. K. Mathews, *J. Biol. Chem.,* 258:5746 (1983).

171. H. Noguchi, G. P. Reddy, and A. B. Pardee, *Cell, 32*:443 (1983).

172. R. Ferone and S. Roland, *Proc. Natl. Acad. Sci. USA, 77*:5802 (1980).

173. T. D. Meek, E. P. Garvey, and D. V. Santi, *Biochemistry, 24*:678 (1985).

174. M. W. McBurney and G. F. Whitmore, *Cell, 2*:173 (1974).

175. B. Shane and E. L. R. Stokstad, *J. Biol. Chem., 251*:3405 (1976).

176. J. Selhub, M. A. Savin, W. Sakami and M. Flavin, *Proc. Nat. Acad. Sci. USA, 68*:312 (1971).

177. R. L. Kisliuk, Y. Gaumont, and C. M. Baugh, *J. Biol. Chem., 249*:4100 (1974).

178. K. Fujii and F. M. Huennekens, *J. Biol. Chem,., 249*:6745 (1974).

179. L. H. Matherly, D. W. Fry, and I. D. Goldman, *Cancer Res., 43*:2694 (1983).

180. C. Wagner, W. T. Briggs, and R. J. Cook, *Biochem. Biophys. Res. Commun., 127*:746 (1985).

181. A. J. Wagner and C. Wagner, *J. Biol. Chem., 256*:4102 (1981).

182. T. Brody and E. L. R. Stokstad, *J. Nutr., 120*:71 (1990).

183. E. L. R. Stokstad and G. M. Vollenweider, *Folic Acid in Animal Feeding*, Fine Chemicals and Technical Bulletin No. 7, American Cyanamid Co., New York, 1955.

184. S. W. Thenen, *J. Nutr., 108*:836 (1978).

185. J. G. Hautvast and M. J. Barnes, *Br. J. Nutr., 32*:457 (1974).

186. E. Kodicek and K. J. Carpenter, *Blood 5*:522 (1950).

187. M. M. Nelson and H. M. Evans, *Proc. Soc. Exp. Biol. Med., 66*:289 (1947).

188. S. W. Thenen, *Nutr. Rep. Int., 19*:267 (1979).

189. V. Herbert, *Trans. Assoc. Am. Physicians, 75*:307 (1962).

190. A. Nirenberg, *Am. J. Nursing, 76*:1776 (1976).

191. H. E. Sauberlich, in *Folic Acid*, National Academy of Sciences, Washington, D. C., 1977, p. 213.

192. B. Shane, T. Tamura, and E. L. R. Stokstad, Clin. Chem. Acta, 100:13 (1980).

193. A. L. Luhby and J. M. Cooperman, *Adv. in Metabolic Disorders, 1*:263 (1964).

194. K. C. Das and V. Herbert, *Br. J. Haematol., 38*:219 (1978).

195. T. D. Luckey, P. R. Moore, C. A. Elvehjem, and E. B. Hart, *Science 103*:682 (1946).

196. C. J. Campbell, R. A. Brown, and A. D. Emmett, *J. Biol. Chem., 152*:483 (1944).

197. M. E. Reid, M. G. Martin, and G. M. Briggs, *J. Nutr., 59*:103 (1956).

198. C. F. Asenjo, *J. Nutr., 36*:601 (1948).

199. E. Kodicek and K. J. Carpenter, *Blood, 5*:540 (1950).

200. V. Herbert, *Arch. Intern Med., 110*:649 (1962).

201. V. Herbert, *New Engl. J. Med., 268*:201, 368 (1963).

202. M. L. Willoughby, *Brit. J. Haematol., 13*:503 (1967).

203. M. L. Willoughby, and F. J. Jewell, *Brit. Med. J., 2*:1568 (1966).

204. I. Chanarin, D. Rothman, A. Ward, and J. Perry, *Brit. Med. J., 2*:390 (1968).

205. I. Chanarin, D. Rothman, J. Perry, and D. Stratfull, *Brit. Med. J., 2*:394 (1968).

206. J. Shapiro, H. Alberts, P. Welch, and J. Metz, *Brit. J. Haematol., 11*:498 (1965).

207. J. Metz and P. Hackland, *Congr. S. Afr. Soc. Haematol. Cape Town* July (1970), cited in *J. Metz, Am. J. Clin. Nutr., 23*:843 (1970).

208. R. Asfour, N. Wahbah, C. Waslien, S. Guindi, and W. Darby, *Am. J. Clin. Nutr., 30*:1098 (1977).

209. Y. Matoth, A. Pinkas, and C. Sroka, *Am. J. Clin. Nutr., 16*:356 (1965).

210. *Recommended Dietary Allowances, Tenth Revised Edition*, Committee on Dietary Allowances Food and Nutrition Board, National Academy of Sciences, Washington, D. C., 1989.

211. J. Jolivet, K. H. Cowan, G. A. Curt, N. J. Clendeninn, and B. A. Chabner, *New Engl. J. Med., 309*:1094 (1983).

212. D. Rothman, *Am. J. Obstetr. Gynecol., 108*:149 (1970).

213. I. H. Rosenberg, B. B. Bowman, B. A. Cooper, C. H. Halsted, and J. Lindenbaum, *Am. J. Clin. Nutr., 36*:1060 (1982).

214. M. E. Weinblatt, J. S. Coblyn, D. A. Fox, P. A. Fraser, D. E. Holdsworth, D. N. Glass, and D. E. Trentham, *New Engl. J. Med., 312*:818 (1985).

215. M. P. Rivey, D. D. Schottelius, and M. J. Berg, *Drug Intelligence and Clinical Pharmacol.,* *18*:292 (1984).
216. D. Kelly, D. Weir, B. Reid, and J. Scott, *J. Clin. Invest., 64*:1089 (1979).
217. C. L. Krumdieck, K. Fukushima, T. Fukushima, T. Shiota, and C. E. Butterworth, *Am. J. Clin. Nutr., 31*:88 (1978).
218. C. H. Halsted, *Am. J. Clin. Nutr., 33*:2736 (1980).
219. O. B. Martinez and D. A. Roe, *J. Nutr., 107*:1157 (1977).
220. A. M. Shojania, *Can. Med. Assoc. J., 126*:244 (1982).
221. C. H. Halsted, *Ann. Rev. Med., 31*:79 (1980).
222. J. Selhub, G. J. Dhar, and I. H. Rosenberg, *Pharmacol. Ther., 20*:397 (1983).
223. M. C. Carey, J. J. Fennelly, and O. Fitzgerald, *Am. J. Med., 45*:26 (1968).
224. V. Herbert and R. Zalusky, *J. Clin. Invest. 41*:1263 (1962).
225. J. Vitale, A. Restrepo, H. Velez, J. B. Riker, and E. E. Hellerstein, *J. Nutr., 88*:315 (1966).
226. B. A. Kochanowski, A. M. Smith, M. F. Picciano, and A. R. Sherman, *J. Nutr., 113*:2471 (1983).
227. V. Herbert, *Lab. Invest., 52*:3 (1985).
228. M. I. Botez, F. Fontaine, and T. Botez, *Eur. Neurol., 16*:230 (1977).
229. J. M. Freeman, J. D. Finkelstein, and S. H. Mudd, *New Engl. J. Med., 292*:491 (1975).
230. P. W. Wong, P. Justice, M. Hruby, E. B. Weiss, and E. Diamond, *Pediatrics, 59*:749 (1977).
231. P. Santiago-Borrero, R. Santini, Periz-Santiago, N. Maldonado, S. Millan, and G. Coll-Camalez, *Pediatrics, 82*;450 (1973).
232. P. Lanzkowsky, M. E. Erlandson, and A. I. Bezan, *Blood, 34*:452 (1969).
233. G. P. Tauro, D. M. Danks, P. B. Rowe, M. B. Van der Weyden, M. A. Schwarz, V. L. Collins, and B. W. Neal, *New Engl. J. Med., 294*:466 (1976).
234. N. Whitehead, F. Reyner and J. Lindenbaum, *J. Am. Med. Assoc., 226*:1421 (1973).
235. C. E. Butterworth, K. D. Hatch, H. Gore, H. Muller, and C. L. Krumdieck, *Am. J. Clin. Nutr., 35*:73 (1982).
236. E. A. Clarke, J. Hatcher, G. E. McKeown-Eyssen, and G. M. Lickrish, *Am. J. Obstet, Gynecol., 151*:612 (1985).
237. D. B. Smith and E. Obbens, in *Folic Acid in Neurology, Psychiatry, and Internal Medicine,* M. I. Botez and E. H. Reynolds (Eds.), Raven Press, New York, 1979, p. 267.
238. S. O. Schwartz, S. R. Kaplan, and B. E. Armstrong, *J. Lab. Clin. Med., 35*:894 (1950).
239. Editorial, *New Engl. J. Med., 237*:713 (1947).
240. E. H. Reynolds, *Lancet, 1*:1376 (1973).
241. E. H. Reynolds, *Lancet 1*:1086 (1967).
242. R. Mattson, B. Gallagher, E. H. Reynolds, and D. Glass, *Arch. Neurol., 29*:78 (1973).
243. T. Spies, R. Hillman, S. Cohlan, B. Kramer, and A. Kanof, in *Diseases of Metabolism,* G. Duncan (Ed.), Saunders, Philadelphia, 1959.
244. B. Horned, R. Cunningham, H. Smith, and M. Clark, *Ann. N.Y. Acad. Sci., 48*:289 (1946).
245. J. Dawson, C. Woodruff, and W. Darby, *Proc. Soc. Exp. Biol. Med., 73*:646 (1950).
246. M. S. Chen and L. Schirch, *J. Biol. Chem., 248*:3631 (1973).
247. J. D. Finkelstein and J. J. Martin, *J. Biol. Chem., 261*:1582 (1976).
248. D. G. Johns and J. R. Bertino, in *Cancer Medicine,* J. F. Holland and E. Frei (Eds.), Lea and Febiger, Philadelphia, 1982, p. 775.
249. J. C. Mendible, O. Villarroel, C. Sánchez, and L. A. Ordóñez, *Acta Cient. Venezolana, 29*:389 (1978).
250. W. Pfender and L. I. Pizer, *Arch. Biochem. Biophys., 200*:503 (1980).
251. E. G. Burton and H. J. Sallach, *Arch. Biochem. Biophys., 166*:483 (1975).
252. J. Paquin, C. M. Baugh, and R. E. MacKenzie, *J. Biol. Chim., 260*:14925 (1985).
253. E. M. Rios-Orlandi, C. G. Zarkadas, and R. E. MacKenzie, *Biochem. Biophys. Acta., 871*:24 (1986).
254. D. J. Cichowicz and B. Shane, *Biochemistry, 26*:513 (1987).

255. W. E. Evans, W. R. Crom, M. Abromowitch, and C.-H. Pui, *New Engl. J. Med.*, *314*:471 (1986).
256. C. J. Allegra, B. A. Chabner, C. U. Tuazon, and H. Masur, *New Engl. J. Med.*, *317*:978 (1987).
257. D. C. Heimburger, C. B. Alexander, R. Birch, C. E. Butterworth, W. C. Bailey, and C. L. Krumdieck, *J. Am. Med. Assoc.*, *259*:1525 (1988).
258. R. W. Erbe, *New Engl. J. Med.*, *293*:807 (1975).
259. K. M. Laurence, N. James, M. H. Miller, G. B. Tennant, and H. Campbell, *Brit. Med. J.*, *282*:1509 (1981).
260. R. W. Smithells, S. Sheppard, C. J. Schorah, M. J. Seller, N. C. Nevin, R. Harris, A. P. Read, and D. W. Fielding, *Lancet, i*:339 (1980).
261. R. W. Smithells, M. J. Seller, R. Harris, D. W. Fielding, C. J. Schorah, N. C. Nevin, S. Sheppard, A.P. Read, S. Walker, and J. Wild, *Lancet, i*:1027 (1983).
262. A. M. Molloy, P. Kirke, I. Hillary, D. G. Weir, and J. M. Scott, *Arch. Disease Childhood*, *60*:660 (1985).
263. J. J. Yunis and A. L. Soreng, *Science, 226*:1199 (1984).
264. J.-C. C. Wang and R. W. Erbe, *Am. J. Med. Genet.*, *17*:303 (1984).
265. D. L. O'Connor, M. F. Picciano, A. R. Sherman, and S. L. Burgert, *J. Nutr.*, *117*:1715 (1987).
266. A. G. Palekar, S. S. Tate, and A. Meister, *J. Biol. Chem.*, *248*:1158 (1973).
267. R. J. Cook, K. S. Misono, and C. Wagner, *J. Biol. Chem.*, *260*:12998 (1985).
268. K. Kvalnes-Krick and M. S. Jorns, *Biochemistry, 26*:7391 (1987).
269. L. H. Matherly, C. K. Barlowe, V. M. Phillips, and I. D. Goldman, *J. Biol. Chem.*, *262*:710 (1987).
270. Y. Natsumeda, T. Ikegami, K. Marayama, and G. Weber, *Cancer Res.*, *48*:507 (1988).
271. R. Kucera and H. Paulus, *Exp. Cell Res.*, *167*:417 (1986).
272. H. Ogawa and M. Fujioka, *Biochem. Biophys. Res. Commun.*, *108*:227 (1982).
273. C. Allegra, J. C. Drake, J. Jolivet, and B. A. Chabner, *Proc. Natl. Acad. Sci. USA*, *82*:4881 (1985).
274. C. C. Y. Ip and A. E. Harper, *J. Nutr.*, *104*:252 (1974).
275. W. D. Cheek and D. R. Appling, *Arch. Biochem. Biophys.*, *270*:504 (1989).
276. L. B. Bailey, C. S. Mahan, and D. Dimperio, *Am. J. Clin. Nutr.*, *33*:1997 (1980).
277. E. Horn, *Brit. Med. J.*, *297*:1325 (1988).
278. A. Zimran and C. Hershko, *Am. J. Clin. Nutr.*, *37*:855 (1983).
279. J. B. Alperin, M. E. Haggard, and W. J. McGanity, *Am. J. Clin. Nutr.*, *22*:1354 (1969).
280. D. Stevens, D. Burman, M. K. Strelling, and A. Morris, *Pediatrics, 64*:333 (1979).
281. H. E. Sauberlich, M. J. Kretsch, J. H. Skala, H. J. Johnson, and P. C. Taylor, *Am. J. Clin. Nutr.*, *46*:1016 (1987).
282. D. W. Horne, D. Patterson, and R. J. Cook, *Arch. Biochem. Biophys.* *270*:729 (1989).
283. J. D. Finkelstein, J. J. Martin, W. E. Kyle, and B. J. Harris, *Arch. Biochem. Biophys.*, *191*:153 (1978).
284. E. P. Frenkel, A. Mukherjee, C. R. Hackenbrock, and P. A. Srere, *J. Biol. Chem.*, *251*:2147.
285. T. Tamura, Y. S. Shin, M. A. Williams, and E. L. R. Stokstad, *Analyt. Biochem.*, *49*:517 (1972).
286. T. Brody, in *Comparative Animal Nutrition*, Vol. 8, A. C. Beynen and C. E. West (Eds.), Karger Medical and Scientific Publ., Basel, in press.
287. T. Brody, *Pteridines, 1*:159 (1989).

13
Vitamin B$_{12}$

Leon Ellenbogen
American Cyanamid Company, Lederle Laboratories
Pearl River, New York

Bernard A. Cooper
McGill University, Royal Victoria Hospital
Montreal, Quebec, Canada

I. HISTORY AND ISOLATION

Vitamin B_{12} (cyanocobalamin), the most recent vitamin discovered, is the most potent of the vitamins. It is best known for its association with Addisonian pernicious anemia. The history of vitamin B_{12} development involves widely divergent investigations into the human deficiency diseases, animal nutrition, and metabolism of microorganisms.

Combe (1), in 1824, ascribed a case of pernicious anemia to a "disorder of the digestive and assimilative organs." In 1855, Addison, an English physician, gave a detailed description of pernicious anemia symptoms (2), but no treatment could be found until the demonstration by Minot and Murphy in 1926 (3) of the successful treatment by liver feeding. In 1929, Castle (4) showed that the intestinal absorption of the antipernicious anemia principle in liver (extrinsic factor) required prior binding to an "intrinsic factor" secreted by the stomach. Biochemists then began a long series of attempts to isolate the active component present in liver concentrates, which was then called the "antipernicious anemia factor." A comprehensive account of the development of the knowledge concerning vitamin B_{12} and pernicious anemia has been published by Castle (5).

In 1948, the isolation of vitamin B_{12} (cyanocobalamin) was reported by Rickes et al. (United States) (6) and by Smith (England) (7). The vitamin was isolated by the U.S. workers by means of a convenient method developed by Shorb and Briggs (8) at the University of Maryland and involving the bacterium *Lactobacillus lactis*. West (9) was the first to show that injections of the vitamin, supplied to him by Rickes et al., induced a dramatic beneficial response in patients with pernicious anemia.

Two crystalline "vitamin B_{12}" preparations were isolated from cultures of *Streptomyces aureofaciens* (10). The first of these had an absorption spectrum similar to that reported for vitamin B_{12} (11,12); the second had a different spectrum and was termed vitamin B_{12b}. Unlike vitamin B_{12} (13), vitamin B_{12b} did not contain cyanide and was named hydroxocobalamin (14). Hydroxocobalamin was indistinguishable from cyanocobalamin in biological activity, including effectiveness against pernicious anemia (15). The cyanide in cyanocobalamin apparently originated from charcoal used in the preparation process.

The isolation of the coenzyme forms of vitamin B_{12} by Barker et al. (16) and Weissbach et al. (17) led to the further recognition that cyanocobalamin is not the naturally occurring form of the vitamin but is rather an artifact that arises from the original isolation procedure. The two *coenzyme* forms of cobalamin found in animals are adenosylcobalamin and methylcobalamin. Humans and other animals contain three main cobalamins: hydroxocobalamin, adenosylcobalamin, and methylcobalamin (18). Cyanocobalamin, however, is the most widely used form of cobalamin in clinical practice because of its relatively greater availability and stability. Most of the metabolic studies utilized cyanocobalamin.

II. CHEMISTRY

A. Structure and Nomenclature

Soon after cyanocobalamin was crystallized, structural studies were initiated by classic degradation experiments and by x-ray crystallography. Considerable knowledge was obtained by degradation studies, but the molecular structures of cyanocobalamin and its coenzyme forms were not definitely established until the brilliant work of Hodgkin and her colleagues (19–21) using x-ray crystallography.

Cyanocobalamin consists of a fundamental portion containing four pyrrole nuclei jointed in a large ring containing six conjugated double bonds, a structure very similar to that of the iron porphyrins. One of the four pyrrole nuclei is completely saturated. The CN group is attached to the cobalt atom, which in turn is linked coordinately to a nitrogen of the 5,6-dimethylbenzimidazole group. As with nucleic acids, vitamin B$_{12}$ contains a nucleotide. However, the base consists of 5,6-dimethylbenzimidazole rather than the various purine or pyrimidine bases of the nucleic acids, and the sugar, ribose, has an α-glycosidic linkage, unlike the β-linkage in the nucleic acids. The D-1-amino-2-propanol moiety of the molecule is esterified to the nucleotide and joined in amide linkage to the porphyrinlike nucleus. The structure of cyanocobalamin, based on the work of Hodgkin et al. (19–21), is shown in Figure 1.

The nomenclature of the corrinoids (1973 recommendations) has been reprinted in detail (22) from the IUPAC-IUB Commission on Biochemical Nomenclature (23–25). They are briefly summarized here:

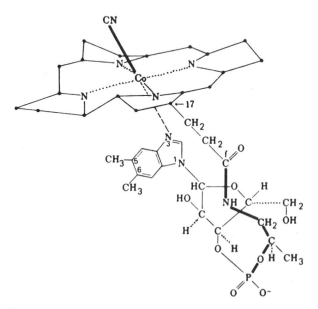

Figure 1   Sketch of vitamin B$_{12}$ (cyanocobalamin). (Based on the work of Hodgkin et al., Refs. 19–21.)

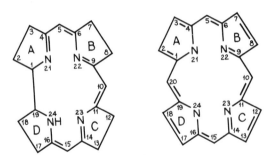

Figure 2 Structural formulas of the corrin (left) and porphyrin (right) nuclei.

1. The name *corrin* is used for the nucleus shown in Figure 2. It is important to note that the number 20 is omitted in numbering the corrin nucleus so that the numbering would correspond to that of the porphyrin nucleus (Fig. 2). The term *corrinoid* is used to cover all compounds containing the corrin nucleus.
2. The name *cobyrinic acid* is used for the structure shown in Figure 3. The terminal carboxyl groups, or amide groups as in the case of vitamin B_{12}, are given letters a to g.
3. The structure shown in Figure 4 is termed cobinic acid, cobinamide, cobamic acid, or cobamide depending upon the R or X grouping, as shown in the formulated figure.
4. The heterocyclic radical of the nucleotide present in most analogs or derivatives, ending in yl, is prefixed to appropriate structures mentioned in 1, 2, or 3.
5. If the cobalt atom is replaced by another metal, the syllable co is replaced by the name of the other metal followed by o or i, according to the valence of the metal. When the cobalt is replaced by hydrogen, the prefix hydrogeno replaces co.
6. Cyanocobalamin is a permissive name for vitamin B_{12}, aquacobalamin for vitamin B_{12b}, and nitrocobalamin for vitamin B_{12c}; however, the term *cobalamin* should not be used in any other sense.

The term *vitamin B_{12}* should be used as the generic descriptor for all corrinoids exhibiting qualitatively the biological activity of cyanocobalamin.

A cobalamin is a cobamide in which 5,6-dimethylbenzimidazole is the aglycon attached by a glycosyl link from its N-1 to the C-1 of the ribose and additionally linked by

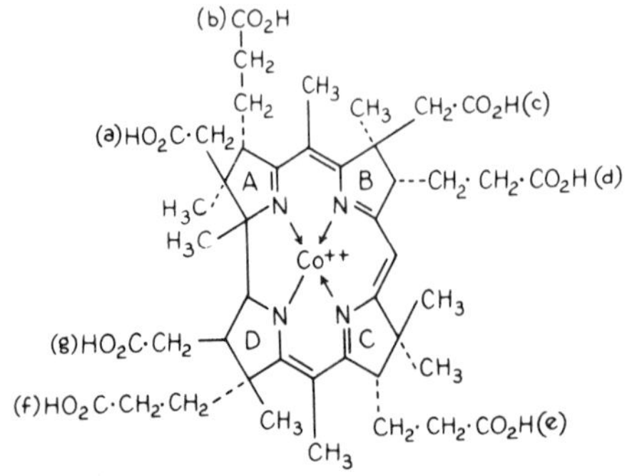

Figure 3 Structural formula of cobyrinic acid.

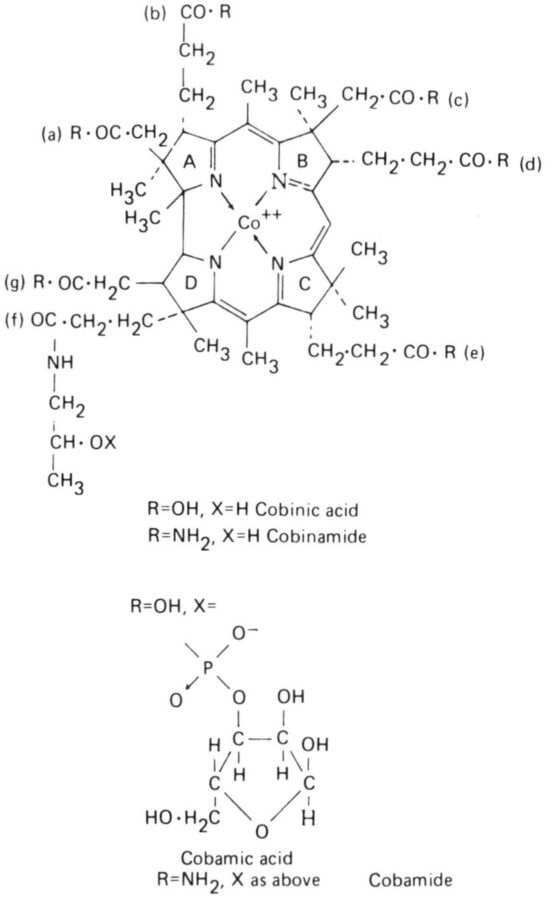

Figure 4 Structural formula of cobinic acid, cobinamide, cobamic acid, or cobamide, depending upon the R or X grouping, as indicated.

a bond between the N-3 and the cobalt (in position α). They may be named as cobamides, as above, or according to the pattern:

(Ligand in Coβ position, if any)-cobalamin (Xb)

Examples:

Coα-[α-(5,6-Dimethylbenzimidazolyl)]-Coα-cyanocobamide, also known as vitamin B$_{12}$, is termed cyanocobalamin.

Coα-[α-(5,6-Dimethylbenzimidazolyl)]-Coα-aquacobamide, also known as vitamin B$_{12a}$, is termed aquacobalamin.

Coα-[α-(5,6-Dimethylbenzimidazolyl)]-Coα-hydroxocobamide, also known as vitamin B$_{12b}$, is termed hydroxocobalamin. (*Note*: Aquacobalamin is the conjugate acid of hydroxocobalamin.)

Coα-[α-(5,6-Dimethylbenzimidazolyl]-Coα-nitritocobamide, also known as vitamin B$_{12c}$, is termed nitritocobalamin.

The permissive term *cobalamin* is used to describe the vitamin B_{12} molecule without the anionic ligand. Examples of the coenzymatic forms of the B_{12} vitamins are:

Coα-[(5,6-Dimethylbenzimidazolyl)]-Coα-adenosylcobamide, or adenosylcobalamin, for the compound formerly known as "coenzyme B_{12}."

Coα-[α-(5,6-Dimethylbenzimidazolyl)]Coα-methylcobamide, or methylcobalamin, for the compound involved in several reactions, including methionine biosynthesis, where a methyl group is ligated to the cobalt in the α position.

Coα-[α(7-adenyl)]-Coα-adenosylcobamide, the coenzymatically active form of "pseudovitamin B_{12}," capable of replacing adenosylcobalamin in many systems.

The coenzymatically active forms of the vitamin possess an organic ligand; either methyl or 5'-deoxy-5'-adenosyl (for brevity, 5'-deoxy-5'-adenosyl may be replaced by adenosyl) attached to the β position of the cobalt by a carbon–cobalt bond, that is, in the position of the CN as shown in Figure 5. The composite structural formula of the various cobalamin analogs is also shown in this figure.

B. Physical Properties

Cyanocobalamin forms red, needlelike, hygroscopic crystals. Its empirical formula is $C_{63}H_{88}N_{14}O_{14}PCo$, and its molecular weight is 1355.

Cyanocobalamin is a neutral, odorless, tasteless compound that is soluble in water (1.2% at 25°C). It is also soluble in alcohol and phenol but is insoluble in acetone,

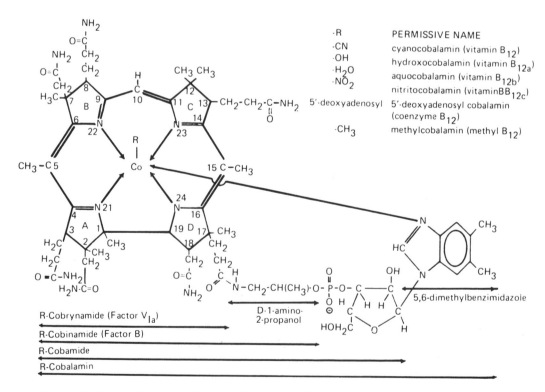

Figure 5   Structural formula of cobalamin analogs. (From Ref. 84.)

chloroform, and ether. Advantage is taken of its insolubility in acetone for crystallization from water–acetone solutions.

The red crystals of cyanocobalamin darken at 210–220 °C and melt above 300 °C. It is levorotatory, and although difficult to measure accurately because of its color, its reported optical activity at 656 nm is −59° and at 643 nm, −100° (26–28).

The absorption spectrum of cyanocobalamin shows three characteristic maxima that are relatively independent of pH. The extinction coefficients (E_{1cm}^M) are: $E_{278} = 16.3 \times 10^3$; $E_{361} = 28.1 \times 10^3$; and $E_{550} = 8.7 \times 10^3$.

C. Chemical Properties

The chemical reactions and properties of cyanocobalamin are numerous and detailed, and some good reviews on this subject have been presented (29,30). Some of the most important properties are given below.

The cyanide group of cyanocobalamin can be replaced by other ions to form hydroxocobalamin, chlorocobalamin, nitrocobalamin, thiocyanatocobalamin, and others (31). All the above-mentioned cobalamins are readily converted to cyanocobalamin after treatment with cyanide. A purple compound formed on addition of excess cyanide to alkaline solutions of cyanocobalamin is called dicyanocobalamin. This compound, which contains two cyanide molecules coordinated to the cobalt atom, is quite unstable. Cyanocobalamin is slowly decomposed by ultraviolet or strong visible light. The cyano group is split off, yielding hydroxocobalamin (32). Prolonged exposure to light causes irreversible decomposition and inactivation (33).

Mild acid hydrolysis of cyanocobalamin induces the removal of the nucelotide (34), whereas more vigorous acid hydrolysis liberates ammonia, 5,6-dimethylbenzimidazole, D-1-amino-2-propanol, and cobyrinic acid (35). Hydrolysis with dilute acids splits the amide group off the side chains, resulting in mono- and polycarboxylic acids (34).

D. Stability

Cyanocobalamin is stable in air and, in dry form, is relatively stable at 100 °C for a few hours. Aqueous solutions at pH 4–7 can be autoclaved at 120 °C. Cyanocobalamin appears to be the most stable of the various analogs studied to date. Crystalline cyanocobalamin is compatible with a wide variety of therapeutic and nutritional substances. In solution, thiamine and nicotinamide, or nicotinic acid, destroy cyanocobalamin slowly (36), whereas the addition of small amounts of iron or thiocyanate appear to protect it (37,38).

E. Analogs and Derivatives

Of the vitamins, cyanocobalamin has the largest and most complex molecule, and so it is not surprising that a multitude of analogs and derivatives have been prepared from it. These analogs are classified according to differences in their structures.

1. Replacement of CN—

Brief mention has already been made of compounds in which an ion or molecule other than the cyano group are coordinated to the cobalt atom. The unstable dicyanocobalamin is not included since it exists only in solution with an excess of cyanide ion.

2. Carboxylic Acids Obtained by Removal of NH₃ on Chains Attached to the Corrin Nucleus

Various carboxylic acids are theoretically possible by hydrolysis of all or part of the amide groups. Most of these have been prepared (38a,b,c). The mono-, di-, and tricarboxylic acid have been prepared, and these arise by hydrolysis of the propionamide chains (34). The hexacarboxylic acid obtained by Cannon, Johnson, and Todd in England was most instrumental for x-ray diffraction work on the structure of cyanocobalamin (39).

3. Lactams and Lactones

Both a lactam and lactone have been prepared from cyanocobalamin. The former was obtained by treatment of the vitamin with alkali, and the latter, by treatment with chloramine T, chlorine, or bromine (30,40).

4. Substituted Amides

A large number of substituted amides have been prepared (41). Smith has listed 18 such substituted amides, many with antivitamin$_{12}$ activity (27) in the microbiological assay with an *Escherichia coli* mutant (42). Baker et al. (43–44) found that some of these amides were inactive as vitamin B_{12} antagonists. These investigators also found that two of the amides and one of the anilide analogs satisfied the nutritional requirements of *Euglena gracilis* and *Lactobacillus leichmannii*, but not those of *E. coli* 113-3 or *Ochromonas malhamenis*. Some of these amides have also been reported by Coates et al. (45) to have antivitamin activity for the growing chick and developing chick embryo. The amides failed, however, to produce cobalamin deficiency in normal chicks, and the analogs did not produce any toxic effects.

5. Bases Other Than 5,6-Dimethylbenzimidazole

Most of the early work with analogs was initiated by Coates and his colleagues at the National Institute for Research in Dairying, England (46). Based on the microbiologic assay (mutant strain of *E. coli*) then available, Coates et al. found that rumen contents and feces of the ruminants had less cyanocobalamin activity for chicks then was expected. Extraction and fractionation of rumen contents and feces led to the identification of three substances resembling cyanocobalamin in structure. They were originally termed factors A, B and C (47–50). At about the same time another analog, termed pseudovitamin B_{12}, was isolated (51,52) and, shortly thereafter, Friedrich and Bernhauer (53) obtained another vitamin B_{12}-like substance, termed factor III, from sewage sludge. The bases in the nucleotides of these various factors are shown in Table 1.

6. Miscellaneous

A corrinoid lacking cobalt was obtained from a photosynthetic bacterium by Toohey (54). This vitamin B_{12} analog, termed factor V_{1a} (cobrynic acid abcdeq hexamide), is shown in Figure 5; it differs from factor B by the absence of the aminopropanol group. Various analogs have been prepared from factor V_{1a} that differ in the amino propanol groupings and in their biological activities.

F. Biological and Microbiological Activities of the Analogs and Derivatives

There are more than 20 naturally occurring analogs and more than 50 analogs produced biosynthetically by *Streptomyces griseus*, *E. coli*, and *Propionibacterium shermanii*, in which different bases have been incorporated. Many of these have been reviewed by Porter (55),

Table 1 Bases of Nucleotides of Various Cobalamin Analogs

Compound	Base of nucleotide
Vitamin B$_{12}$ (cyanocobalamin)	5,6-Dimethylbenzimidazole
Factor A	2-Methyladenine
Factor B	None
Factor C	Guanine
Factor III	5-Hydroxybenzimidazole
Pseudovitamin B$_{12}$	Adenine

Smith (30), Coates and Kon (56), and Heinrich et al. (57). The latter review includes some studies on derivatives obtained by substitution in the D-isopropanol moiety and/or alteration of the phosphate linkage to the ribose moiety.

The naturally occurring analogs are active in several microorganisms, and it is for this reason that they were not recognized until more specific biological and microbiological tests were available and until studies were initiated in humans. Many of the naturally occurring analogs were eventually found to be inactive in animals, whereas many of the analogs obtained by biosynthesis were active. In humans, one is confronted again with two types of analog activity. Some analogs, such as α-(5,6-chlorobenzimidazolyl)cobamide dichloride, α-(5-hydroxybenzimidazolyl)cobamide cyanide (factor III), and α-(benzimidazolyl)cobamide cyanide, are inferior to cyanocobalamin when administered orally, whereas all are equally effective pareneterally (58–61).

For many of the analogs, there is good correlation between the activity in the human and that in the chick (62).

G. Cobalamin Antagonists

Antimetabolites prepared by modification of the cyanocobalamin structure may function by interfering with (30):

The uptake of cobalamins
The formation of the coenzyme forms
The biochemical action of the coenzymes

Modification in or substitution of the nucleotide base produces forms inhibitory to certain bacteria (*M. tuberculosis, L. lactus*) (63,64). Woolley and Stewart (65) reported that the analog containing 2,2-dimethyl-4,5-diaminobenzene caused some regression of spontaneous tumors in the mouse. Timmis and Epstein (66) and Epstein (67) studied more than 100 benzimidazolelike compounds for their effect on the growth of the vitamin B$_{12}$–dependent green alga, *Euglena gracilis*. Several compounds were found that inhibited the growth of the organism at levels as low as 10–50 μg. Antagonists may be produced by changes in the vitamin B$_{12}$ molecule, particularly if these affect the (31):

Hydroxyl groups of the ribose of the nucleotide
Conversion of propionamide chains to substituted amides
Modification of the alkanolamine bridge

The changes may result in faulty cobalamin absorption or in inhibition of cell growth.

It is difficult to distinguish between a positive inhibitory and a more passive interference with the uptake of cyanocobalamin. The effective antagonists were prepared by Smith and colleagues by hydrolyzing at least one of the propionamide groups in the vitamin molecule. The inhibitory activity was increased by converting the acids into substituted amides of methylamine or some other amine. The necessary acids were made either by deliberate hydrolysis of cyanocobalamin with dilute hydrochloric acid or from by-product fractions arising in the manufacture of cyanocobalamin. Competitive inhibition was demonstrated in rat-growth tests (32).

Several antagonists at oral doses of 0.1–3 μg/day were found to depress the growth rate of depleted rats receiving either no cyanocobalamin or suboptimal amounts, compared with controls receiving no antagonist. Latner (33) has shown that one of the antagonists, the "ethylamide," effectively competes with cyanocobalamin for uptake by the gut.

Several substituted amide, lactone, and lactam analogs of cyanocobalamin competed with the vitamin for its binding to intrinsic factor and depressed absorption of the vitamin in humans (68,69). The lactone and ethylamide analogs interfered with gastrointestinal absorption of cyanocobalamin in rats and with the uptake of the vitamin by intact segments of rat gut (70,71). The growth of HeLa cells in tissue culture was inhibited by the methylamide analog (68).

The anilide analog was shown to have antivitamin B_{12} activity in the growing chick embryo only when the analog was derived from hens relatively deficient in cobalamin (72). Some analogs in which the aminopropanol portion was altered were able to inhibit the growth of *E. coli* and chick embryos (73).

In conclusion, despite extensive studies of antagonists, at present there are no known clinically useful antagonists (antimetabolites) of cyanocobalamin.

H.   Coenzyme Antagonists

A large series of analogs of adenosylcobalamin, modified either in the upper or the lower ligand or in the corrin macrocycle, have been tested for their ability to replace or to inhibit the action of the coenzyme in the ribonucleotide reductase, the dioldehydrase, the glycrerol dehydratase, and the ethanolamine ammonia-lyase reactions (73a,b,c,d).

Analogs in which the propionamide side chains (b,d, and e) are hydrolyzed are only marginally active as coenzymes and are poor inhibitors of ribonucleotide reduction. The generation of a negative charge on the periphery of the ring clearly interferes with the binding of the coenzyme, indeed blocking the negative charge of adenosylcobalamin e-carboxylic acid by amidation even with the bulky 2,4-dinitroaniline moiety, restores coenzyme activity. Adenosylepicobalamin in which the e-propionamide side chain is inverted is completely inactive as a coenzyme in the ribonucleotide reductase system, but functions as a coenzyme in the dioldehydrase reaction.

Studies with analogs modified in the base of the nucleoside ligand have demonstrated that neither the 6-amino group nor N-7 of purine ring are essential for activity, since both nebularylcobalamin and tubercidylcobalamin are able to function as coenzymes.

Studies with analogs modified in the ribofuranose ring indicate that, although neither the 2' or 3' hydroxyl nor the ribose ring oxygen are essential for the catalytic process, even small changes in the ribose moiety have a profound effect on coenzyme function.

In the ribonucleotide reductase reaction all analogs that are active as coenzymes, but surprisingly also several inactive analogs, are degraded to enzyme-bound cob(II)alamin and presumably a 5'-deoxynucleoside.

Similarly, in the dioldehydrase system, complexes of the apoenzyme with active analogs show cob(II)alaminlike absorption spectra in the presence of 1,2-propanediol.

Analogs in which two extra methylene groups are interposed between the 5'-deoxyadenosyl moiety and the cobalt atom or in which the ribose moiety is replaced by two or more methylene carbons are very potent inhibitors of all the enzymatic systems tested.

Evidence that human plasma contains a number of cobalamin analogs has been presented (74a). These analogs have lower relative affinities for intrinsic factor than R protein. The origins and structures of these newly recognized cobalamin analogs are unknown but are clearly different from the most common cobalamin analogs synthesized by microorganisms. They could represent either degradation products of these cobalamin analogs or other cobalamin analogs that are synthesized by microorganisms in trace amounts.

The activities or inhibitory properties of these newly recognized cobalamin analogs for the two animal cobalamin-dependent enzymes and the enzymes that convert cobalamin to its coenzyme forms are also unknown. It is unlikely that they possess full cobalamin activity, however, because they have all decreased growth-promoting activity for *E. gracilis* or *L. leichmannii*.

I. Synthesis

The similarities between the corrinoids and porphyrins, such as their similar ring systems, suggest that these two groups of substances have common biosynthetic features.

Most of the progress in this area has been made during the last 10 years. As with heme synthesis, the δ-aminolevulinic acid is first converted into porphobilinogen (PBG). Four molecules of porphobilinogen are required for the biosynthesis of cobyrinic acid. Two enzymes are required to catalyze the conversion of four molecules of the monopyrrole (PBG) into uroporphyrinogen III. They are PBG-deaminase and uroporphyrinogen-III cosynthetase. Four units of PBG are assembled head-to-tail by deaminase, starting with ring A and building around to ring D.

The seven C-methyl groups that are introduced into cobrynic acid are transferred intact from S-adenosylmethionine (the S-adenosylmethione is derived from methionine). Much of this progress depended heavily on the use of precursors labeled with carbon-13. Detailed reviews have been published (75). Krasna and associates (76) showed that L-threonine can be the precursor of the 1-amino-2-propanol moiety that links the corrin ring to the nucleotide. The initial action is a decarboxylation of the threonine. The route of incorporation of the L-threonine into corrinoids remains to be elucidated.

It is not yet known how and when cobalt is incorporated into the corrin ring. One certainty is that cobalt is inserted before amidations of the side chains, since cobyrinic acid, the simplest corrinoid isolated from *P. shermanii*, contains cobalt. The recently observed cell-free *P. shermanii* extract that catalyzes the conversion of δ-aminolevulinic acid to cobyrinic acid clearly contains the cobalt-inserting system, but details are not yet available (77,78).

Corrinoid biosynthesis represents a coalescence of variations on biosynthetic themes from the fields of amino acid, vitamin, pyrrole, nucleotide, and metal biochemistry (79). A more detailed review of the biosynthesis of cobalamins as recently been published (79).

Extracts of *Clostridium tetanomorphum* and *Propionibacterium shermanii* can convert cyanocobalamin to its coenzyme form (adenosylcobalamin) (80,81). Adenosine triphosphate (ATP) is required, and isotopic studies have shown that the adenosine of ATP is incorporated into the nucleoside of the coenzyme (82).

The brilliant work of Woodward and Eschenmoser led to the total chemical synthesis of vitamin B_{12}. Their work required the efforts of about 100 workers from several countries. The details of this complicated chemical method have been published (82a). The synthetic vitamin B_{12} has been well identified and characterized through the use of physical methods. Some of the biological properties of this synthetic vitamin remain to be determined. It showed, however, full biological activity in the *L. leichmanii* assay.

J. Commercial Forms

Commercially available stable forms of cyanocobalamin for therapy are cyanocobalamin and hydroxocobalamin. These drugs share the cobalamin molecular structure but differ in the group attached to the cobalt atom. The most commonly used oral form of cobalamin is cyanocobalamin. In rare cases, such as tobacco amblyopia and optic neuropathy, hydroxocobalamin has proven therapuetic advantage over cyanocobalamin (83).

When administered parenterally, hydroxocobalamin produces a more sustained increase of plasma cobalamin levels than does cyanocobalamin. However, at *intervals of 1 month*, usually used for parenteral maintenace therapy of pernicious anemia, the plasma cobalamin levels achieved after administration of hydroxycobalamin fall to the same levels as after cyanocobalamin (84).

Hydroxocobalamin has been used successfully to prevent nitroprusside-induced cyanide toxicity (85). Sodium nitroprusside is widely used to treat severe hypertension, to induce surgical hypotension, and to decrease myocardial oxygen demand after myocardial infarction or congestive heart failure. It has also been used to treat cerebral vasospasm. However, the usefulness of sodium nitroprusside therapy is limited by the toxicity of the cyanide, the major metabolite of nitroprusside degradation. Hydroxocobalamin combines with cyanide to form cyanocobalamin, which is excreted unchanged in the urine.

III. ASSAY

A. Clinical

Before cyanocobalamin was first isolated and crystallized, the antipernicious anemia factor (APA), as it was then called, was assayed with difficulty and with only semiquantitative precision in human subjects with pernicious anemia. Potency of APA was determined by the magnitude of the increase in red blood cell count, hemoglobin, and the rise in reticulocyte percentage.

Doses of crystalline cyanocobalamin are now expressed in terms of weight. The unit of weight generally used is the microgram (μg) because of the very low levels needed in clinical use. Human serum levels of cobalamins are measured in picograms per milliliter (pg/ml; 10^{-12} g/ml). The normal values range from 200 to 900 pg/ml, and values below 100 pg/ml are diagnostic of cobalamin deficiency (86).

B. Chemical

1. Spectrophotometric

This rapid and accurate method for the assay of cyanocobalamin depends upon the absorption of cyanocobalamin at 361 nm. As little as 25 μg/ml can be determined. Many of the cobalamin analogs have absorption maxima at 361 nm also, and therefore the usefulness of the assay is limited for the most part to pure samples of cobalamin.

2. Colorimetric

A sensitive assay method for cyanocobalamin is used on the cyanide content (87,88). Cyanide is liberated by reduction or by photolysis and is measured by a sensitive colorimetric procedure. Of course, this technique does not differentiate cyanocobalamin from other analogs containing cyanide. An alternate method has been proposed based on the difference in the spectrum of cyanocobalamin and its purple dicyanide complex (89).

Other colorimetric methods are based on the presence of 5,6-dimethyl-benzimidazole (90) and on the hydrolysis products resulting from treatment of cyanocobalamin with strong hydrochloric acid (91,92).

Chemical methods, although very sensitive and accurate, are time consuming and tedious and therefore are not amenable to routine assays of many samples.

C. Microbiological

Microbiological assays for cyanocobalamin are sensitive and can be applied to crude materials. They have been widely used, principally for determining the vitamin content in a large number of blood and other tissue samples. However, there is a problem of specificity, since cobalamin analogs give varying responses in microorganisms.

1. Lactobacillus

The first microbiologic assay for cyanocobalamin utilized *L. lactis* (93,94). This assay was very difficult to carry out, and a more stable organism *L. leichmannii* 313 (American Type Culture Collection [ATCC] 7830) was found to respond well (95,96). Another strain of this organism (ATCC 4797) has also been used (97,98). In the approved technique of the U.S. Pharmacopoeia, ATCC 7830 is used.

Lactobacilli respond to various cobalamin analogs, as well as to thymidine and other deoxyribonucleosides. For many problems, particularly serum analyses, response to deoxyribonucleosides is not serious, since *L. leichmannii* requires about 1000 times more deoxyribonucleosides than cyanocobalamin for growth.

2. Escherichia coli

Several assays based on the use of this organism (strain 113-3) have been used successfully (99–102). This organism is slightly less sensitive than *L. leichmannii* and responds to many analogs, but it does not respond to deoxyribonucleosides. Methionine at comparatively much higher levels will substitute for cobalamins.

3. Euglena gracilis

Of all the organisms tested, *E. gracilis* appears to offer the greatest sensitivity in assaying for cyanocobalamin (103). The conditions of this assay have been improved and further developed by Hutner and associates (104). The disadvantage of this organism is that it grows slowly, requiring about 5 days for optimal growth.

Microbiological assays are painstaking procedures that require sterile technique and several days to perform and that cannot be used if patients are taking drugs such as antibiotics that interfere with the growth of the organism.

4. Ochromonas malhamensis

Ochromonas malhamensis, a chrysomonad, was discovered by Hutner et al. (105); the assay method was subsequently developed (106). The response of this organism to cobalamin analogs, which is one of the most specific, parallels the discrimination shown by humans toward cobalamins. This organism is also a slow grower.

D. Biological

Cyanocobalamin assays involving higher animals are somewhat more difficult and time consuming than microbiological assays. The large stores of cobalamins found in young, growing animals reared from normal mothers present the biggest problem. Some of these objections have been overcome by including stress factors to intensify depletion or by feeding diets that increase the requirements for cobalamin (107–110). The chick assay has been the most widely used of the biological assays (111,112).

E. Isotope Dilution

1. Radioisotope Dilution

These assays measure the extent to which cobalamin, after first being liberated from bound materials, competes with radioactively labeled cyanocobalamin for binding sites on a protein.

The development of radiodilution assays, particularly for the measurement of serum cobalamin levels, has met the need for a rapid and simple method and has made the determination of blood levels in humans more generally available. Radiodilution assays of blood involve extraction of bound cobalamin from a sample of serum, the conversion of the cobalamin to cyanocobalamin, and, after mixing with a known quantity of radioactive cyanocobalamin, the association with a cobalamin ligand with high affinity for the vitamin. Dilution of the radioactive cyanocobalamin by endogenous cobalamin allows calculation of the concentration of the vitamin extracted from the serum (113,114).

The specificity of the cobalamin ligand (binding protein) is crucial to the accuracy of the assay. The ligand, or binder, is usually intrinsic factor. It is important to use purified intrinsic factor as the binder when performing radiodilution assay for serum cobalamin, since human plasma contains cobalamin analogs that may mask cobalamin deficiency. These biologically inactive analogs are present in serum in sufficient concentrations to interfere substantially with a radiodilution assay for cobalamin when nonpurified intrinsic factor is used as the binding protein (115–117). The less purified preparations of intrinsic factor contain, in addition to intrinsic factor, proteins that can bind the inactive cobalamin analog (118). In the absence of pure intrinsic factor, nonradioactive cobinamide (a vitamin B_{12} analog) can be added to saturate the non–intrinsic-factor proteins prior to addition of cobalamin.

The isotope dilution methods for the assay of cobalamins have been replacing the microbiologic methods in the past few years, and at present they are more widely used than most other methods.

Further comment on the reliability of cobalamin assays has recently been published (118a). These authors maintain that commerical radiodilution kits for the assay of serum cobalamin, which are in widespread use as screening tests, may give erroneously high results.

In another recent study, England and Linnell reported on the results of a U.K. quality control program in which participating laboratories assayed serum cobalamin in a single sample by radiodilution and microbiological methods (118b). The sample, assayed at 95 ng/liter by the reference laboratories, showed levels ranging from 50 to 730 g/liter by the microbiological assay, and from 50 to 1750 ng/liter by the radiodilution assay.

The authors say all current methods of serum cobalamin assay are unreliable. They contested the theory that nonspecific binding causes erroneous radiodilution results, since "there is no evidence to support the contention that cobalamin analogues circulate in man." They suggested that the nature of cobalamin binding in serum meant that most of the cobalamin assayed by present methods is metabolically inactive.

Over 90% of cobalamin assays are performed by radiodilution. As a result of earlier reports of unreliable results, the U.S. National Committee for Clinical Laboratory Standards (NCCLS) published a standard, which was ratified by the Food and Drug Administration earlier in 1980, recommending that all radiodilution kits for cobalamin should contain purified intrinsic factor as the cobalamin-binding protein (118c). All manufacturers wishing to market such kits in the United States must now comply with these recommendations.

IV. SOURCES OF COBALAMINS

Until recently, the occurrence in nature of cobalamin was considered to be limited to bacteria and animal tissues. In 1962, Fries (118d) reported that peas, cultivated under aseptic conditions, produced corrin that supported the growth of the B$_{12}$-requiring organisms, *E. coli* (strain 113-3), *E. gracilis*, and *Goniotrichum elegans*. In 1964, Katake and Ono (118e) reported low amounts of cobalamins in several plants. In 1967, Laties and Hoelle (118f) reported that slices of potato tubers catabolized labeled proprionate in a manner consistent with the participation of the coenzyme B$_{12}$-dependent enzyme methylmalonyl-CoA mutase. In 1969, Petrosyan et al. (118g) detected vitamin B$_{12}$ by microbiological assay in bean plants. Poston (118h) reported the presence of coenzyme B$_{12}$-dependent leucine 2,3-aminomutase in beans, ryegrass, and potato tubers. Excellent sources of cobalamins are animal organ meats, especially the liver, kidney, and heart (119,120). Table 2 gives the dietary sources of cobalamin. Cobalamins originate from the ingestion of vitamin-containing tissues of animals and from an animal's own digestive tract. Herbivorous animals obtain all their cobalamins from that produced by the intestinal flora, and by coprophagy. In carnivorous animals and humans, intestinal synthesis of cobalamins is not sufficient, and dietary cobalamins are required. The cobalamin distribution in the organs of humans is discussed in the next section.

V. METABOLISM

A. Absorption

1. Methods of Determining Cobalamin Absorption in Humans

Before the introduction of the use of labeled cyanocobalamin, estimates of absorption were based mostly on indirect evidence. Microbiological assays were used to measure deposition of the absorbed vitamin in tissues. Qualitatively, the degree of hematopoietic response in cobalamin-deficient patients was used as an index of absorption. Because of the synthesis of cobalamins by bacteria in the intestine, it has not been possible to measure microbiologically the unabsorbed cyanocobalamin from an unlabeled oral dose.

Five different methods involving various radioactive isotopes of cobalt (^{56}Co, ^{57}Co, ^{58}Co, and ^{60}Co) are available for determining the absorption of an oral dose of radioactive cyanocobalamin in humans. The five methods are discussed briefly here; detailed reviews of these techniques have been presented elsewhere (121–123).

Urinary excretion test.   Introduced by Schilling (124), the urinary excretion method of measuring cyanocobalamin absorption, frequently called the Schilling test, or UET, is

Table 2 Dietary Sources of Cobalamins

High (50–500 μg/100 g)	Medium (5–50 μg/100 g)	Low (0.2–5 μg/100 g)
Kidney, lamb	Kidney	Fish
	Rabbit	Cod
	Beef	Flounder
		Haddock
Liver	Liver	Sole
Lamb	Rabbit	Halibut
Beef	Chicken	Lobster
Calf		Scallop
Pork	Heart	Shrimp
	Beef	Swordfish
Brain, beef	Rabbit	Tuna
	Chicken	
	Egg yolk	Beef
	Clams	Lamb
	Oysters	Pork
	Crabs	Chicken
	Sardines	Egg (whole)
	Salmon	Cheese
		American
		Swiss
		Milk (cow)

the most widely used. After a small, single oral dose of radioactive cyanocobalamin (0.5–2.0 μg), no urinary radioactivity is detected in normal or pernicious anemia subjects.

However, if a parenteral injection (i.e., a "flushing dose") of 1000 μg of nonradioactive cyanocobalamin is given simultaneously or within 2 hr after the oral dose, a significant amount of radioactivity is excreted by normal individuals, but very little is found in pernicious anemia subjects. Excretion of substantial radioactivity in the urine of pernicious anemia patients occurs only when oral intrinsic factor is given. Not all the absorbed radioactivity is flushed into the urine by the parenteral cyanocobalamin; approximately one-third of the absorbed dose is recovered in the urine in 24 hr (125–127). If a second parenteral injection of unlabeled cyanocobalamin is given 24 hr after the oral test dose, an additional amount equivalent to as much as 50% of the first day's excretion may be recovered (128). Because of the delayed excretion of radioactivity observed in some normal and pernicious anemia subjects and in patients with renal disease, it is desirable to use two flushing doses and to collect two 24-hr urine specimens after each oral dose of labeled cyanocobalamin (128–131). It is absolutely necessary to use at least two flushing doses when testing intrinsic factor preparations consecutively in the same patient. The second injection also serves to eliminate further radioactivity from the body.

A shortened procedure that measures the absorption of cyanocobalamin in the presence and absence of intrinsic factor simultaneously has been proposed (132). Two different isotopes of cobalt are required, one bound to intrinsic factor and the other free. This procedure has been used successfully and was found to be acceptable to both patients and clinicians. It is extremely important to mix the intrinsic factor and labeled cyanocobalamin before administration. The administration of two separate capsules, one containing the labeled cyanocobalamin and the other a preparaton of intrinsic factor, may lead to spuriously low results (133).

Many sensitive counting techniques and a large quantity of special equipment have been developed so that relatively large urine volumes may be counted with maximum precision. The advantages of the urinary excretion test are that: (1) results can be obtained in 24–48 hr; (2) as much as 50% of the absorbed radioactivity can be flushed from the body; (3) the method is suitable for use with outpatients; (4) it is possible to test the greatest number of samples on the sample patient in the shortest time; and (5) with the flushing dose the patient receives treatment during the test. The disadvantages are that it is an indirect method requiring quantitative urine collections and that increased tissue levels of cobalamins resulting from larger parenteral doses may affect the results of the test (125,128,134).

Fecal excretion test.   The fecal excretion test, described by Heinle et al. (135), was the first isotopic method used for the study of cyanocobalamin absorption. The difference between the dose and the amount excreted in the feces represents the quantity of cobalamin absorbed. Normal subjects absorb from 50 to 60% of a 1.0 μg oral dose, whereas pernicious anemia subjects absorb less than 10%. When the same dose is given to pernicious anemia patients together with a fully active intrinsic factor preparation, absorption is increased to normal levels. The agreements of the results obtained by this method with those obtained by the hepatic uptake and urinary excretion tests are very good (136).

The fecal excretion technique is in theory the most accurate and quantitative means of determining absorption since it yields a direct result. Its disadvantages are that: (1) 7–10 days are required to collect all unabsorbed fecal radioactivity; (2) it is the least pleasant of the methods; (3) because only a small percentage of a large dose is absorbed, it cannot be used to measure accurately absorption of doses much above 5–10 μg; and (4) fecal radioactivity does not represent exclusively unabsorbed cyanocobalamin, since it has been shown that some absorbed vitamin is excreted into the feces by the bile.

Hepatic uptake method.   The hepatic uptake technique, described by Glass et al. (137), is concerned with the measurement of absorbed cyanocobalamin deposited in the liver. Subjects with pernicious anemia, in contrast to normal subjects, show no hepatic uptake of radioactivity after an oral dose of cyanocobalamin unless it is accompanied by the administration of intrinsic factor. By placing a directional scintillation counter over the surface projection of the liver, a semiquantitative estimate of the amount of cobalamins deposited and, indirectly, the amount absorbed can be obtained. The increase in radioactivity in the liver is slow; the peak concentration is reached 2–4 days after the oral dose. For measuring intestinal absorption by hepatic uptake, a more rapid quantitative method with the use of a double label (^{57}Co and ^{60}Co) has also been proposed (138).

Excellent correlation has been found beween the hepatic uptake and the fecal and urinary excretion methods (136,139). It is a decided advantage of the hepatic uptake method that patient cooperation is unnecessary. On the other hand, special equipment is required, and the procedure does not lend itself to consecutive assays of intrinsic factor on the patient. In addition, inhibition of uptake is observed in liver disease.

Blood plasma radioactivity: The blood plasma radioactivity method, introduced by Booth and Mollin (139) and Doscherholmen et al. (140), depends on the presence of a peak of radioactivity in the blood 8–12 hr after giving an oral test dose. Pernicious anemia subjects, unless given intrinsic factor with the labeled dose, have very little plasma radioactivity at any time. Because in normal subjects less than 5% of the oral dose appears in the total plasma at peak concentration, this method requires the use of labeled cyanocobalamin with very high specific activity. This method shows good correlation with the urinary excretion method (141).

Whole-body counting: Whole body counting is similar to the hepatic uptake method, but radioactivity of the whole body is measured instead of liver radioactivity (142). Whole-body counting makes use of equipment that is expensive and not generally available. Typical values of the amount of radioactivity measured after a test dose of labeled cyanocobalamin with and without a potent source of intrinsic factor are given in Table 3. Absorption tests have been of great value in diagnosing cobalamin deficiencies, especially in differentiating between Addisonian pernicious anemia and cobalamin malabsorption of intestinal origin (143). The administration of intrinsic factor usually corrects impaired absorption of cobalamin in patients with pernicious anemia but not in those with intestinal malabsorption.

The assimilation of cobalamins from food involves both digestive and absorptive processes (see Sec. V.A.3). The absorption tests use labeled crystalline cyanocobalamin, which is not always physiological, since it circumvents the digestive process. The importance of this digestive process is seen by the recent observations that some patients do not absorb labeled cobalamins satisfactorily if they are incorporated into food, even though they absorb crystalline cyanocobalamin normally (144,145).

2. Site of Cobalamin Absorption

The absorption of physiological doses of cobalamin in the human alimentary tract takes place almost exclusively in the ileum. This conclusion is based on defective cobalamin absorption in diseases of the lower ileum or after resection of the ileum, measurement of intestinal radioactivity after oral administration of radioactive cyanocobalamin, and installation of radioactive cyanocobalamin in various segments of intestine. Impaired absorption of cobalamins is found in patients who have undergone resection of the ileum, but not after resection of the duodenum or jejunum (143,146–150). The addition of intrinsic factor or antibiotics could not correct the impaired cobalamin absorption.

Various investigators have studied the site of cobalamin absorption by following instillation of cyanaocobalamin and cyanocobalamin–intrinsic factor complex. Direct instillation of cobalamins in the jejunum only (segment closed at proximal and distal ends) did not result in any significant cyanocobalamin absorption (151). Cobalamin is absorbed, whether it is instilled in the duodenum, jejunum, or ileum. The cobalamin instilled in the upper intestine probably moved down to the ileum before it was absorbed. In pernicious

Table 3 Typical Values of Radioactive Cyanocobalamin in Pernicious Anemia Patients With and Without Intrinsic Factor by Five Different Methods

Assay method	Percentage of oral dose of cyanocobalamin detected in patients	
	Without intrinsic factor	With intrinsic factor
Urinary excretion test	0–7	10–30
Fecal excretion	80–100	30–60
Hepatic uptake	0–1	40–50
Blood radioactivity	0–1	3–5
Total body radioactivity	0–20	30–60

anemia patients, the ileum absorbed cyanocobalamin only when intrinsic factor was added. Similar experiments conducted by Best et al. (152) and Johnson and Berger (153), implicated the ileum as the site of absorption after the use of delayed-relapse capsules containing labeled cyanocobalamin. With polyethylene glycol as a marker in a test meal containing labeled cyanocobalamin, samples of intestinal juice from different parts of the intestine also lead to the conclusion that most of the absorption occurred in the terminal portion of the small intestine (150).

3. Mechanism of Absorption

Cobalamins can be absorbed by two different mechanisms:

An active mechanism (intrinsic factor mediated). The active mechanism is mediated by intrinsic factor, a glycoprotein secreted by the partietal cells of the gastric mucosa. It is of primary importance in the absorption of physiological doses of cobalamin (approximately 1–5 μg).
A diffusion-type mechanism (nonintrinsic factor mediated). The diffusion-type mechanism is operative when the amount of vitamin is large, usually in excess of the amount available from the diet (154).

Active mechanism (intrinsic factor–mediated): The events that take place in the intestine after the ingestion of physiological amounts of cobalamin require about 8–10 hr for the completion of the absorption of the vitamin in humans. The sequence of events can be classified as: (1) removal of cobalamin from combination with other dietary sources: (2) binding of cobalamin to intrinsic factor; (3) intestinal transit through the small intestine to the ileum; (4) attachment of cobalamin–intrinsic factor complex to specific receptors on the absorptive surface of the ileum; (5) transfer of cobalamin across the small intestinal epithelial absorptive cell to the portal plasma; and (6) release of the vitamin from cobalamin–intrinsic factor complex.

Removal of Cobalamins from Combination with Other Dietary Sources—Essentially all dietary cobalamin is present in coenzyme form. Unless cyanocobalamin in medicinal form is ingested, the main cobalamins in food are adenosylcobalamin and hydroxocobalamin (155). Significant amounts of the coenzymes are converted to hydroxocobalamin during the preparation of food (155,156). Most studies of cobalamin absorption have been performed with cyanocobalamin. The absorption of cyanocobalamin is essentially the same as that of hydroxocobalamin (156,158). The cobalamins are released from attachment to protein in vitro by heating, acid, and proteolytic enzymes (159,160). In contrast to cobalamin–intrinsic factor complexes, pancreatic proteases readily release cobalamin from protein linkage.

Binding of Cobalamin to Intrinsic Factor—A prerequisite for the intestinal absorption of physiological amounts of cobalamin is binding to intrinsic factor. Upon its release, cobalamin is bound to intrinsic factor.

The intrinsic factor molecule probably has at least two functional sites, a cobalamin-binding site and a receptor site that attaches to a receptor mechanism on the surface of the intestinal mucosa (161–166). There is excellent evidence that the bound vitamin is protected against enzymatic digestion and heating (167–169). The presence of the vitamin also diminishes or prevents inactivation of human intrinsic factor by various means (170,171). It protects intrinsic factor against autodigestion during transport from the stomach to the ileum, where the intrinsic factor can then promote the uptake of the bound vitamin. Intrinsic factor also probably protects cobalamin from uptake by intestinal bacteria.

Transit Through the Small Intestine—The cobalamin–intrinsic factor complex is carried to the ileum by peristalsis. The complex is resistant to enzymatic hydrolysis by various enzymes, as mentioned above. In vitro, very few enzymes can split off cobalamins from the complex or digest the complex, whereas the free intrinsic factor is more labile, as well as more susceptible to enzymatic breakdown (163–165). In view of the fact that the intrinsic factor molecule dimerizes, it would appear that the polymerization causes some conformational change that prevents the enzymes from attacking susceptible bonds (50,51,170–175). In addition, the dimerization apparently also protects the vitamin from bacterial utilization.

Attachment of Cobalamin to Ileal Receptors—The cobalamin–intrinsic factor complex is transiently attached to an ileal receptor (118). The proximal small intestine does not have the ability to enhance absorption of the vitamin; only the ileum has this property. Free cobalamin is attached to the ileal receptors only weakly, if at all. This uptake is also specific for intrinsic factor. Cobalamin-binding proteins of serum, saliva, colostrum, and tears do not enhance the uptake of cobalamin (176).

Several other characteristics of this attachment to ileal receptor have been found:

1. Energy supply or a specific enzymatic step is probably not required (177).
2. Intrinsic factor enhancement of cobalamin uptake is not affected by changes in temperature from 7 to 37 °C (177), suggesting that the attachment of intrinsic factor-bound vitamin, although specific, results from absorption and not from a specific energy-requiring enzymatic process.
3. Attachment of the complex to the receptor occurs preferentially at a pH between 6.0 and 8.0 (153,155,177–179). Maximal binding between human intrinsic factor-cobalamin complex and ileal mucosal homogenates has been reported to occur in the pH range of 6.5–9.5. These results are in good agreement with those of studies in other species (180).
4. Divalent cations are required for attachment. Removal of calcium ion or addition of a chelating agent to the medium in vitro reduces intrinsic factor uptake of cobalamin (178,181).

The precise nature of the ileal receptor is unknown. The receptor is probably antigenic and is specific for the distal end of the small intestine.

Good progress has been made recently in attempts to solubilize and purify ileal receptors from human tissue (180,182–185). The characteristics of these purified receptors appear to be the same (temperature independence divalent cation requirement, and pH optimum near neutrality) as previously reported with less pure preparations. It has been speculated that the receptor may be a glycoprotein or a mucopolysaccharide, since glycoproteins or mucopolysaccharide or both are present at the absorptive surface of the intestinal cell (177).

Transport of Cobalamin Across the Intestinal Epithelial Cell—In contrast to the attachment of cobalamin to receptors on the brush borders, entry of cobalamin into the epithelial cell is a slow, endergonic process (159,186,187). The attachment of cobalamin to the receptors occurs between 2 and 3 hr after ingestion. An additional 3–4 hr are required before significant amounts of the vitamin appear in the blood in humans. Peak blood levels are reached 8–12 hr after ingestion in humans (188). This indicates that a slow and probably complex mechanism is involved in the transport of cobalamins across the cell membrane. Prolonged interaction between the cobalamin–intrinsic factor complex and the membrane receptor would explain the slow rate of absorption of the vitamin (189).

Release of Cobalamin from Cobalamin–Intrinsic Factor Complex—Cobalamin is bound to intrinsic factor when it reaches the ileum, and it probably is bound to intrinsic factor when it is attached to the ileal brush borders. However, when it enters the portal blood it is no longer bound to intrinsic factor but to specific transport proteins called transcobalamins. At some point in the absorption process, the vitamin must separate from intrinsic factor, since intrinsic factor is not absorbed (187,190–192). This release probably is the last phase of cobalamin asborption, and unequivocal evidence for its presence has not yet been presented. That the vitamin in blood is bound to a molecule that has neither the biological nor the immunological characteristics of intrinsic factor and that intrinsic factor is not absorbed provide strong evidence that some process is occurring that separates cobalamin from intrinsic factor.

Role of the Pancreas—A considerable number of patients with pancreatic insufficiency absorb crystalline cyanocobalamin poorly, and this malabsorption is completely corrected by the administration of pancreatic enzymes or purified trypsin and partially corrected by the administration of bicarbonate (193,194). Recent evidence suggests that the primary defect in cobalamin absorption in pancreatic insufficiency is an inability to degrade partially a nonintrinsic factor (R protein)–cobalamin complex because of a deficiency of pancreatic proteases (195–197). Since cobalamin is bound preferentially to these R proteins in the acid milieu of the stomach, rather than to intrinsic factor, the cobalamin remains bound to R protein in the slightly alkaline environment of the intestine until pancreatic proteases partially degrade the R proteins and thereby enable cobalamin to become bound exclusively to intrinsic factor. The partial correction of cobalamin malabsorption observed with bicarbonate is due to neutralization of gastric acid, since slightly alkaline pH intrinsic factor can partially compete with R protein for the initial binding and retention of cobalamin.

Toskes and associates have been unable to conform these observations, and they suggest that the mechanism of cobalamin malabsorption in chronic pancreatitis remains undefined (198,199). Data from the Toskes laboratory suggest that the pancreas secretes a specific factor found in preparations of serine proteases that correct cobalamin malabsorption in patients with chronic pancreatitis. These workers have suggested that the pancreatic factor modified the gastric intrinsic factor in an as yet undefined manner.

Nonintrinsic factor–mediated absorption of cobalamin: A passive mechanism (not mediated by intrinsic factor) is operative when the amount of administered vitamin is large, usually in excess of the amount available from a normal diet. Absorption probably occurs by diffusion. About 1% of an oral dose of 100–500 μg of cobalamin is absorbed in pernicious anemia patients (200). The site of cobalamin absorption with large pharmacological doses is nonspecific (201); some absorption of the vitamin occurs through the nasal mucosa, rectal mucosa, and skin (201–203). The amount of cobalamin that can be absorbed from a single oral dose in normal and pernicious anemia subjects is shown in Tables 4 and 5, respectively. It appears from these data that the average maximum absorption is about 1.5 μg in normal subjects regardless of the size of the dose. If doses in excess of 100–300 μg are given orally to pernicious anemia patients, significant amounts of cobalamin are absorbed. Serum cobalamin levels in the pernicious anemia patients receiving these high doses are in the normal range (204). Since intrinsic factor is absent or deficient in pernicious anemia, large doses must be absorbed by a mechanism independent of intrinsic factor.

The patterns of plasma radioactivity after the administration of small and large oral doses of labeled cyanocobalamin have been studied (139,140,146,147). The level of radioactivity in the blood starts to increase 3–6 hr after oral administration of physiological doses and reaches a peak at 8–12 hr after ingestion; patients receiving large doses show an

Table 4 Absorption of a Single Oral Dose of Cyanocobalamin in Normal Human Subjects

Oral dose	Amount of cyanocobalamin absorbed	
(μg)	μg	Percentage of oral dose
0.1	0.08	80
0.25	0.19	76
0.5	0.35	70
1.0	0.56	56
2.0	0.92	46
5.0	1.4	28
10.0	1.6	16
20.0	1.2	6
50.0	1.5	3

Source: Data from various authors and summarized by Chanarin (121).

early rise in radioactivity 1–2 hr after ingestion, with peak values 4–6 hr after the dose (205). In addition, some of the cobalamin appears in the lymph, in contrast to the results obtained with small physiological doses (206,207).

In contrast to the intrinsic factor–mediated absorption, the nonintrinsic factor–mediated absorption of cobalamin does not appear to require calcium ions (159,208,209) and is independent of pH (159). Beyond these data, the mechanism of the nonintrinsic factor–mediated absorption is not well defined. It is not certain whether receptors for large amounts of cobalamin exist in the intestine.

Intestinal absorption of cobalamin analogs: Except for hydroxocobalamin and possibly adenosylcobalamin, most of the other corrinoids tested, which are not normally found in foods or dietary supplements, are poorly absorbed compared to cyanocobalamin (65). A detailed review of the absorption of cobalamin analogs has been published (118).

Table 5 Absorption of a Single Oral Dose of Cyanocobalamin in Pernicious Anemia Subjects

Oral dose	Amount of cyanocobalamin absorbed	
(μg)	μg	Percentage of oral dose
1	0.057	5.7
3	0.108	3.6
10	0.260	2.6
100	1.1	1.1
200	2.0	1.0
400	4.0	1.0
800	8.8	1.1
5000	50.0	1.0

Source: From Ref. 208.

B. Transport

1. Plasma

Following absorption in humans, most of the cobalamins are found in the plasma attached to specific proteins. There are at least two classes of cobalamin-binding proteins, which were initially distinguished by their electrophoretic mobilities (210–212). The binding proteins were found in the α- and β-globulin fractions.

Two binders studied extensively by Hall and Finkler (213–215) and by Hall (216), by means of DEAE-cellulose and CM-cellulose chromatography, were named transcobalamin I and transcobalamin II, respectively (213–216).

Evidence for a third binding (transcobalamin III) in normal human serum has been presented by several investigators (217–223). This protein seems to resemble transcobalamin II in its behavior on DEAE-cellulose and its electrophoretic mobility and transcobalamin I in its antigenic characteristics, behavior on Sephadex G-150, and its inability to stimulate uptake of cobalamin by reticulocytes (222,223).

Transcobalamin I and III, part of a class of proteins that is antigenically cross-reactive, heterogenous in carbohydrate composition, and present in many body tissues and fluids, are designated as "R binders." The term *R. binder* was originally used by Grasbeck (224) to denote a cobalamin-binding protein (from human gastric juice) that was devoid of intrinsic factor activity and had a rapid electrophorectic mobility. The R-type cobalamin-binding proteins from other sources do not show rapid mobility. Transcobalamin II is chemically and immunologically distinct from transcobalamin I and III and other R binders. Transcobalamin I, and α-glycoprotein of molecular weight 60,000, carries the majority of cobalamins found in plasma. Transcobalamin II has a molecular weight of 38,000 and is the chief transport protein for the newly absorbed vitamin. The function of R proteins has not been unequivocally established, whereas transcobalamin II is known to facilitate the uptake of cobalamin by a large number of tissues.

A deficiency of transcobalamin I causes no apparent abnormality in cobalamin metabolism (225). In contrast to transcobolamin I, transcobalamin II is necessary for normal cellular maturation of the hematopoietic system. Transcobalamin II deficiency occurs as a rare inborn error of protein metabolism that is inherited as an autosomal recessive condition (226–228).

The cobalamin entering the blood after oral ingestion appears to be bound to transcobalamin II (214). More than 8 hr after administration, an increasing proportion of the labeled vitamin becomes bound to transcobalamin I. However, the uptake of cobalamin by transcobalamin II is probably still going on at 24 hr (216). Since most people usually ingest food several times a day, a small but constant amount of transcobalamin II–cobalamin complex is circulating. The amount of vitamin absorbed to transcobalamin II probably never exceeds 20 pg/ml plasma (216).

2. Transport of Cobalamins to Tissues

Transcobalamin II facilitates cobalamin uptake by a number of different cells in vivo and in vitro. For example, cobalamin uptake by HeLa cells in tissue culture is increased by transcobalamin II, and liver uptake of cobalamin from plasma occurs more readily when the vitamin is bound to transcobalamin II than to transcobalamin I (229). Transcobalamin II promotes the cobalamin uptake of erythrocyte suspensions in which there is a higher than normal proportion of reticulocytes (230). Transport of cobalamins into L1210 murine leukemic cells, L51784 murine leukemic cells, human bone marrow cells, isolated rat liver mitochondria, and cultured human fibroblast is also mediated by transcobalamin II

(231,232). This process is biphasic, consisting of an initial step, in which the transcobalamin II–cobalamin complex binds to the cell surface, and a second step, in which the cobalamin enters the cell.

The primary step is the binding of the complex to the external membrane of the cell. This step is insensitive to temperature, depends on calcium ions, and is inhibited by ethylaminediaminetetracetate (EDTA). Specific receptors have been identified that probably mediate this transcobalamin binding (233,234). The second step appears to involve transport of the vitamin into the cell.

Entry of cobalamin into the cytoplasm of the cell requires 1–6 h after the transcobalamin II–cobalamin complex interacts with the receptor of the cell surface. Transport appears to be by endocytosis (234a) with final processing of the transcobalamin II–cobalamin complex occurring in lysozomes where the transcobalamin II is digested and its fragments leave the cell. The residual cobalamin in the lysozome is not associated with a detectable binder (234b), and it rapidly enters the cytoplasm. Cultured cells incubated in agents which prevent generation of low pH in endosomes or of maturation of lysozomes do not transport cobalamin into the cytoplasm, do not digest the transcobalamin II, and accumulate transcobalamin II–cobalamin in vesicles (234a). Transport of cobalamin from intestine to portal blood may also be by endocytosis (234c).

These major intracellular cobalamin-binding proteins are the two cobalamin-dependent apoenzymes-methylmalonyl-CoA mutase and methyltetrahydrofolate methyltransferase. They are associated with mitochondria and cytoplasm, respectively (235,236).

The transcobalamin II–cobalamin complex is degraded in the lysosome, freeing the cobalamin, and some of the cobalamin is used to synthesize methylcobalamin in the cytosol. Mammalian cells require cobalamin as a cofactor for two enzymes: N^5-methyltetrahydrofolate: homocysteine methyltransferase (5-methyltetrahydropteroyl-L-glutamate: L-homocysteine 5-methyltransferase, EC 2.1.1.13), which catalyzes the conversion of homocysteine to methionine, and methylmalonyl-CoA mutase (methylmalonyl CoA: CoA-carbonyl mutase, EC 5.4.99.2), which catalyzes the rearrangement of methylmalonyl CoA to succinyl CoA (see also Sec. VI). Cyanocobalamin is converted within cells to either methylcobalamin, a coenzyme for methyltransferase, or adenosylcobalamin, the coenzyme for mutase (235,236). For more details, see recent reviews (232,237).

C. Tissue Distribution and Storage

After the isolation of cyanocobalamin, it was assumed that serum cobalamin was either cyanocobalamin or a mixture of hydroxocobalamin and cyanocobalamin. In retrospect, the light sensitivities of the coenzyme forms and the vitamin and the conversion of these compounds to hydrocobalamin account for the delay in discovering the coenzyme forms. In addition, the finding that inorganic cyanide facilitated the recovery of the vitamin from extracts ensured that cyanocobalamin was the form most likely to be isolated.

It is now known that most of the cobalamins in humans occur as the two coenzymatically active forms, adenosylcobalamin and methylcobalamin.

Methylcobalamin constitutes 60–80% of the total plasma cobalamin. In pernicious anemia subjects, methylcobalamin is disproportionately reduced in relation to the other major components, so that the ratio of methylcobalamin to hydroxocobalamin falls to less than 1.0 (238) (Table 6).

More recently, the cobalamin distribution of the various transcobalamins has been determined (239,240). Transcobalamin II contained about equal amounts of methylcobalamin and adenosylcobalamin, whereas methylcobalamin accounted for most

Table 6 Plasma Cobalamins in Normal Subjects and Pernicious Anemia Patients

| Subjects | No. subjects | Plasma cobalamins (pg/ml) | | | | Ratio of Me:CO-OH B$_{12}$ | CN-B$_{12}$ (% of total) |
		Total B$_{12}$ plasma	Me-B$_{12}$	CN-B$_{12}$[a]	CO-OH B$_{12}$[a]		
Normal subjects	28	522 ± 34	364 ± 25	3.2 ± 1.8	155 ± 16	2.9 ± 0.3	0–8
Pernicious anemia patients	29	64 ± 4.8	9.0 ± 1.9	7.2 ± 1.8	48.8 ± 4.3	0.22 ± 0.05	0–41

[a]Me-B$_{12}$, methylcobalamin; CN-B$_{12}$, cyanocobalamin; CO-OH B$_{12}$, mixture of deoxyadenosylcobalamin and hydroxocobalamin.
Source: From Ref. 238.

of the cobalamin attached to the other transcobalamins. Adenosylcobalamin was the next most abundant cobalamin on transcobalamin I and III. No hydroxocobalamin was observed attached to transcobalamin II. Traces of cyanocobalamin were found to be attached to all the transcobalamins.

In normal human subjects, cobalamins are found principally in the liver (241–242); the average amount is 1.5 mg. The kidneys, heart, spleen, and brain each contain about 20–30 μg (241). The total cobalamin content in the liver of a 3-week-old premature infant was found to be 28 μg (241). A steady increase was found in total cobalamin content in the liver with increase in age (244). Mean values for the total body content calculated for human adults range from 2 to 5 mg (241,242).

The pituitary gland in humans, dogs, rats, and rabbits has the greatest concentration per gram of tissue of any organ (243). Adenosylcobalamin is the major cobalamin in all the cellular tissues, constituting about 60–70% in the liver and about 50% in the other organs. A more detailed review of the fate and storage of cobalamins has been published (244).

D. Excretion

The urinary, biliary, and fecal routes are the main excretion pathways. Urinary excretion by glomerular filtration of free cobalamin is minimal, varying from 0. to 0.25 μg/day. The total loss from the body ranges between 2 and 5 μg daily (245). In pernicious anemia and other conditions associated with cobalamin deficiency, urinary excretion of cobalamin is reduced. Though the origin of urinary cobalamin is uncertain, it is thought that some cobalamin is derived from the tubular epithelial cells and the lymph (246). It is only the unbound plasma cobalamin that is available for urinary excretion.

Cyanocobalamin is excreted much more rapidly after intravenous than after intramuscular injection. Following parenteral or intravenous administration of 0.1–1.0 mg cyanocobalamin, 50–90% of the dose is excreted in the urine within 48 hr. Patients with renal disease excrete cyanocobalamin, administered parenterally, more slowly than normal subjects. Owing to its greater binding in most patients, less hydroxocobalamin than cyanocobalamin is excreted after injection of the same dose of each (245).

Approximately 0.5–5 μg of cobalamin is secreted into the alimentary tract daily, mainly in the bile (246). Of this, at least 65–75% is reabsorbed in the ileum by means of the intrinsic factor mechanism. This efficient conservation of the vitamin helps explain why pure vegetarians who eat almost no vitamin B_{12} take decades to develop a deficiency. Those subjects who fail to secrete intrinsic factor are unable to reabsorb biliary cobalamin, and therefore, a cobalamin deficiency may then develop. A normal enterohepatic circulation is vital to the conservation of biliary cobalamin. In subjects who have a reduced ability to absorb cobalamin via the intestine, a cobalamin deficiency develops relatively rapidly.

VI. BIOCHEMICAL FUNCTION

The specific biochemical reactions in which the cobamide coenzymes participate are of two types: (1) those that contain 5'-deoxyadenosine linked covalently to the cobalt atom (adenosylcobalamin), and (2) those that have a methyl group attached to the central cobalt atom (methylcobalamin).

The conversion of cyanocobalamin to its coenzyme form is catalyzed by an enzyme system, vitamin B_{12} coenzyme synthetase, present in a large number of different microorganisms and in human tissue (247–250). The vitamin undergoes a reduction, presumably to B_{12}s or Co^{1+} form, and then reacts with a deoxyadenosyl moiety derived from ATP. In addition to ATP, the reaction requires diol or dithiol, a reduced flavin or reduced ferredoxin as the biological alkylating agent (249–251).

A. Reactions Requiring Adenosylcobalamin

All but one of the reactions requiring adenosylcobalamin can be classifed as rearrangement reactions. The exception is the adenosylcobamide-dependent reduction of ribonucleotide triphosphate to deoxyribonucleotide triphosphates.

In the rearrangement reactions, a hydrogen atom moves from one carbon atom to an adjacent one in an exchange for an alkyl, acyl, or electronegative group, which migrates in the opposite direction:

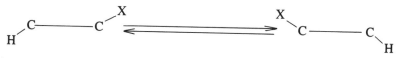

In all these rearrangement reactions, adenosylcobalamin is an intermediate hydrogen carrier; the migrating hydrogen atom attaches to the 5′ carbon of the adenosyl group before it is transferred to the product.

To date, 10 such rearrangements have been reported (Table 7). The enzymes catalyzing the reactions can be classified in terms of the group that trades place with a hydrogen atom during the course of the rearrangement. The three classifications are:

1. Interconversion between branched-chain and straight-chain compounds by coenzyme-dependent migration of alkyl or acyl group (reactions 1–3, Table 7).
2. Migration of an OH or NH$_2$ group to a carbon atom already bearing a hydroxyl group. Elimination of water or ammonia occurs, and an aldehyde is formed (reactions 4–6, Table 7).
3. Migration of an NH$_2$ group from a terminal carbon atom to an adjacent methylene group, the rearrangement resulting in the conversion of a primary amine to a secondary amine (reactions 7–10, Table 7).

The mechanism of the group X migration is poorly understood (see Refs. 252–254 for detailed review of the studies of the mechanism of the rearrangements).

All the above-mentioned rearrangements occur in bacteria where each constitutes a step in their energy pathways.

As yet only one of these reactions has been identified in mammals, namely, the conversion of methylmalonyl coenzyme A to succinyl coenzyme A. This reaction is a step in the pathway for the catabolism of propionic coenzyme A, derived from the breakdown of valine and isoleucine. As mentioned, methylmalonic aciduria is sometimes useful as a sensitive index of cobalamin deficiency except in the rare cases in which it is due to an inborn metabolic error. However, a normal methylmalonic acid excretion does not rule out the presence of cobalamin deficiency.

Ribonucleotide reduction is the single adenosylcobamide-dependent reaction that is not a rearrangement reaction (253,255–259). In the ribonucleotide reduction reaction, the 2′-hydroxyl group is replaced by the hydrogen with retention of configuration at the 2′-carbon atom. This reaction provides the building blocks for the synthesis of DNA. Interestingly, the ribonucleotide reductase reaction has so far been demonstrated only in prokaryotic organisms and the Euglenophyta (259a–e). It has been anticipated that cells in which DNA synthesis is impaired by cobalamin deficiency would be found to contain a cobamide-dependent ribonucleotide reductase (see Sec. VI.B). It is therefore ubiquitous

Table 7 Adenosylcobalamin-Coenzyme Dependent Rearrangements

Enzyme	Reaction catalyzed[a]
1. Glutamate mutase	
2. Methylmalonyl-CoA mutase	
3. α-Methyleneglutarate mutase	
4. a. Dioldehydrase	
b. Dioldehydrase	

5. Glyceroldehydrase

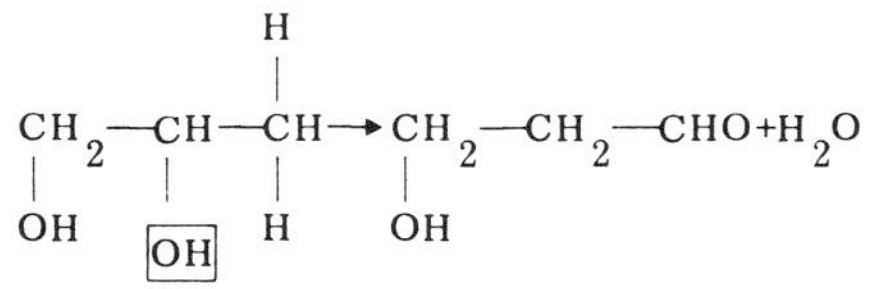

$$CH_2-CH \rightarrow CH_2-CH_2-CHO + H_2O$$

with substituents $-OH$, $\boxed{OH}$, $-OH$, H

6. Ethanolamine ammonia-lyase

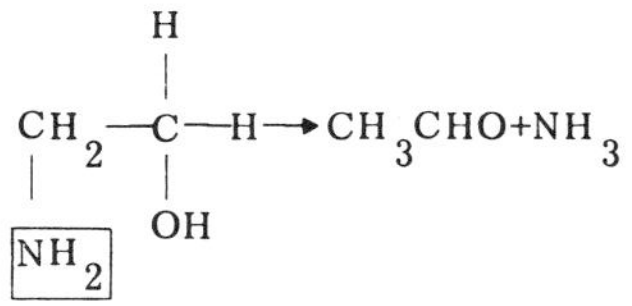

$$CH_2-C-H \rightarrow CH_3CHO + NH_3$$

with substituents $\boxed{NH_2}$, $-OH$, H

7. L-β-Lysine mutase

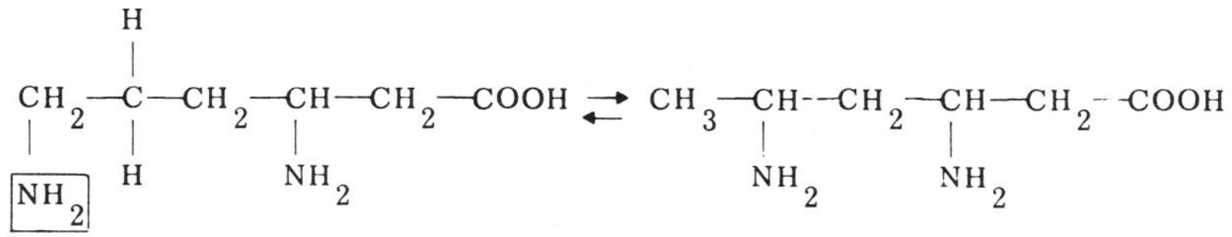

$$CH_2-C-CH_2-CH_2-COOH \rightleftharpoons CH_3-CH-CH_2-CH-CH_2-COOH$$

with substituents $\boxed{NH_2}$, H, $-NH_2$ and products $-NH_2$, $-NH_2$

8. D-α-Lysine mutase

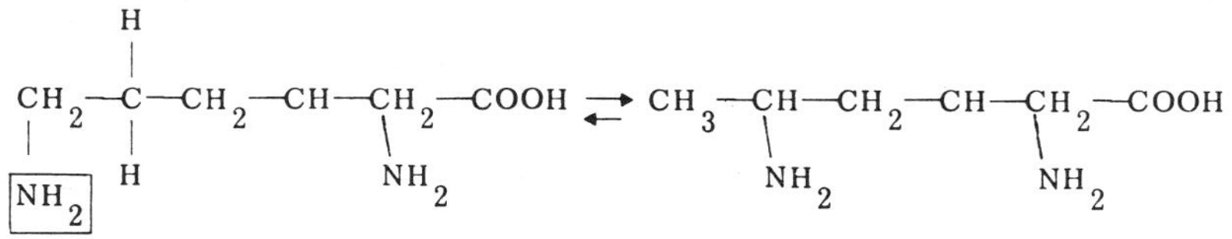

$$CH_2-C-CH_2-CH_2-COOH \rightleftharpoons CH_3-CH-CH_2-CH_2-COOH$$

with substituents $\boxed{NH_2}$, H, $-NH_2$ and products $-NH_2$, NH_2

9. Ornithine mutase

$$CH_2-C-CH_2-COOH \rightleftharpoons CH_3-CH-CH_2-CH-COOH$$

with substituents $\boxed{NH_2}$, H, $-NH_2$ and products $-NH_2$, $-NH_2$

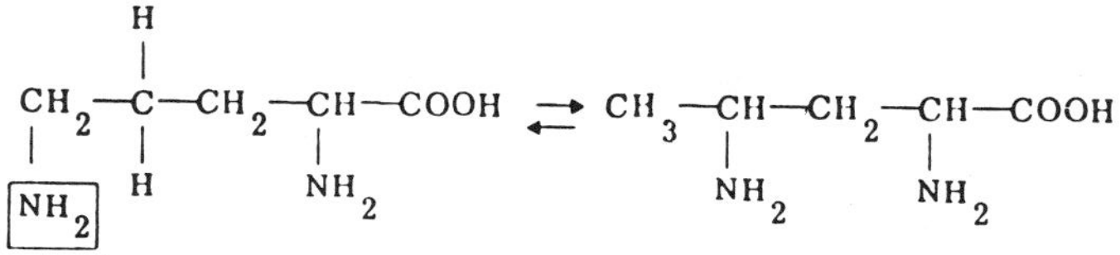

10. L-β-Leucine aminomutase

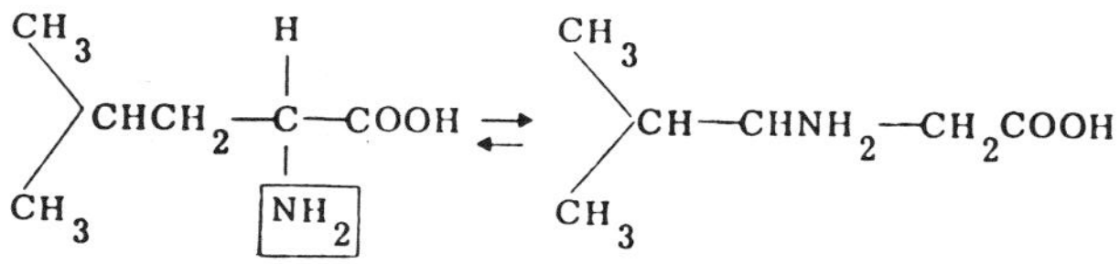

$$CH_3-CH-CHCH_2-C-COOH \rightleftharpoons CH_3-CH-CH-CHNH_2-CH_2COOH$$

with substituents CH_3, $\boxed{NH_2}$, H and products CH_3, CH_3

a $\boxed{}$ = group X, which migrates.

in living organisms. In most species, including mammalian, the enzyme is an iron-containing protein that requires no cofactor and that uses ribonucleotide diphosphates as substrates. In certain organisms, however, such as the flagellate *E. gracilis*, and a number of bacteria, such as *L. leichmannii*, ribonucleotide reduction is accomplished by an iron-free adenosylcobamide-requiring enzyme that uses the nucleoside triphosphates as substrates. The electron donor for the ribonucleotide reductase reaction is thioredoxin or glutaredoxin (259f–h), a small protein found in both bacterial and mammalian systems; it is used as the reducing agent by both the cobamide-requiring and the iron-requiring enzymes.

B. Reactions Requiring Methylcobalamin (Methylcobamides)

The reactions requiring methylcobalamin (Table 8) have been reviewed in detail by Stadtman (260) and Poston and Stadtman (261). These reactions require a protein-bound corrinoid. Again, only one of these reactions has been demonstrated in mammals, namely, that catalyzed by n^5-methyltetrahydrofolate homocysteine methyltransferase. An enzyme-bound methylcobalamin is formed as an intermediate in the transfer of the methyl moiety of N^5-methyltetrahydrofolate to homocysteine by the cobalamin-dependent methyltransferase. Free methylcobalamin can be used as an alternative substrate for the methylation of homocysteine in many instances, although not all cobalamin-dependent methyltransferases appear to exhibit activity with this donor.

In essence, the methyltransferase reaction can be viewed as the sum of two half-reactions, consisting of the successive methylation and demethylation of cobalamin bound to the enzyme:

$$N^5\text{-Methyltetrahydrofolate + enzyme} \cdot \text{cobalamin} \longrightarrow$$
$$\text{tetrahydrofolate + enzyme} \cdot \text{methylcobalamin} \tag{1}$$
$$\text{Enzyme} \cdot \text{methylcobalamin + homocysteine} \longrightarrow$$
$$\text{enzyme} \cdot \text{cobalamin + methionine} \tag{2}$$

The biosynthesis of methane also requires a cobalamin–protein complex. The methyl group is transferred to the cobalt atom of the cobalamin compound to form an enzyme-bound methylcobalt derivative followed by a reductive cleavage to yield methane; coenzyme M is involved (261a, b).

Another strictly anaerobic process in which acetate rather than methane is the final fermentation product also appears to require a cobalamin enzyme as an essential catalyst. These bacteria meet growth requirements by converting a mixture of hydrogen and carbon dioxide to acetic acid.

The exact mechanisms of the biosynthesis of methane and acetate await more detailed investigation.

Table 8 Reactions Requiring Methylcobalamin

Enzyme	Reaction catalyzed
1. N^5-Methyltetrahydrofolate homocysteine methyltransferase (methionine synthetase)	CH_3-THFA + $HSCH_2CH_2CH(NH_2)$ COOH $\longrightarrow$ $CH_3SCH_2CH_2CH(NH_2)$ COOH + THFA[a]
2. Methane synthetase	$2CH_3OH + H_2 \longrightarrow CH_4 + 2H_2O$
3. Acetate synthetase	$2CO_2 + 4H_2 \longrightarrow CH_3COOH + 2H_2O$

[a]THFA = Tetrahydrofolic acid.

VII. DEFICIENCY

Detailed reviews dealing with various aspects of cobalamin deficiency have been published (84,262–268). Factors that may contribute to this deficiency are as follows.

A. Lack of Intrinsic Factor Secretion

This is the most common cause of cobalamin malabsorption.

1. Pernicious Anemia

Adult pernicious anemia is the most commonly acquired cause of failure to assimilate cobalamins. The inability to secrete intrinsic factor results in the failure of the subject to absorb cobalamins. It may take as long as 5–7 years after the cessation of intrinsic factor secretion before any outward signs of pernicous anemia are evident, because body stores of cobalamins are sufficient during this period.

Pernicious anemia, inherited as an autosomal dominant trait, chiefly affects persons past middle age. The incidence of pernicious anemia in the general population is 1–2 per 1000 and about 25 per 1000 among relatives of pernicious anemia probands (269). Pernicious anemia has also been described in a few children, usually late in childhood.

In addition to megaloblastic anemia, the most prominent signs and symptoms of vitamin B$_{12}$ deficiency are weakness, tiredness, pale and smooth tongue, dyspnea, splenomegaly, leukopenia, thrombocytopenia, achlorhydria, paresthesia, neurological changes, loss of appetite, loss of weight, and low serum cobalamin levels. Disturbed division and nuclear maturation of proliferating epithelial cells is sometimes demonstrable in buccal mucosal scrapings and intestinal biopsies. It is extremely rare to find patients with pernicious anemia who have free acid and serum cobalamin levels above 100 pg/ml. The gastric mucosal atrophy characteristic of pernicious anemia is a diffuse lesion involving the fundus and the entire body of the stomach; involvement of the antral mucosa is normal.

There is a rare hereditary form of congenital pernicious anemia caused by lack of gastric intrinsic factor. This congenital condition usually appears clinically early in life. Rarely, onset may be delayed past 3 years of age. This failure of intrinsic factor secretion is isolated and is associated with normal gastric histology and ability to secrete hydrochloric acid and pepsin.

2. Gastrectomy

Total gastrectomy in humans always produces cobalamin deficiency, since it completely removes the site and source of intrinsic factor secretion. Afer 5–7 years without receiving adequate vitamin therapy, clinical signs of cobalamin deficiency will appear. With the passage of time, other less extensive types of gastric resection may also result in defects of cobalamin assimilation. Approximately 1–20 years following resection of about 60% of the stomach for peptic ulcer, about 30% of the patients develop defective cobalamin absorption as determined with labeled cyanocobalamin. Approximately 6% develop megaloblastic anemia.

3. Destruction of Gastric Mucosa

The ingestion of corrosive agents, such as strong acids or alkalis, either accidentally or with suicidal intent, can destroy the gastric mucosa. Many of these patients invariably come to surgery for either partial or total gastrectomy.

B.   Competitive Utilization of Cobalamins

Surgically produced *blind* loop
Strictures
Anastomoses
Diverticula
Diphyllobothrium latum (tapeworm) infestation

Observations on patients with lesions such as blind loops, stenoses, strictures; or small bowel diverticula have demonstrated that an inappropriate bacterial overgrowth in stagnant areas may introduce into the intestinal stream sufficient organisms to absorb all or adsorb much of the dietary cobalamin passing by. Apparently only competitive uptake and no gross injury to the bowel wall are involved. In many of the above-mentioned instances, cobalamin malabsorption can be corrected by antibiotic therapy.

Cobalamin malabsorption existing in some of the people in Finland who ingested raw fish containing the broad tapeworm *Diphyllobothrium latum* is not particularly prevalent today. Because of the proximal location of the intestinal worm, effective release of the vitamin from food and its binding to the intrinsic factor may not occur in time to prevent the vitamin from reaching the parasite.

C.   Small Intestine Defect

Celiac spruce
Tropical sprue
Gräsbeck-Imerslund syndrome
Resection of the ileum
Ileitis

Patients with small intestine defects do not have deficiency of intrinsic factor. The gastric juice of these patients contains normal amounts of intrinsic factor, and exogenous intrinsic factor cannot restore the absorption to normal.

An unknown defect in the ileum appears to be responsible for the failure of cobalamin absorption. In sprue or celiac disease, the upper intestine is usually more severely affected, and consequently, malabsorption of folic acid and other nutrients often precedes cobalamin deficiency.

Impaired absorption of cobalamin is a regular manifestation of tropical sprue. Like celiac sprue, tropical sprue is a small bowel mucosal disease. The malabsorption in some patients with tropical sprue disappears following treatment with broad-spectrum antibiotics.

In the Gräsbeck-Imerslund syndrome, usually manifest before the age of 3 years, there is a defect in the ability of the distal ileum to absorb the cobalamin–intrinsic factor complex despite its normal absorption to the surface microvilli and the normal appearance of epithelial cells in light and electron microscopy.

Cobalamin malabsorption also ensues when ileal receptors specific for intrinsic factor–bound vitamin are lost or damaged by disease involving the ileal mucosa. Malabsorption of the vitamin takes place immediately after resection of the ileum, whereas ileitis may or may not result in malabsorption of the vitamin, depending on the severity of damage to the absorptive cells.

D. Miscellaneous Causes of Cobalamin Deficiency

1. Inborn Errors of Cobalamin Metabolism

Deficiency of transcobalamin I has been observed in six patients in five families (234a,269a,b,c). In these patients, R binder (transcobalamin I + III) was decreased in or absent from plasma, saliva, and leukocytes. In two of the patients (269b,c) neurological disease was noted. The relationship between the R binder deficiency and the neurological disease is unclear, but it has been suggested that it might be caused by cobalamin analog which are ineffectively cleared into the bile due to the R binder deficiency.

Patients deficient in transcobalamin II develop manifestations of cobalamin deficiency (234b). In most, plasma cobalamin level has been normal or low, and in most, deficiency has appeared early in life (half of the patients have developed symptoms within the first postnatal month). A total of 27 proved cases have been described in 20 families. Several cases have been the asymptomatic siblings of symptomatic cases. Abnormal excretion of methylmalonic acid has been described in two of the four cases in whom it was measured before therapy, but homocystinuria has not been observed in the three patients examined for this before therapy. Three of 10 published cases had neurological abnormalities. Patients have responded to folate therapy, but two of the five so treated developed neurological abnormalities. Patients have been effectively controlled with large doses of vitamin B$_{12}$ (usually hydroxocobalamin) given by injections of 500 μg once or twice weekly, or 3-7 times per week by mouth.

Several errors of tissue metabolism have been described:

Cobalamin A and B (234b): Defects in generation of 5′deoxyadenosyl cobalamin in mitochondria, causing methylmalonic aciduria, acidosis, and a variety of secondary defects defined as "nonketotic hyperglycinemia." In cobalamin B patients, the adenosyl transferase required to add the 5′-deoxyadenosyl group to cobalamin is defective. Cobalamin B patients have responded less frequently to treatment with large doses of cobalamin than have cobalamin. A patients (269d). Only 1 of 12 cobalamin A patients died of the disease, whereas three of 10 reported cobalamin B patients died despite therapy.

Cobalamin C and D (234b,269a): Cobalamin C patients appear to be unable to accumulate cobalamin in the cytoplasm and mitochondria despite apoenzyme forms of methionine synthase and MMA-Coa mutase which should bind the cobalamin. Methionine synthase has been reported not to bind cobalamin with Co^{3+}. Failure of an unidentified cobalamin Co^{3+} reductase has been postulated as the cause of these defects. Transcobalamin II–cobalamin is assimilated by cultured fibroblasts grown from these patients, but cells remain cobalamin–deficient, suggesting that free cobalamin enters the cytoplasm from lysozymes and is lost to the exterior, or leaks out of endosomes during the assimilation process. The clinical phenotypes of C and D are identical, but only one family with two cobalamin D members has been described, whereas 14 families with at least 18 cobalamin C patients have been described and documented. Of 11 cobalamin C or D patients who became symptomatic during infancy, all but one had evidence of neurological impairment, whereas delirium or psychosis was found in all 3 symptomatic patients who were detected as adults. At least 4 cobalamin C and one cobalamin D patients were asymptomatic. In 3 patients, a characteristic retinal abnormality was reported.

Treatment with large doses of cobalamin (usually hydroxocobalamin) has been effective in many of the patients. In several, betaine administration has been effective to reduce plasma homocysteine and increase plasma methionine.

Cobalamin E and G (234b,269g): In these patients, methionine synthase is ineffective, whereas methylmalonyl-Coa mutase activity is normal. Patients with cobalamin G disease appear to have ineffective methionine synthase enzyme. The enzyme appears to bind cobalamin but generation of methyl-cobalamin is ineffective. Methionine synthase activity from cobalamin E cells is normal in extracts, but inactive within the cell. A reducing activity which may be required to maintain cobalamin as C^{2+} has been postulated. These defects have characteristically been observed in infants and young children with homocystinuria and megaloblastic anemia. Treatment is with large doses of cobalamin (usually hydroxocobalamin) plus betaine to correct homocystinemia and low levels of methionine.

Cobalamin F: Two children (269h,i) have been detected whose cells cannot incorporate cobalamin, despite accumulation of cobalamin in lysozomes. Transcobalamin II-cobalamin is assimilated by the cells, and, unlike in cells treated with chloroquine, the transcobalamin II is digested and lost, leaving free cobalamin in lysozomes, which does not enter the cell. One child died, but the other has responded to treatment with large doses of hydroxocobalamin.

2. Zollinger-Ellison Syndrome

Impaired absorption of cobalamin has been observed in patients with massive gastric hypersecretion associated with gastrin-producing islet-cell tumors of the pancreas. The malabsorption is not improved with intrinsic factor administration. It has been postulated that the impaired absorption may be due to intraluminal pH or increased association of cobalamins with R binders at lowered intestinal pH.

3. Drugs and Cobalamin Deficiency

The absorption of cobalamins is impaired by *para*-aminosalicylic acid, colchicine, and neomycin. In the case of colchicine, it appears that the drug alters the histology and enzyme activity of the intestine, which then results in malabsorption (270).

The biguanidines metformin and phenformin have been used in the treatment of diabetes since 1957. Weight loss, associated with malabsorption, occurs as a side effect of these drugs, and a number of patients on long-term metformin therapy have developed cobalamin malabsorption. Once the metformin therapy is terminated, blood vitamin levels revert to normal in most patients (271). This malabsorption is due, not to lack of intrinsic factor, but probably to the competitive inhibition of vitamin absorption in the distal ileum or to the inactivation of the enzyme system involved in the absorption of cobalamin.

Recent studies indicate that potassium chloride can cause a reduced absorption of the vitamin in some patients (272).

A study of the incidence of megaloblastic change after ventilation with nitrous oxide suggests that nitrous oxide oxidizes cyanocobalamin in vitro and probably also in vivo when a premixed 50% nitrous oxide/50% oxygen mixture is given (273).

Methylcobalamin synthesis is markedly depressed by nitrous oxide, whereas adenosylcobalamin synthesis is not. This selective effect on methylcobalamin synthesis and hence on the methionine synthetase pathway suggests that megaloblastosis is probably secondary to methylcobalamin deletion (274,274a).

Table 9 summarizes the vitamin B_{12}-drug interrelationships.

E. Nutritional Deficiency

Cobalamin stores in the human body exceed the daily requirement by about 1000-fold. This reserve helps explain why clinical cobalamin deficiency due to dietary insufficiency

Table 9 Cobalamin–Drug Interactions

Drug	Result of interaction
Aminosalicyclic acid (PAS)	Decreased absorption
Colchicine	Malabsorption
Neomycin	Malabsorption
Guanidines	Decreased absorption
Metformin	Decreased absorption
Phenformin	Decreased absorption
Potassium chloride	Decreased absorption
Nitrous oxide	Interferes with B$_{12}$ metabolism
Fiber	Enhances excretion

is not often seen. Moreover, the small intestine contains microflora that can synthesize significant amounts of cobalamin. Nevertheless, a completely vegetarian diet, one devoid of meat, eggs, and dairy products, can produce cobalamin deficiency, if consumed for several years.

Recently, the number of persons ingesting purely vegetarian diets has grown (274–281). There have been recent reports of cobalamin deficiency in infants breast-fed by strictly vegetarian mothers (274,279–281). The mother's breast milk, with its low concentration of cobalamin, provides the infant with its only source of cobalamins. The occurrence of severe deficiency of cobalamin in infants whose nursing mother's tissues are depleted of cobalamin indicates the importance of the vitamin to the growing organism.

There are also sizable numbers of young people and adults who consume diets that are largely or exclusively vegetarian (280,282). Many of these people have low plasma cobalamin levels; some develop anemia if they are not supplemented with medicinal cobalamin.

High intakes of certain fibers could aggravate a precarious vitamin balance in individuals with a history of poor dietary intake. It has been shown that the inclusion of either cellulose or pectin in a fiber-free basal diet increased the rate of fecal excretion of cobalamin (283).

F. Tests for Deficiency or Defective Absorption

A common procedure for the measurement of deficiency has been the determination of the serum levels. Low serum levels are associated with low body content of the vitamin (262,264,267,284). Microbiological assay methods or radioisotopic dilution techniques, such as previously described, may be used for this purpose.

The inability of the patient to secrete hydrochloric acid in response to an injection of histamine stimulant is strong evidence of the failure to secrete intrinsic factor (262,264,267,284). Intrinsic factor can be measured directly in gastric juice by an isotope dilution technique.

The most commonly employed clinical procedure for defining the nature of cobalamin malabsorption is the urinary excretion test (Schilling test) (see Sec. V.A).

Deficiency of cobalamin or folate would be expected to interfere with the synthesis of methionine. Homocysteine in plasma is coupled to proteins by —S—S—bonds, and is undetectable in plasma extracts unless it is released from these bonds. Using such an approach, homocystinemia has been observed in the majority of patients with significant deficiency of cobalamin or folate. Measurement of plasma methylmalonic acid using GLC-mass spectroscopy has also improved recognition of patients deficient in cobalamin (284a). It has been reported that using these techniques, one-third of patients with significant deficiency of cobalamin may have plasma cobalamin levels greater than 100 pg/ml, and in 2–5%, plasma cobalamin levels may be within the normal range. Such measurements have revolutionized the recognition of deficiency of cobalamin in the absence of megaloblastic anemia and will be especially useful in detection of cobalamin deficiency induced neurological disease.

G. Therapy

The various types of cobalamin deficiences have been referred to in previous sections. For these deficiences, cyanocobalamin is administered with or without the intrinsic factor, depending on the specific needs of the patient (262).

1. Vitamin B_{12} Without Intrinsic Factor

Single, large oral doses (1000 μg) of vitamin B_{12} without intrinsic factor have been proven effective in the treatment of pernicious anemia. This has been substantiated by a number of investigators (297,298). The absorption of a small amount of cobalamins from massive doses is independent of the action of intrinsic factor and is believed to occur by a "mass-action" effect, resulting in diffusion of some cobalamin. An oral dose of at least 150μg a day is deemed necessary to maintain the pernicious anemia patient. Single weekly oral doses of 1000 μg satisfactorily maintain some pernicious anemia patients. Oral therapy is, however, not often recommended. Crosby, however, has recently found this type of therapy useful in treating pernicious anemia (299).

2. Vitamin B_{12} With Intrinsic Factor

Since intrinsic factor deficiency results in the inability to absorb vitamin B_{12} and consequently produces pernicious anemia, it appears that the ideal and more physiological form of therapy is the oral administration of intrinsic factor. However, this form of therapy has never received enthusiastic support, as some patients fail to take the prescribed oral medication daily or fail to return to their physicians for periodic evaluation.

A number of investigative reports show that a variable percentage of pernicious anemia patients become refractory to intrinsic factor preparations after prolonged treatment. Recent evidence indicates that the reduced ability of certain pernicious anemia patients to absorb cobalamins may be an autoimmune phenomenon rather than an acquired tolerance. On the basis of available evidence, it appears that oral treatment with intrinsic factor and cyanocobalamin can be used successfully instead of injection therapy when patients are regularly checked for their ability to continue to absorb cobalamins.

3. Parenteral Therapy

Most patients can be maintained with monthly injections of about 60–100 μg cyanocobalamin. Saturation of body stores of this vitamin is accomplished more rapidly with parenteral treatment. Thus, it is apparent that correction of cobalamin deficiency in pernicious anemia can be accomplished by various means. As Dr. Damashek has remarked, "Whereas there was nothing but systemic care for the fatal disease pernicious anemia, we are now faced with the embarrassment of riches."

VIII. NUTRITIONAL REQUIREMENTS

Daily cobalamin requirements have been estimated from three different types of studies: (1) the amount necessary to treat megaloblastic anemia from cobalamin deficiency, (2) the comparison of blood and liver concentration in normal and cobalamin-deficient subjects, and (3) the body stores and turnover rates of the vitamin.

The intramuscular injection of as little as 0.1 μg daily in patients with pernicious anemia produces a suboptimal reticulocyte response and an increase in hemoglobin concentration (285). However, parenteral doses of about 1.0 μg/day seem necessary to maintain patients with pernicious anemia in complete hematological and neurological remission (286,287). In patients who have a normal secretion of intrinsic factor, such as vegans, 1.0–1.5 μg orally is sufficient to raise serum cobalamin levels and produce a reticulocytosis (288,289).

The normal turnover rate of cobalamin by humans is about 2.5 μg/day (287,290). These estimates are compatible with clinical observations concerning the length of time required for the deficiency signs to develop in patients who either have undergone total gastrectomy or have had cyanocobalamin therapy withdrawn (291). Megaloblastic anemia occurs on an average in about 4 years in humans whose total body stores are about 2–3 mg. Based on these studies and those on the efficacy of absorption the Joint FAO/WHO Expert Group in 1970 recommended a daily intake of 2 μg for the normal adult (292).

In 1989, the Food and Nutritional Board of the National Academy of Sciences recommended a daily intake of 2.0 μg for adults (293). The recommended intakes in infancy are 6.3 μg up to 6 months of age and 0.5 μg from 6 months to 1 year of age. The recommendation for infants is based on the average concentration of the vitamin in human milk.

The recommended allowance during pregnancy and lactation has been increased from 2.2 to 2.6 μg/day. The fetal demand on maternal stores has been estimated to be about 0.3 μg/day, and the elevated metabolic demands of pregnancy an additional 0.3 μg daily (292).

IX. TOXICITY

The Select Committee on Generally Recognized as Safe (GRAS) Substances of the Federation of American Society for Experimental Biology has concluded that "the addition of vitamin B$_{12}$ to food in amounts far in excess of need or of absorbability appears to be without hazard." Cyanocobalamin has caused no toxicity in animals at levels several thousand times their nutritional requirements.

Injections of crystalline cyanocobalamin are usually painless and rarely cause untoward local or allergic reactions.

No reports are known attributing carcinogenic or mutagenic properties to cyanocobalamin (294). Several reports also indicate that cyanocobalamin does not possess any teratogenic potential (295), and according to the FDA (296):

There is no evidence in the available information on (cyanocobalamin) that demonstrates, or suggests reasonable grounds to suspect, a hazard to the public when it is used at levels that are now current and in the manner now practiced, or that might reasonably be expected in the future.

ACKNOWLEDGMENTS

The author is grateful to Dr. Harry P. C. Hogenkamp and Dr. Bernard M. Babior for their helpful criticisms of the manuscript, and to Dr. Blanche Ried for her valuable assistance in the many chores incident to the final preparation of the manuscript.

REFERENCES

1. J. S. Combe, *Trans. Med.-Chirurg. Soc. (Edinburg)*, *1*:194 (1824).
2. T. Addison, *On the Constitutional and Local Effects of Disease of the Suprarenal Capsules*, Samuel Highley, London, 1855, p. 2.
3. G. R. Minot and W. P. Murphy, *JAMA, 91*:923 (1926).
4. W. B. Castle, *Am. J. Med. Sci., 178*:748 (1929).
5. W. B. Castle, in *Cobalamin: Biochemistry and Pathophysiology*, B. M. Babior (Ed.), John Wiley and Sons, New York, 1975, p. 1.
6. E. L. Rickes, N. G. Brink, F. R. Koniuszy, T. R. Wood, and K. Folkers, *Science, 107*:396 (1948).
7. E. L. Smith, *Nature (Lond.), 161*:638 (1948).
8. M. S. Shorb and G. M. Briggs, *J. Biol. Chem., 176*:1463 (1948).
9. R. West, *Science, 107*:398 (1948).
10. J. V. Pierce, A. C. Page, E. L. R. Stokstad, and T. H. Jukes, *J. Am. Chem. Soc., 71*:2952 (1949).
11. B. Ellis, V. Petrow, and G. R. Snook, *J. Pharm. Pharmacol., 1*:60 (1949).
12. N. G. Brink, D. E. Wolf, E. Kaczka, E. L. Rickes, F. R. Koniuszy, T. R. Wood, and K. Folkers, *J. Am. Chem. Soc., 71*:1854 (1949).
13. N. G. Brink, F. A. Kuehl, Jr., and K. Folkers, *Science, 112*:354 (1950).
14. T. H. Jukes and E. L. R. Stokstad, *Vitam. Horm., 9*:1 (1951).
15. H. Lichtman, J. Watson, V. Ginsberg, J. V. Pierce, E. L. R. Stokstad, and T. H. Jukes, *Proc. Soc. Exp. Biol. Med., 72*:643 (1949).
16. H. A. Barker, H. Weissbach, and R. D. Smyth, *Proc. Natl. Acad. Sci. USA, 44*:1093 (1958).
17. H. Weissbach, J. I. Toohey, and H. A. Barber, *Proc. Natl. Acad. Sci. USA, 44*:1095 (1958).
18. J. C. Linnel, A. V. Hoffbrand, H. A. Hussein, I. J. Wise, and D. M. Matthews, *Clin. Sci. Mol. Med., 46*:163 (1974).
19. D. C. Hodgkin, J. Pickworth, J. H. Robertson, K. N. Trueblood, R. J. Prosen, J. G. White, R. Bonnett, J. R. Cannon, A. W. Johnson, I. Sutherland, A. Todd, and E. L. Smith, *Nature (Lond.), 176*:325 (1955).
20. P. G. Lenhert and D. C. Hodgkin, *Nature (Lond.), 102*:937 (1961).
21. D. C. Hodgkin, *Science: 150*:979 (1965).
22. The Nomenclature of Corrinoids (1973 Recommendations), *Biochemistry, 13*:1555 (1974).
23. IUPAC-IUB Commission on Biochemical Nomenclature, *Biochemistry, 11*:1726 (1972) (and in other journals).
24. IUPAC-IUB Commission on Biochemical Nomenclature, *Biochemistry, 11*:942 (1972), (and in other journals).
25. IUPAC-IUB Commission on Biochemical Nomenclature, *Biochemistry, 9*:4022 (1970).
26. N. G. Brink, D. E. Wolf, E. Kaczka, E. L. Rickes, F. R. Koniuszy, J. R. Wood, and K. Folkers, *J. Am. Chem. Soc., 71*:1854 (1949).
27. K. H. Fantes, J. E. Page, L. F. J. Parker, and E. L. Smith, *Proc. R. Soc. [Biol.],136*:592 (1949).
28. D. C. Hodgkin, M. W. Porter, and R. C. Spiller, *Proc. R. Soc. [Biol.], 136*:592 (1949).
29. K. Folkers, in *Vitamin B_{12} und Intrinsic Factor 1*, Europaisches Symposium, Hamburg, 1956, H. C. Heinrich (Ed.), F. Enke, Stuttgart, 1957, p. 9.
30. E. L. Smith, *Vitamin B_{12}*, Methuen, London, 1965.

31. E. Kaczka, D. E. Wolf, F. A. Kuehl, and K. Folkers, *J. Am. Chem. Soc.*, *73*:3569 (1951).
32. W. L. C. Veer, J. H. Edenhauser, H. G. Wijmenga, and J. Lens, *Biochim. Biophys. Acta*, *6*:225 (1950).
33. L. J. De Merre and C. Wilson, *J. Am. Pharm. Assoc. Sci. Ed.*, *45*: 129 (1956).
34. J. B. Armitage, J. R. Cannon, A. W. Johnson, L. F. J. Parker, E. L. Smith, W. H. Stafford, and A. R. Todd, *J. Chem. Soc.*, *71*:3849 (1953).
35. N. G. Brink and K. Folkers, *J. Am. Chem. Soc.*, *72*:4442 (1950).
36. M. Blitz, E. Egen, and E. Gunsberg, *J. Am. Pharm. Assoc. Sci. Ed.*, *43*:651 (1960).
37. S. L. Mukheyee and S. P. Pen, *J. Pharm. Pharmacol.*, *9*:759 (1957).
38. S. Kawajiri, U. S. Patent No. 2,959,520 (1960).
38a. V. K. Berhauer, H. Vogelmann, and F. Wagner, *Hoppe-Seylers Z. Physiol. Chem.*, *349*:1281 (1968).
38b. V. K. Bernauer, H. Vogelmann, and F. Wagner, *Hoppe-Seylers Z. Physiol. Chem.*, *349*:1271 (1968).
38c. D. L. Anton, H. P. C. Hogenkamp, T. E. Walker, and N. A. Matwiyoff, *J. Am. Chem. Soc.*, *102*:2215 (1980).
39. J. R. Cannon, A. W. Johnson, and A. R. Todd, *Nature (Lond.)*, *174*:168 (1954).
40. E. L. Smith, in *Vitamin B$_{12}$ und Intrinsic Factor 1*, Europaisches Symposion, Hamburg, 1956, H. C. Heinrich (Ed.), F. Enke, Stuttgart, 1957, p. 1.
41. E. L. Smith, L. F. S. Parker, and D. E. Gant, *Biochem. J.*, *62*:14P (1956).
42. W. F. J. Cuthbertson, J. Gregory, P. O'Sullivan, and H. F. Pegler, *Biochem. J.*, *62*:15P (1956).
43. H. Baker, O. Frank, I. Pasher, S. H. Hutner, V. Herbert, and H. Sabotka, *Proc. Soc. Exp. Biol. Med.*, *100*:825 (1959).
44. H. Baker, O. Frank, I. Parker, S. H. Hutner, and H. Sobotka, *Proc. Soc. Exp. Biol. Med.*, *104*:33 (1960).
45. M. E. Coates, M. K. Davies, and G. F. Harrison, *Arch. Biochem. Biophys.*, *87*:93 (1960).
46. M. E. Coates, J. E. Ford, G. F. Harrison, S. K. Kon, J. W. G. Porter, W. F. J. Cuthbertson, and H. F. Pegler, *Biochem. J.*, *49*:LXII (1951).
47. J. E. Ford, S. K. Kon, and J. W. G. Porter, *Biochem J.*, *50*:IX (1952).
48. M. E. Coates, J. E. Ford, G. H. Harrison, S. K. Kon, and J. W. G. Porter, *Bichem. J.*, *51*:VI (1952).
49. J. E. Ford, S. K. Kon, and J. W. G. Porter, *Biochem. J.*, *52*:VIII (1952).
50. J. E. Ford and J. W. G. Porter, *Biochem. J.*, *51*: V(1952).
51. J. J. Pfiffner, D. G. Calkins, R. C. Peterson, O. D. Bird, V. McGlohon, and R. N. Stipek, in *Abstr. Papers 120 Meeting Am. Chem. Soc., New York, Sept. 3–7, 1951*, 1951, pp. 22C-23C.
52. H. W. Dion, D. G. Calkins, and J. J. Pfiffner, *J. Am. Chem. Soc.*, *74*:1108 (1952).
53. W. Friedrich and K. Bernhauer, *Angew. Chem.* *65*:27 (1953).
54. J. I. Toohey, *Proc. Natl. Acad. Sci. USA*, *54*:934 (1965).
55. J. W. G. Porter, in *Vitamin B$_{12}$ and Intrinsic Factor 1*, Europaisches Symposion, Hamburg, 1956, H. C. Heinrich (Ed.), F. Enke, Stuttgart, 1957, p. 43.
56. M. E. Coates and S. K. Kon, in *Vitamin B$_{12}$ and Intrinsic Factor 1*, Europäisches Symposion, Hamburg, 1956, H. C. Heinrich (Ed.), F. Enke, Stuttgart, 1957, p. 72.
57. H. C. Heinrich, W. Friedrich, E. Gabbe, S. P. Manjrekar, and M. Staak, in *Abstr. 5th Intern. Congr. Nutrition*, Washington, D. C., 1960, p. 62.
58. C. Rosenblum, D. T. Woodbury, J. P. Gilbert, K. Okuda, and B. F. Chow, *Proc. Soc. Exp. Biol. Med.*, *89*:63 (1955).
59. C. Rosenblum, R. S. Yamamoto, R. Wood, D. T. Woodbury, K. Okuda, and B. F. Chow, *Proc. Soc. Exp. Biol. Med.*, *91*:364 (1956).
60. C. Rosenblum and B. F. Chow, *Proc. Soc. Exp. Biol. Med.*, *95*:30 (1957).
61. E. K. Blackburn, H. T. Swan, G. R. Tudhope, and G. M. Wilson, *Br. J. Haematal.*, *3*:429 (1957).

62. M. E. Coates, M. K. Davies, R. Dawson, G. F. Harrison, E. S. Holdsworth, S. K. Kon, and J. W. G. Porter, *Biochem. J.*, *64*:682 (1956).

63. L. N. Hallenger, R. Silber, and G. Neumann, *Proc. Soc. Exp. Biol. Med.*, *85*:624 (1954).

64. D. Hendlin and M. H. Soass, *J. Bacteriol.*, *62*:633 (1951).

65. D. W. Woolley and J. M. Stewart, *Biochem. Pharmacol.*, *11*:1163 (1962).

66. G. Timmis and S. S. Epstein, *Nature (Lond.)*, *184*:1383 (1955).

67. S. S. Epstein, *Nature (Lond.)*, *188*:143 (1960).

68. E. L. Smith, in *Vitamin B$_{12}$ and Intrinsic Factor 2*, Europäisches Symposion Hamburg, 1961, H. C. Heinrich (Ed.), F. Enke, Stuttgart, 1962, p. 226.

69. M. B. Bunge and R. F. Schilling, *Proc. Soc. Exp. Biol. Med.*, *96*:587 (1957).

70. A. L. Latner and L. C. D. P. Raine, *Nature (Lond.)*, *180*:1197 (1957).

71. A. L. Latner and L. C. D. P. Raine, *Biochem., J.*, *68*:592 (1958).

72. M. E. Coates, M. K. Davies, and G. F. Harrison, *Arch. Biochem. Biophys.*, *87*:93 (1960).

73. H. C. Heinrich, W. Friedrich, and P. Riedel, *Biochem Z.*, *334*:284 (1961).

73a. H. P. C. Hogenkamp, in *Vitamin B$_{12}$*, B. Zagalak and W. Fredrich (Eds.), W. De Gruyter, Berlin, 1979, p. 490.

73b. T. Toraya, T. Shirakashi, S. Fukui, and H. P. C. Hogenkamp, *Biochemistry*, *14*:3949 (1975).

73c. T. Toraya, K. Ushio, S. Fuku, and H. P. C. Hogenkamp, *J. Biol. Chem.*, *252*:963 (1977).

73d. G. N. Sando, R. L. Blakeley, H. P. C. Hogenkamp, and P. J. Hoffman, *J. Biol. Chem.*, *250*:8774 (1975).

74. J. F. Kolhouse, H. Kondo, N. C. Allen, E. Podels, and R. H. Allen, *N. Engl. J. Med.*, *299*:785 (1978).

74a. H. Kondo, J. F. Kolhouse, and R. H. Allen, *Proc. Natl. Acad. Sci. USA*, *77*:817 (1980).

75. A. R. Battersby, C. J. R. Fookes, G. W. J. Matcham, and E. McDonald, *Nature*, *285*:17 (1980).

76. A. I. Krasna C. Rosenblum, and D. B. Sprinson, *J. Biol. Chem.*, *225*:745 (1947).

77. A. L. Scott, B. Yagen, and E. Lee, *J. Am. Chem. Soc.*, *95*:5761 (1973).

78. A. I. Scott, *Science*, *184*:760 (1974).

79. H.C. Friedman, in *Cobalamin: Biochemistry and Pathophysiology*, B. M. Babior (Ed.), John Wiley and Sons, New York, 1975, p. 75.

80. H. Weissbach, B. Redfield, and A. Peterkovsky, *J. Biol. Chem.*, *236*:40P (1961).

81. R. O. Brady and H. A. Barker, *Biochem. Biophys. Res. Commun.*, *4*:464 (1961).

82. A. Peterkovsky, B. Redfield, and H. Weissbach, *Biochem. Biophys. Res. Commun.*, *5*:213 (1961).

82a. R. B. Woodward, in *Vitamin B$_{12}$*, B. Zagalak and W. Friedrich (Eds.), W. deGruyter, Berlin, 1979, p. 37.

83. J. A. Chisolm, J. Bronte-Stewart, and W. S. Foulds, *Lancet*, *2*:450 (1967).

84. V. Herbert, in *The Pharmacological Basis of Therapeutics*, 5th Ed., L. S. Goodman and A. Gilman (Eds.), MacMillian, New York, 1975, p. 1324.

85. J. Cottrell, P. Casthely, J. Brodie, K. Patel, A. Klein, and H. Turndorf, *N. Engl. J. Med.*, *298*:809 (1978).

86. W. B. Castle and H. A. Godwin, in *Gastroenterology*, 3rd Ed., H. L. Bockus (Ed.), W. B. Saunders, Philadelphia, 1976, p. 95.

87. G. E. Boxer and J. C. Richards, *Arch. Biochem. 30*:372 (1951).

88. G. E. Boxer and J. C. Richards, *Arch. Biochem.*, *30*:382 (1951).

89. G. O. Rudkin, Jr., and R. J. Taylor, *Anal. Chem.*, *24*:1155 (1952).

90. G. E. Boxer and J. C. Richards, *Arch. Biochem.*, *29*:75 (1950).

91. K. H. Fantes and D. M. Ireland, *Biochem. J.*, *46*:XXXIV (1950).

92. H. C. Heinrich, *Z. Anal. Chem.*, *135*:251 (1952).

93. M. S. Shorb, *J. Biol. Chem.*, *169*:455 (1947).

94. M. S. Shorb, *Science*, *107*:397 (1948).

95. C. E. Hoffmann, E. L. R. Stokstad, A. L. Franklin, and T. H. Jukes, *J. Biol. Chem.*, *176*:1465 (1948).

96. C. E. Hoffman, E. L. R. Stokstad, B. L. Hutchings, A. C. Dornbush, and T. H. Jukes, *J. Biol. Chem.*, *181*:635 (1949).

97. L. D. Wright, H. P. Skeggs, and J. W. Huff, *J. Biol. Chem.*, *176*:1467 (1948).

98. H. P. Skeggs, H. M. Nepple, K. A. Valentine, J. W. Huff, and L. D. Wright, *J. Biol. Chem.*, *184*:211 (1950).

99. B. D. Davis and E. S. Mingioli, *J. Bacteriol.*, *60*:17 (1950).

100. P. R. Burkholder, *Science, 114*:459 (1951).

101. E. Harrison, K. A. Lees, and F. Wood, *Analyst, 76*:696 (1951).

102. K. A. Lees and J. P. R. Toutill, *Analyst, 80*:531 (1955).

103. S. H. Hutner, L. Provasoli, E. L. R. Stokstad, C. E. Hoffmann, M. Belt, A. L. Franklin, and T. H. Jukes, *Proc. Soc. Exp. Biol. Med.*, *70*:118 (1949).

104. S. H. Hutner, M. K. Bach, and G. I. M. Ross, *J. Protozool, 3*:101 (1956).

105. S. H. Hutner, L. Provasoli, and J. Filfus, *Ann. N.Y. Acad. Sci.*, *56*:852 (1953).

106. J. E. Ford, *Br. J. Nutr.*, *7*:299 (1953).

107. D. K. Bosshardt, W. J. Paul, K. O'Doherty, J. W. Huff, and R. H. Barnes, *J. Nutr.*, *37*:21 (1949).

108. C. A. Nichol, L. S. Dietrich, W. W. Cravens, and C. A. Elvehjem, *Proc. Soc. Exp. Biol. Med.*, *70*:40 (1949).

109. D. C. Hill and H. D. Branion, *Poult. Sci.*, *31*:892 (1952).

110. W. F. J. Cuthbertson and D. M. Thornton, *Br. J. Nutr.*, *6*:170 (1952).

111. M. E. Coates, G. F. Harrison, and S. K. Kon, *Biochem. J.*, *46*:VII (1950).

112. W. L. Williams, A. S. Stiffey, and T. H. Jukes, *J. Agric. Food Chem.*, *4*:364 (1956).

113. D. L. Mollin, B. B. Anderson, and J. F. Burman, *Clin. Haematol.*, *5*:521 (1976).

114. C. Gottlieb, K. S. Lau, L. R. Wasserman, and V. Hebert, *Blood, 25*:875 (1965).

115. J. F. Kolhouse, *N. Engl. J. Med.*, *299*:785 (1978).

116. B. A. Cooper and V. M. Whitehead, *N. Engl. J. Med.*, *299*:816(1978).

117. R. M. Donaldson, Jr., *N. Engl. J. Med.*, *299*:827 (1978).

118. L. Ellenbogen, in *Cobalamin: Biochemistry and Pathophysiology*, B. M. Babior (Ed.), John Wiley and Sons, New York, 1975, p. 215.

118a. K. L. Cohen and R. M. Donaldson, Jr., *JAMA, 244*:1942–1945 (1980).

118b. J. M. England and J. C. Linnell, *Lancet, 2*:1072–1074 (1980).

118c. NCCLS Proposed Standard : PSLA Guidelines for Evaluating a B$_{12}$ (cobalamin) Assay, U. S. National Committee for Clinical Laboratory Standards, March, 1980.

118d. L. Fries. *Physiol. Plantarum, 15*:566 (1962).

118e. Y. Katake and T. Ono, *Shokukin Eiseigku Zara, 5*:39 (1964).

118f. G. G. Laties and C. Hoelle, *Phytochemistry, 6*:49 (1967).

118g. A. P. Petrosyan, L. A. Abramyan, and M. B. Sarkisyan, *Vopr. Mikrobiol.*, *4*:181 (1969).

118h. J. M. Poston, *Science, 195*:301 (1977).

119. H. Lichtenstein, A. Beloran, and E. W. Murphy, Home Economics Research Report No. 13, USDA, Washington, D. C.

120. L. J. Bogert, G. M. Briggs, and D. H. Calloway, *Nutrition and Physical Fitness*, W. B. Saunders, Philadelphia, 1973.

121. I. Chanarin, *The Megaloblastic Anemias*, Blackwell, Oxford, 1968.

122. L. Ellenbogen, in *Newer Methods of Nutritional Biochemistry*, A. Albanese (Ed.), Academic Press, New York, 1963, p. 272.

123. D. L. Mollin, *Br. Med. Bull.*, *15*:8 (1959).

124. R. F. Schilling, *J. Lab. Clin. Med.*, *42*:860 (1953).

125. S. T. Callender and J. R. Evans, *Clin. Sci.*, *14*:387 (1955).

126. W. R. Best, W. F. White, K. C., Robbins, W. A. Landmann, and S. L. Steelman, *Blood 1*:338 (1956).

127. L. D. Mac Lean and H. S. Block, *Proc. Soc. Exp. Biol. Med.*, *87*:171 (1954).
128. L. Ellenbogen, W. L. Williams, S. F. Rabiner, and H. C. Lichtman, *Proc. Soc. Exp. Biol. Med.*, *89*:357 (1955).
129. F. E. Bull, D. C. Campbell, and C. A. Owen, Jr., *Fed. Proc.*, *15*:509 (1956).
130. C. E. Rath, P. F. McCuroy, and B. J. Duffy, *N. Engl. J. Med.*, *256*:111 (1957).
131. A. L. Dunn, J. R. Walsh, and J. M. Holthaus, *Arch. Intern. Med.*, *101*:927 (1958).
132. J. H. Katz, J. Dimase, and R. M. Donaldson, Jr., *J. Lab. Clin. Med.*, *61*:266 (1963).
133. J. W. D. McDonald, R. M. Barr, and W. B. Barton, *Ann. Intern. Med.*, *83*:827 (1975).
134. S. J. Baker and D. L. Mollin, *Br. J. Haematol.*, *1*:46 (1955).
135. R. W. Heinle, A. D. Welch, A. Scharf, G. C. Meacham, and W. Prusoff, *Trans. Assoc. Am. Physicians*, *65*:214 (1952).
136. M. Pollycove and L. Apt, *N. Engl. J. Med.*, *255*:207 (1956).
137. G. B. J. Glass, L. J. Boyd, G. A. Gellin, and L. Stephanson, *Arch. Biochem. Biophys.*, *51*:251 (1954).
138. H. Weisberg and G. B. J. Glass, *J. Lab. Clin. Med.*, *68*:163 (1966).
139. C. C. Booth and D. L. Mollin, *Br. J. Haematol.*, *2*:223 (1956).
140. A. Doscherholmen, P. S. Hagen, and M. Liu, *Blood*, *12*:336 (1957).
141. A. Doscherholmen and D. Ripley, *Arch. Intern. Med.*, *134*:1019 (1974).
142. H. C. Heinrich, in *Kunstkishe Radioactive Isotope in Physiologie Diagnostik and Therapie*, H. Schwieg and F. Turba (Eds.), Springer, Berlin, 1961, p. 660.
143. P. A. McIntyre, M. V. Sachs, J. F. Krevans, and C. L. Conley, *Arch. Intern. Med.*, *98*:541 (1956).
144. A. Doscherholmen and W. R. Swaim, *Gastroenterology*, *64*:913 (1973).
145. C. King, J. Leibach, and P. Toskes, *Gastroenterology*, *64*:1080 (1977).
146. C. C. Both and D. L. Mollin, *Lancet*, *2*:1007 (1957).
147. W. T. Cooke, E. U. Cox, M. J. Meynell, and R. Gaddie, *Lancet*, *2*:123 (1959).
148. A. C. L. Clarke and C. C. Booth, *Arch. Dis. Child*, *35*:595 (1960).
149. G. N. Cornell, H. Gilder, F. Moody, C. Frey, and J. M. Beal, *Bull. N.Y. Acad. Med.*, *37*:675 (1961).
150. E. Allock, *Gastroenterology*, *40*:81 (1961).
151. Y. Citrin, C. De Rosa, and J. A. Halsted, *J. Lab. Clin. Med.*, *50*:667 (1957).
152. W. R. Best, J. H. Frenster, and M. M. Zolot, *J. Lab. Clin. Med.*, *50*:793 (1957).
153. P. C. Johnson and E. S. Berger, *Blood*, *13*:457 (1958).
154. V. Ronnov-Jessen and J. Hansen, *Blood*, *25*:224 (1965).
155. J. Farquharson and J. F. Adams, *Br. J. Nutr.*, *36*:127 (1976).
156. I. L. Craft, D. M. Matthews, and J. C. Linnell, *J. Clin. Pathol.*, *24*:449 (1971).
157. J. J. Chosy, A. Killander, and R. F. Schilling, in *Vitamin B_{12} and Intrinsic Factor 2*, Europäisches Symposion, Hamburg, H. C. Heinrich (Ed.), F. Enke, Stuttgart, 1961, p. 668.
158. J. F. Adams, F. McEwan, and A. Wilson, *Br. J. Nutr.*, *29*:65 (1973).
159. B. A. Cooper and W. B. Castle, *J. Clin. Invest.*, *39*:199 (1960).
160. S. G. Schade and R. F. Schilling, *Am. J. Clin. Nutr.*, *20*:636 (1967).
161. M. B. Bunge and R. F. Schilling, *Proc. Soc. Exp. Biol. Med.*, *96*:587 (1957).
162. R. Grasbeck, *Acta Chem. Scand.*, *12*:142 (1958).
163. G. B. J. Glass, L. Stephason, M. Rich, and R. W. Laughton, *Br. J. Haematol.*, *3*:401 (1957).
164. R. Grasbeck, *Acta Physiol. Scand.*, *45*:88 (1959).
165. R. Grasbeck, *Acta Physiol. Scand.*, *45*:116 (1959).
166. V. Herbert, *J. Clin. Invest.*, *38*:102 (1959).
167. K. Okuda and T. Fujii, *Arch. Biochem. Biophys.*, *115*:302 (1966).
168. L. Ellenbogen and D. R. Highley, *Fed. Proc.*, *29*:633 (1970).
169. R. Grasbeck, I. Kantero, and M. Siurala, *Lancet*, *1*:234 (1959).
170. W. W. Bromer and E. O. Davisson, *Biochem. Biophys. Res. Commun.*, *4*:61 (1961).
171. J. Abels and R. F. Schilling, *J. Lab. Clin. Med.*, *64*:375 (1964).

172. R. Grasbeck, K. Simons, and I. Sinkkonen, *Biochim. Biophys. Acta, 127*:47 (1966).

173. L. Ellenbogen and D. R. Highley, *J. Biol. Chem., 242*: 1004 (1967).

174. R. H. Allen and C. S. Mehlman, *J. Biol. Chem., 248*: 3660 (1973).

175. R. H. Allen and C. S. Mehlamn, *J. Biol. Chem., 248*:3670 (1973).

176. K. Simons, *Soc. Sci. Fenn Comment Biol. 27*:5 (1964).

177. R. M. Donaldson, Jr., I. L. Mac Kenzie, and J. S. Tier, *J. Clin. Invest., 46*:1215 (1967).

178. V. Herbert and W. B. Castle, *J. Clin. Invest., 40*:1978 (1961).

179. L. W. Sullivan, V. Herbert, and W. B. Castle, *J. Clin. Invest., 42*:1443 (1963).

180. D. C. Hooper, D. H. Alpers, R. L. Burger, C. S. Mehlman, and R. H. Allen, *J. Clin. Invest., 52*:3074 (1973).

181. R. Grasbeck and W. Nyberg, *Scand. J. Clin. Lab. Invest., 10*:448 (1958).

182. M. Katz and B. A. Cooper, *Br. J. Haematol., 26*:569 (1974).

183. R. Cotter, S. P. Rothenberg, and J. P. Weiss, *Biochim. Biophys. Acta, 490*:19 (1977).

184. M. Katz, S. K. Lee, and B. A. Cooper, *N. Engl. J. Med., 287*:425 (1972).

185. M. Katz, C. S. Mehlman, and R. H. Allen, *J. Clin. Invest., 53*:1274 (1974).

186. E. W. Strauss, T. H. Wilson, and A. Hotchkiss, *Am. J. Physiol., 198*:103 (1960).

187. J. D. Hines, A. Rosenberg, and J. W. Harris, *Proc. Soc. Exp. Biol. Med., 129*:653 (1968).

188. A. Doscherholmen, P. S. Hagen, and L. Olin, *J. Lab. Clin. Med., 54*:434 (1959).

189. R. M. Donaldson, Jr., D. M. Small, S. Robins, and V. I. Mathan, *Biochim. Biophys. Acta, 311:477 (1973).*

190. *T. J. Peters and A. V. Hoffbrand, in The Cobalamins*, H. R. V. Arnstein and R. J. Wrighton (Eds.), Churchill-Livingstone, Edenburgh, 1971, p. 61.

191. N. Yamaguchi, W. S. Rosenthal, and G. B. J. Glass, *Am. J. Clin. Nutr., 23*:156 (1970).

192. R. F. Schilling and L. L. Scholesser, in *Vitamin B₁₂ und Intrinsic Fact 1*, Europäisches Symposion, Hamburg, 1956, H. C. Heinrich (Ed.), F. Enke, Stuttgart, 1957, p. 194.

193. P. P. Toskes, J. Hansell, J. Cerda, and J. J. Deren, *N. Engl. J. Med., 286*:627 (1971).

194. P. P. Toskes, J. J. Deren, J. Fruiterman, and M. E. Conrad, *Gastroenterology, 65*:199 (1973).

195. G. V. von der Lippe, *Scand. J. Gastroenterol., 12*:257 (1977).

196. R. H. Allen, B. Seetharam. E. Podell, and D. H. Alpers, *J. Clin. Invest., 61*:47 (1978).

197. R. H. Allen, B. Seetharam, N. C. Allen, E. R. Podell, and D. H. Alpers, *J. Clin. Invest., 61*:1628 (1978).

198. W. Steinberg, P. Toskes, C. Curington, and R. Shah, *Gastroenterology, 78*:1270 (1980).

199. W. Steinberg, C. Currington, and P. Toskes, *Gastroenterology, 76*:1255 (1979).

200. W. K. Shinton and A. K. Singh, *Br. J. Haematol., 13*:75 (1967).

201. R. W. Monto and J. W. Rebuck, *Arch. Intern. Med., 93*:219 (1954).

202. R. W. Monto and J. W. Rebuck, *Blood, 10*:1151 (1955).

203. M. C. G. Israels and S. Shubert, *Lancet, 1*:341 (1954).

204. J. N. M. Chalmers and N. D. Shinton, *Lancet, 2*:1069 (1958).

205. A. Doscherholmen, P. S. Hagen, M. Liu, and L. Olin, *J. Clin. Invest., 36*:1551 (1957).

206. P. G. Reizenstein, E. P. Cronkite, L. M. Meyer, E. Usenik, and D. Driscoll, *Proc. Soc. Exp. Biol. Med., 105*:233 (1960).

207. K. B. Taylor and J. E. French, *Q. J. Exp. Physiol., 45*:72 (1960).

208. V. Herbert, *J. Clin. Invest., 38*:102 (1959).

209. B. A. Cooper, W. Paranchych, and L. Lowenstein, *J. Clin. Invest., 41*:370 (1962).

210. W. R. Pitney, M. F. Beard, and E. J. Van Loon, *J. Biol. Chem., 207*:143 (1954).

211. A. Miller and J. F. Sullivan, *J. Clin. Invest., 37*:556 (1958).

212. H. C. Heinrich, L. S. Erdmann-Oehlecker, L. Sommer, and G. Radel, *Clin. Chim. Acta., 1*:311 (1956).

213. C. A. Hall and A. E. Finkler, *Biochim. Biophys. Acta. 78*:233 (1963).

214. C. A. Hall and A. E. Finkler, *J. Lab. Clin. Med., 65*:459 (1965).

215. C. A. Hall and A. E. Finkler, *Proc. Soc. Exp. Biol. Med., 123*:56 (1966).

216. C. A. Hall, *Br. J. Haematol., 16*:429 (1969).

217. B. L. Hom and H. Olesen, *Scand. J. Clin. Lab. Invest., 19*:269 (1967).

218. C. Lawrence, *Blood, 33*:899 (1969).

219. E. J. Gizis, M. F. Dietrich, G. Ohoi, and L. M. Meyer, *J. Lab. Clin. Med., 75*:673 (1970).

220. F. J. Bloomfield and J. M. Scott, *Br. J. Haematol., 22*:33 (1972).

221. R. Carmel, *Br. J. Haematol., 22*:53 (1972).

222. R. L. Burger, C. S. Mehlman, and R. H. Allen, *J. Biol. Chem., 250*:7700 (1975).

223. R. L. Burger, R. J. Schneider, C. S. Mehlman, and R. H. Allen, *J. Biol. Chem., 250*:7707 (1975).

224. R. Grasbeck, *Prog. Hematol., 6*:233 (1969).

225. R. Carmel and V. Herbert, *Blood, 33*:1 (1969).

226. N. Hakami, P. E. Neiman, G. P. Canellos, and J. Lazerson, *N. Engl. J. Med., 285*:1163 (1971).

227. C. R. Scott, N. Hakami, C. C. Teng, and R. N. Sagerson, *J. Pediatr., 81*:1106 (1972).

228. W. H. Hitzig, V. Dohmann, H. J. Pluss, and D. Vischer, *J. Pediatr., 85*:622 (1974).

229. A. E. Finkler and C. A. Hall, *Arch. Biochem. Biophys. 120*:79 (1967).

230. F. P. Retief, C. W. Gottleib, and V. Herbert, *J. Clin. Invest., 415*:1907 (1966).

231. W. Paranchych and B. A. Cooper, *Biochim. Biophys. Acta, 60*:393 (1962).

232. M. J. Mahoney and L. E. Rosenberg, in *Cobalamins: Biochemistry and Pathophysiology,* B. M. Babior (Ed.), John Wiley and Sons, New York, 1975, p. 369.

233. C. Fiedler-Nagy, C. R. Rowley, J. W. Coffey, and D. N. Miller, *Br. J. Haematol., 31*:311 (1975).

234. P. A. Friedman, M. A. Shea, and J. K. Wallace, *J. Clin Invest., 59*:51 (1977).

234a. P. Youngdahl-Turner, and L. E. Rosenberg, *J. Clin. Invest., 61*:1331 (1978).

234b. B. A. Cooper and D. S. Rosenblatt, *Ann. Rev. Nutr., 7*:291 (1987). C. R. Kapadia, D. Serfilippi, K. Voloshin, and R. M. Ddonaldson, Jr., *J. Clin. Invest, 71*:440 (1983).

234c. R. Carmel, *Blood, 59*:152 (1982).

235. I. S. Mellman, P. Youngdahl-Turner, W. F. Willard, and L. E. Rosenberg, *Proc. Natl. Acad. Sci. USA, 74*:916 (1977).

236. J. F. Kolhouse and R. H. Allen, *Proc. Natl. Acad. Sci. USA, 74*:921 (1977).

237. L. Ellenbogen, in *International Review of Biochemistry, Biochemistry of Nutrition,* Part A, Vol. 27, A. Neuberger and T. H. Jukes (Eds.). University Park Press, Baltimore, 1979, p. 45.

238. J. C. Linnell, A. V. Hoffbrand, T. J. Peters, and D. M. Matthews, *Clin. Sci., 40*:1 (1971).

239. N., Nexø, *Scand. J. Haematol., 18*:358 (1977).

240. C. M. L. A. Mac Donald, A. Farquharson, R. G. Bessent, and J. F. Adams, *Clin. Sci. Mol. Med., 52*:215 (1977).

241. G. I. M. Ross and D. L. Mollin, in *Vitamin B$_{12}$ und Intrinsic Factor 1,* Europäisches Symposion, Hamburg, 1956, H. C. Heinrich (Ed.), F. Enke, Stuttgart, 1957, p. 437.

242. G. B. J. Glass, L. J. Boyd, and G. A. Gellin, *Blood, 10*:95 (1955).

243. J. M. Cooperman, A. L. Luhby, D. N. Teller, and J. F. Marley, *J. Biol. Chem., 235*:191 (1960).

244. J. C. Linnel, in *Cobalamin: Biochemistry and Pathophysiology,* B. M. Babior (Ed.), John Wiley and Sons, New York, 1975, p. 287.

245. N. K. Shinton, *Br. Med. J., 1*:557 (1972).

246. J. C. Linnell, in *Cobalamin: Biochemistry and Pathophysiology,* B. Babior (Ed.), John Wiley and Sons, New York,1975, p.287.

247. H. A. Barker, *Biochem. J., 105*:1 (1967).

248. J. Pawelkiewicz, M. Gorna, W. Fenrych, and S. Magas, *Ann. N.Y. Acad. Sci, 112*:641 (1964).

249. M. J. Mahoney and L. E. Rosenberg, *J. Lab. Clin. Med., 78*:302 (1971).

250. S. S. Kerwar, C. Spears, B. McAuslan, and H. Weissbach, *Arch. Biochem. Biophys., 142*:231 (1971).

251. E. Vitols, G. A. Walker, and F. M. Huennekens, *Biochem. Biophys. Res. Commun., 15*:372 (1964).

252. J. S. Krouwer and B. B. Babior, *Mol. Cell. Biochem., 15*:89 (1977).

253. B. M. Babior, in *Cobalamin: Biochemistry and Pathophysiology*, B. M. Babior (Ed.), John Wiley and Sons, New York, 1975, p. 141.

254. B. M. Babior and J. S. Krouwer, *CRC Crit. Rev. Biochem., 35*, March (1979).

255. R. L. Blakley, *J. Biol. Chem., 240*:2173 (1965).

256. W. S. Beck and J. Hardy, *Fed. Proc., 24*:421 (1965).

257. M. Dowling, A. Adams, and L. Helleuga, *Biochim. Biophys. Acta., 108*:233 (1965).

258. R. Abrams and S. Duraiswami, *Biochem. Biophys. Res. Commun., 18*:409 (1965).

259. R. L. Blakey and H. A. Barker, *Biochem. Biophys. Res. Commun., 16*:391 (1964).

259a. P. K. Tsai and H. P. C. Hogenkamp, *J. Biol. Chem., 255*:1273 (1980).

259b. G. N. Sando and H. P. C. Hogenkamp, *Biochemistry, 12*:3316 (1973).

259c. F. K. Gleason and H. P. C. Hogenkamp, *Biochim. Biophys. Acta, 27u*:466 (1972).

259d. F. Stutzenberger, *J. Gen. Microbiol., 81*:501 (1974).

259e. H. P. C. Hogenkamp and G. N. Sando, *Struct. Bond., 20*:23 (1974).

259f. V. Pigiet and R. R. Conley, *J. Biol. Chem., 253*:1910 (1978).

259g. A. Holmgren, *J. Biol. Chem., 253*:424 (1978).

259h. A. Holmgren, *Proc. Natl. Acad. Sci. USA, 73*:2275 (1976).

260. T. C. Stadtman, *Science, 171*:859 (1971).

261. J. M. Poston and T. C. Stadtman, in *Cobalamin: Biochemistry and Pathophysiology*, B. M. Babior (Ed.), John Wiley and Sons, New York, 1975, p. 111.

261a. R. P. Gunsalus and R. S. Wolfe, *J. Bacteriol., 135*:851 (1978).

261b. G. D. Taylor and R. S. Wolfe, *J. Biol. Chem., 249*:4879 (1974).

262. S. J. Baker and E. M. DeMaeyer, *Am. J. Clin. Nutr., 32*:368 (1979).

263. W. Beck, in *Cobalamin: Biochemistry and Pathophysiology*, M. Babior (Ed.), John Wiley and Sons, New York, 1975, p.403.

264. I. Chanarin, *The Megaloblastic Anemias*, Blackwell Scientific Publications, Oxford, 1969.

265. W. B. Castle, *Am. J. Med., 48*:541 (1970).

266. V. Herbert, N. Colman, and E. Jacob, *The Year in Hematology*, A. Gordon, R. Silber, and J. La Bue (Eds.), Plenum Press, New York, 1977, Ch. 17.

267. W. Castle and H. Godwin, in *Gastroenterology*, Vol. 2, H. Bockus (Ed.), W. B. Saunders, Philadelphia, 1976, p. 95.

268. R. Donaldson, in *Cobalamin: Biochemistry and Pathophysiology*, M. Babior (Ed.), John Wiley and Sons, New York, 1975, p. 335.

269. P. A. McIntyre, R. Hahn, C. L. Conley, and B. Glass, *Bull. Johns Hopkins Hosp., 104*:309 (1959).

269a. R. Carmel and V. Herbert, *Blood 33*:1 (1969).

269b. S. Shinnar, H. S. Singer, *N. Engl. J.Med., 311*:451 (1984).

269c. S. M. Matsui, M. J. Mahoney, and L. E. Rosenberg, *N. Engl. J. Med., 308*:857 (1983).

269d. H. F. Willard, R. S. Mehlman, and L. E. Rosenberg, *Am. J. Hum. Genet. 30*:1 (1978).

269e. G. A. Mitchell, D. Watkins, S. B. Melancon, D. S. Rosenblatt, G. Geoffroy, et al. *J. Pediatr. 108*:110 (1986).

269f. D. Watkins and D. S. Rosenblatt, *J. Clin. Invest., 81*:1690 (1988).

269g. D. S. Rosenblatt, R. Laframboise, J. Pichette, P. Langevin, B. A. Cooper, T. Costa, *Pediatrics, 78*:51 (1986).

269h. D. S. Rosenblatt, A. Hosack, N. V. Matiasuk, and B. A. Cooper, *Science, 228*:1319 (1985).

269i. S. P. Stabler, P. D. Marcell, E. R. Podell, and R. H. Allen *J. Clin. Invest., 810*:4660 (1988).

270. S. Yosselson, *Drug Intell. Clin. Pharm., 10*:8 (1976).

271. D. Roe, *Drug Ther., 279*, April (1973).

272. D. Roe, *Drug-Induced Nutritional Deficiencies* Avi. Publishing, Westport, Connecticut, 1976.

273. J. A. L. Amess, G. M. Rees, J. F. Burman, D. G. Nancekievill, and D. L. Mollin, *Lancet, 1*:339 (1978).

274. M. C.Wighton, J. Manson, M. Speed, E. Robertson, and E. Robertson, and E. Chapman, *Med. J. Aust.*, 1, July, (1979).

274a. I. Chanarin, *J. Clin. Pathol.*, *35*:909 (1980).

275. R. Carmel, *Ann. Mt. Med.*, *88*:67 (1978).

276. E. Zmora, R. Gorodisher, and B. Jacob, *Am. J. Dis. Child.*, *133*: 141 (1979).

277. L. Finberg, *Am. J. Dis. Child.*, *133*:129 (1979).

278. J. Dwyer, W. Dietz, G. Hass, and R. Suskind, *Am. J. Dis. Child.*, *133*:134 (1979).

279. M. Higginbottom, L. Sweetman, and W. Nyhan, *N. Engl. J. Med.*, *299*:317 (1978).

280. M. C. Wighton, J. I. Manson, M. B. Speed, E. Robertson, and E. Chapman, *Med. J. Aust.*, 2:1 (1979).

281. J. R. Short, J. Tiernan, and S. Hawgood, *Med. J. Aust.*, 2:483 (1979).

282. S. Winawer, R. Streiff, and N. Lamcheck, *Gastroenterology, 53*:310 (1967).

283. Dietary fiber and vitamin B_{12} balance, *Nutr. Rev.*, 37:116 (1979).

284. Harvard Pathophysiology Series, in *Hematology*, W. S. Beck (Ed.), M.I.T. Press, Cambridge, Massachusetts, 1973, p.106.

284a. J. Lindenbaum, E. B. Healton, D. G. Savage, J. C. M. Brust, T. J. Garrett, E. R. Podell, P. D. Marcell, S. P. Stabler, and R. H. Allen, *N. Engl. J. Med.*, *318*:1720 (1988).

285. L. W. Sullivan and V. Herbert, *N. Engl. J. Med.*, *272*:340 (1965).

286. V. Herbert, in *Modern Nutrition in Health and Disease: Dietotherapy*, 5th Ed., R. S. Goodhart and M. E. Shils (Eds.), Lea and Febiger, Philadelphia, 1973.

287. R. M. Heyssel, R. C. Bozias, W. J. Darby, and M. C. Bell, *Am. J. Clin. Nutr.*, *18*:176 (1966).

288. S. J. Winawer, R. R. Streff, and N. Zamcheck, *Gastroenterology, 53*:130 (1967).

289. J. S. Stewart, P. L. D. Roberts, and A. V. Hoffbrand, *Lancet*, 2: 542 (1970).

290. V. Herbert, *Am. J. Clin. Nutr.*, *21*:743 (1968).

291. W. J. Darby, E. Jones, S. L. Clark, Jr., W.J. McGanity, J. D. de Oliveira, C. Perez, J. Kevany, and J. Le Brocquy, *Am. J. Clin. Nutr.*, *6*:513 (1958).

292. Joint FAO/WHO Expert Group, 1970, *Requirements of Ascorbic Acid and Vitamin D, Vitamin B_{12}, Sulfate and Iron*, WHO Tech. Rep. Ser. No., 452, 1970, pp. 34–43.

293. Food and Nutrition Board, National Research Council, *Recommended Dietary Allowances*, 10th edition, National Academy Press, Washington, D. C., 1989.

294. Environment Mutagen Information Center, *EMIC/Gras Lit Review*, Report ORNL-EMIC-1, Oakridge National Laboratory, Oakridge, Tennessee, 1973.

295. L. Richardson and R. Brock, *J. Nutr.*, *58*:135 (1956).

296. U. S. Department of Commerce National Technical Information Service P. B. 289–922, FDA, Washington, D. C. 1978, p. 17.

297. C. C. Ungley, *Br. Med. J.* 2:905 (1950).

298. C. L. Conley, *Am. J. Med.*, *13*:284 (1952).

299. W. H. Crosby, *Arch. Intern. Med.*, *140*:1582 (1980).

14
Choline

Mabel M. Chan
New York University
New York, New York

I. INTRODUCTION

Choline is a nutrient known to be essential for mammalian organisms other than humans, since its discovery and isolation in 1862 (1). Although present in food, it is also synthesized by many animal species (2). Recent studies indicate that there are certain clinical conditions and disorders where choline may be deficient and supplementation of dietary choline may be beneficial (3). However, owing to the lack of knowledge concerning the biosynthesis and utilization in human beings and the lack of confirmatory experimental and clinical evidence of choline deficiency in humans, its essentiality as a vitamin for humans cannot be established yet.

II. CHOLINE

A. History

Choline was found to be a component of the sinapin of mustard seed by Von Babo and Hirschbrunn in 1952 and as a component of the lecithin of ox bile by Strecker in 1862 (2). Early studies of choline as a nutrient follow closely the discovery in insulin by Banting and Best in 1922. It was first noted that the administration of insulin helped mobilize excess lipids in the livers of diabetic depancreatized dogs. Subsequent studies (4–6) on the metabolism of depancreatized dogs demonstrated that choline is the active constituent of dietary lecithin that provides the lipotropic activity. Betaine, a dietary precursor of choline, was found to have similar effects in rats and dogs. In 1932, Best and Huntsman (7) reported the development of fatty livers in rats fed a low-choline, high-fat diet, which was prevented by choline supplementation. These experiments led to studies on the role of choline in nutrition.

Commercially, choline salts are generally synthesized from trimethylamine and ethylene chlorhydrin and ethylene oxide (2). Biocolinea, Hepacholine, and Liportil are trade names for choline chloride (8). Choline chloride and choline bitartrate are both choline salts listed in the code of Federal Regulations as nutrients and/or dietary supplements that are generally recognized as safe (GRAs) (9).

B. Chemical Properties and Analytical Procedures

Choline (trimethyl-β-hydroxyethylammonium), $(CH_3)_3H^+CH_2CH_2OH$, is a strong organic base and decomposes in alkaline solution with the release of trimethylamine. It is hygroscopic and freely soluble in water and alcohol, but insoluble in ether and chloroform. It appears as colorless or white crystals or crystalline powder (2,10).

Choline determination is complicated by the various forms in which it may be present in the sample. Free choline may be extracted with water or alcohol, but more exacting procedures must be used for the extraction of total choline. Precautions have to be taken for the preparation of biological tissues, which contain enzymes that rapidly hydrolyze phosphate esters of choline in nervous tissues when animals are killed. For example, when post-mortem enzymatic hydrolysis of choline in nervous tissues is minimized by microwave irradiation (11), better estimates of choline in nervous tissues have been obtained (12).

The reineckate method, which involves the precipitation of choline as a reinecke salt in a colorimetric reaction (13), is the classical and has been the most widely used method for quantitative determination of choline. Microbiological assay employing *Neurospora crassa* cholineless-1 (14) or *Torulopis pintolopessi* (15,16) has also been used to estimate choline activity in various tissues. Procedures involving enzymatic, fluorometric, gas chromatographic, photometric, and polarographic methods have been developed (17). Enzymatic radioisotope assay and gas chromatography provide high sensitivity and specificity and have been most widely used in recent studies (18–27). These methods are being continuously adapted and modified to provide more rapid, sensitive, and economical measurements.

C. Bioassasy

Chemical analyses primarily provide values that denote choline availability, as differentiated from bioassays that provide information on the available choline in food (28).

Earlier determination of choline by biological assay was based on the conversion of choline to acetylcholine, which was estimated by its pharmacological effect on tissues such as rectus abdominis muscle of the frog and the isolated intestine of the rabbit (29). The accuracy was greatly influenced by the presence of interfering substances, such as potassium salts, histamine, and other constituents in the tissues. Later, bioassay methods made use of growth response of animals, such as chicks, to additional choline as the criterion of choline bioavailability (28,30). Such assays make the assumption that choline is the first limiting nutrient and that growth response is linearly proportional to the levels of choline added to the diet. The validity of the assumption has recently been tested (31). The result suggests that growth is influenced by other constituents in choline-limiting diets, such as dietary protein and methionine level; therefore, such assays may not be reliable measures of the choline content of foodstuffs.

D.   Content in Food

Choline is widely distributed in foods and is ingested mainly in the form of lecithin (phosphatidylcholine). Less than 1% of the choline occurs in foods as the free base (32). Choline is also present in many processed foods and food supplements since it is used commercially as an additive or ingredient in the form of lecithin (32). Lecithin and choline are not analogous terms. Commercial forms of lecithin are actually mixtures of phosphatides, containing as little as 20% phosphatidylcholine. Therefore, it has been recommended that the use of the trivial name lecithin in the scientific literature be restricted to the commercial products, to differentiate it from the chemical term of phosphatidylcholine (33).

Choline chloride and choline bitartrate are added to infant formulas and milk products to assure the presence of choline in an amount of approximately that present in milk (34). The Infant Formula Act of 1980 sets choline chloride at 7 mg per 100 cal as a requirement for non–milk base infant formula (35). A recent study reported that the choline concentration in samples of commercial infant formula varied widely from 100.3 to 647.5 μM and was significantly lower than the amounts stated on the labels (36).

Table 1 presents some typical foods containing high, medium, and low choline chloride levels (32,34). The richest food sources of choline are egg yolk, liver, soybean, wheatgerm, and peanut. The brain, which is not commonly consumed, is also high in choline. Other animal tissues and vegetables contain significant amounts of choline and lecithin. Detailed lists of choline chloride content in a variety of food products have been published (2,32). However, most of these data are based on early studies and shold be considered as estimates only. Reexamination of choline content of foods by updated methodology to provide more accurate and reliable data is needed.

Owing to the presence of choline in many processed foods as lecithin and the availability of lecithin in health food stores, it is difficult to obtain a reliable assessment of the daily intake of choline in the American diet because of the uncertainty in the average daily consumption of such products. Estimates of total choline intake, as lecithin and free choline, ranged between 250–500 mg per day (32,34). However, the actual intake can be affected by many factors that specifically influence food habits. Until more reliable food composition information is available, an accurate determination of current consumption cannot be established.

Table 1 Choline Chloride Contents of Some Food Products[a]

High: > 200 mg/100g		Medium: 100–200 mg/100 g		Low: < 100 mg/100 g	
egg yolk	1713	rolled oats	151	trout muscle	84
beef liver	630	peanut butter	145	cauliflower	78
defatted wheatgerm	423	barley	139	cabbage	46[b]
beef brain	410	asparagus	128	lettuce	18[b]
beef kidney	333	rice polish	126	milk	10.1[b]
soybeans	237	pork ham	120	carrots	9.5[b]

[a]Based on freshweight.
[b]Average value.
Source: Adapted from Refs. 32 and 34.

E. Metabolism

Lecithin is the most abundant choline-containing compound in the diet. Less than 10% of choline is present either as the free base or sphingomyeline (32). About 50% of the lecithin ingested enters the thoracic duct intact. The rest is degraded to glycerophosphoryl choline (lysolecithin) in the intestinal mucosa and then to choline in the liver. Human plasma choline is reflective of the lecithin intake, thus, the consumption of a meal high in lecithin elevates plasma choline levels (37–39).

When choline is ingested, approximately two-thirds is metabolized by intestinal microorganisms to trimethylamine (which produces the fishy odor when choline is taken orally), which is excreted in the urine (40,41) 6–12 hours after consumption. The remaining one-third appears to be absorbed intact, probably by a Na^+-dependent carrier mechanism (42). By contrast, when an equivalent amount of choline is consumed in the form of lecithin, less urinary trimethylamine is excreted, with the majority of the metabolite appearing in the urine 12–24 hours after ingestion (43). The use of antimicrobial agents to suppress intestinal flora decreased urinary trimethylamine excretion from choline ingestion(44,45).

When choline is administered intravenously, insignificant amounts of trimethylamine appear in the urine (40). These results indicate that degradation of choline to trimethylamine is restricted to the microflora of the gastrointestinal tract.

Choline is stored in the animal tissues such as brain, kidney, and liver primarily as phosphatidylcholine (lecithin) in the form of diacylester (Fig. 1) and sphingomyelin, an ester of phosphocholine and a ceramide (Fig. 2) (46).

F. Function

Choline serves as a source of labile methyl groups for the biosynthesis of other methylated compounds. It is the precursor of acetylcholine, a neurotransmitter, and a major component of phospholipids, lecithin, and sphingomyelin.

The formation of betaine from choline provides an important source of labile methyl groups for transmethylation reactions (47,48). Oxidation of choline to betaine is a principle pathway for choline metabolism that is active in many tissues, in particular liver and kidney (49). This reaction proceeds in the following sequence:

$$(CH_3)-H^+CH_2CH_2OH \longrightarrow (CH_3)_3N^+CH_2CHO \longrightarrow (CH_3)_3N^+CH_2COOH$$
$$\text{Choline} \qquad\qquad\qquad \text{betaine aldehyde} \qquad\qquad\qquad \text{betaine}$$

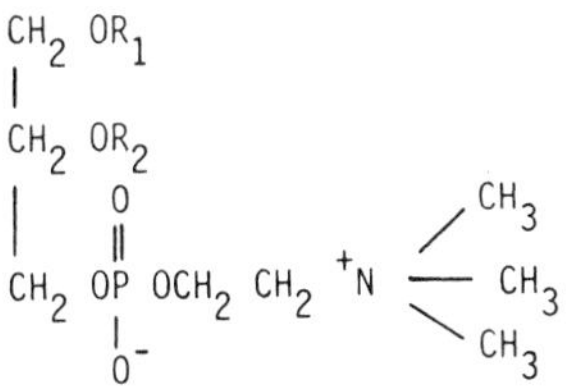

CH₂ OR₁
|
CH₂ OR₂
| O
| ‖
CH₂ OP OCH₂ CH₂ ⁺N ⟨ CH₃ — CH₃ ⟨ CH₃
|
O⁻

Figure 1 A phosphatidylcholine. R_1 and R_2 represent fatty acyl groups.

Choline dehydrogenase, a mitochondrial enzyme, catalyzes the dehydrogenation of choline to betaine aldehyde. Betaine aldehyde dehydrogenase, a soluble enzyme, then oxidizes the aldehyde to betaine. Betaine can transfer a methyl group to homocysteine to form methionine and dimethylglycine (Fig. 3). These reactions do not require vitamin B_{12} and folic acid. Hence, when rats were fed a methionine-deficient diet in the absence of folic acid and vitamin B_{12}, the rats responded to choline (50). Such transmethylation reactions allow choline to be synthesized *de novo* by ethanolamine, as outlined in Figure 3. The active form of methionine S-adenosylmethionine, provides the methyl groups. Therefore, choline may be replaced in the diet without incurring a deficient state, if methionine or homocysteine, betaine, and certain ethanolamines are adequate (2,47).

Choline is the physiological precursor of acetylcholine, a mediator of synaptic transmission. Biosynthesis of acetylcholine requires choline acetyltransferase (CAT):

$$(CH_3)_3N^+CH_2CH_2OH + CH_3COCoA \xrightarrow{\text{CAT}} (CH_3)_3N^+CH_2OH_2OOCCH- + CoA$$
$$\text{Choline} \qquad\qquad \text{acetyl CoA} \qquad\qquad\qquad \text{acetylcholine}$$

There is a considerable amount of interest in the role of choline as a precursor of acetylcholine. As discussed in the section on the pharmacological use of choline, exogenous administration may be beneficial in the treatment of several neurological disorders.

The formation of phosphatidylcholine (lecithin) from choline is another biochemical function of choline. Lecithin is a major lipid component of most cell membranes. Its biosynthesis can occur in two different pathways. The principal pathway involves the metabolism of choline in the mitochondria to form lecithin in the following reactions (49):

Choline + ATP ⟶ phosphocholine + ADP   (1)

Cytidine triphosphate + phosphocholine ⟶
         Cytidine diphosphate-choline + PPi   (2)

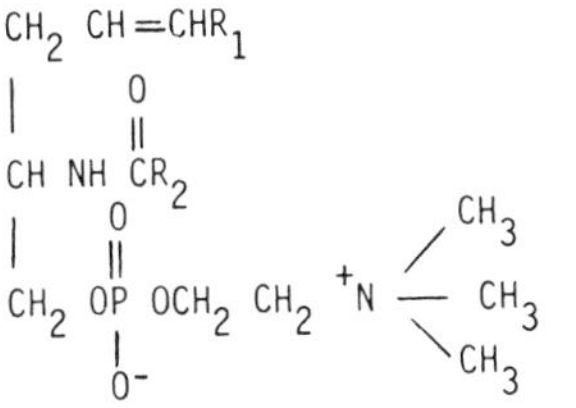

CH₂ CH=CHR₁
| O
| ‖
CH NH CR₂
| O
| ‖
CH₂ OP OCH₂ CH₂ ⁺N ⟨ CH₃ — CH₃ ⟨ CH₃
|
O⁻

Figure 2 Sphingomyelin R_1 and R_2 represent fatty acyl groups.

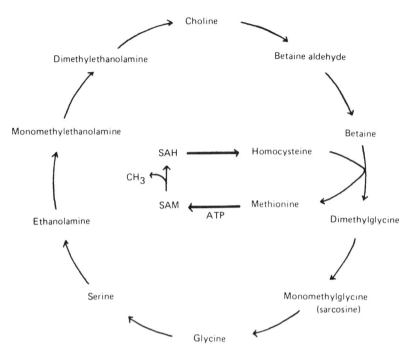

Figure 3 The role of choline in methylation. SAM = S-adenosylmethionine; SAH = S-adenosylhomoserine.

Cytidine diphosphate-choline + 1,2-diacylglycerol $\longrightarrow$
  phosphatidyl choline (lecithin) + cytidine monophosphate   (3)

The enzymes for these reactions are widely distributed in most tissues, such as liver, brain, heart, and kidney. The second pathway involves the sequential methylation of phosphatidylethanolamine by the methyl group donor S-adenosylmethionine (50). A microsomal enzyme, phosphatidylethanolamine methyl transferase, catalyzes this three-step process (51). A summary of the recent progress on the regulation of phosphatidylcholine biosynthesis has been reviewed (52).

Owing to the basic function of choline in membrane structure, the lack of choline is manifested in a variety of phospholipid-related functions such as fatty liver and lesions of the kidney (see Sec. II.G) and impairment of lipoprotein metabolism (53). Choline acts as a lipotrophic agent, which is described by Best et al. (54) as "a substance which decreases the rate of deposition and accelerates the rate of removal of liver fat." In the absence of dietary choline, fats and cholesterol ester accumulate in the liver. The addition of choline to the ration can reverse the trend (8). The incidence of experimental atherosclerosis has been shown to be reduced by choline, which may act by intervening in the conversion of cholesterol to bile acids (8). A soy phosphatidylcholine diet has been reported to be a more potent hypocholesterolemic agent than corn oil by reducing the absorption of dietary cholesterol and increasing the excretion of neutral sterols in rats (55). Studies on the efficacy of lecithin feeding in patients with hyperlipidemia, however, have yielded in consistent results (56,57).

G. Deficiency Signs

The lesions associated with choline deficiency have been reviewed in detail. The most common signs of choline deficiency are fatty liver and hemorrhagic kidney necrosis (2,58). In general, the severity of the lesions in animal species is influenced by other dietary factors, such as methionine, vitamin B_{12}, and folic acid, which are involved in methylation process, the nature of dietary fat and protein (59), as well as the sources of choline (60,61). If food intake and, consequently, growth are depressed by the deficient diet, the severity of choline deficiency is reduced. The inconsistency in such dietary modifying factors has result in controversy in regard to choline deficiency in animal species.

1. Animals

The primary lesion of choline deficiency that has been observed in most animal species studied is fatty liver. Stainable fat can be detected in hepatocytes within hours after a choline-deficient diet has been fed to rats (59), and accumulation of triacylglycerols has been shown to occur with 24 hours (62), probably due to the lack of choline for the CDP-choline pathway, coupled with a reduction of the transmethylase pathway (63). In rats, dogs, and monkeys, prolonged choline deficiency may result in cirrhosis (58), which may be associated with reduced oxidative drug metabolism and cytochrome p-450 isozymes (64). The pathogenesis of fatty liver in choline deficiency is not completely understood. The suggested probable cause involves a defect in lipoprotein secretion from the liver (65,66) and the sequestration of triacylglycerols into a potential enlarged hepatic pool (67). Liver cell proliferation occurs when rats are fed a diet deficient in choline and methionine for as short a period of time as 1–2 weeks (68,69), perhaps induced by hepatitis, cell loss, and necrosis (70). It has been suggested that antioxidants or vitamin E may have a protective effect in hepatic fibrous proliferation (71).

Hemorrhagic kidney degeneration is another major alteration observed in several animal species, including rat, mouse, rabbit, calf, and pig. Histological examination of the kidneys affected showed massive tubular necrosis, which is probably the initial lesion (72). Interstitial hemorrhage developed (73), followed by complete renal failure, which may result in death. Several hypothesis have been proposed to account for this lesion (58). For example, lysosomal changes in prenecrotic and early necrotic stages may play an important role in renal changes of choline-deficient weanling rats (74); the excess of catecholamines in the kidney forming an imbalance between sympathetic and parasympathetic systems may account for the pathogenesis of renal injury (75). It appears that impairment in phospholipid function in membranes is at least indirectly, if not basically, responsible.

Secondary lesions, resulting from faulty lipid transport and function, including hypolipidemia, perosis, hemorrhagic lesions, cardiovascular dysfunctions, hypertension, impaired clotting, and thymus regression, have also been reported (58).

The mechanism(s) involved is unclear. Impaired phospholipid interconversion was observed (76). Similar to inositol deficiency, choline deficiency alters lipoprotein synthesis and transport, which may be the principal causal factors for these disorders.

Other problems related to choline deficiency include impaired immune response (77), vascular damage and elevated free radical formation in liver, kidney, and heart (78,79); alteration in the synthesis of lung surfactant (80–82); and failure of pregnant rats to reach parturition (83). In choline-deficient rats, thermoregulation has also been shown to be less efficient. This symptom is probably related to the decrease in lipid deposits in kidney and liver (83). Choline deficiency has also been found to exert promoting and/or carcinogenic effects (84–86). A combination of metabolic alterations, such as changes in cell membrane lipid composition (87,88) and peroxidation (89) as a result of choline deficiency, may enhance the susceptibility of liver cells to tumor formation.

2. Humans

The effect of choline deficiency in humans has been reviewed by Turkii (90). Most of the studies on choline deficiency in humans have focused on disease states that produce liver cirrhosis or fatty livers, suggesting a probable involvement of choline in the pathogenesis of liver diseases in humans. However, the results are inconclusive. Clinical signs that resemble dietary choline deficiency in animals have not been reported in humans. Recent investigations in patients in total parenteral nutrition (TPN) showed that abnormal liver function in these patients may be associated with choline deficiency (91–95). Further observations showed that free plasma choline levels fell during TPN therapy (96,97) and coincided with the increase in serum glutamate pyruvate transaminase (SGPT), which is indicative of hepatic damage (97). These studies indicate that patients undergoing treatment with TPN have depleted choline reserves and choline deficiency may become evident.

H. Nutritional Assessment

Plasma choline levels in humans reflect dietary consumption (38). After the consumption of 3 g choline chloride in a meal, serum choline rose by 86% over the mean fasting level of 11.7 nmol/ml.

Since choline is ubiquitously present in food, there appears to be insignificant clinical concern for choline deficiency, and routine assessment of choline status is rarely practiced. However, care must be taken when patients are maintained on TPN, which could represent a form of iatrogenic malnutrition. Burt and co-workers (97) compared the plasma levels of free choline in 23 healthy volunteers (6–10 nmol/ml) to those of 15 patients on TPN. They suggested that the fall of free plasma choline below normal range may be related to a choline deficiency state and one reason for the transient liver function abnormalities observed during total parenteral nutrition.

I. Nutritional Requirements

1. Animals

It has been demonstrated that under some conditions, several animal species may require dietary choline. For example, when intake of precursors or accessory factors, such as methionine, vitamin B_{12}, or folacin is insufficient, dog, cat, monkey, pig, rabbit, and trout have been shown to require exogenous choline (2,59). The young animals also show a higher need for choline than adults (9).

Reported estimates of dietary choline levels in various animal species have been compiled by Wilson (58) and Marks (98). Table 2 presents the reported estimates of dietary choline levels for several animal species. Amounts typically fed to laboratory and farm animals range from 1 to 1.5 g/kg diet. Most semipurified diets have been supplemented with choline to ensure optimal growth and reduce the possibility of marginal choline deficiency in many animal species.

2. Humans

Choline is classified as one of the nutrients "known to be essential for certain higher animals, but for which no proof exists for a dietary need by humans" (1). It appears that the average intake from foods is adequate for health.

Table 2 Reported Estimates of Dietary Choline Levels for Various Animal Species

Species	g/kg diet	Other units
Calves	—	260 mg/l milk
Cats	1.5	—
Chicks, broiler-starting	1.5	—
Chicks, broiler-growing	13.0	30.6 mg/day[a]
Dogs	1.0	55 mg/kg/day
Fish (trout)	1.5	—
Guinea Pig	1.0–1.5	—
Hamster	1.0	—
Hens, Ducks (laying and breeding)	1.1	—
Horses		
foals	0.15	—
race and breeding	0.6	
working and saddle	0.45	—
yearlings	0.3	—
Mink and Foxes	1.0	100–500 mg/day
Mouse	1.5	—
Piglets		
starting	1.2	—
fatting	0.9	—
growing	1.0	—
Rabbit	2.0	—
Sows, breeding	0.9	—
Swine, young	1.0	—

[a]From Ref. 28.

Source: Adapted from Refs. 58 and 98.

J. Factors That Influence Choline Status and Groups That Are at Risk of Deficiency

Since choline can be synthesized in vivo by methylation of ethanolamine, the intake of methionine and other methyl donors (betaine) and precursors (vitamin B_{12} and folacin) may influence the dietary need for choline (2,59). For example, when young swines were fed diets low in methionine, the choline requirement was increased (99). Dietary choline and inorganic sulfury supplementation appeared to exert a sparing effect on methionine need in human diets (100).

Studies on alcoholics with liver cirrhosis have suggested that choline status may be affected by alcohol intake. Animal studies have demonstrated that ethanol increased the requirement of choline in the liver by accelerating the oxidative degradation of choline (101–105). Ethanol may also enhance choline requirement by brain, since it reduced the incorporation of choline into acetylcholine (106) and the stimulated release of acetylcholine from brain slices (107). Acara (108) showed that in perfusion studies with isolated kidney, ethanol increased choline excretion by the renal tubules. However, there is no evidence that choline need is higher in alcohol-treated animals, since supplementation is as effective as a well-balanced diet in relieving the liver disorders (101). In fact, massive choline supplementation has failed to prevent alcohol-induced liver fibrosis and may be hepatotoxic (109).

In addition, mice experiments suggest that certain behavioral changes that occur with aging may be related to choline (110,111). Senile mice were observed to improve passive avoidance retention with choline ingestion. A survey of healthy elderly subjects reported that serum choline increases with age, but serum choline was correlated neither to the levels of intake nor to cognitive function (112).

Although it has not been shown that choline is required by infants, the young of all animal species studied appear to be most susceptible to deficient choline intakes (9). To ensure optimal growth, commercially prepared infant formulas and milk products have been supplemented with choline to assure the presence of choline in an amount approximating that naturally occurring in milk (34).

Recent reports on patients undergoing total parenteral nutrition (TPN) suggest that this group may be at risk for developing liver abnormalities as a result of the lack of choline in the TPN formula (93–97). Malnourished patients undergoing TPN therapy had significantly lower plasma choline concentration than well-nourished control subjects. When these patients were treated with lipid emulsion and an amino acid–glucose solution, their plasma choline level increased (96). Choline status of patients on TPN should, therefore, be monitored, since these patients appear to be susceptible to choline deficiency.

Other conditions that have been suggested to bear a relationship to choline status include a number of neurotransmitter diseases, depression (113), hypoglycemic stupor (114), and memory storage (115).

K. Efficacy of Pharmacological Doses

Choline is a component of the neurotransmitter acetylcholine, and the ingestion of choline can affect the concentration of this compound in the brain (116,117).

It had been shown that the administration of free choline by injection (118,119), stomach tube (120), or dietary supplementation (121,122) increased not only serum choline levels, but also brain choline and acetylcholine concentrations in rats. Furthermore, oral administration of choline, as well as lecithin, was demonstrated to be effective in increasing serum choline levels in humans (38) and brain and adrenal acetycholine levels in rats (123). These findings indicate that choline loading may be beneficial to patients with disease related to a deficiency of cholinergic neurotransmission. The therapeutic strategy is based on the pharmacological action of large doses of choline or lecithin to increase brain choline above normal levels by a mass action effect, thereby stimulating acetylcholine synthesis within nerve terminals.

Davis et al. (124) reported a patient with tardive dyskinesia (a movement disorder generally associated with the intake of antipsychotic medication) who showed marked improvement of the disorder following the oral ingestion of large doses of choline. Subsequent clinical trials with tardive dyskinesia patients using choline and lecithin have met with considerable success. Other disorders or symptoms associated with inadequate cholinergic transmission that have been treated with choline or lecithin include Huntington's chorea, Alzheimer's disease, mania, Gilles de la Tourette, and ataxia. A list of clinical traits employing choline or lecithin preparations is presented in Table 3. Based on current evidence, it appears that diet therapy with choline or lecithin has met with the most success in the treatment of tardive dyskinesia. The efficacy of choline or lecithin loading in other disorders or symptoms has not been convincing.

Table 3 Clinical Trials of Choline and Lecithin in Neurotransmitter-Related Syndromes and Disorders

Syndrome or Disorder	Dosage	g/day	Result[a]	Reference
Tardive dyskinesia	choline	(16)	1/1	124
	choline	(12–14)	5/5	125
	choline	(12–20)	3/4	126
	choline	(18)	2/4	127
	choline	(0.15–0.20[b])	9/20	128
	choline	(20)	2/5	129
	choline	(10)	1/2	130
	lecithin	(4–49)	2/2	131
	lecithin	40–80)	3/3	132
	lecithin	(105)	3/3	125
	lecithin	(50)	6/6	133
	lecithin	(8–24)	1/1	134
	choline	(6)	5/5	135
	choline	(0.2–3[b])	7/11	136
	lecithin	(25)	0/8	137
	lecithin	(25–30)	4/4	138
	lecithin	(31.5–50[c])	0/9	139
	lecithin	(15–30)	0/1	140
	lecithin	(30)	0/17	141
Huntington's chorea	choline	(20)	2/4	126
	choline	(20)	3/8	129
	choline	(10)	2/4	130
	lecithin	(4–49)	0/3	131
Alzheimer's disease	choline	(5–10)	0/7	142
	choline	(8)	0/3	143
	choline	(9)	0/10	144
	choline	(9)	2/8	145
	choline	(12)	5/5[d]	146
	choline	(3.6)	0/5[e]	147
	lecithin	(35)	0/10	148
	lecithin	(30)	0/10	149
	lecithin	(15–30)	0/10	150
	lecithin	(15[c])	0/6	151
	lecithin	(25)	positive[f]	152
	lecithin	(25)	negative[g]	153
Ataxia	choline	(10)	6/6	130
	choline	(4)	1/14	154
	choline	(5)	1/1	155
	lecithin	(4–49)	10/16	131
Mania	lecithin	(15–30)	7/8	156
Gilles de la Tourette	choline	(10)	1/3	130
	lecithin	(0.512)	0/5	157
Memory impairment	choline	(16)	0/8[h]	158
	choline	(12–20)	0/14	159

[a]Each ratio indicates the number of patients improved to the number of patients studied.
[b]Grams per kilogram body weight per day.
[c]Grams per 70 kilogram body weight per day.
[d]The response from subjects were found to be significantly improved.
[e]All five patients performed slightly worse than baseline.
[f]Significant difference between placebo ($n = 14$) and lecithin group ($n = 16$).
[g]No significant difference between placebo ($n = 17$) and lecithin group ($n = 18$).
[h]No significant improvement in memory performance.

An evaluation of the efficacy of the pharmacological doses of choline is complicated by a number of factors. In early studies, choline was seldom tolerated due to the fishy odor produced from the microbial degradation of choline to trimethylamine in the gastrointestinal tract. Later trials used lecithin preparations, which do not undergo microbial metabolism, thus eliminating the unpleasant odor associated with choline. In addition, lecithin was shown to be more effective than choline (160): in equivalent doses (2.3 g free base), oral lecithin elevated plasma choline levels by 265%, compared with an 86% increase with choline chloride. Oral administration of large quantities of choline and lecithin produced adverse effects, including diarrhea, nausea, salivation, and depression. Part of these side effects was attributed to impurities occurring in the extraction of lecithin from sources like soy products and may be lessened with the improvement in the purification of lecithin preparations. Most lecithin preparations contain about 50% lipids. Thus, the caloric contribution, when administered in high dose, is another factor that needs to be considered.

A survey of clinical studies reveals a lack of standardization of dosages and the need to objectively assess parameters, such as improving memory in the aged. Other variables that complicate the comparison from study to study include reliable patient history and duration of treatment (161). Nevertheless, these data do provide some positive evidence supporting the efficacy of precursor loading technique in the treatment of neurological diseases, such as tardive dyskinesia, associated with insufficient cholinergic tone (162,163). This same technique has had limited effect on Alzheimer's disease, which is thought to be a disorder involved with multiple neurotransmitter deficits, rather than acetylcholine alone (164–167). The current clinical approach to the treatment of symptoms, such as senile dementia of the Alzheimer type, has focused on the combined administration of lecithin and piracetam, a metabolic enhancer. This regimen has been reported to be more effective than either agent alone (161,168,169). Based on the finding that there was a consistent and severe loss of nicotinic receptors in Alzheimer's disease, the use of nicotinic agonists is a new strategy proposed for Alzheimer's disease therapy (170).

L. Hazards of High Doses

Despite the potential of choline as a therapeutic agent for brain disorders, it is important not to slight the possible hazards of high dosages. Estimates of the oral LD_{50} of choline chloride from rats vary from 3.4 to 6.7 g/kg (34).

Although no adverse effect occurs with a single dose of 10 g (171) the use of pharmacological doses of choline up to 20 g/day have resulted in symptoms related to excessive cholinergic stimulation, such as increased salivation and sweating, nausea, dizziness, diarrhea, depression, and a longer P-R interval in electrocardiograms (33,126,130,156).

Experimental animal toxicity data on the symptoms of choline overdosage include salivating, trembling, jerking, cyanosis, convulsion, and respiratory paralysis (34,172). Ball(173) recently reported that when rats were exposed perinatally to 22 mg of soy lecithin preparation daily, sensorimotor development and brain cell maturation were altered.

REFERENCES

1. National Academy of Sciences, *Recommended Dietary Allowances*, National Research Council, Washington, D. C., 1980.
2. W. H. Griffith and J. F. Nyc, Choline—Chemistry, in *The Vitamins: Chemistry, Physiology, Pathology, Methods*, 2nd Ed., Vol. 3, W. H. Sebrell and R. S. Harris (Eds.), Academic Press, New York, 1971, pp. 3–15.

3. A. Barbeau, J. H. Growdon, and R. J. Wurtman (Eds.), Choline and lecithin in brain disorders, in *Nutrition and the Brain*, Vol. 5, Raven Press, New York, 1979.

4. F. N.Allan, D. J. Bowie, J. J. R. MacLeod, and W. L. Robinson, Behavior of depancreatized dogs kept alive with insulin, *Br. J. Exp. Pathol., 5*:75–83 (1924).

5. J. M. Hershey, Substitution of "lecithin" for raw pancreas in the diet of the depancreatized dog, *Am. J. Physiol., 93*:657–658 (1930).

6. C. H. Best and J. M. Hershey, Further observations on the effects of some component of crude lecithin in depancreatized animals, *J. Physiol.* (Lond.), *75*:49–55 (1932).

7. C. H. Best and M. E. Huntsman, The effects of the components of lecithin upon the deposition of fat in the liver, *J. Physiol.* (Lond.), *75*:405–412 (1932).

8. Federation of the American Society for Experimental Biology, *Evaluation of the Health Aspects of Choline Chloride and Choline Bitartrate as Food Ingredients*, NTIS PB-252654, 1975.

9. Office of the Federal Register, General Services Administration, Choline Bitartrate and Choline Chloride, Section 121.101(d)(5), in *Code of Federal Regulations*, Title 21, Food and Drugs, Parts 10 to 129, Rev., U.S. Government Printing Office, Washington, D.C., 1974.

10. B. L. Oser, *Hawk's Physiological Chemistry*, 14th Ed., McGraw-Hill, New York, 1965.

11. W. B. Stavinoha, and S. T. Weintraub, Choline content of rat brain, *Science, 183*:964–965 (1974).

12. D. R. Haubrich, and T. J. Chippendale, Regulation of acetylcholine synthesis in nervous tissue, *Life Sci., 20*:1465–1478 (1977).

13. Association of Official Agricultural Chemists, *Official Method of Analysis*, Washington, D. C., 1984.

14. E. Lied and O. R. Braekkan, Determination of total choline in biological materials, *Int. J. Vitam. Nutr. Res., 45*:438–447 (1975).

15. H. Baker, O. Frank, D. J. Tuma, A. J. Barak, M. F. Sorrell, and S. H. Hutner, Assay for free and total choline of rats and man with *Torulopsis pintolopessi, Am. J. Clin. Nutr., 31*:532–540 (1978).

16. S. H. Zeisel, Free and choline assay, *Am. J. Clin. Nutr., 31*:1978–1980 (1978).

17. I. Hanin, *Choline and Acetylcholine: Handbook of Chemical Assay Methods*, Raven Press, New York, 1974.

18. I. Hanin, Methods for the analysis and measurement of acetylcholine: An overview, in *Modern Methods in Pharmacology*, S. Spector and N. Back (Eds.), Alan R. Liss, New York, 1982, pp. 29–38.

19. F. P. Bymaster, K. W. Perry, and D. T. Wong, Measurement of acetylcholine and choline in brain by HPLC with electrochemical detection, *Life Sci., 37*:1775–1781 (1985).

20. L. Campanella, M. Mascini, G. Palleschi, and M. Tomassetti, Determination of choline-containing phospholipids in human bile and serum by a new enzyme sensor, *Clin. Chem. Acta, 151*:71–83 (1985).

21. I. Das, J. de Belleroche, C. J. Moore, and F. C. Rose, Determination of free choline in plasma and erythrocyte samples and choline derived from membrane phosphatidylcholine by chemiluminescence method, *Anal. Biochem., 152*:178–182 (1986).

22. G. Damsma, B. H. C. Westerink, and A. S. Horn, A simple, sensitive, and economic assay for choline and acetylcholine using HPLC, an enzyme reactor, and an electrical detector, *J. Neurochem., 45*:1649–1652 (1985).

23. Y. Irarashi, T. Sasahara, and Y. Maruyama, Determination of choline and acetylcholine levels in rat brain regions by liquid chromatography with electrochemical detection, *J. Chromatogr., 322*:191–199 (1985).

24. K. E. McMahon and P. M. Farrell, Measurement of free choline concentrations in maternal and neonatal blood by micropyrolysis gas chromatography, *Clin. Chim. Acta, 149*:1–12(1985).

25. N. A. Muma and P. P. Rowell, A sensitive and specific radioenzymatic assay for the simultaneous determination of choline and phosphatidylcholine, *J. Neurosci. Meth., 12*:249–157 (1985).

26. P. E. Potter, J. L. Meek, and N. H. Neff, Acetycholine and choline in neuronal tissue measured by HPLC with electrochemical detection, *J. Neurochem.*, *41*:188–194 (1983).

27. A. K. Singh and L. Drewes, Improved analysis of acetylcholine and choline in canine brain and blood samples by capillary gas. Chromatography-mass spectometry, *J. Chromatogr.*, *339*:170–174 (1985).

28. B. A. Molitoris and D. H. Baker, Assessment of the quantity of biologically available choline in soybean meal, *J. Anim. Sci.*, *42*:481–489 (1976).

29. H. C. Chang and J. H. Gaddum, Choline esters in tissue extracts, *J. Physiol.* (Lond.), 79:255–285 (1933).

30. E. P. Berry, C. W. Carrick, R. E. Roberts, and S. M. Hagne, A deficiency of available choline in soybean oil and soybean oil meal, *Poult. Sci.*, *22*:442–445 (1943).

31. G. M. Pesti, N. J. Benevenga, A. E. Harper, and M. L. Sunde, Factors influencing the assessment of the availability of choline in feedstuffs, *Poult. Sci.*, *60*:188–196 (1981).

32. J. J. Wurtman, Sources of choline and lecithin in the diet, in *Nutrition and the Brain*, A. Barbeau, J. H. Growden, and R. J. Wurtman (Eds.), Raven Press, New York, 1969, pp. 73–82.

33. J. L. Wood and R. G. Allison, Effects of consumption of choline and lecithin on neurological and cardiovascular systems. *Fed. Proc.* 41:3015–3021 (1982).

34. Informatics, Inc., *Scientific Literature Reviews on Generally Recognized As Safe (GRAS) Food Ingredients, Choline Salts*, NTIS PB-223845, 1973.

35. Infant Formula Act of 1980, 96th Congress of the United States, Public Law 96-359, 1980.

36. S. H. Zeisel, D. Char, and N. F. Sheard, Choline, phosphatidylcholine, and sphingomyelin in human and bovine milk and infant formulas, *J. Nutr.*, *116*:50–58 (1986).

37. R. J. Wurtman, M. J. Hirsch, and J. H. Growdon, Lecithin consumption raises free choline levels, *Lancet,* 2:68–69 (1977).

38. M. J. Hirsch, J. H. Growdon, and R. J. Wurtman, Relations between dietary choline of lecithin intake, serum choline levels, and various metabolic indices, *Metabolism,27*:953–960 (1978).

39. R. J. Branconnier, An analysis of dose-response of plasma choline to oral lecithin, *Biol. Psychiatr.*, *19*:765–770 (1984).

40. J. De La Huerga and H. Popper, Urinary excretion of choline metabolites following choline administration in normals and patients with hepatobiliary diseases *J. Clin. Invest.*, *30*:463–470 (1951).

41. S. Lowis, M.A. Eastwood, and W. G. Brydon, The influence of creatinine, lecithin, and choline feeding on aliphatic amine production and excretion in the rat, *Br. J. Nutr.*, *54*:43–51 (1985).

42. E. Hegazy and M. Schwenk, Choline uptake by isolated enterocytes of guinea pig, *J. Nutr.*, *114*:2217–2220 (1984).

43. J. De La Huerga and H. Popper, Factors influencing choline absorption in the intestinal tract, *J. Clin. Invest.*, *31*:598–603 (1952).

44. A. Asatoor and M. Simenhoff, The origin of urinary dimethylamines, *Biochim. Biophys. Acta, 111*:384–392 (1965).

45. D. R. Haubrich, N. H. Gerber, and A B. Pflueger, Choline availability and the synthesis of acetylcholine, in *Nutrition and the Brain*, A. Barbeau, J. H. Growdon, and R. J. Wurtman (Eds.), Raven Press, New York, 1979, pp. 57–71.

46. U. M. T. Houtsmuller, Metabolic fate of dietary lecithin, in *Nutrition and the Brain*, A. Barbeau, J. H. Growdon, and R. J. Wurtman (Eds.), Raven Press, 1979, pp. 83–93.

47. T. H. Jukes, Metabolic relationships in the transfer of methyl groups, *Fed. Proc.*, *30*:155–159 (1971).

48. W. H. Griffith and H. M. Dyer, Present knowledge of methyl groups in nutrition, *Nutr. Rev.*, *26*:1–4 (1968).

49. A. L. Lehninger, *Biochemistry*, Worth Publishers, New York, 1975.

50. C. Artom, Enzymes for the formation of lecithins by transmethylation in the livers of developing rats, *Proc. Soc. Exp. Biol. Med.*, *132*:1025–1030 (1969).

51. J. Bremer and D. M. Greenberg, Methyl transferring enzyme of microsomes in the biosynthesis of lecithin (phosphatidylcholine), *Biochim. Biophys. Acta.*, *46*:205–216 (1961).

52. S. L. Pelech and D. E. Vance, Regulation of phosphatidylcholine biosynthesis, *Biochim. Biophys. Acta.*, *779*:217–251 (1984).

53. S. Mookerjea, Action of choline in lipoprotein metabolism, *Fed. Proc.*, *30*:143–149 (1971).

54. C. H. Best, C. C. Lucas, J. H. Ridout, and J. M. Patterson, Dose response curves in the estimation of potency of lipotropic agents, *J. Biol. Chem.*, *196*:317–329 (1950).

55. J. E. O'Mullane, A comparison of the effects of feeding linoleic acid-rich lecithin corn oil on cholesterol absorption and metabolism in the rat, *Atherosclerosis*, *45*:81–90 (1982).

56. S. H. Zeisel, Dietary choline: Biochemistry, physiology, and pharmacology, *Ann. Rev. Nutr.*, *1*:95–121 (1981).

57. Y. A. Kesaniemi, and S. M.Grundy, Effects of dietary polyenylphosphatidyl-choline on metabolism and triglycerides in hypertriglyceridemic patients, *Am. J. Clin. Nutr.*, *43*:98–107 (1986).

58. R. B. Wilson, Nutrient deficiencies in animals: Choline, in *CRC Handbook Series in Nutrition and Food*, Section E, Nutritional Disorders, Vol. 2, M. Rechcigl, Jr. (Ed.), CRC Press, West Palm Beach, FL, 1978, p. 95–121.

59. C. C. Lucas, and J. H. Ridout, Fatty livers and lipotropic phenomena, in *Progress in the Chemistry of Fats and Other Lipids*, Vol. 10, Pergamon Press, London, 1967, pp. 1–150.

60. M. Y. Jenkins and G. V. Mitchell, Influence of three dietary sources of choline on liver lipids in rats fed animal or plant protein, *Nutr. Res.*, *5*:473–485 (1985).

61. K. Imaizumi, K. Mawatari, M. Murata, I. Ikeda, and M. Sugano, The contrasting effect of dietary phosphatidylethanolamine and phosphatidylcholine on serum lipoproteins and liver lipids in rats. *J. Nutr.*, *113*:2403–2411 (1983).

62. B. Rosenfeld and J. M. Lang, Diurnal changes in liver and plasma lipids of choline-deficient rats, *J. Lipid Res.*, *7*:10–16 (1966).

63. R. Pascale, L. Pirisi, L. Diano, S. Zanetti, A. Satta, E. Bartoli, and F. Feo, Role of phosphatidylethanolamine methylation in the synthesis of phosphatidylcholine by hepatocytes isolated from choline-deficient rats, *FEBS Letters*, *145*:293–297 (1982).

64. M. Murray, L. Zaluzny, and G. C. Farrell, Drug metabolism in cirrhosis. Selective changes in cytochrome P-450 isozymes in choline-deficient rat model, *Biochem. Pharmacol.*, *35*:1817–1824 (1986).

65. B. Lombardi and A. Oler, Choline deficiency fatty liver, *Lab. Invest.*, *17*:308–321 (1967).

66. B. Lombardi, P. Palni, and F. F. Schlunk, Choline deficiency fatty liver: Impaired release of hepatic triglycerides, *J. Lipid Res.*, *9*:437–446 (1968).

67. A. Chalvardjian, Mode of action of choline. II. The fate of intravenously administered labelled fatty acids in choline-deficient rats, *Can. J. Biochem.*, *47*:207–218 (1969).

68. P. M. Newberne and A. E. Rogers, Aflatoxin B, carcinogenesis in lipotrope-deficient rats, *Cancer Res.*, *29*:1965–1972 (1969).

69. S. E. Abanobi, B. Lombardi, and H. Shinozuka, Stimulation of DNA synthesis and cell proliferation in the liver of rats fed a choline-devoid diet and their suppression by phenobarbitol, *Cancer Res.*, *42*:412–415 (1982).

70. A. K. Ghoshal, M. Ahluwalia, and E. Farber, The rapid induction of liver cell death in rats fed a choline deficient methionine low diet, *Am. J. Pathol.* *113*:309–314 (1983).

71. R. B. Wilson, P. M. Newberne, and N. S. Kula, Protection by antioxidants against sclerosis of chronic choline deficiency, *Exp. Mol. Pathol.*, *21*:118–122 (1974).

72. M. M. de Oca, J. C. Perazzo, A. J. Monserrat, and E. E. Arrizurieta de Muchnik, Acute renal failure induced by choline deficiency structural-functional correlations, *Nephron*, *26*:41–48 (1980).

73. I. C. Wells, Hemorrhagic kidney degeneration in choline deficiency, *Fed. Proc.*, *30*:151–154 (1971).

74. A. J. Monserrat, F. Hamilton, A. K. Ghoshal, E. A. Porta, and W. S. Hartroft, Lysosomes in the pathogenesis of the renal necrosis of choline-deficient rats. *Am. J. Pathol.*, *68*:113–146 (1972).

75. R. R. Costa, M. A. Rossi, and J. S. M. Oliveira, Pathogenesis of the renal injury in choline deficiency: The role of catecholamines and acetylcholine, *Br. J. Exp. Pathol.*, *60*:613–619 (1979).

76. J. L. Beare-Rogers, Time sequence of liver phospholipid alterations during deprivation of dietary choline, *Can. J. Physiol. Pharmacol.*, *49*:171–177 (1970).

77. H. McCoy, L. Williams, and C. Caroll, Interaction of dietary fat and route of immunization in the immune response of the rat, *Nutr. Rep. Int.*, *19*:289–298 (1979).

78. R. B. Wilson, N. S. Kula, P. M. Newberne, and M. W. Conner, Vascular damage and lipid peroxidation in choline-deficient rats, *Exp. Mol. Pathol.*, *18*:357–368 (1973).

79. T. H. Rushmore, Rapid lipid peroxidation in the nuclear fraction of rat liver induced by diet deficient in choline and methionine, *Cancer Letters*, *24*:251–255 (1984).

80. S. L. Katyal and B. Lombardi, Effects of dietary choline and N,N-dimethylaminoethanol on lung phospholipid and surfactant of newborn rats, *Ped. Res.*, *12*:952–955 (1978).

81. K. E. McMahon and P. M. Farrell, Effects of choline deficiency on lung phospholipid concentrations in the rat, *J. Nutr.*, *116*:936–943 (1986).

82. R. W. Yost, A. Chander, and A. B. Fisher, Differential response of lung and liver of juvenile rats to choline deficiency, *J. App. Physiol.*, *59*:738–742 (1985).

83. Anonymous, Fat deposition in coronary arteries of rats exposed to cold, *Nutr. Rev.*, *14*:284–285 (1956).

84. D. H. Copeland and W. D. Salmon, The occurrence of neoplasms in the livers, lungs, and other tissues of the rat as a result of prolonged choline deficiency, *Am. J. Pathol.* 22:1059–1067 (1946).

85. A. K. Ghoshal and E. Farber, Induction of liver cancer by a dietary deficiency in choline and methionine without added carcinogens, *Carcinogenesis*, *5*:1367–1370 (1984).

86. J. Locker, T. V. Reddy, and B. Lombardi, DNA methylation and hepatocarcinogenesis in rats fed a choline-devoid diet, *Carcinogenesis*, *7*:1309–1312 (1986).

87. S. Yokoyama, M. A. Sells, T. V. Reddy, and B. Lombardi, Hepatocarcinogenesis and promoting action of a choline-devoid diet in the rat. *Cancer Res.*, *45*:2834–2842 (1985).

88. J. M. Betschart, M. A. Virji, M. I. R. Perera, and H. Shinozuka, Alterations in hepatocyte insulin receptors in rats fed a choline-deficient diet, *Cancer Res.*, *46*:4425–4430 (1986).

89. M. I. R. Perera, A. J. Demetris, S. L. Katyal, and H. Shinozuka, Lipid peroxidation of liver microsome membranes induced by choline deficient diet and its relationship to diet induced promotion of the induction of r-glutanyl transpeptidase positive foci, *Cancer Res.*, *45*:2533–2538 (1985).

90. P. R. Turkki, Effect of nutrient deficiencies in man: Choline, in *CRC Handbook Series in Nutrition and Food*, Vol. 1, M. Rechcigl, Jr. (Ed.), CRC Press, West Palm Beach, FL, 1978, pp. 45–53.

91. G. F. Sheldon, S. R. Petersen, and R. Sanders, Hepatic dysfunction during hyperalimentation, *Arch. Surg.*, *113*:504–508 (1978).

92. B. V. MacFadyen, S. J. Dudrick, G. Baquero, and E. T. Gum, Clinical and biological changes in liver function during intravenous hyperalimentation, *J. Parent. Enter. Nutr.*, *3*:438–443 (1979).

93. I. Tulikoura and K. Huikuri, Morphological fatty changes and function of liver, serum free fatty acids and triglycerides during parenteral nutrition, *Scand. J. Gastroenterol.*, *17*:177–185 (1982).

94. W. W. Wagner, A. C. Lowry, and H. Silberman, Similar liver function abnormalities occur in patients receiving glucose-based and lipid-based parenteral nutrition, *Am. J. Gastroenterol.*, *78*:199–202 (1983).

95. J. R. Poley, Liver and nutrition: Hepatic complications of total parenteral nutrition, in *Textbook of Gastroenterology and Nutrition in Infancy*, E. Lebenthal (Ed.), Raven Press, New York, 1981, pp. 743–763.

96. N. F. Sheard, J. A. Tayek, B. R. Bistrian, G. L. Blackburn, and S. H. Zeisel, Plasma choline concentration in humans fed parenterally, *Am. J. Clin. Nutr., 43*:219–224 (1986).

97. M. E. Burt, I. Hanin, and M. F. Brennan, Choline deficiency associated with total parenteral nutrition, *Lancet, 2*:638–639 (1980).

98. J. Marks, *A Guide to the Vitamins, Their Roles in Health and Disease*, Medical and Technical Publishing, Lancaster, England, 1977.

99. J. C. Russet, J. L. Krider, T. R. Cline, H. L. Thacker, and L. B. Underwood, Choline-methionine interactions in young swine, *J. Anim. Sci., 49*:708–714 (1979).

100. M. K. D. Vemury, C. Kies, and H. M. Fox, L-methionine/choline/inorganic sulfur interrelationships in soy-based diets fed to human adults, *Nutr. Rep. Int., 22*:369–382 (1980).

101. Anonymous, Influence of alcohol and choline deficiency upon rat liver uptake of choline, *Nutr. Rev., 29*:237–239 (1971).

102. D. J. Tuma, A. J. Barak, D. F. Schafer, and M. F. Sorrell, Possible interrelationship of ethanol metabolism and choline oxidation in the liver, *Can. J. Biochem., 51*:117–120 (1973).

103. A. J. Barak, D. J. Tuma, and M. F. Sorrell, Relationship of ethanol to choline metabolism in the liver: A review, *Am. J. Clin. Nutr., 26*:1234–1241 (1973).

104. J. A. Thompson and R. C. Reitz, Studies of the acute and chronic effects of ethanol ingestion on choline oxidation, *Ann. N.Y. Acad. Sci. 273*:194–204 (1976).

105. A. J. Barak, D. J. Tuma, and H. C. Beckenhauer, Ethanol, the choline requirement, methylation, and liver injury, *Life Sci., 37*:789–791 (1985).

106. A. K. Rawat, Brain levels and turnover rats of presumptive neurotransmitters as influenced by administration and withdrawal of ethanol in mice, *J. Neurochem., 22*:915–922 (1974).

107. J. W. Clark, H. Kalant, and F. J. Carmichael, Effect of ethanol tolerance on release of acetylcholine and norepinephrine by rat cerebral cortex, *Can. J. Physiol. Pharm., 55*:758–768 (1977).

108. M. Acara, Effect of ethanol on the renal excretion and metabolism of choline in the isolated perfused rat kidney, *Drug. Metab. Dispos., 7*:113–117 (1979).

109. C. S. Lieber, M. A. Leo, K. M. Mak, L. M. De Carli, and S. Sato, Choline fails to prevent liver fibrosis in ethanol-fed baboons but causes toxicity, *Hepatology, 5*:561–572 (1985).

110. R. T. Bartus, R. L. Dean, J. A. Goas, and A. S. Lippa, Age-related change in passive avoidance retention: Modulation with dietary choline, *Science, 209*:301–303 (1980).

111. R. T. Bartus, R. L. Dean, D. Beer, and A. S. Lippa, The cholinergic hypothesis of geriatric memory dysfunction, *Science, 217*, 408–417 (1982).

112. C. J. Sanchez, E. Hooper, P. J. Garry, J. M. Goodwin, and J. S. Goodwin, The relationship between dietary intake of choline, choline serum levels, and cognitive function in healthy elderly persons, *J. Am. Geriat. Soc., 32*:208–212 (1984).

113. D. S. Janowsky, M. K. El-Yousef, and J. M. Davis, Acetylcholine and depression, *Psychosom. Med., 36*:248–257 (1974).

114. J. M. Gorell, C. P. Navarro, and P. W. Shwendner, Regional CNS levels of acetylcholine and choline during hypoglycemic stupor and recovery, *J. Neurochem., 36*:321–324 (1981).

115. C. H. Rauca, E. Kammerer, and H. Matthies, Choline uptake and permanent memory storage, *Pharmac. Biochem. Behav., 13*:21–25 (1980).

116. J. H. Growdon and R. J. Wurtman, Dietary influences on the synthesis of neurotransmitters in the brain, *Nutr. Rev., 37*:129–136 (1979).

117. M. H. Fernstrom, Lecithin, choline, and cholinergic transmission, in *Nutritional Pharmacology*, G. Spiller (Ed.), Alan R. Liss, New York, 1981, pp. 5–29.

118. E. L. Cohen and R. J. Wurtman, Brain acetylcholine: Increase after systemic choline administration, *Life Sci., 16*:1095–1102 (1975).

119. D. R. Haubrich, P. W. Wedeking, and P. F. L. Wang, Increase in tissue concentration of acetylcholine in guinea pigs in vivo induced by administration of choline, *Life Sci., 14*:921–927 (1974).

120. M. H. Fernstrom and R. J. Wurtman, Increase in striatal choline acetyltransferase activity after choline administration, *Brain Res., 165*:358–361 (1979).

121. E. L. Cohen and R. J. Wurtman, Brain acetylcholine: Control by dietary choline, *Science, 191*:561–562 (1976).

122. D. R. Haubrich and A. B. Pflueger, Choline administration: Central effect mediated by stimulation of acetylcholine synthesis, *Life Sci., 24*:1083–1090 (1979).

123. M. J. Hirsch and R. J. Wurtman, Lecithin consumption increases acetylcholine concentrations in rat brain and adrenal gland, *Science, 202*:223–225 (1978).

124. K. L. Davis, P. A. Berger, and L. E. Hollister, Choline for tardive dyskinesia, *N. Engl. J. Med., 293*:152–153 (1975).

125. A. J. Gelenberg, J. C. Doller-Wojcik, and J. H Growdon, Choline and lecithin in the treatment of tardive dyskinesia: Preliminary results from a pilot study, *Am. J. Psychiatr., 136*:772–776 (1979).

126. K. L. Davis, L. E. Hollister, J. D. Barchas, and P. A. Berger, Choline in tardive dyskinesia and Huntington's disease, *Life Sci., 19*:1507–1515 (1976).

127. C. A. Tamminga, R. C. Smith, S. E. Erickson, S. Chang, and J. M. Davis, Cholinergic influences in tardive dyskinesia, *Am. J. Psychiatr., 134*:769–774 (1977).

128. J. H. Growdon, M. J. Hirsch, R. J. Wurtman, and W. Wiener, Oral choline administration to patients with tardive dyskinesia, *N. Engl. J. Med., 297*:524–527 (1977).

129. K. L. Davis, L. E. Hollister, P. A. Berger, and A. L. Vento, Studies on choline chloride in neuropsychiatric disease: Human and animal data, *Psychopharmacol. Bull., 14*:56–58 (1978).

130. A. Barbeau, Emerging treatment: Replacement therapy with choline or lecithin in neurological diseases, *Can. J. Neurol. Sci. 5*:157–160 (1978).

131. A. Barbeau, Lecithin in neurologic disorders, *N. Engl. J. Med. 299*:200–201 (1978).

132. J. H. Growdon, A. J. Gelenberg, J. Doller, M. J. Hirsch, and R. J. Wurtman, Lecithin can suppress tardive dyskinesia, *N. Engl. J. Med. 298*:1029–1030 (1978).

133. I. V.Jackson, E. A. Nuttall, I. O. Ibe, and J. Perez-Cruet, Treatment of tardive dyskinesia with lecithin, *Am. J. Psychiatr., 136*:1458–1460 (1979).

134. K. Wilbur, A. V. Kulik, and T. C. Brecht, Lecithin for tardive dyskinesia, *Am. J. Psychiatr., 139*:1375 (1982).

135. R. Ray, N. Ramakrishnan, and B. S. S. Rao, Oral choline in tardive dyskinesia, *Ind. J. Med. Res., 76*:628–631 (1982).

136. H. A. Nadrallah, F. J. Dunner, R. E. Smith, M. McCalley-Whitters, and A. D. Sherman, Variable clinical response to choline in tardive dyskinesia, *Psychol. Med., 14*:697–700 (1984).

137. M. H. Branchey, L. B. Branchey, N. M. Bark, and M. A. Richardson, Lecithin in the treatment of tardive dyskinesia, *Commun. Psychopharmacol., 3*:303–307, (1979).

138. J. Perez-Cruet, I. Menendez, and J. Alvarez- Ghersi, Double-blind study of lecithin in the treatment of persistent tardive dyskinesia, *Bol. Assoc. Med. P.R., 73*:531–537 (1981).

139. B. G. Anderson, D. Reker, M. Ristich, E. Friedman, M. Banay-Schwartz, and J. Volarka, Lecithin treatment of tardive dyskinesia—a progress report, *Psychopharmacol. Bull., 18*:87–88 (1982).

140. D. V. Jeste and R. J. Wyatt, *Understanding and Treating Tardive Dyskinesia*, Guilford Press, New York, 1982.

141. E. F. Domino, W. W. May, S. Demetrion, B. Matthews, S. Tait, and B. Kovacic, Lack of clinically significant improvement in patients with tardive dyskinesia following phosphatidylcholine therapy, *Biol. Psychiatr., 20*:1189–1196 (1985).

142. W. D. Boyd, J Graham-White, G. Blackwood, I. Glen, and J. McQueen, Clinical effects of choline in Alzheimer senile dementia, *Lancet, 2*:711 (1977).

143. P. Etienne, S. Gauthier, G. Johnson, B. Collier, T. Mendis, D. Dastoor, M. Cole, and H. F. Muller, Clinical effects of choline in Alzheimer's disease, *Lancet, 1*:508–509 (1978).

144. C. M. Smith, M. Swase, A. N. Exton-Smith, M. J. Phillips, P. W. Overstall, M. E. Piper, and M. R. Bailey, Choline therapy in Alzheimer's disease, *Lancet, 2*:318 (1978).

145. A. Whiteley, J. L. Signoret, Y. Agid, and F. L'Hermitte, Action de la choline sur les troubles mnésiques de la maladie d'Alzheimer, *Rev. Neurol. (Paris), 135*:8–9 (1979).

146. P. Fovall, M. W. Dysken, L. W. Lazarus, J. M. Davis, R. L. Kahn, R. Jope, S. Finkel and P. Rattan, Choline bitartrate treatment of Alzheimer-type dementias, *Commun. Psychopharmacol., 4*:141–145 (1980).

147. B. H. Peters and H. S. Levin, Effects of physostigmine and lecithin on memory in Alzheimer disease, *Ann. Neurol., 6*:219–221 (1979).

148. G. Vroulis, R. C. Smith, J. C. Schoolar, G. Dahlen, E. Katz, and C. H. Misra, Reduction in cholesterol risk factors by lecithin in patients with Alzheimer's disease, *Am. J. Psychiatr., 139*:1633–1634 (1982).

149. N. L. Canter, M. Hallett, and J. H. Growdon, Lecithin does not affect EEG spectral analysis or P_{300} in Alzheimer disease, *Neurology (N.Y.), 32*:1260–1266 (1982).

150. M. W. Dysken, P. Fovall, C. M. Harris, and J. M. Davis, Lecithin administration in Alzheimer's dementia [letter], *Neurology (N.Y.), 32*:1203–1204 (1982).

151. N. Pomara, E. F. Domino, H. Yoon, S. Brinkman, C. Tamminga, and S. Gershon, Failure of single dose lecithin to alter aspects of central cholinergic activity in Alzheimer's disease, *J. Clin. Psychiatr., 44*:293–295 (1983).

152. R. Levy, A. Little, P. Chuaqui, and M. Reith, Early results from double-blind placebo controlled trial of high dose phosphatidylcholine in Alzheimer's disease, *Lancet, 1*:987–988 (1983).

153. A. Little, R. Levy, P. Chuaqui-Kidd, and D. Hand, A double-blind placebo controlled trial of high dose lecithin in Alzheimer's disease, *J. Neurol. Neurosurg. Psychiatr., 48*:736–742 (1985).

154. C. M. Lawrence, P. Millac, G. S. Stout, and J. W. Ward, The use of choline chloride in ataxic disorders, *J. Neurol. Neurosurg. Psychiatr., 43*:452–454 (1980).

155. N. J. Legg, Oral choline in cerebellarataxia, *Br. Med. J., 2*:1403–1404 (1978).

156. B. M. Cohen, A. L. Miller, J. F. Lipinski, and H. G. Pope, Lecithin in mania: A preliminary report, *Am. J. Psychiatr., 137*:242–243 (1980).

157. H. Moldofsky and P. Sandor, Lecithin in the treatment of Gilles de la Tourette's syndrome, *Am. J. Psychiatr., 140*:1627–1629 (1983).

158. R. C. Mohs, K. L. Davis, J. R. Tinklenberg, L. E. Hollister, J. A. Yesavage, and B. S. Kopell, choline chloride treatment of memory deficits in the elderly, *Am. J. Psychiatr., 136*:1275–1277 (1979).

159. S. H. Ferris, G. Sathananthan, B. Reisberg, and S. Gershon, Long-term choline treatment of memory-impaired elderly patients, *Science, 205*:1039–1040 (1979).

160. R. J. Wurtman, W. J. Hirsch, and J. H. Growdon, Lecithin consumption raises serum-free choline levels, *Lancet, 2*:68–69 (1977).

161. J. H. Growdon, Clinical evaluation of compounds for the treatment of memory dysfunction, *Ann. N.Y. Acad. Sci., 444*:3437–3449 (1985).

162. G. S. Rosenberg and K. L. Davis, The use of cholinergic precursors in neuropsychiatric diseases, *Am. J. Clin. Nutr., 36*:709–720 (1982).

163. J. H. Growdon, Phosphatidylcholine and tardive dyskinesia [letter], *Biol. Psychiatr., 21*:702–704 (1986).

164. P. Davies, R. Katzman, and R. D. Terry, Reduced somatostatin-like immunoreactivity in cerebral cortex from cases of Alzheimer's disease and Alzheimer senile dementia, *Nature, 288*:279–280 (1980).

165. D. Bowen, Biochemical assessment of neurotransmitter and metabolic dysfunction and cerebral atrophy in Alzheimer's disease, in *Biological Aspects of Alzheimer's Disease*, R. Katzman (Ed.), Banbury Report 15, Cold Spring Harbor, New York, 1983, pp. 219–231.

166. Y. Ichimiya, H. Arai, K. Kosaka, and R. Iizuka, Morphological and biochemical changes in the cholinergic and monoaminergic systems in Alzheimer-type dementia, *Acta Neuropath.* (Berl.), *70*:112–116 (1986).

167. T. J. Crook, Clinical drug trials in Alzheimer's disease, *Ann. N.Y. Acad. Sci., 444*:428–436 (1985).

168. T. Samorajski, G. A. Vroulis, and R. C. Smith, Piracetam plus lecithin trials in senile dementia of the Alzheimer's type, *Ann. N.Y. Acad. Sci., 444*:478–481 (1985).

169. R. T. Bartus, R. L. Dean, and B. Beer, Cholinergic precursor therapy for geriatric cognition: Its past, its present, and a question of its future, in *Nutrition in Gerontology*, J. M. Ordy, D. Harman, and R. Alfin-Slater (Eds.), Raven Press, New York, 1984, pp. 191–225.

170. P. J. Whitehouse, A. M. Martino, P. G. Antuono, P. R. Lowenstein, J. T. Coyle, D. L. Price, and K. J. Kellar, Nicotinic acetylcholine binding sites in Alzheimer disease, *Brain Res., 371*:146–151 (1986).

171. A. G. Goodman, L. S. Goodman, and A. Gilman, *The Pharmacological Basis of Therapeutics*, 6th Ed., MacMillan, New York, 1970, pp. 1574–1576.

172. M. Byington, Effect of nutrient toxicities in animals and man: Choline, in *CRC Handbook Series in Nutrition and Food*, Section E, Vol. 3, M. Rechcigl, Jr. (Ed.), CRC Press, West Palm Beach, FL, 1978.

173. J. M. Bell, Perinatal dietary supplementation with a commercial soy lecithin preparation: Effects on behavior and brain biochemistry in the developing rat, *Devel. Psychobio., 18*:383–394 (1985).

15
Carnitine

Peggy R. Borum
University of Florida
Gainesville, Florida

I. HISTORY

The compound carnitine was isolated from meat extracts and identified during the first decade of this century. It was a compound with no known function until the 1950s, when it was shown to be a required growth factor for the mealworm *Tenebrio molitor*. Since it was a small water-soluble compound required in the diet of *Tenebrio molitor*, it was given the name vitamin BT (1). Although carnitine is clearly a vitamin for the mealworm, there is no data to suggest that carnitine is a vitamin for the healthy human adult. There is some data indicating that carnitine is a conditionally essential nutrient for some segments of the population who would be under the care of a physician. Table 1 lists the types of pathophysiology that might result in a patient requiring carnitine in the diet. However,

Table 1 Patients Who May Require Supplementary Carnitine

Altered biosynthesis	Altered transport	Increased excretion
Malnutrition	Malnutrition	Immaturity
Immaturity	Immaturity	Organic aciduria
Genetic carnitine deficiency	Genetic carnitine deficiency	Genetic carnitine deficiency
Liver disease	Liver disease	Liver disease
Renal disease		Renal disease
		Treatment with certain drugs such as valproate

certain businesses are marketing carnitine to the public as vitamin BT or vitamin B_7 in such a manner that the customer would assume that it is a vitamin for humans.

There has been an enormous increase in the basic science research and clinical research interest in carnitine during the sixth, seventh, and eighth decades of this century. In 1964 a symposium entitled "Recent Research On Carnitine, Its Relation To Lipid Metabolism," a symposium in 1979 entitled "Carnitine Biosynthesis, Metabolism and Functions," and a symposium in 1985 entitled "Clinical Aspects of Human Carnitine Deficiency" were convened and the proceedings published (2–4). Carnitine has been the subject of several recent review articles (5–9).

II. CHEMICAL PROPERTIES AND ANALYTICAL PROCEDURES

Carnitine (β-hydroxy-λ-trimethylaminobutyrate) is a very hygroscopic quaternary amine compound with a molecular weight of 161.2 daltons. Many of the functions of carnitine are dependent upon the formation of an ester at the hydroxyl group with a carboxylic acid.

The most commonly used methodology to determine the carnitine concentration in biological samples is the radioenzymatic assay first described in 1972 (10) and modified by several investigators (11–13). The assay is both accurate and sensitive for the determination of total carnitine. However, carnitine is found in biological samples both as the free carnitine and as the ester of a wide variety of acyl compounds. Many research and clinical activities would greatly benefit from the identification and quantitation of each acylcarnitine in the sample. Mass spectroscopy assay can identify a particular acylcarnitine, but it is not practical methodology for routine screening (14).

III. CONTENT IN FOOD

Carnitine is found in food products obtained from animals (15, 16). Milk from all mammalian species contains carnitine, but meat is the major source of carnitine in the diet of the adult. The carnitine concentration increases in the order of fish, poultry, pork, beef, and lamb. In general, the redder the meat, the higher the concentration of carnitine. Table 2 lists the carnitine content in a typical serving of different types of meat.

Since plants contain little or no carnitine, vegetarians consume little carnitine. During the fermentation process of temph preparation, the mold produces carnitine. A serving of temph has approximately the same concentration of carnitine as a serving of

Table 2 Carnitine Content of Different Meats

Meat Serving	μmol Carnitine
Fish sandwich	9
Fried chicken breast	13
Fried chicken legs	29
Roast pork	215
Hamburger	466
Ground round	798

white fish. Nutrition formulations such as infant formulas made from plant products contain no endogenous carnitine (17). In recent years all infant formula prepared from soy protein or other protein sources containing no endogenous carnitine have been supplemented with carnitine to provide a carnitine concentration similar to human milk.

Several laboratories are investigating the transport of carnitine across the small intestine (18, 19). Little is known concerning the bioavailability of carnitine in different foods or of crystalline carnitine dissolved in an aqueous solution and administered orally.

IV. METABOLISM

Carnitine is synthesized predominantly in the liver and the kidney of the human from the essential amino acids lysine and methionine (Fig. 1.). The nutrients iron, ascorbate, niacin, and vitamin B_6 are also required for carnitine biosynthesis (20, 21). Thus, a diet limiting in any of these essential nutrients or an abnormally functioning liver or kidney may impair the ability of the body to synthesize carnitine.

Tissues such as cardiac muscle and skeletal muscle require carnitine for normal fuel metabolism but cannot synthesize carnitine and are totally dependent on the transport of carnitine from other tissues. Several transport systems have been identified in different tissues, but much more research is needed to elucidate the metabolic compartmentation of carnitine.

V. FUNCTIONS

It is well established that carnitine functions in the transport of long-chain fatty acids from the cytosol into the matrix of the mitochondria, which is the site of β oxidation. Carnitine is required to transport any carbon chain at the coenzyme A level across a membrane (22). Acyl CoA compounds, such as palmitoyl CoA, are high-energy compounds which cannot penetrate any membrane. Palmitoyl CoA can be converted to palmitoyl carnitine, which is also a high-energy compound but can be transported across membranes by the action of a translocase. The palmitoryl carnitine can be converted to palmitoyl CoA in its new location without the need for the hydrolysis of ATP or some other high-energy compound. If the thiokinase is located in one compartment of the cell and converts the carbon chain to the coenzyme A level, the acyl CoA cannot be transported across membranes into another compartment where it is needed without the action of carnitine and the associated transferases and translocase. Carnitine functions in the translocation of acyl CoA without the expenditure of large amounts of metabolic energy. Carnitine facilitates the β oxidation of long-chain fatty acids in the mitochondria by transporting the substrate into the mitochondria. Carnitine appears to facilitate the β oxidation of very long-chain fatty acids

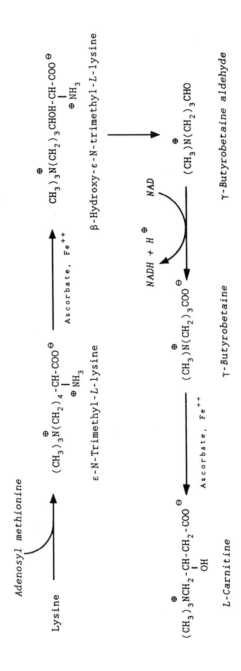

Figure 1

in the peroxisomes by transporting the medium-chain fatty acid product out of the peroxisomes. Carnitine appears to facilitate the oxidation of the ketoacids of the branched-chain keto acids by transporting out of the mitochondria an intermediate that inhibits the pathway. Carnitine facilitates the removal of acyl CoA compounds that can accumulate to toxic concentrations by transporting the compounds out of the cell and permitting their excretion in the urine.

VI. DEFICIENCIES

The first carnitine-deficient patient was described in the early 1970s. During that decade, the terms primary carnitine deficiency and secondary carnitine deficiency were often used clinically. Very few patients have been clearly demonstrated to have a metabolic defect in either the biosynthetic pathway or the transport of carnitine from one tissue to the another (23). Most patients have been described as having a secondary carnitine deficiency. These are often patients with an identified inborn error of metabolism that results in the accumulation of acyl compounds in the body and perhaps an organic aciduria. Several patients have been described with carnitine palmitoyltransferase deficiency. Both the terms carnitine deficiency and carnitine palmitoyltransferase deficiency describe at least two families of syndromes (24).

VII. NUTRITIONAL STATUS

Assessment of the carnitine status of a particular individual is difficult because plasma carnitine concentrations and urinary carnitine excretion are not good indicators of tissue carnitine status. A patient with low carnitine concentrations in plasma may have normal carnitine concentrations in muscle or liver. A patient with normal plasma carnitine concentrations may have low carnitine concentrations in muscle or liver. Thus, caution must be exercised in using plasma carnitine concentrations to assess the carnitine status of a patient (25). It is also difficult to know how low a carnitine concentration must be before it is pathological. Much more work is needed to improve our ability to assess carnitine status.

VIII. NUTRITIONAL REQUIREMENTS

There are no established nutritional requirements for carnitine. The growing body of data indicating the importance of carnitine in the diet of infants has led infant formula manufacturers in the United States to supplement carnitine-free formulas to obtain a concentration of carnitine that is similar to that of breast milk. However, there are no data defining a dietary requirement of carnitine for any patient population.

IX. FACTORS THAT MAY INFLUENCE CARNITINE STATUS AND GROUPS AT GREATER RISK OF DEFICIENCY

Factors such as prematurity, certain severe metabolic stresses, inborn errors of metabolism, malnutrition, and impaired liver or renal function may increase the risk for carnitine deficiency (26) (see Table 1). The liver of the premature neonate may not have a fully developed biosynthetic capacity, and the neonatal kidney may not have a fully developed capability to resorb carnitine. Extremely preterm neonates with a variety of metabolic stresses and maintained on carnitine-free total parenteral nutrition have been shown to have very low tissue carnitine concentrations (27). Certain inborn errors of metabolism as well as various types of metabolic stress may lead to the increased production of acyl compounds that are excreted in the urine as acylcarnitine and thus are a continuous drain on the body pool of carnitine. Some drugs such as valproic acid also increase the excretion of carnitine in the urine as acylcarnitine. Patients with liver disease or renal disease may not have the normal carnitine biosynthetic pathway and be at risk for deficiency.

X. PHARMACOLOGICAL USE OF CARNITINE

Several hundred patients have been given carnitine supplementation at dosages that far exceed the usual dietary intake of carnitine (28). Oral dosages such as 100 mg per kg body weight per day for infants and children with failure to thrive and 1–3 g of carnitine per day for adults with muscle weakness have been frequently used. Some patients may experience diarrhea if supplementation is begun at these dosaes but if they are started at smaller dosages and then increased gradually, there is usually little problem with diarrhea. Only the physiological L-carnitine should be used. There is some indication that administration of the D-isomer may interfere with the normal functions of the L-isomer. The health effects of the oral administration of carnitine at the dosages listed above have been reviewed (29).

REFERENCES

1. S. Friedman and G. S. Fraenkel. New and Unidentified Growth Factors. III. Carnitine. In *The Vitamins*, Vol 5, W. H. Sebrell, Jr. and R. S. Harris (Eds.), Academic Press, New York, 1972, pp. 329–355.
2. G. Wolf (Ed.), *Recent Research on Carnitine, Its Relation to Lipid Metabolism*, M.I.T. Press, Cambridge, MA, 1965.
3. Rene A. Frenkel and J. Denis McGarry (Eds.), *Carnitine Biosynthesis, Metabolism, and Functions*, Academic Press, New York, 1980.
4. Peggy R. Borum (Ed.), *Clinical Aspects of Human Carnitine Deficiency*, Pergamon Press, New York, 1986.
5. P. R. Borum, Carnitine, *Ann. Rev. Nutr.*, 3:233–259 (1983).
6. C. J. Rebouche and D. J. Paulson, Carnitine metabolism and function in humans, *Ann. Rev. Nutr.*, 6:41–66 (1986).
7. J. Bremer, Carnitine—metabolism and functions. *Physiological Reviews*, 63:1420–1480 (1983).
8. L. L. Bieber, Carnitine, *Ann. Rev. Biochem.*, 57:261–283 (1988).
9. H. R. Sholte and P. C. de Jonge, Metabolism, Function and Transport of Carnitine in Health and Disease. In *Carnitin in der Medizin*, R. Gitzelmann, K. Baerlocher, and B. Steinmann (Eds.), Schattauer, New York, 1987, pp. 21–59.
10. G. Cederblad and S. Lindstedt, A method for the determination of carnitine in the picomole range, *Clinica Chimia Acta*, 37:235–243 (1972).
11. J. D. McGarry and D. W. Foster, An improved and simplified radioisotopic assay for the determination of free and esterified carnitine, *J. Lipid Res.* 17:277–281 (1976).
12. R. C. Fishlock, L. L. Bieber, and A. M. Snoswell, Sources of error in determinations of carnitine and acylcarnitine in plasma, *Clin. Chem.*, 30:316–318 (1984).
13. C. Rossle, K. P. Kohse, H.-E. Franz, and P. Furst, An improved method for the determination of free and esterified carnitine, *Clinica Chimica Acta*, 149:263–268 (1985).
14. A. L. Yergey, D. J. Liberato, and D. S. Millington, Thermospray liquid chromatography/mass spectrometry for the analysis of L-carnitine and its short-chain acyl derivatives, *Anal Biochem.*, 139:278–283 (1984).

15. M. E. Mitchell, Carnitine metabolism in human subjects. I. Normal metabolism, *Am. J. of Clin. Nutr.*, *31*:293–306 (1978).

16. P. R. Borum, Carnitine content of hospital diets, *Fed. Proc.*, *39*:4103 (1980).

17. P. R. Borum, C. M. York, and H. P. Broquist, Carnitine content of liquid formulas and special diets, *Am. J. Clin. Nutr.*, *32*:2272–2276 (1979).

18. C. J. Gross, L. M. Henderson, and D. A. Savaiano, Uptake of L-carnitine, D-carnitine and acetyl-L-carnitine by isolated guinea-pig enterocytes, *Biochimica et Biophysica Acta*, *886*:25–433 (1986).

19. B. U. K. Li, M. L. Lloyd, A. L. Shug, and W. A. Olsen, Jejunal carnitine (C) levels and absorption in humans, *Ped. Res.*, *21* (1987).

20. V. Tanphaichitr, D. W. Horne, and H. P. Broquist, Lysine, a precursor of carnitine in the rat, *J. Biol. Chem.*, *246*:6364–6366 (1971).

21. C. J. Rebouche and A. G. Engel, Tissue distribution of Carnitine biosynthetic enzymes in man, *Biochim. Biophys. Acta*, *630*:22–29 (1980).

22. P. R. Borum, Role of carnitine in lipid metabolism. In *Lipids in Modern Nutrition*, 1987, pp. 51–58.

23. W. R. Treem, C. A. Stanley, D. N. Finegold, D. E. Hale, and P. M. Coates, Primary carnitine deficiency due to a failure of carnitine transport in kidney, muscle, and fibroblasts, *New Engl. J. Med.*, *319*:1331–1336 (1988).

24. C. Angelini, C. Trevisan, G. Isaya, G. Pegolo, and L. Vergani, Clinical varieties of carnitine and carnitine palmitoyltransferase deficiency, *Clin. Biochem*, *20*:1–7 (1987).

25. P. R. Borum, T. O. Rumley, and E. Taggart, *Caution Required in Clinical Use of Plasma Carnitine Concentration for Assessment of Carnitine Status.* Presented at ESPEN, Paris, 1986.

26. P. R. Borum, Carnitine—who needs it? *Nutrition Today*: 4–6 (1986).

27. D. Penn, E. Schmidt-Sommerfeld, and F. Pascu, Decreased Tissue carnitine concentrations in newborn infants receiving total parenteral nutrition, *J. Pediatrics*, *98*:976–978 (1981).

28. K. L. Goa and R. N. Brogden, L-carnitine. A preliminary review of its pharmacokinetics, and its therapeutic use in ischaemic cardiac disease and primary and secondary carnitine deficiencies in relationship to its role in fatty acid metabolism, *Drugs*, *34*:1–24 (1987).

29. P. R. Borum and F. D. Fisher (Eds.), *Health Effects of Dietary Carnitine*, Life Sciences Research Office, Bethesda, MD, 1983.

16
Substances Without Vitamin Status

Mildred M. Cody
Georgia State University
Atlanta, Georgia

I. INTRODUCTION

The term *vitamin* has been applied to many chemical substances that do not meet the criteria for vitamins. Many compounds described as vitamins in the scientific literature of the 1930s and 1940s have since proven to be identical to other essential nutrients or to be mixtures of many compounds; examples of these would be vitamins M, B_{11}, T, and B_c, which have folacin activity; vitamin G, which is identical to riboflavin; vitamin F, which was confirmed to be *cis,cis*-linoleic acid; and vitamin V, which is $NAD^+/NADH + H^+$. Some compounds, such as inositol and bioflavonoids, exhibit biological activity without being dietary essentials for humans and occasionally have been accorded vitamin status. A third group of substances are called vitamins by promoters for profit; these substances, including

565

pangamate, laetrile, gerovital, and orotic acid, are not dietary essentials and are more properly called pseudovitamins.

II. VITAMIN NAMES DISCARDED DURING THE YEARS OF DISCOVERY

Research conducted during the 1930s and 1940s resulted in the chemical and biological characterization of many compounds. As chemical syntheses and isolations were confirmed, it became clear that a single compound might bear several names, depending on its described function(s) or its source(s). Additionally, compounds required by one species were not always required by other species; generally, vitamin status is designated for those nutrients considered dietary essentials for humans. For these reasons, many of the substances referred to as "vitamins," "growth factors," or "accessory factors" in early research literature are no longer considered to be vitamins.

A. Vitamins M, B_c, B_{10}, B_{11}, T, and B_x

Investigations of vitamins M, B_c, B_{10}, B_{11}, and B_x converged in the mid-1940s with the synthesis of pteroylglutamic acid (PGA) and the isolation of vitamin B_{12}. Prior to these structural confirmations, extracts of liver, yeast, vegetables, and insects were found to have various biological activities in different animal species, and each finding was investigated and reported independently. Since purification of extracts was generally incomplete and since the many conjugated forms of PGA have varying biological activities, it took several years to determine that many of these vitamins required the fundamental pteroylglutamic acid unit for activity and could be given the group name of *folacin*.

1. VITAMIN M

The name vitamin M was given by Day et al. to a semipurified yeast extract that prevented nutritional macrocytic anemia in monkeys. This complex was later more narrowly defined to be the folacin compounds pteroylglutamic acid, pteroyltriglutamate, and pteroylheptaglutamate and was successfully used in the clinical treatment of macrocytic anemias resulting from dietary folacin deficiency, sprue, and pregnancy (1,2).

2. VITAMIN B_c

Hogan and Parrott reported a macrocytic anemia and reduced growth in chicks fed a semipurified diet. These observations were confirmed by Pfiffner et al., who showed that these symptoms could be alleviated by feeding vitamin B_c, an extract from liver. Vitamin B_c deficiency symptoms were alleviated by folacin, and vitamin B_c crystallized from liver was shown to be identical to synthetic pteroylglutamate (1,2).

3. VITAMINS B_{10} AND B_{11}

Vitamins B_{10} and B_{11}, which were extracted from liver or from *Mycobacterium tuberculosis* grown in the presence of *para*-aminobenzoic acid, were described by Briggs et al. as the chick "feather factor" and the chick "growth factor," respectively (3). The reduced feathering and feather depigmentation symptomatic of reported vitamin B_{10} deficiencies were symptoms of vitamin B_{12} deficiency and were alleviated by administration of vitamin B_{12} (2). Folic acid optimized the growth rate depressed by reported deficiency of vitamin B_{10} (2).

4. VITAMIN T

Vitamin t—termitin, penicin, torutilin, insectine, hypomycin, mycoine, or the sesame seed factor—was an extract from yeast, sesame seeds, or insects. Early claims were that vitamin T increased weights and growth rates for guppies, golden hamsters, suckling pigs, chicks, mice, insects, and humans; improved wound healing in white mice; accelerated insect development; and had a favorable influence on human skin disorders (4). However, the addition of vitamin T to a diet adequate in known factors had no effect on the growth rate of young rats or on their feed utilization (5). Subsequent purification revealed vitamin T to be a varied mixture of folacin, vitamin B_{12}, desoxyribosides, and amino acids (5).

5. VITAMIN B_x

Para-aminobenzoic acid, a component of pteroylglutamate formerly called vitamin B_x, was found to be a provitamin for some bacteria, but it does not have vitamin activity in humans because humans lack the ability to synthesize folacin from it (6).

B. Vitamin B_4

Chicks and rats maintained on autoclaved cereals without nutritional supplements exhibit retarded growth and develop general muscular weakness leading to paralysis (7). These symptoms could be alleviated by feeding a factor from yeast or liver extract that Reader termed *vitamin B_4* (8). Early reports identified vitamin B_4 as adenine (9), but the apparent vitamin B_4 deficiency was not alleviated by the addition of adenine to the diet (10). Other workers cured apparent vitamin B_4 deficiency in the rat by feeding thiamin and cured vitamin B_4 deficiency in chicks by supplementing vitamin B_4–deficient diets with glycine, arginine, and cystine. The existence of vitamin B_4 was never confirmed, since all purported vitamin B_4 deficiency symptoms could be alleviated by known nutritional factors (2).

C. Vitamin L

Vitamin L was the name given by Nakahara et al. in the 1930s to two distinct factors his group reported to be essential for lactation in the rat (11). Vitamin L_1, extracted from bovine liver, was later confirmed to be anthranilic acid (12). Vitamin L_2, extracted from yeast, was later confirmed to be adenylthiomethylpentose (12). Reports of a rat lactation factor were not confirmed by other laboratories (13), and neither of these purified compounds is a dietary essential for humans.

III. NONESSENTIAL, BIOLOGICALLY ACTIVE FOOD COMPONENTS

A. Inositol

1. HISTORY

Scherrer isolated inositol from muscle in 1850 (14). Almost a century later, Wooley described an inositol-deficiency syndrome in mice characterized by inadequate growth, alopecia, and eventual death. Wooley's work was later challenged on the basis that the diets were deficient in several of the B-complex vitamins and that the levels of inositol from impure diets, gastrointestinal microfloral synthesis, and endogenous synthesis were not quantified (15).

2. CHEMISTRY AND ANALYTICAL PROCEDURES

There are nine isomers of inositol; however, the only biologically active isomer, myoinositol, is *cis*-1,2,3,5-*trans*-4,6-cyclohexanehexol (Fig. 1)(16). It is an optically inactive,

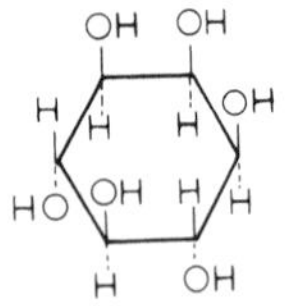

Figure 1 Myoinsitol. (*Source* From Ref. 16.)

sweet, odorless, crystalline powder that is water soluble, slightly alcohol soluble, and ether insoluble (16). Myoinositol is obtained commercially from an aqueous (0.2% sulfur dioxide) extract of corn kernels by precipitation and hydrolysis of crude phytate (17).

Turbidometric measurement of the growth of myoinositol-requiring *Saccharomyces carlsbergensis* or *S. cerevisiae* is the traditional assay for myoinositol. This traditional microbiological method is being replaced by more rapid gas-liquid, paper, and thin-layer chromatographic methods. Pretreatment with concentrated acid is used to release bound forms of myoinositol prior to analysis, depending on the nature of the sample and the method selected (14).

3. CONTENT IN FOOD

The 2500 kcal average American diet has been estimated to contain approximately 900 mg myoinositol (18). All plants and animals contain measurable amounts of myoinositol (19). The most concentrated dietary sources of myoinositol are foods that consist of seeds— beans, grains, and nuts; cantaloupe and citrus fruits are also good plant sources (19). Most inositol from plant sources occurs bound to phosphate as phytate. Better animal sources are the organ meats, which contain myoinositol in free form or as a component of phospholipids (16). The myoinositol contents of 487 common foods have been measured and tabulated by Clements and Darnell (19).

Levels of myoinositol in human colostrum have been reported in the range of 200–500 mg/liter (17,20,21). The level in human milk is 100–200 mg/liter (17,20). In comparison, cow's milk contains 30–80 mg/liter (20,21).

The GRAS (Generally Recognized as Safe) status of myoinositol has been reaffirmed by the Select Committee on GRAS Substances (16):

> There is no evidence in the available information on inositol that demonstrates, or suggests reasonable grounds to suspect, a hazard to the public when it is used at levels that are now current or that might reasonably be expected in the future.

Its only uses as a food additive are in infant formulas and in special dietary foods as a nutritional supplement.

Some losses of myoinositol result from processing and preparation procedures (19). However, these losses are not large, especially when compared to the normal variations of myoinositol contents of foods.

4. METABOLISM

Over 99% of ingested myoinositol is absorbed by rats and by humans (14,16,18). Absorption is slow in both species, with a dose of 0.5 g myoinositol per kg body weight causing moderate diarrhea in humans (16). Absorption of myoinositol by dogs is inefficient (16). Absorption of myoinositol from phytate is decreased from over 90% absorption to less than 50% absorption by high levels of dietary calcium, which chelates the phytate to produce insoluble salts (22). Phytase, an enzyme capable of hydrolyzing these salts occurs naturally in some plant and animal tissues. The dietary calcium level has no effect on the absorption of unbound myoinositol (22).

In most of the mammalian systems examined, myoinositol is absorbed by active (electrogenic) transport; notable exceptions are its apparent nonmediated transport in dogs and in rat skeletal muscle (23–27). D-Glucose has been reported to inhibit the transport of myoinositol by depolarizing membrane potential (24,25,27). This inhibition of myoinositol transport in the presence of large amounts of glucose has special significance in untreated diabetics, who exhibit impaired myoinositol transport into tissues and who excrete large amounts of myoinositol in urine (18). A defect in myoinositol transport, resulting in total efflux of myoinositol from lens tissue, is responsible for cataract formation in a strain of mice with the hereditary error (26).

Myoinositol has been isolated from mammalian tissue as free myoinositol, phosphatidylinositol, mono- and disubstituted phosphates of phosphatidylinositol (phosphatidylinositol 4-phosphate and phosphatidylinositol 4,5-biphosphate, respectively), and as the disaccharide, 6-O-β-D-galactopyranosyl-myoinositol (28). Inositol may be absorbed from dietary sources or may be synthesized de novo from glucose in a reaction requiring NAD^+ (29). Most mammalian cellular myoinositol exists in membrane phospholipids as phosphatidylinositol with a characteristic 1-steroyl,2-arachidonyl fatty acid pattern (30). De novo synthesis of phosphatidylinositol occurs largely in the endoplasmic reticulum; phosphorylation of the inositol headgroup by kinase is apparently a plasma membrane phenomenon (21). Highest concentrations of phosphatidylinositol are found in the kidney and in neural tissues. The disaccharide 6-O-β-D-galactopyranosyl-myoinositol is a unique rat mammary metabolite (28).

Myoinositol is catabolized in the kidney, where it is converted to glucose and metabolized via the pentose phosphate cycle to CO_2 (14,22). In rats, over 50% of ingested myoinositol is metabolized to CO_2 in 48 hours (22). Myoinositol ingested by fasting rats is effective in reducing ketosis.

Normal myoinositol clearance by adults is 2.8 ml/min (31,32). This clearance is increased in normal adults by oral myoinositol loading to increase plasma myoinositol levels (14,24). In diabetics and in uremics, myoinositol clearance is typically elevated (18,24,32). Although kidney function impairment is common in diabetics, this impairment is not the sole reason for the elevated myoinositol clearance, since glucose loading in normal adults has also produced elevated myoinositol clearance (24).

5. BIOCHEMICAL FUNCTIONS

The biochemical functions of myoinositol are probably related to its roles as a phospholipid component of membranes and lipoproteins. Many lipodystrophies caused by dietary and/or physiological stresses can be reduced by myoinositol administration (33–38). This lipotrophic role of inositol probably relates to its function as a lipoprotein component, since secretion of lipoproteins by the liver depends on an adequate supply of myoinositol (15,30). Myoinositol's lipotropic activity is usually synergistic with that of choline (14,16), another lipoprotein component.

Michell (30) and Holub (39,40) have reviewed many of the functions of myoinositol associated with its role as a membrane component. In addition to the general role of maintaining selective permeability of plasma membranes, phosphatidylinositol and its highly charged phosphorylated forms regulate cell-surface phenomena and act as secondary messengers.

Mobilization of intracellular calcium is another major role of myoinositol. An increased turnover of membrane phosphatidylinositol, the "PI effect," has consistently been shown to result in an increased level of intracellular calcium (41). The calcium-mobilizing system, as described by Berridge and Irvine (41), begins as a hormone or other agonist binds to a receptor site on the plasma membrane, activating a phosphodiesterase which hydrolyzes phosphatidylinositol 4,5-biphosphate, yielding the diacylglycerol and myoinositol 1,4,5-triphosphate. The myoinositol triphosphate then binds to a receptor site on the endoplasmic reticulum, causing the release of calcium; up to 50% of the stored calcium can be released upon exposure to myoinositol triphosphate. Calcium then serves to regulate the activities of regulatory enzymes. The reuptake of calcium occurs when myoinositol triphosphate is hydrolyzed by triphosphatase (42). The disappearance of phosphatidylinositol, which was the first clue for the involvement of inositol derivatives in calcium flux, is probably related to the replacement of the metabolized phosphatidylinositol 4,5-biphosphate by the phosphatidylinositol.

6. DEFICIENCIES

Myoinositol deficiency is characterized by various lipodystrophies, which can be produced in intact laboratory animals under dietary or physiological stress. Major examples of these lipodystrophies include abnormal intestinal laurate-rich triglyceride accumulation and hypolipidemia in female gerbils fed diets high in laurate and myristate (33,34); fatty livers in female gerbils or in castrated male gerbils fed diets high in fat and deficient in myoinositol (36); fatty livers in myoinositol-deficient lactating rats (35,37,38).

These lipodystrophies are apparently the result of impaired lipid transport from the affected tissue, resulting from reduced lipoprotein formation or secretion (15,33–37,43). In rats, release of triglycerides to plasma was three times slower in myoinositol-deficient dams than in controls (37); lipoprotein release was similarly delayed (37), and liver phospholipid was about half that of controls (35). In gerbils, lipodystrophies are characterized by a reduced lipoprotein secretion (36) and reduced plasma levels of lipoproteins (33,43). The removal of about one-third of the accumulated lipid from intestines of myoinositol-deficient female gerbils by an 18-hour fast (33) is also consistant with a reduced lipid transport. Additionally, gerbils fed low-fat or high-carbohydrate diets do not accumulate intestinal lipids, even in myoinositol deficiency (34).

The mechanism controlling this impaired lipid transport is unclear. Phosphatidylinositol-rich, very-low-density lipoproteins (VLDL) are required to transport saturated fatty acids from the intestine. Secretion of VLDL is decreased in myoinositol-deficient gerbils (36). The phosphatidylethanolamine that replaces phosphatidylinositol in myoinositol deficiency may not function as well in lipid transport as a component of lipoproteins (15,35). Changes in dietary lipid may also affect lipoprotein function; arachidonate and linoleate are decreased in phosphatidylinositol in lipodystrophic gerbils (33,44). Additionally, lipase activity in lipodystrophic, myoinositol-deficient gerbils is decreased to 70% of control levels (43).

Myoinositol deficiency in dams had no deleterious effect on pup growth in rats (44). However, decreasing myoinositol in diet did decrease myoinositol in milk (38). Neonatal rats fed myoinositol-deficient diets from 6 to 72 days of age exhibited no apparent deficiency signs or symptoms, except for reduced free myoinositol levels in some tissues (45).

No deficiency of inositol has been reported in humans (14). This is probably due to the availability of inositol from dietary sources, from endogenous synthesis, and from bacterial synthesis.

7. NUTRITIONAL ASSESSMENT

Plasma levels of myoinositol in normal adults have been reported in the range of 0.8–1.2 mg per 100 ml (24). However, plasma and/or tissue levels of myoinositol are not commonly analyzed, since myoinositol status is not generally a clinical concern.

8. NUTRITIONAL REQUIREMENTS

Exogenous myoinositol is essential for the gerbil (6). However, dietary essentiality has not been demonstrated for humans, and no RDA has been established for myoinositol (6). Synthesis of myoinositol by the human kidney has been estimated to be 2 g/day, providing 4 g myoinositol per day in the binephric human (46). This is significantly above the estimated 1 g/day intake from dietary sources. Myoinositol is not considered to be a vitamin for humans because it is readily synthesized endogenously (6,16). Its universal occurrence in phospholipids (14), its occurrence at high levels in human milk (15,16,20,21), and its specific requirement by all studied human cell lines in culture (15) point to its biochemical importance, but its endogenous synthesis and readily available exogenous sources make deficiency unlikely. Requirements of human cell culture may be different from requirements in humans; cell cultures may lose their capacity to synthesize myoinositol, or cell needs for myoinositol as a membrane component may greatly exceed needs of intact humans. Since myoinositol is present at rather high levels in human milk and since we know very little of the role of myoinositol in growth and development, myoinositol is added to infant formulas to ensure against deficiency during early development, when need may be greatest (16).

9. FACTORS THAT MAY AFFECT INOSITOL STATUS

Administration of antibiotics, dietary stress, and physiological stress may influence the need for myoinositol. Antibiotics kill inositol-producing gut flora, reducing the exogenous supply of myoinositol to the body. Increasing levels of dietary saturated fatty acids may stress inositol-requiring lipid transport systems; additionally, dietary saturated fatty acids and linolenate are not good substrates for phospholipid synthesis. Lactation stress in rats also increases the need for myoinositol.

Impaired myoinositol metabolism occurs in diabetics, uremics, and premature infants. Untreated human diabetics excrete large amounts of myoinositol in urine and exhibit increased plasma myoinositol levels and altered transport into such tissues as nerves and adipose (18,47,48); insulin therapy restores myoinositol metabolism toward normal (18,47). Premature infants and uremic adults excrete more myoinositol than they ingest and exhibit increased plasma myoinositol levels. Impaired kidney function has been implicated as a causative factor in the reduced metabolism of myoinositol in all three clinical conditions (18,24,32,49); untreated diabetics have the additional stress of hyperglycemia, which may affect myoinositol absorption (24,25,27).

10. EFFICACY OF PHARMACOLOGICAL DOSES

Therapeutic administration of myoinositol has resulted in small reductions in plasma cholesterol levels in hypercholesterolemic patients given 2 g/day for 6–10 weeks and in decreased liver lipid in patients with gastrointestinal cancers given a single 280-mg dose (16). Doses of 1–3 g/day for 12 days were unsuccessful in treating tone deafness and alopecia and resulted in minor elevations in serum cholesterol (14,16).

Diabetics exhibit decreased nerve content of myoinositol, and incorporation of myoinositol into the sciatic nerves of diabetic rats is reduced one-third compared with controls (50). Insulin administration improves myoinositol utilization by diabetic rats (50), and oral loading of myoinositol to further improve peripheral nerve function in diabetics is being considered (18,48). In preliminary experiments, 500 mg myoinositol administered orally twice daily for 2 weeks in human diabetics increased action potentials in median (76%), sural (160%), and popliteal (40%) nerves, but conduction velocities were unaffected (24).

11. EFFECT OF HIGH DOSES

Oral administration of 1–2 g myoinositol per day for a period of 2 months or 15 mg myoinositol 1 day followed by 30 mg myoinositol per day for 3 days resulted in no apparent adverse reactions except mild diarrhea and increased excretion of creatinine for several days (14,16). Intravenous administration of 4 g myoinositol (approximately 67 mg myoinositol per kg body weight) resulted in no apparent adverse reactions, except a 15–25% reduction in BMR (14,16). No long-term tests have been reported, but large doses tend to be excreted in urine.

Administration of myoinositol to rats at 1% of diet (approximately 2 g myoinositol per kg body weight) for 60 days prior to mating had no effect on reproductive performance, litter size, or viability of offspring (16). Feeding myoinositol at a level of 50 mg/day to weanling rats resulted in a slight growth retardation (14). Di- and triphosphorylated myoinositol (phytate metabolites) bind calcium in the gut to potentially reduce mineralization (22).

B. Bioflavonoids

1. HISTORY

In 1936 Szent-Gyorgyi and his co-workers reported that crude extracts of vitamin C from lemon juice or red peppers were more effective than purified ascorbic acid in treating scorbutic guinea pigs (51). "Citrin" was subsequently isolated from lemon juice extracts and was variously designated vitamin P (permeability vitamin) or vitamin C_2 (synergist of vitamin C) (52,53). "Citrin" was later determined to be a mixture of flavonoids (54). Although a number of flavonoids exhibit biological activities, including reduction of capillary fragility and protection of biologically important compounds through antioxidant activity, none of the flavonoids has been demonstrated to be essential for humans or to be capable of causing deficiency syndromes when they are removed from the diet (6,54). Since they are nonessential food constituents that exhibit biological effects, the Joint Committee on Biochemical Nomenclature of the American Society of Biological Chemists and the American Institute of Nutrition recommended that the term *vitamin P* be replaced by the more general designation *bioflavonoids* (1950) (55), and the Committee on Dietary Allowances of the Food and Nutrition Board has designated the bioflavonoids as pharmacological agents instead of as nutritional agents (1980) (6).

2. CHEMISTRY

Flavonoids are colored phenolic substances found in all higher plants; over 3000 different flavonoids have been isolated from plant extracts (56). They are the major sources of red, blue, and yellow pigments, except for carotenoids, in the plant kingdom, and in their purified forms they are usually described as colored crystals that are weakly soluble in hot water and in solvents that are miscible in water (57).

Most of the flavonoids share the basic structure 1,4-benzopyrone substituted with a phenyl group at the 2 position (Fig. 2). The flavonoids have been subdivided into 12 structural groups—flavones, flavanones, flavonols, flavanonols, isoflavones, anthocyanins,

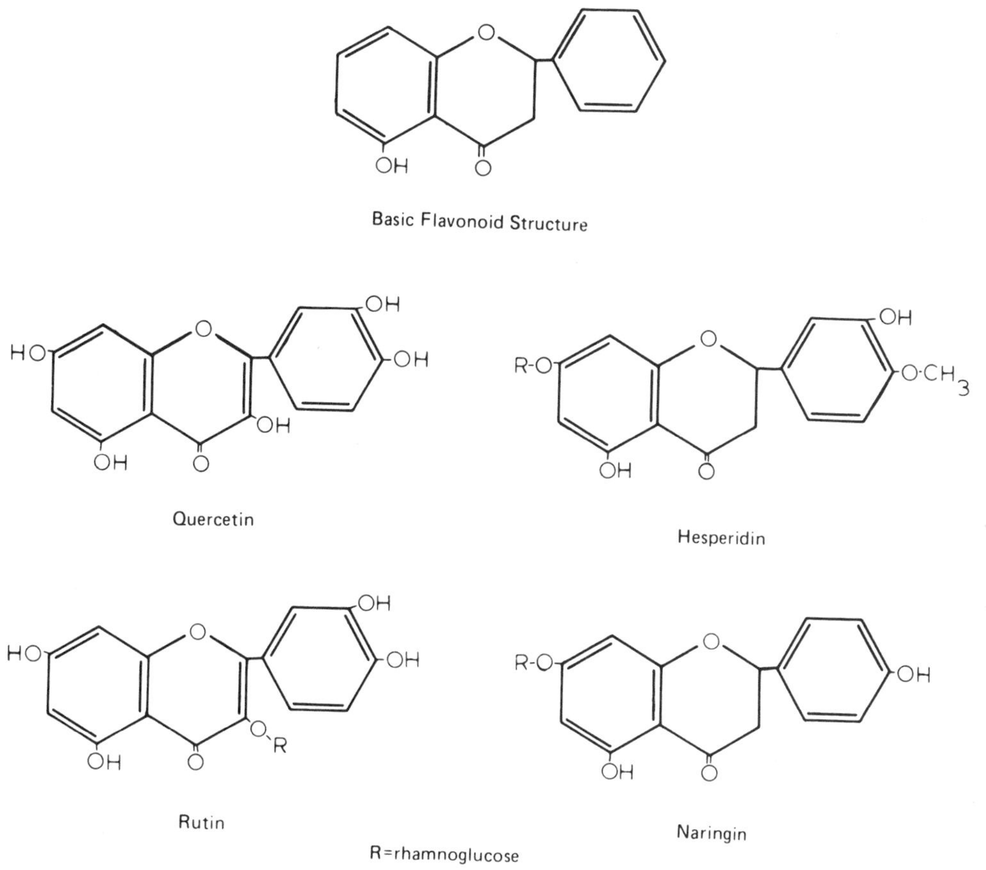

Basic Flavonoid Structure

Quercetin

Hesperidin

Rutin

Naringin

R=rhamnoglucose

Figure 2 Bioflavonoids. (*Source* From Ref. 54).

anthocyanidins, leucoanthycyanins, chalcones, dihydrochalcones, aurones, and catechins—largely determined by differences in the oxidation of the pyrone moiety. Individual flavonoids within groups differ in the number and positions of substitutions in the aromatic rings. The hydroxyl groups in the molecules enable flavonoids to form glycosides by binding with sugars, and most naturally occurring flavonoids are present as glycosides (54). Some commonly occurring flavonoids are described in Figure 2. Note that structurally related aglycones and their glycosides may not share names (for example, rutin and quercetin).

Flavonoids from plant extracts can be separated effectively by high pressure liquid chromotography (HPLC) (56,58). Coupling the HPLC system to a photodiode array detector allows spectra to be recorded for each compound separated during elution.

3. CONTENT IN FOOD

Flavonoids are ubiquitous throughout the plant kingdom, with higher flavonoid concentrations being found in colored exterior tissues, such as peels and skins, than in interior tissues (59,60). Accurate data are not available for concentrations of individual flavonoids in most of the plants commonly consumed by humans; however, Kuhnau has estimated that the average American per capita flavonoid consumption from a mixed diet is 1 g/day (59). The greatest source of flavonoids in the diet is fruit juice, with orange juice supplying approximately 22 mg hesperidin per capita per day and grapefruit juice supplying approximately 5.6 mg naringin per capita per day (54).

Although the largest contributor of flavonoids to the American diet is naturally occurring in fruits and vegetables, the natural extracts of many citrus fruits have GRAS status for use in food and animal feed (54). The individual flavonoids in these extractives are not specified, but hesperidin and naringin are major constituents. Additionally, naringin is listed separately as GRAS (54). Consumption of flavonoids from additive usage is less than 0.025 mg per capita per day, which is much lower than consumption from naturally occurring sources (54).

Flavonoids in food are subject to oxidative decomposition, to enzymatic degradation, and to polymerization during storage, cooking, and processing. Additionally, the water-soluble compounds are commonly leached into cooking liquids.

4. METABOLISM

Flavonoid glycosides must be hydrolyzed prior to their absorption in the small intestine. The enzymes required to hydrolyze the glycosides are not in human digestive secretions or in the intestinal wall but are supplied by gut microflora (54,57). After absorption, the flavonoids are bound in the liver as glucuronides and/or sulfate conjugates prior to degradation and/or excretion (54,57). Most of the absorbed flavonoid is degraded to phenolic compounds, the specific compound(s) depending on the flavonoid and the animal species, and excreted in urine within 24 hours (54,57). A smaller amount is excreted in bile for reabsorption or excretion in feces (51,57).

5. BIOCHEMICAL FUNCTIONS

Many different biological effects of bioflavonoids have been reported (57,61,62). Since there are many different flavonoids, each with its own chemical and biochemical characteristics, many different responses to flavonoid administration have been reported. One consistent finding is that some bioflavonoids and bioflavonoid mixtures reduce capillary fragility and/or reduce capillary permeability, possibly by antioxidant "sparing" of vitamin C, which is directly involved with maintaining vascular integrity (54). Many of the flavonoids chelate metal ions, especially copper and iron, to form metallic complexes. This characteristic may be responsible for their antioxidant activities in hydrophilic and lipophilic systems (54).

Different flavonoids have been reported to activate or inhibit the cytochrome P450–dependent monooxygenase system, which is responsible for the metabolism of many drugs, steroids, bile acids, and fatty acids (63). In addition, flavonoids have been reported to inhibit cyclic nucletide phosphodiesterases (64,65); this would have the effect of amplifying the effects of cAMP and cGMP second messenger systems in such processes as cell division, cardiac contraction, immunological response, blood platelet aggregation, and energy production (65).

One of the most studied flavonoids in metabolic systems is quercetin. In vitro inhibition by quercetin and related bioflavonoids has been reported for many enzymes, including O-methyltransferase, the enzyme that normally inactivates epinephrine and norepinephrine (66); and aldose reductase (66,67), an enzyme that is apparently involved in cataract formation by diabetics and galactosemics. Quercetin has been reported to inhibit arachidonate metabolism at several steps: phospholipase A_2, the enzyme responsible for the hydrolysis and release of arachidonic acid from membrane phospholipids (64); lipoxygenase, which is important in the biosynthesis of proinflammatory arachidonic acid metabolites (68); and cyclooxygenase, an enzyme that is important for biosynthesis of prostaglandins from arachidonate (64). Quercetin also inhibits the release of histamine and other allergic-mediators from mast cells (68,69) and exhibits antiviral activity (69,70). Significance of these reactions in vivo has not been determined.

6. EFFICACY OF PHARMACOLOGICAL DOSES

Although bioflavonoids exhibit a number of potentially useful properties, there are no currently accepted therapeutic roles of bioflavonoids. Many folk remedies have been based on flavonoid extractives from plants, but scientifically designed clinical trials must be conducted to determine efficacy. In addition, flavonoids must be selected for specificity in each treatment to reduce side effects. For example, quercetin, which can reduce the cellular component of inflammation through its inhibition of lipoxygenase, affects many other metabolic systems, which may result in unwanted side effects.

7. SAFETY

Bioflavonoids, at levels consumed from traditional American diets, are generally considered to be nontoxic. In rats, the ED_{50} values for various bioflavonoids administered intraperitoneally or intravenously ranged from 50 to 4000 mg/kg (57). In humans, doses of several grams of hesperidin per day administered for months have not proven toxic (45). Tannins, which are a major flavonoid in red wines, beans, and sorghum, have been shown to bind proteins and reduce growth rates in animals; epidemiologically, they have been linked to cancer of the esophagus in humans (71). Quercetin, the aglycone of rutin, a bioflavonoid constituent of citrus peel, is mutagenic in microbial systems (54) and caused intestinal and bladder cancers in rats ingesting it at a 0.1% level (72); MacGregor (73) and Ueno et al. (74) have reviewed other genotoxicity and carcinogenicity studies.

IV. PSEUDOVITAMINS

A. Vitamin B_{17} (Laetrile)

1. HISTORY

In his public statement on Laetrile (75), then–FDA Commissioner Kennedy labeled Laetrile the "unproven cancer remedy of the 1970's." First broadly promoted as a cancer remedy in the early 1950s, it rose to national prominence in the 1970s with promotion by Dr. E. T. Krebs, Jr. and the organization of a group called "The Committee for Freedom of Choice in Cancer Therapy." The label *Vitamin B_{17}* enhanced its image of being a natural curative. Since evidence supporting the safety and efficacy of Laetrile had never been submitted to FDA, FDA had always prohibited its shipment via interstate commerce. In 1977, as a response to *Rutherford* v. *United States*, a case in which a Kansas resident sought legal permission to use Laetrile, FDA was ordered to evaluate Laetrile as a drug. In his July 29, 1977, statement, then–FDA Commissioner Kennedy confirmed that, "There is no basis in law or in fact for the use of Laetrile or related substances in the treatment of cancer," upholding the prohibition by interstate commerce of the substance.

2. CHEMISTRY AND ANALYTICAL PROCEDURES

The term *laetrile* is often used interchangeably with the terms Laetrile, amygdalin, and vitamin B_{17}. Laetrile is a specific chemical entity having the chemical name 1-mandelonitrile-β-glucuronic acid (Fig. 3) (76). Amygdalin (Fig. 4) is a β-cyanogenic glucoside

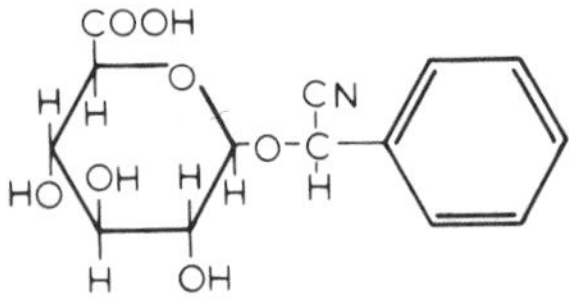

Figure 3 Laetrile. (*Source* From Ref. 75.)

occurring naturally in the kernels or seeds of most fruits (77). Amygdalin is the most common constituent of samples labeled as "Laetrile" (77–79).

Separation and quantification of epimers of amygdalin and their hydrolysis products by reversed-phase high pressure liquid chromotography has been reported (80). This procedure can be used to prepare purified quantities of D-amygdalin, the form of amygdalin which can be metabolized by β-glucosidases, for biologic evaluation.

3. METABOLISM

Mandelonitrile (Fig. 5) is the common end product of laetrile and amygdalin metabolism in humans. Intestinal β-glucuronidase hydrolyzes orally administered Laetrile to glucuronic acid and mandelonitrile (75,76). Amygdalin can be degraded by bacterial β-glucosidases in the intestine to mandelonitrile + glucose (81–83), or, through the activity of amygdalase in the mucosal brush border cells, amygdalin can be metabolized to prunasin + glucose (84,85). Prunasin (Fig. 6) is rapidly absorbed and efficiently cleared by the liver and kidney (84), but some prunasin is converted to mandelonitrile + glucose in the intestine by prunase (86).

Animal cells do not contain enzymes required to release cyanide from mandelonitrile (75,76). However, gut microflora may be able to release free cyanide from mandelonitrile (81,82). This observation is supported by elevated concentrations of cyanide in the bloodstream and increased levels of thiocyanate in urine following oral, but not intravenous, administration of laetrile or amygdalin (81,82,87) and by studies with gnotobiotic animals (83).

4. NUTRITIONAL REQUIREMENTS

United States and Canadian drug authorities do not recognize Laetrile or amygdalin (or any similar cyanogenic glucosides) as vitamins and do not recognize a "vitamin B_{17}" (6,75). Additionally, there is no documented function for laetrile or amygdalin in human metabolic systems.

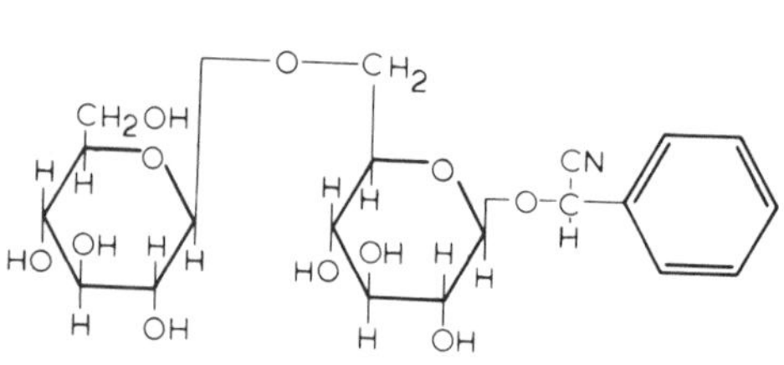

Figure 4 Amygdalin. (*Source* From Ref. 75.)

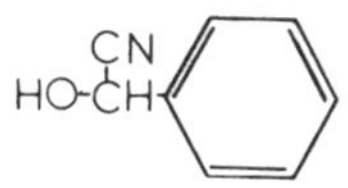

Figure 5 Mandelonitrile. (*Source* From Ref. 75.)

5. EFFICACY OF PHARMACOLOGICAL DOSES

Although many unsupported claims have been made for the therapeutic benefit of laetrile treatment, the most publicized claims are for its use in treating cancer. In these claims the two major lines of argument that have been advanced are that the cyanide in laetrile acts specifically to destroy cancer cells and that cancer is a disease of nutritional deficiency of laetrile which requires treatment exclusively by dietary control. Extensive animal and clinical trials have not supported these claims (75,76,88,89).

6. TOXICITY

Purified amygdalin and laetrile are essentially nontoxic in humans unless the cyanide they contain is released by enzymatic activity. Apricot kernels contain β-glucosidases, which hydrolyze amydgalin to form two molecules of glucose and one molecule of mandelonitrile, and oxynitrilase, which will hydrolyze mandelonitrile to cyanide and benzaldehyde. These enzymes come in contact with the amygdalin only when the kernels are crushed prior to consumption; otherwise, the apricot kernels will pass through the digestive tract intact (76). Cyanide poisoning, resulting in death from consumption of crushed apricot kernels and from consumption of Laetrile preparations containing enzymes which could release cyanide, has been reported (76). Oral administration of laetrile, amygdalin, and prunasin during pregnancy in hamsters have been reported to result in skeletal malformations in offspring; this teratogenic effect is apparently caused by increased cyanide concentrations, since intravenous administration did not result in the abnormalities and since administration of thiosulfate, which detoxifies cyanide, protected the offspring from teratogenic effects of orally administered chemicals (86).

B. Vitamin B$_{15}$ (Pangamic Acid)

Pangamate is not recognized as a vitamin by Canadian or U.S. drug authorities (6,90). It is not a chemically defined substance. Preparations marketed in the United States as

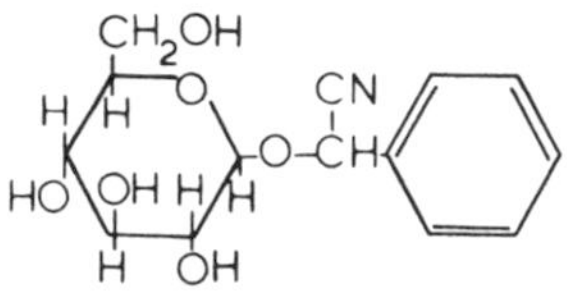

Figure 6 Prunasin. (*Source* From Ref. 75.)

"pangamate" or as "vitamin B_{15}" have been chemically analyzed by the U.S. Food and Drug Administration and have been found to contain one or more of the following compounds: calcium gluconate, glycine, N,N-dimethylglycine, N,N-diisopropylamine dichloroacetate (91). Of these compounds, N,N-diisopropylamine dichloroacetate is the only one with pharmacological activity; it has been shown to decrease blood pressure and body temperature in rats, resulting in death from respiratory failure in acute toxicity (90). Diisopropylamine dichloroacetate also demonstrates mutagenicity in the Ames Salmonella/mammalian microsome mutagenicity test (92). Since the compositions of "pangamate" preparations are undefined, adequate clinical studies to test the curative claims made for "pangamate" have not been conducted, and reported evidence is anecdotal. Claims for the use of commercial pangamate preparations by athletes as an ergogenic aid have been examined, with no reported advantage over placebo administration (93). In laboratory studies of rats injected with commercial pangamate preparations and with purified components of pangamate preparations (15 mg preparation/0.5 ml saline, pH 7) no improvement in physiological or biochemical parameters associated with exercise were noted (94). There is no scientific evidence that "pangamate" preparations have vitamin activity or offer therapeutic benefit.

C. Vitamin B_{13} (Orotic Acid)

In 1948 Novak and Hauge (95) isolated a compound from distillers' dried solubles that was provisionally called vitamin B_{13}. The purified compound is orotic acid, an intermediate in pyrimidine metabolism. Bovine milk, which contains approximately 80 μg/ml of orotic acid, is the only food known to contain appreciable amounts of preformed orotic acid (96), but all amino acids are capable of contributing to the orotic acid pool (97).

Many claims have been made for the use of orotic acid supplements in the treatment and prevention of circulatory, gastrointestinal, and hepatic disorders. These claims are based largely on the finding that rats fed orotic acid at dietary levels of 1% exhibit decreased serum cholesterol levels (98,99). However, this effect has been found to be species specific; mice, guinea pigs, hamsters, and monkeys do not exhibit these changes (99,100). Reports of slight hypocholesteremic effects in humans following oral administration of 6 g orotic acid/week without other dietary change were not supported by a more controlled clinical study in which 1 g orotic acid/day was administered orally to 12 hospital outpatients in a weight reduction program (101). Oral administration of orotic acid has consistently been shown to increase the urinary excretion of urate and decrease serum urate levels (101–103). This may suggest a role for orotic acid in the treatment of gout, although clinical studies would need to be conducted to determine efficacy.

No acute or chonic effects from oral administration of orotic acid at 6 g/day for 3 weeks or at 3 g/day for 8 months in humans have been noted (101). The induction of fatty livers by orotic acid in rats (98) has not been found in other species, possibly because other species excrete excess orotic acid more efficiently (100,104).

Orotic acid is not recognized as a vitamin by Canadian or U.S. drug authorities (6). It has no known coenzyme function. Humans have not exhibited any dietary requirement for it, and no deficiency in humans or other mammals has been reported.

D. Vitamin H_3 (Gerovital)

Gerovital, also named vitamin H_3 or vitamin GH_3, is a buffered solution of procaine hydrochloride, better known as Novocain, a painkiller used by dentists (105). As the name indicates, gerovital is promoted as a nutritional substance that alleviates symptoms of diseases associated with aging. These claims have not been supported by scientific studies, and gerovital is not recognized as a vitamin by Canadian or U.S. drug authorities (6).

E. Vitamin U

The methylsulfonium salts of methionine, which are naturally occurring in cabbage and other green vegetables, in milk, and in green (unfermented) teas (106), have been called "antipeptic ulcer factors" and vitamin U by researchers who reported that their oral administration reduced incidence and/or severity of experimentally induced peptic ulcers in guinea pigs (107–109). These claims were not supported by later clinical trials (110), and the compounds are not recognized as vitamins by Canadian or U.S. drug authorities (6,41).

V. POTENTIAL NEW VITAMIN

Pyrroloquinoline quinone (PQQ) and copper are cofactors for lysyl oxidase, an enzyme required for crosslinking of collagen and elastin (111). In response to dietary deprivation of PQQ, mice exhibited a lathyritic friability of skin, a sign also reported for mice fed copper-deficient diets. Pregnant mice fed chemically defined diets apparently devoid of PQQ exhibited reproductive failure, as well. PQQ is ubiquitous in dietary components, including water, and may be produced in mammalian cells at less than optimal levels, making it difficult to assess its status as an essential nutrient. Since its absence from the diet apparently results in severe defects that threaten life, normal growth, and reproductive success, further work with PQQ may result in its establishment as a vitamin.

VI. CONCLUSION

The term *vitamin* denotes dietary need. Although many substances have been called vitamins historically, today the list of substances recognized as vitamins is much shorter. This is because dietary requirements have not been confirmed for these substances. The human body does need myoinositol for normal functioning; however, myoinositol is not a vitamin by definition because it is not a dietary essential for normal humans consuming normal diets. The human body does not have a demonstrated need for bioflavonoids, Laetrile, pangamate, orotic acid, or gerovital. Use of the term *vitamin* to describe these compounds is a health fraud, since it is an implicit promise for a "natural curative" that has no scientific basis.

REFERENCES

1. W. J. Darby, in *Vitamins and Hormones: Advances in Research and Applications*, Vol. 5, R. S. Harris and K. V. Thimann (Eds.), Academic Press, New York, 1947.
2. F. A. Robinson, *The Vitamin B Complex*, John Wiley and Sons, New York, 1951.
3. G. M. Briggs, Jr., T. D. Luckey, C. A. Elvehjem, and E. B. Hart, *J. Biol. Chem.*, *148*:163 (1943).
4. W. Goetsch, *Experientia*, *3*:326 (1947).
5. A. Bender and E. Tunnah, *J. Sci. Food Agric.*, *4*:331 (1953).
6. National Academy of Sciences, *Recommended Dietary Allowances*, National Research Council, Washington, D.C., 1989.

7. O. Kline, C. Elvehjem, and E. Hart, *Biochem. J.*, *30*:780 (1936).

8. V. Reader, *Biochem. J.*, *24*:1827 (1930).

9. R. Tschesche, *Ber.*, *66B*:581 (1933).

10. C. Chen, *Bull. Agric. Chem. Soc. Jpn.*, *10*:105 (1934).

11. W. Nakahara, F. Inukai, S. Ugami, and Y. Nagata, *Proc. Jpn. Acad.*, *22*:139 (1946).

12. S. Ugami, *J. Jpn. Chem.*, *1*:50 (1947).

13. S. J. Folley, E. W. Ikin, S. K. Kon, and H. M. S. Watson, *Biochem. J.*, *32*:1988 (1938).

14. Informatics, Inc., *Scientific Literature Reviews on Generally Recognized as Safe (GRAS) Food Ingredients—Inositol*, NTIS #PB223861, 1973.

15. A. Kukis and S. Mookerjea, *Nutr. Rev.*, *36*:233 (1978).

16. Select Committee on GRAS Substances, *Evaluation of the Health Aspects of Inositol as a Food Ingredient*, NTIS #PB262660, 1975.

17. Inositol: Proposed Affirmation of GRAS Status as a Direct Human Food Ingredient, *Federal Register*, *43*:22056–22058, 1978.

18. R. S. Clements, Jr. and R. Reynertson, *Diabetes*, *26*:215 (1977).

19. R. S. Clements, Jr. and B. Darnell, *Am. J. Clin. Nutr.*, *33*:1954 (1980).

20. K. Ogasa, M. Kuboyama, I. Kiyosawa, T. Suguki, and M. Itoh, *J. Nutr. Sci. Vitaminol.*, *21*:129 (1975)

21. J. Matsuyama, M. Ezawa, M. Kimura, J. Seimiya, and T. Nagasawa, *Tamagawa Daigaku Nogakubu Kenkju Hokoku*, *1979*:13 (1979).

22. A. Nahapetian and V. R. Young, *J. Nutr.*, *110*:1458 (1980).

23. B. A. Molitoris, I. E. Karl, and W. H. Daughaday, *J. Clin. Invest.*, *65*:783 (1980).

24. M. R. Hammarman, B. Sacktor, and W. H. Daughaday, *Am. J. Physiol.*, *239*:F113 (1980).

25. W. F. Caspary and R. K. Crane, *Biochim. Biophys. Acta*, *203*:308 (1970).

26. E. Wada, T. Takenawa, and T. Tsumita, *Biochim. Biophys. Acta*, *554*:145 (1979).

27. J. Lerner and R. Smajula, *Comp. Biochem. Physiol.*, *62A*:939 (1979).

28. W. F. Naccarato, R. E. Ray, and W. W. Wells, *J. Biol. Chem.*, *250*:1872 (1975).

29. C. H.-J. Chen and F. Eisenberg, Jr., *J. Biol. Chem.*, *250*:2963 (1975).

30. R. H. Michell, *Biochim. Biophys. Acta*, *415*:81 (1975).

31. L. M. Lewin, S. Melmed, J. H. Passwell, Y. Yannai, M. Brush, S. Orda, H. Boichis, and H. Bank, *Pediatr. Res.*, *12*:3 (1978).

32. S. Melmed, L. M. Lewin, and H. Bank, *Am. J. Med. Sci.*, *274*:55 (1977).

33. S.-H. Chu and D. M. Hegsted, *J. Nutr.*, *110*:1209 (1980).

34. S.-H. Chu and D. M. Hegsted, *J. Nutr.*, *110*:1217 (1980).

35. L. E. Burton and W. W. Wells, *J. Nutr.*, *107*:1871 (1977).

36. G. A. Hoover, R. J. Nicolosi, J. E. Corey, M. El Lozy, and K. C. Hayes, *J. Nutr.*, *108*:1588 (1978).

37. L. E. Burton and W. W. Wells, *J. Nutr.*, *109*:1483 (1979).

38. L. E. Burton and W. W. Wells, *J. Nutr.*, *106*:1617 (1976).

39. B. J. Holub, *Annu. Rev. Nutr.*, *6*:563 (1986).

40. B. J. Holub, *Nutr. Rev.*, *45*:65 (1987).

41. M. J. Berridge and R. F. Irvine, *Nature*, *312*:315 (1984).

42. M. A. Seyfred, L. E. Farrell, and W. W. Wells, *J. Biol. Chem.*, *259*:13204 (1984).

43. S.-H. Chu and R. P. Geyer, *Biochim. Biophys. Acta*, *664*:89 (1981).

44. M. N. Woods and D. M. Hegsted, *J. Nutr.*, *109*:2146 (1979).

45. L. E. Burton, R. A. Ray, J. R. Bradford, J. P. Orr, J. A. Nickerson, and W. W. Wells, *J. Nutr.*, *106*:1610 (1976).

46. R. S. Clements, Jr. and A. G. Diethelm, *J. Lab. Clin. Med.*, *93*:210 (1979).

47. D. J. Heaf and D. J. Galton, *Clin. Chim. Acta*, *63*:41 (1975).

48. J. G. Salway, J. A. Finnegan, D. Barnett, L. Whitehead, A. Karunanayaka, and R. B. Payne, *Lancet*, *2*:1280 (1978).

49. C. Servo and E. Pitkanen, *Diabetologia*, *11*:575 (1975).

50. J. S. Hothersall and P. McLean, *Biochim. Biophys. Acta*, *88*:477 (1979).

51. A. Szent-Gyorgyi and A. Rusznyak, *Nature* (Lond.), *138*:27 (1936).

52. A. Bentsath, S. Rusznyak, and A. Szent-Gyorgyi, *Nature* (Lond.), *138*:198 (1936).

53. M. Gabe and J. L. Parrot, *J. Physiol.* (Lond.), *40*:63 (1948).

54. Select Committee on GRAS Substances, *Tentative Evaluation of the Health Aspects of Hesperidin, Naringin, and Citrus Bioflavonoid Extracts as Food Ingredients* (hearing draft), 1980.

55. Joint Committee on Nomenclature, *Science*, *112*:628 (1950).

56. J. B. Harborne, in *Plant Flavonoids in Biology and Medicine*, V. Cody, E. Middleton, Jr., and J. B. Harborne (Eds.), Alan R. Liss, Inc., New York, 1986.

57. Informatics, Inc., *Monograph on Bioflavonoids*, NTIS #PB289600, 1978.

58. K. Hostettmann and A. Marston, in *Plant Flavonoids in Biology and Medicine*, V. Cody, E. Middleton, Jr., and J. B. Harborne (Eds.), Alan R. Liss, Inc., New York, 1986.

59. J. Kuhnau, *World Rev. Nutr. Diet.*, *24*:117 (1976).

60. K. Herrmann, *J. Food Technol.*, *11*:433 (1976).

61. V. Cody, E. Middleton, Jr., and J. B. Harborne (Eds.), *Plant Flavonoids in Biology and Medicine*, Alan R. Liss, Inc., New York, 1986.

62. L. Farkas, M. Gabor, and F. Kallay (Eds.), *Flavonoids and Bioflavonoids*, Elsevier, New York, 1985.

63. A. W. Wood, D. S. Smith, R. L. Chang, M.-T. Huang, and A. H. Conney, in *Plant Flavonoids in Biology and Medicine*, V. Cody, E. Middleton, Jr., and J. B. Harborne (Eds.), Alan R. Liss, Inc., New York, 1986.

64. S. G. Laychock, in *Plant Flavonoids in Biology and Medicine*, V. Cody, E. Middleton, Jr., and J. B. Harborne (Eds.), Alan R. Liss, Inc., New York, 1986.

65. A. Beretz, R. Anton, J.-P. Cazenave, in *Plant Flavonoids in Biology and Medicine*, V. Cody, E. Middleton, Jr., and J. B. Harborne (Eds.), Alan R. Liss, Inc., New York, 1986.

66. S. D. Varma and J. H. Kinoshita, *Biochem. Pharmacol.*, *25*:2505 (1976).

67. S. D. Varma, in *Plant Flavonoids in Biology and Medicine*, V. Cody, E. Middleton, Jr., and J. B. Harborne (Eds.), Alan R. Liss, Inc., New York, 1986.

68. A. F. Welton, L. D. Tobias, C. Fiedler-Nagy, W. Anderson, W. Hope, K. Meyers, and J. W. Coffey, in *Plant Flavonoids in Biology and Medicine*, V. Cody, E. Middleton, Jr., and J. B. Harborne (Eds.), Alan R. Liss, Inc., New York, 1986.

69. E. Middleton, Jr., H. Faden, G. Drzewiecki, and D. Perrissoud, in *Plant Flavonoids in Biology and Medicine*, V. Cody, E. Middleton, Jr., and J. B. Harborne (Eds.), Alan R. Liss, Inc., New York, 1986.

70. J. W. T. Selway, in *Plant Flavonoids in Biology and Medicine*, V. Cody, E. Middleton, Jr., and J. B. Harborne (Eds.), Alan R. Liss, Inc., New York, 1986.

71. L. G. Butler, J. C. Rogler, H. Mehansho, and D. M. Carlson, in *Plant Flavonoids in Biology and Medicine*, V. Cody, E. Middleton, Jr., and J. B. Harborne (Eds.), Alan R. Liss, Inc., New York, 1986.

72. A. M. Pamukcu, S. Yalciner, J. F. Hatcher, and B. T. Bryan, *Cancer Res.*, *40*:3468 (1980).

73. J. T. MacGregor, in *Plant Flavonoids in Biology and Medicine*, V. Cody, E. Middleton, Jr., and J. B. Harborne (Eds.), Alan R. Liss, Inc., New York, 1986.

74. I. Ueno, K. Haraikawa, M. Kohno, T. Hinomoto, H. Ohya-Nishiguchi, T. Tomatsuri, and K. Yoshihira, in *Plant Flavonoids in Biology and Medicine*, V. Cody, E. Middleton, Jr., and J. B. Harborne (Eds.), Alan R. Liss, Inc., New York, 1986.

75. *Laetrile: The Commissioner's Decision*, HEW Publication #77-3056, Washington, D.C., 1977.

76. V. Herbert, *Am. J. Clin. Nutr.*, *32*:1121 (1979).

77. M. D. Holzbecher, M. A. Moss, and H. Ellenberger, *J. Toxicol.: Clin. Toxicol.*, *22*:341 (1984.).

78. T. Cairns, J. E. Froberg, S. Gonzales, W. S. Langham, J. J. Stamp, J. K. Howie, and D. T. Sawyer, *Anal. Chem.*, *50*:317 (1978).

79. J. P. Davignon, L. A. Trissel, and L. M. Kleinman, *Cancer Treat. Rep.*, *62*:99 (1978).

80. D. J. Smith and J. D. Weber, *J. Chromatog. Sci.*, *22*:94 (1984).

81. R. T. Dorr and J. Paxinos, *Ann. Intern. Med.*, *89*:389 (1978).

82. C. G. Moertel, M. W. Ames, J. S. Kovach, T. P. Moyer, J. R. Rubin, J. H. Tinker, *J. Am. Med. Assoc.*, *245*:591 (1981).

83. J. H. Carter, M. A. McLarfferty, and P. Goldman, *Biochem. Pharmacol.*, *29*:301 (1980).

84. A. G. Rauws, M. Olling, A. Timmerman, *J. Toxicol.: Clin. Toxicol.*, *19*:851 (1983).

85. A. G. Rauws, M. Olling, and A. Timmerman, *Arch. Toxicol.*, *49*:311 (1982).

86. C. C. Willhite, *Science*, *215*:1513 (1982).

87. S. R. A. Adewusi and O. L. Oke, *Can. J. Physiol. Pharmacol.*, *63*:1080 (1985).

88. C. G. Moertel, T. R. Fleming, J. Rubin, L. K. Kvols, G. Sarna, R. Koch, V. E. Currie, C. W. Young, S. E. Jones, and J. P. Davignon, *N. Engl. J. Med.*, *306*:201 (1982).

89. M. P. Chitnis, M. K. Adwankar, and A. J. Amonkar, *J. Cancer Res. Clin. Oncol.*, *109*:208 (1985).

90. V. Herbert, *Am. J. Clin. Nutr.*, *32*:1534 (1979).

91. J. W. Turczan, United States Food and Drug Administration Laboratory Information Bulletin #2005A, 1978.

92. M. D. Gelernt and V. Herbert, *Nutr. Cancer*, *3*:129 (1982).

93. M. E. Gray and L. W. Titlow, *Med. Sci. Sports and Exercise*, *14*:424 (1982).

94. G. L. Dohm, S. Debnath and W. R. Frisell, *Biochem. Med.*, *28*:77 (1982).

95. A. F. Novak and S. M. Hauge, *J. Biol. Chem.*, *174*:235 (1948).

96. B. L. Larson and H. M. Hegarty, *J. Dairy Sci.*, *62*:1641 (1979).

97. L. C. Hatchwell and J. A. Milner, *J. Nutr.*, *108*:578 (1978).

98. R. P. Durschlag and J. L. Robinson, *J. Nutr.*, *110*:816 (1980).

99. K. K. Harden and J. L. Robinson, *J. Nutr.*, *114*:411 (1984).

100. R. P. Durschlag and J. L. Robinson, *J. Nutr.*, *110*:822 (1980).

101. J. L. Robinson and D. B. Dombrowski, *Nutr. Res.*, *3*:407 (1983).

102. W. N. Kelley, M. L. Greene, I. H. Gox, F. M. Rosenbloom, R. I. Levy, and J. E. Seegmiller, *Metab.*, *19*:1025 (1970).

103. J. L. Robinson, D. B. Dombrowski, L. R. Tauss, and L. R. Jones, *Am. J. Clin. Nutr.*, *41*:605 (1985).

104. W. J. Visek and J. D. Shoemaker, *J. Am. College of Nutr.*, *5*:153 (1986).

105. A. Hecht, *FDA Consumer*, *14*:16 (1980).

106. Ohtsuki, M. Kawabata, K. Taguchi, H. Kokura, and S. Kawamura, *Agric. Biol. Chem.*, *48*:2471 (1984).

107. G. Cheney, *J. Am. Diet. Assoc.*, *26*:668 (1950).

108. K. Seri, T. Matsuo, M. Asano, R. Sato, and T. Kato, *Arzneimilttelforsch.*, *28*:1711 (1978).

109. E. Adami, *Atti, Soc. Lombarda. Sci. Med. Biol.*, *10*:60 (1955).

110. B. Colombo, *Minerva Med.*, 2944 (1959).

111. J. Killgore, C. Smidt, L. Duich, N. Romero-Chapman, D. Tinker, K. Reiser, M. Melko, D. Hyde, and R. Rucker, *Science*, *245*:850 (1989).

Index

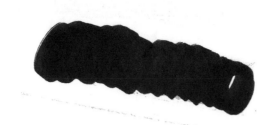